ULT CALORIE COUNTER
& DIET JOURNAL

- ✔ Wine, Liquor & Beer
- ✔ Calories, Fat & Carbs
- ✔ 30-Week Diet Journal
- ✔ Most & Least Healthy

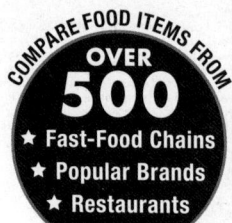

COMPARE FOOD ITEMS FROM **OVER 500**
- ★ Fast-Food Chains
- ★ Popular Brands
- ★ Restaurants

By Alex A. Lluch
Health & Fitness Expert
Author of Over 3 Million Books Sold!

WS Publishing Group
San Diego, California 92119

ULTRA SIMPLE CALORIE COUNTER & DIET JOURNAL

By Alex A. Lluch

Published by WS Publishing Group
San Diego, California 92119
Copyright © 2011 by WS Publishing Group

Nutritional and fitness guidelines based on information provided by the United States Food and Drug Administration, Food and Nutrition Information Center, National Agricultural Library, Agricultural Research Service, and the U.S. Department of Agriculture.

Photo Credits:
Front cover image: © iStockphoto/Nicole S. Young
Food icons: © iStockphoto/stdemi (dairy, meats, bread, grains, seafood, etc.)
Food icons: © iStockphoto/Jane Norton (condiments)
Food icons: © iStockphoto/Viviyan (fast foods, donuts, coffee, cupcakes, pizza)
Food icons: © iStockphoto/Kristina Smirnova (alcoholic beverages)
Food icons: © iStockphoto/RoccoMontoya (jam)
Food icons: © iStockphoto/totallyjamie (ice cream, candy and donut)
Food icons: © iStockphoto/DimensionsDesigns (taco and burrito)

For inquiries:
Log on to www.WSPublishingGroup.com
E-mail info@WSPublishingGroup.com

ISBN-13: 978-1-936061-15-0

Printed in China

TABLE OF CONTENTS

RESTAURANTS & FAST-FOOD CHAINS

TABLE OF CONTENTS

RESTAURANTS & FAST-FOOD CHAINS

RESTAURANTS & FAST-FOOD CHAINS

POPULAR BRANDS BY CATEGORY   **475**

TABLE OF CONTENTS

FOOD ITEMS BY CATEGORY (CONT.)

FOOD ITEMS BY CATEGORY (CONT.)

COMPLETE LIST OF NAME BRANDS

A

A-1 Steak Sauce

Accelerade

Act II Microwave Popcorn

Allen's

Alouette

Alta Dena

American Almond

American Roland Food Co.

Annie's Naturals

Apple Time

Aquafina

Arrowroot

Athenos

Aunt Jemima

Azteca Foods

B

B&G Foods

Baker's Chocolate and Coconut

Balance Bar

Ball Park Franks

Banquet

Barnum's Animal Crackers

Baskin Robbins

Bays English Muffins

Beech-Nut Baby Food

Ben and Jerry's

Berstein's Dressings

Best Foods

Betty Crocker

Bisquick

Blue Bunny Ice Cream

Blue Diamond Almonds

Boboli

Boca Meatless

Breakstone's

Bruce Food Products

Brummel & Brown

Bugles

Bumblebee Tuna

Bush's Beans

Butterball

C

Cadbury's

California Pizza Kitchen

California Sun Dry

Campbell's Soups

Canola Information Service

Capri Sun

Carl Buddig

TABLE OF CONTENTS

COMPLETE LIST OF NAME BRANDS (CONT.)

COMPLETE LIST OF NAME BRANDS (CONT.)

COMPLETE LIST OF NAME BRANDS (CONT.)

COMPLETE LIST OF NAME BRANDS (CONT.)

COMPLETE LIST OF NAME BRANDS (CONT.)

Log on to

WSPublishingGroup.com

for other best-selling diet
and fitness books!

Introduction

By purchasing this book you have taken the first and most important step to lose weight, stay in shape, feel better, and have more energy than you ever thought possible. Research has shown, again and again, that the best way to accomplish your health and weight-loss goals is to track the calories, fat, and carbs in the foods you eat on a daily basis.

THE BENEFITS OF LOSING WEIGHT

Losing weight has major benefits that can improve your way of life. Weight loss can lower the risk of numerous diseases, including heart disease, stroke, cancer, and diabetes.

However, it is difficult in today's society to make the right choices regarding your health and diet. Our jobs promote sedentary lifestyles, our days are busier than ever, and fast-food, while usually unhealthy, is convenient and inexpensive. Many food companies use larger portions as a selling point, making the claim that bigger is better. It then becomes the consumer's responsibility to monitor what and how much he or she eats.

We know how difficult it can be to choose wisely when you are eating out, dining with friends, and planning meals at home. Portions at restaurants are larger than ever, and meals are often cooked with unhealthy sauces, dressings, and breading. It is extremely hard to locate a healthy option on many restaurant menus. Additionally, it has been scientifically proven that most people will consume hundreds of extra calories when dining in a group or social setting.

Think back to the last dinner you attended with a group of friends: Did you order an extra cocktail, partake in a fatty appetizer, or share a large dessert? The answer is probably yes. But have you ever thought about how many extra calories you are consuming during these get-togethers?

What about when you plan meals at home or make a grocery list? Do you know which are the most nutritious options? When you aren't sure of the nutritional content of different foods, it can be difficult to plan meals and grocery shop for healthy items. Perhaps you never realized that eating a seemingly healthy salad with vegetables can actually contain more calories and fat and less fiber and protein than a cheeseburger, if you coat the salad in ranch dressing!

The wonderful thing about *Ultra Simple Calorie Counter & Diet Journal* is that it takes the guesswork out of ordering or preparing a healthy meal. The book's portable size makes it easy to put in your purse or car so you can quickly and conveniently look up the nutritional values for any food item.

Ultra Simple Calorie Counter & Diet Journal is the most comprehensive book on the market, providing nutritional information and serving sizes for over 300 national brands and over 200 restaurants and fast-food chains.

USING THIS BOOK WHEN DINING OUT

Refer to this book when planning to eat out and you will be able to determine the restaurant that best suits your needs. For instance, if you are in the mood for a hamburger, you can browse this book and choose a restaurant that has the healthiest burger choices.

If you have decided where to go, you can use the information provided in this book to choose the best options from the restaurant's menu. For example, you may find that the steak and potato entrée has fewer calories than a chicken salad made with high-fat mayonnaise-based dressing. Wouldn't it be nice to enjoy the steak dish you crave, knowing that you're making the healthy choice?

Or, perhaps you will refer to the section on mixed drinks, wine, and spirits and learn that one piña colada contains 440 calories. This knowledge can help you decide between having the piña colada or a dessert at the end of your meal.

As you can see, this book allows you to plan ahead and make trade-offs when dining out, so you eat and drink within your daily limits.

USING THIS BOOK WHEN MAKING A GROCERY LIST AND PLANNING MEALS AT HOME

Use this book when writing your grocery list. You will be able to plan healthy, hearty meals and buy only items or national brands that contribute to eating smart, losing weight, and feeling better.

For instance, while using this book, you may realize that the muffin you usually eat for breakfast has a whopping 500 calories, 24 grams of fat, and 60 grams of carbs! An alternative meal might be an omelet with 1 large egg, ½ ounce of cheese, and ½ ounce of ham, as well as a whole wheat english muffin. The nutritional totals for this hearty breakfast option come to only 284 calories, 12 grams of fat, and 26 grams of carbohydrates. Although a ham-and-cheese omelet and english muffin may sound like more food than the muffin, that meal is actually better for you. Throw in an apple for good measure— it has just 55 calories, no fat, and all-natural carbs!

USING THE DIET JOURNAL PAGES

Studies show that people who keep track of what they eat by using a diet journal lose twice as much weight as those who don't. That is because a diet journal forces you to stay accountable for every bite of food and sip of a drink you put in your mouth. You will quickly realize that you are probably eating too much food, and that there are some simple places to cut back on calories, such as eliminating soda or sugary foods from your diet.

This book is wonderful because it combines nutritional information with your diet journal. Use it when you are cooking or dining out to easily record the calories, fat and carbs for the foods you eat right in the journal.

By using *Ultra Simple Calorie Counter & Diet Journal* you can stop relying on fad diets or depriving yourself of the things you love to eat. With this handy book, you can easily compare and contrast foods to make the best selections, even while dining out or on-the-go. You will find that by monitoring and recording what you eat and drink in the journal pages you will lose weight and feel great, almost effortlessly.

Congratulations, and happy eating!

Your Weight & Health Status

The most important reasons to start a weight-loss program are to look and feel great, and to reduce the risk of health complications such as heart disease and diabetes. Before you start, however, it is important to assess your health status. There are three methods to determine your overall physical condition: your height and weight measurements, waist size, and Body Mass Index (BMI). Another consideration is your family history.

For adults 18 years and older, the first step is to measure your height and weight. Use those two numbers to find your BMI on the following page. If your BMI falls within the range of 19 to 24, you are considered healthy. If your BMI lands from 25 to 29, then you have an increased risk of developing health problems. If your BMI is 30 or above, you could be considered obese. If you fall into the last two categories, it is essential to plan and manage your weight-loss program.

The second factor in evaluating your weight is your waist size. Use a tape measure to calculate your waist circumference below your rib cage and above your belly button. You have an increased health risk for developing serious chronic illness if your waist size is more than 35 inches for women and 40 inches for men.

Your personal history and family background can shed additional light on possible health risks. Be aware of increased potential problems if your family history includes arthritis, high blood pressure, high cholesterol, high blood sugar, death at a young age, heart problems, cancer, or respiratory illness. A history of family illness doesn't mean these conditions are destined to be a part of your future, but it is yet another reason to get started on the road to good health and physical fitness.

BODY MASS INDEX - BMI

The most common way to determine whether or not a person is obese is through Body Mass Index, or BMI. This is a ratio of a person's height and weight. When a person's BMI is over 25, he or she can be considered overweight. Unfortunately, BMIs over 25 are an increasing trend in America's health statistics. We are a nation whose waistline is expanding and will continue to grow unless we take control of our eating habits.

Body composition can vary greatly from individual to individual. Two people who possess the same height and weight can have different bone structure and varying percentages of muscle and fat. Therefore, your weight alone is not the only factor in assessing your risk for weight-related health issues. Your BMI can help indicate whether or not your health is at risk.

Calculating your BMI: Locate your height in the left-hand column of the chart. Then move across the row to your weight. The number at the very top of the column is your BMI.

BMI	19	20	21	22	23	24	25	26	27	28	29	30	31	32	33	34	35
Height							**Weight in pounds**										
4'10"	91	96	100	105	110	115	119	124	129	134	138	143	148	153	158	162	167
4'11"	94	99	104	109	114	119	124	128	133	138	143	148	153	158	163	168	173
5'	97	102	107	112	118	123	128	133	138	143	148	153	158	163	168	174	179
5'1"	100	106	111	116	122	127	132	137	143	148	153	158	164	169	174	180	185
5'2"	104	109	115	120	126	131	136	142	147	153	158	164	169	175	180	186	191
5'3"	107	113	118	124	130	135	141	146	152	158	163	169	175	180	186	191	197
5'4"	110	116	122	128	134	140	145	151	157	163	169	174	180	186	192	197	204
5'5"	114	120	126	132	138	144	150	156	162	168	174	180	186	192	198	204	210
5'6"	118	124	130	136	142	148	155	161	167	173	179	186	192	198	204	210	216
5'7"	121	127	134	140	146	153	159	166	172	178	185	191	198	204	211	217	223
5'8"	125	131	138	144	151	158	164	171	177	184	190	197	203	210	216	223	230
5'9"	128	135	142	149	155	162	169	176	182	189	196	203	209	216	223	230	236
5'10"	132	139	146	153	160	167	174	181	188	195	202	209	216	222	229	236	243
5'11"	136	143	150	157	165	172	179	186	193	200	208	215	222	229	236	243	250
6'	140	147	154	162	169	177	184	191	199	206	213	221	228	235	242	250	258
6'1"	144	151	159	166	174	182	189	197	204	212	219	227	235	242	250	257	265
6'2"	148	155	163	171	179	186	194	202	210	218	225	233	241	249	256	264	272
6'3"	152	160	168	176	184	192	200	208	216	224	232	240	248	256	264	272	279
	Healthy					**Overweight**						**Obese**					

HEALTH RISKS AND YOUR WEIGHT

For most adults, BMI and waist size are fairly reliable indicators of whether or not you are overweight. These two indicators are also effective in assessing your risk of weight-related health issues.

Your waist measurement determines whether or not you have the tendency to carry fat around your midsection. A higher waist size may indicate a greater risk for weight-related health issues such as high blood pressure, type 2 diabetes and coronary artery disease. Typically, the higher your Body Mass Index, the greater risk to your health. This risk also increases if your waist is greater than 35 inches for women or 40 inches for men.

If your weight indicates that you are at a higher risk for health problems, consult your primary care physician to determine safe and effective ways to improve your health. Even moderate amounts of weight loss, around 5 to 10 percent of your weight, can have long-lasting health benefits.

Risk of Associated Disease According to BMI and Waist Size			
Body Mass Index		Waist less than or equal to 40" Men 35" Women	Waist greater than 40" Men 35" Women
18 or less	Underweight	N/A	N/A
19-24	Normal	N/A	N/A
25-29	Overweight	Increased	High
30-35	Obese	High	Very High
Over 35	Obese	Very High	Very High

IDENTIFY YOUR EATING PATTERNS

Changing your eating habits requires adjusting your attitude toward food. Begin by understanding the situations and emotional triggers that lead to overeating. Let's take a look at some common behaviors:

Are you compelled to eat as an emotional response to your thoughts and feelings? If you eat when you're upset, frustrated, angry, lonely, or tired, the answer most likely is yes. Food feels like the perfect temporary solution that is, until it is finished, and then guilt sets in because the food choice may not have been healthy. Try to choose other behaviors as an emotional response, such as taking a walk or calling a friend.

Do you eat when you are not hungry because you think you should? Sometimes the time of day is enough encouragement to eat a meal or a quick snack, despite a lack of actual physical hunger. Instead, learn to listen to your body. If you are not hungry, you shouldn't eat.

Do you feel guilty leaving food on your plate? Perhaps when you were a child, you were told to finish all of the food on your plate. This sense of guilt should no longer gauge how much food you should eat. It is acceptable to stop eating when you feel full.

Do you make poor food choices because of peer pressure? It is far easier to go with the flow when those around you are eating unhealthy foods. It takes self-control and determination to follow your weight-loss plan at social gatherings or all-you-can-eat buffets. Congratulate yourself when you stick to your plan and successfully fend off unhealthy snacking urges.

Do you eat out of boredom? Food can become a time-filler when you are bored. Don't fall into this trap! Try to motivate yourself and choose a fun and interesting activity as an alternative to snacking. If you are otherwise occupied with an activity where food is not involved, it will be easier to wait for your regularly scheduled meal.

PERSONAL SUCCESS

Reaching your personal goals for weight-loss and health starts with the desire for success. You've started on the path to success by buying this book and honestly assessing your eating habits.

Motivation: Your journey takes on a new challenge as you look at the reasons behind your desire for personal success. The first component is to discover your source of motivation. What are your top three reasons for pursuing your weight-loss goal? Write them down in a journal and read them often as a reminder and a source of inspiration. They will help you stay focused on your future goals.

Realistic Timelines: The second component is to set realistic goals for yourself. Using this book to monitor what you eat is the best way to lose weight and stay healthy. However, promises of instant weight loss are too good to be true and are most likely unhealthy and even dangerous. Just keep track of what you eat, make healthy decisions, and stick to a realistic timeline. General guidelines for healthy weight loss suggest losing 1 to 2 pounds per week.

Celebrating Success: The third component is to focus on the positive aspects of your weight loss. Try to celebrate small achievements along the way to keep yourself motivated toward your long-term goal. These personal achievements will help you keep a positive attitude. For instance, if you turned down a caloric dessert in favor of a fiber-filled piece of fruit, pat yourself on the back! Acknowledge your accomplishments, no matter if they are baby steps or huge leaps of progress.

Visualization: A mental picture is worth a thousand words. In your mind's eye, envision your weight loss before it happens. Visualize all aspects of the new you, from your appearance to your improved health. Remember, if you can see it, chances are very good that you can make that healthy visual a reality.

Maintenance: The fifth and final component is maintaining your weight loss long after you have achieved your goal. Remember to stick with the healthy behaviors, habits, and attitudes that led you to your goal. Refer to this book each time you join go out for dinner, attend a party, write a grocery list, or make a meal at home. Keep up the good work, for there is nothing more gratifying than maintaining an ideal weight and a healthy lifestyle!

Secrets to Losing Weight

SUGGESTED DAILY CALORIES FOR WEIGHT MAINTENANCE

Your total daily calories should be based on your age, gender, body type, and level of physical activity. Active men should consume approximately 2,800 calories per day to maintain their ideal weight. Active women and sedentary men should eat 2,200 calories. Sedentary women and older adults should strive for 1,600 calories. If you are not sure of how many daily calories you should consume, consult your primary care physician for a recommendation.

Suggested Daily Calories for Weight Maintenance

Sedentary women and older adults should consume approximately 1,600 calories daily.	Most children, teenage girls, active women and sedentary men should consume approximately 2,200 calories daily. Pregnant or breast-feeding women may need to consume more.	Most teenage boys and active men and some very active women should consume approximately 2,800 calories daily.

SUGGESTED DAILY CALORIES FOR WEIGHT LOSS

The total number of daily calories for a weight-loss plan will depend on the number of pounds you wish to lose. Once you have determined the daily number of calories that you should eat to maintain your weight (based on the chart above), you should decrease your total caloric intake by an average of 500 calories per day for a moderate weight loss. To proceed in a safe and healthy manner, you can eliminate those 500 calories simply by decreasing the amount of sugars, refined carbohydrates, and alcohol in your diet, most of which provide calories with little nutritional value.

RECOMMENDED DAILY AMOUNT FROM EACH FOOD GROUP

The United States Department of Agriculture is known for its Food Guide, which is a nutritional reference for many health groups and dietary plans. The USDA Food Guide separates the foods you should eat into six different categories: 1) grains, 2) vegetables, 3) fruits, 4) fats and oils, 5) milk and dairy products, and 6) meat, beans, fish, eggs, and nuts. The suggested amounts have been developed to help you select the proper amount of food to eat from each group on a daily basis. Each group provides you with a different set of essential nutrients. By following the recommended serving sizes, you can be assured that you are getting the proper amounts of protein, fats, carbohydrates, fiber, vitamins, and minerals. This guide can be adjusted to suit your personal needs.

The USDA Food Guide separates the foods you should eat into six different categories:

1. **GRAINS**
   (6-11 SERVINGS)

2. **VEGETABLES**
   (3-5 SERVINGS)

3. **FRUITS**
   (2-4 SERVINGS)

4. **MILK & DAIRY PRODUCTS**
   (2-3 SERVINGS)

5. **MEAT, BEANS, FISH, EGGS & NUTS**
   (2-3 SERVINGS)

6. **FATS & OILS**
   (USE SPARINGLY)

DAILY AMOUNT OF FOOD FROM EACH GROUP

Daily Calorie Level	1,200	1,400	1,600	1,800	2,000	2,200	2,400	2,600	2,800	3,000
Grains	4 oz.	5 oz.	5 oz.	6 oz.	6 oz.	7 oz.	8 oz.	9 oz.	10 oz.	10 oz.
Vegetables	1.5 C (3 srv)	1.5 C (2 srv)	2 C (4 srv)	2.5 C (5 srv)	2.5 C (5 srv)	3 C (6 srv)	3 C (6 srv)	3.5 C (7 srv)	3.5 C (7 srv)	4 C (8 srv)
Fruits	1 C (2 srv)	1.5 C (3 srv)	1.5 C (3 srv)	1.5 C (3 srv)	2 C (4 srv)	2 C (4 srv)	2 C (4 srv)	2 C (4 srv)	2.5 C (5 srv)	2.5 C (5 srv)
Milk	2 C	2 C	3 C	3 C	3 C	3 C	3 C	3 C	3 C	3 C
Meat, Beans, Fish & Nuts	3 oz.	4 oz.	5 oz.	5 oz.	5.5 oz.	6 oz.	6.5 oz.	6.5 oz.	7 oz.	7 oz.
Fats & Oils	17 g	17 g	22 g	24 g	27 g	29 g	31 g	34 g	36 g	44 g

Food group amounts shown in cups (C) or ounces (oz.), with number of servings (srv) in parentheses. Oils are shown in grams.

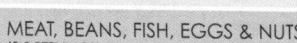
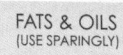

THE NUTRITION FACTS LABEL

Most packaged foods have a nutrition facts label. Use this information to make healthy choices quickly and easily.

Nutrition Facts

Serving Size 1 cup (228g)
Servings Per Container 2

Amount per Serving	
Calories 250 Calories from Fat 110	
	% Daily Value*
Total Fat 12g	18%
Saturated Fat 3g	15%
Trans Fat 3g	
Cholesterol 30mg	10%
Sodium 470mg	20%
Total Carbohydrate 31g	10%
Dietary Fiber 0g	0%
Sugars 5g	
Protein 5g	
Vitamin A	4%
Vitamin C	2%
Calcium	20%
Iron	4%

* Percent Daily Values are based on a 2,000 calorie diet. Your Daily Values may be higher or lower depending on your calorie needs.

	Calories:	2,000	2,500
Total Fat	Less than	65g	80g
Sat Fat	Less than	20g	25g
Cholesterol	Less than	300mg	300mg
Sodium	Less than	2,400mg	2,400mg
Total Carbohydrate		300g	375g
Dietary Fiber		25g	30g

LABEL AT A GLANCE

Start Here: Check the serving size and servings per container.

Calories: 400+ calories per serving is considered high. Note the calories from fat.

Daily Values: 5%=low, 20%=high.

Limit These Nutrients: Eating too much fat, saturated fat, trans fat, cholesterol, or sodium may put you at an increased health risk for diseases such as heart disease, some cancers, or high blood pressure.

Get Enough of These Nutrients: Most Americans do not receive the proper amount of fiber, vitamins A and C, calcium or iron from their diets. Eating enough of these nutrients can limit your risk of diseases such as osteoporosis and heart disease.

Daily Values Footnote: This footnote makes recommendations for key nutrients based on diets of 2,000 and 2,500 daily calories.

A Breakdown Of The Nutrition Facts Label: The first place to look when selecting foods at the market is the product label. Check out the Nutrition Facts for the ingredient list, serving size, calories, amounts, nutrients, portions, and percentage of daily nutritional values. Often you will see "enriched" food sources for wheat or pasta. This is an indication that vitamins or minerals have been added for nutrition. Commonly added nutrients are calcium, thiamin, riboflavin, niacin, iron, and folic acid. The ingredient list tells you exactly what is in the food, including nutrients and whether fat or sugar have been added. The ingredients are also listed in descending order by weight.

What is a Serving Size?: When hunger strikes and a type of food calls out to you, it is important to look at the label for serving size information. The Nutrition Facts label indicates the quantity of food per portion and the number of servings in the package. Serving sizes are now standardized to make it easier to compare foods in familiar units like cups, pieces, grams, or metric amounts. According to the sample label on the previous page, 1 serving of food equals 1 cup containing 250 calories. If you ate the whole package, you would have consumed 2 cups or 500 calories.

All Calories Are Not Created Equal: Calories provide a concrete measure of how much energy you receive from a serving size of a selected food. If you are overweight, chances are you consume more calories than your body needs on a daily basis. You should also be aware of how many calories per serving come from fat. In the sample label, there are 250 calories in a serving, and 110 of those come from fat. That means almost half of the calories are from fat. If you ate 2 servings or 500 calories, 220 would come from fat, which is 44 percent. To lose weight, select foods with 20 percent or less of its calories per serving coming from fat. These can be from proteins, dairy products, and whole grain breads, cereals, and pasta. Most fresh fruits and vegetables are naturally low in fat.

Keep Tabs on Cholesterol: Cholesterol is a fat-like substance present in all animal foods, such as meat, poultry, fish, milk and milk products, and egg yolks. It's a good idea to select lean meats, avoid eating the skin of poultry, and use low-fat milk products. Egg yolks and organ meats, like liver, are high in cholesterol. Plant foods, such as fruit and vegetables, do not contain cholesterol. Why is this important information? Eating foods high in dietary cholesterol increases blood cholesterol in many people, which increases their risk for heart disease. Most health authorities suggest dietary cholesterol should be limited to 300 mg or less per day.

Salt and Sodium: It's important to include some salt in your diet, but it should be limited to 2,400 mg per day. You can keep track of your daily intake by looking at the Nutrition Facts label. Go easy on luncheon and cured meats, cheeses, canned soups and vegetables, and soy sauce. Look for no-salt-added products at your supermarket. Be cautious and avoid adding table salt to your food. Each teaspoon of salt adds 2,000 mg of sodium to your diet. So put down the salt shaker and retrain your taste buds.

Sugar – How Sweet It Isn't: Sugar is an ingredient that is found in almost every food product. If you are counting calories, it is important to look at the list of ingredients to identify all sources of sugar. Obvious foods that add sugar are jams, ice cream, canned fruit and chocolate milk. You will also find it in cereals, sauces, frozen foods, and salad dressings. Here's a list of common sweeteners that are essentially sugar: white sugar, honey, sucrose, fructose, maltose, lactose, syrup, corn syrup, high fructose corn syrup, molasses, and fruit juice concentrate. If these terms are found in the first four listings on the label, that food is likely to be very high in sugar. Hint: labels are listed in grams. Consider 4 grams to equal 1 teaspoon of sugar. The total daily intake for all added sugar sources not found naturally in the food itself should be a maximum 6 teaspoons a day.

Carbohydrates: Breads, cereals, rice, and pasta provide carbohydrates, which are excellent sources of energy. If you are on a weight-loss plan, it is important to include them in your diet because they provide vitamins, minerals, and fiber. One serving of carbohydrates equals one slice of bread, one ounce of ready-to-eat cereal, or 1/2 cup cooked cereal, rice or pasta. Focus on complex carbohydrates, such as whole grain breads, cereals, and brown rice. Keep these foods healthy by not adding additional butter, margarine, cream, cheese, sugar, oils, and fat. Limit refined carbohydrates, such as white flour and sugar, as well as processed foods like prepackaged candy, cookies, cakes, and chips.

Fruits & Vegetables: Fruits and vegetables can be works of art if you select a rainbow of nine colorful choices throughout your day. For example, eat a yellow banana, green broccoli, orange carrots, a red apple, purple cabbage, and blueberries. Rotate your selections to get the most from your foods. Fruits and vegetables provide vitamins A and C, and folate. They also contain minerals like iron, potassium, and magnesium. Keep in mind that it is important to eat these foods as fresh as possible, preferably raw, and avoid adding butter, salt, and high-fat salad dressings. When possible, choose the actual piece of fruit, like an apple, over juice.

Protein: The USDA Food Guide suggests eating cooked lean meat as a source of protein for optimum health. Protein provides an essential supply of B vitamins, zinc, and iron. Make sure you get enough of these nutrients by combining a variety of choices, such as lean cuts of beef, pork, veal, lamb, chicken, turkey, fish, and shellfish. Other protein possibilities are eggs, beans, nut butters, tofu, dried nuts, and seeds. Try to choose lean cuts of meat, remove the skin from poultry, trim away all visible fat, go easy on egg yolks, and eat nuts and seeds sparingly.

Fat: As a food source, fat supplies energy and essential fatty acids to your body. Fat-soluble vitamins like A, D, E and K and carotenoids need fat to be absorbed into the body. Not all types of fat are healthy, however, especially saturated fats found in whole milk, butter, ice cream, poultry skin, and palm oil. Unsaturated fats, found mainly in vegetable oils, do not increase blood cholesterol.

A third category called trans fat is formed when liquid oils are made into solid fats, like shortening and hard margarine. This type of fat is dangerous because it raises blood cholesterol and increases the risk of coronary heart disease, which is one of the leading causes of death in the United States. Foods high in trans fat are processed foods made with partially hydrogenated vegetable oils, such as vegetable shortenings. These oils can be found in crackers, cookies, candies, snack foods, fried foods, and baked goods. It is difficult to avoid all foods with trans fat, so the ideal goal would be to limit your intake of processed foods as much as possible.

Foods With Healthy Sources of Fat: Try choosing vegetable oils like olive, canola, soybean, sunflower, and corn. Avoid coconut and palm kernel oils. Consider adding fish to your menu twice a week. Salmon and mackerel have omega-3 fatty acids, which offer protection against heart disease. Choose lean meats like skinless chicken, lean beef, and pork. Avoid all fried foods. Watch your fat calories because they contain 9 calories per gram, compared to carbohydrates and protein, which have only 4 calories per gram.

THE DIFFERENT TYPES OF FATS

FATS & THEIR SOURCES

Saturated Fats: Limit these fats. Saturated fats tend to raise blood cholesterol. Foods that contain higher amounts of saturated fats include high fat dairy products (like cheese, whole milk, cream, and regular ice cream), butter, fatty meats, lard, palm oil, and coconut oil.

Trans fatty acids: Limit these fats. Foods that are high in trans fatty acids tend to raise blood cholesterol as well. These foods include those high in partially hydrogenated vegetable oils, such as hard margarine and shortenings. Foods with a high amount of this type of fat include some commercially fried foods and some baked goods.

Dietary Cholesterol: Limit cholesterol. Foods that are high in cholesterol also tend to raise blood cholesterol. These foods include liver and other organ meats, egg yolks, and dairy fat.

Unsaturated Fats: Unsaturated fats and oils do not raise blood cholesterol. These types of fats occur in vegetable oils such as olive, canola and corn oils, most nuts, avocados, and fatty fish like salmon. Some fish, such as salmon, tuna, and mackerel, contain omega-3 fatty acids that may offer protection against heart disease. This is the best type of fat to include in your diet. Just be sure to avoid excess calories.

EXERCISE AND WEIGHT CONTROL

Carrying around too much body fat is a nuisance. Many people fight the "battle of the bulge" through diet alone because exercise is not always convenient. Few of today's occupations require physical activity, and many people spend hours behind desks and computers. In addition, much of our leisure time is spent in sedentary pursuits. To reverse this trend, it is important to adjust your attitude and find time to exercise each day. Some of the most common reasons people use to avoid physical activity include:

1. "I don't have the time."
2. "I'm too tired and I don't feel like it."
3. "I'm not very good at exercising."
4. "It's not convenient to get to my workout place."
5. "I'm afraid and embarrassed."

Overweight or Overfat?: Being overweight and being overfat are two different dilemmas. Some people, such as athletes, have a muscular physique and weigh more than average for their age and height. But their body composition, which is the amount of fat versus lean body mass (muscle, bone, organs and tissue), is within an acceptable range. Others can weigh within the range of U.S. guidelines, yet they can carry around too much fat. Use exercise as a way to balance your body fat percentage. An easy self-test is to pinch the thickness of fat at your waist and abdomen. If you can pinch more than an inch of fat, excluding muscles, chances are you have too much body fat.

Energy Balance and Counting Calories: Losing weight boils down to a simple mathematical formula: consume fewer calories than you burn. Learn how to balance energy intake (food) with energy output (calories burned through physical activity). If you take in more calories than your body needs to perform your day's activities, it will be stored as fat. Therefore, the only solution is to consume the proper amount of calories that your body needs to maintain good health. Then exercise so that your body can utilize the stored fat. The end result will be your desired weight loss.

CALORIES BURNED BY TYPICAL PHYSICAL ACTIVITIES

LIGHT ACTIVITIES: 150 or less	CAL/HR.
Billiards	140
Lying down/sleeping	60
Office work	140
Sitting	80
Standing	100

MODERATE ACTIVITIES: 150-350	CAL/HR.
Aerobic dancing	340
Ballroom dancing	210
Bicycling (5 mph)	170
Bowling	160
Canoeing (2.5 mph)	170
Dancing (social)	210
Gardening (moderate)	270
Golf (with cart)	180
Golf (without cart)	320
Grocery shopping	180
Horseback riding (sitting trot)	250
Light housework/cleaning, etc.	250
Ping-pong	270
Swimming (20 yards/min)	290
Tennis (recreational doubles)	310
Vacuuming	220
Volleyball (recreational)	260
Walking (2 mph)	200
Walking (3 mph)	240
Walking (4 mph)	300

VIGOROUS ACTIVITIES: 350 or MORE   CAL/HR.

Aerobics (step)	440
Backpacking (10 lb load)	540
Badminton	450
Basketball (competitive)	660
Basketball (leisure)	390
Bicycling (10 mph)	375
Bicycling (13 mph)	600
Cross country skiing (leisurely)	460
Cross country skiing (moderate)	660
Hiking	460
Ice skating (9 mph)	384
Jogging (5 mph)	550
Jogging (6 mph)	690
Racquetball	620
Rollerblading	384
Rowing machine	540
Running (8 mph)	900
Scuba diving	570
Shoveling snow	580
Soccer	580
Spinning	650
Stair climber machine	480
Swimming (50 yards/min.)	680
Water aerobics	400
Water skiing	480
Weight training (30 sec. between sets)	760
Weight training (60 sec. between sets)	570

Favorite Alcoholic Drinks

ALCOHOL, BEER AND WINE

Eating smarter and losing weight doesn't have to mean having to skip out on events, parties and drinks with friends. Alcohol, in moderation, can still be a part of a healthy diet. In fact, studies have shown that moderate drinking (about 12 ounces of beer or 5 ounces of wine per day) can improve cardiovascular health and lower the risk of stroke and high blood pressure.

In this section, calorie, fat and carb information for beer, cocktails, liqueur, liquor, shooters and wine will help you avoid high-calorie drinks and enjoy alcoholic beverages that are within your daily calorie allotment.

Be aware that alcohol may increase appetite, induce cravings for high-calorie or salty foods, and decrease self-control. Always drink alcohol in moderation and monitor your intake while drinking when food is present at events, barbecues or happy hours.

FAVORITE ALCOHOLIC DRINKS

	Cal	Fat	Cbs
BEERS			
Light			
Amstel Light, 1 bottle	100	0	5
Bud Light, 12 fl oz	110	0	7
Coors Light, 12 fl oz	102	0	5
Corona Light, 1 bottle	105	0	5
Kirin Light, 12.2 fl oz	100	0	7
• Michelob Ultra, 1 bottle	73	0	2
Miller Lite, 12 fl oz	96	0	3
Milwaukee's Best Light, 12.2 fl oz	98	0	4
Natural Light, 12 fl oz	95	0	3
• Samuel Adams Light, 12 fl oz	119	0	10
Regular			
Blue Moon, 12 fl oz	171	0	14
Budweiser , 12 fl oz	145	0	11
Corona Extra, 1 bottle	148	0	13
Guinness, Stout, 1 pint	170	0	6
• Heineken, 1 bottle	140	0	11
Kirin,12.2 fl oz	145	0	10
Miller Genuine Draft,12 fl oz	143	0	13
Newcastle, 12 fl oz	140	0	12
• Samuel Adams, 12 fl oz	180	0	18
Stella Artois, 11.2 fl oz	154	0	6
Non-Alcoholic			
Beck's Non-Alcoholic, 12 fl oz	90	0	20
• Coors Non-Alcoholic, 1 bottle	65	0	14
O'Douls, 12 fl oz	70	0	15
Old Milwaukee NA, 1 can	71	0	15
• St. Pauli Girl NA, 12 fl oz	95	0	22
COCKTAILS			
Alexander, 1 cocktail	170	2	8
Black Russian, 1 cocktail	240	0	16
Bloody Mary, 1 cocktail	115	0	5
Bourbon & Soda, 1 cocktail	105	0	0
Daiquiri, 1 cocktail	113	0	4
Gin & Tonic, 1 cocktail	197	0	16
Grasshopper, 1 cocktail	222	4	22
High Ball, 1 cocktail	107	0	2
Lemon Drop Martini, 1 cocktail	150	0	32
Long Island Ice Tea, 1 cocktail	140	0	11
Mai Tai, 1 cocktail	264	0	23
Manhattan, 1 cocktail	136	0	2
Margarita, 1 cocktail	159	0	6
Mint Julep, 1 cocktail	188	0	4
• Mojito, 1 cocktail	100	0	21

• MOST HEALTHY   • LEAST HEALTHY

FAVORITE ALCOHOLIC DRINKS	Cal	Fat	Cbs
• Piña Colada, 1 cocktail	440	9	26
Rum and Coke , 1 cocktail	150	0	15
Sangria, 1 cocktail	165	0	23
Screwdriver, 1 cocktail	171	0	18
Seabreeze, 1 cocktail	170	0	20
Seven and Seven , 1 cocktail	180	0	16
Singapore Sling, 1 cocktail	230	0	12
Tequila Sunrise, 1 cocktail	175	0	15
Tom Collins, 1 cocktail	156	0	3
Whiskey Sour, 1 cocktail	139	0	5
White Russian, 1 cocktail	253	1	17

LIQUEURS

	Cal	Fat	Cbs
99 Apples - 49.5% (99 prf), 1 oz.	72	0	8
Alize - 16.0% (32 prf), 1 oz.	103	0	11
• Amaretto - 28.0% (56 prf), 1 oz.	110	0	17
Barenfang - 40.0% (80 prf), 1 oz.	103	0	11
Continental - 17.5% (35 proof), 1 oz.	85	2	9
Crème de Cassis - 20.0% (40 proof), 1 oz.	80	0	11
Crème de Coconut - 17.0% (34 prf), 1 oz.	103	0	11
DeKuyper Grape Schnapps, 1 oz.	70	0	10
Forbidden Fruit - 50.0% (100 proof),1 oz.	103	0	11
Godiva - 17.0% (34 proof),1 oz.	103	0	11
Hypnotiq - 17.5% (35 proof), 1 oz.	103	0	11
Jagermeister - 35.0% (70 proof), 1 oz.	103	0	11
Jubilee - 24.0% (48 proof), 1 oz.	72	0	6
Kahlua- 26.5% (53 proof), 1 oz.	90	0	11
Maui Blue Hawaiian - 15.0% (30 prf), 1 oz.	72	0	10
Midori - 23.0% (46 proof), 1 oz.	79	0	11
Sour Puss - 15.5% (31 proof), 1 oz.	103	0	11
• Tequila Rose - 17.0% (34 proof), 1 oz.	69	0	7
Tia Maria - 27.0% (54 proof), 1 oz.	92	0	10
Zwack - 43.0% (86 proof),1 oz.	87	12	9

LIQUORS

	Cal	Fat	Cbs
Brandy - 40.0% (80 proof), 1 oz.	69	0	2
Gin - 40.0% (80 proof), 1 oz.	69	0	0
Rum - 40.0% (80 proof), 1 oz.	69	0	0
Tequila - 40.0% (80 proof), 1 oz.	69	0	0
Vodka - 40.0% (80 proof), 1 oz.	69	0	0
Whiskey - 40.0% (80 proof), 1 oz.	69	0	0

SHOOTERS

	Cal	Fat	Cbs
Buttery Nipple, 1.5 fl oz	130	2	14
Chocolate Cake Shot, 1 shot	85	0	6
Fuzzy Navel, 1.5 fl oz	120	0	7
Kamikazi, 1.5 fl oz	150	0	2
Purple Hooter, 1.5 fl oz	90	0	6
Red-Headed Slut, 2 oz	164	0	18

• MOST HEALTHY • LEAST HEALTHY

FAVORITE ALCOHOLIC DRINKS	Cal	Fat	Cbs
• Soco Lime, 2 oz	167	0	15
• Vodka Lemon Drop, 1 oz	38	0	2
Washington Apple, 3 oz	140	0	10
WINE			
Dry Dessert Wine, 1 fl. oz.	45	0	3
Red Table Wine, 1 fl. oz.	25	0	1
• Sweet Dessert Wine, 1 fl. oz.	47	0	4
• White Table Wine, 1 fl. oz.	25	0	1

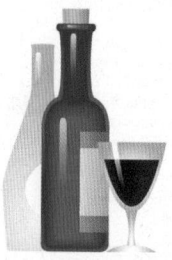

• MOST HEALTHY   • LEAST HEALTHY

Restaurants & Fast-food Chains

RESTAURANTS & FAST-FOOD CHAINS

With complete calorie, fat and carb information for more than 200 restaurants and fast-food chains, you will easily be able to choose a place to eat out without wrecking your diet. Many people trying to eat smarter say that dining out is the number one thing that prevents them from losing weight. Finding a healthy option can be difficult at many restaurants and fast-food locations. That's where this section will come in handy. Nutritional information for every salad, side, entrée, appetizer, dessert and beverage at hundreds of restaurants will help you decide where to eat and what to order when you're dining out. You will save hundreds of calories and dozens of grams of fat and carbohydrates by referring to this chapter.

Losing weight and eating better can still include a delicious dinner at a restaurant or a meal from the drive-thru — you just need to know what your healthy options are. Keep this book close by when you are dining out and you'll be well on your way to dropping unwanted pounds!

A&W RESTAURANT

	Cal	Fat	Cbs
Hot Dogs			
• Coney (Chili) Cheese Dog, 117 g	380	23	28
Coney (Chili) Dog, 88 g	340	20	26
• Dog (plain), 53 g	310	19	23
Sandwiches & Strips			
Cheeseburger, 169 g	420	21	37
Chicken Strips- 3 pieces, 159 g	500	29	32
Crispy Chicken Sandwich 213 g	550	25	52
Grilled Chicken Sandwich, 207 g	400	15	31
• Hamburger, 155 g	380	19	33
Original Bacon Cheeseburger, 217 g	530	30	39
• Original Bacon Double Chz burger, 297 g	760	45	45
Original Double Cheeseburger, 282 g	680	38	44
Papa Burger, 282 g	690	39	44
Papa Single Burger, 206 g	470	25	38
Sides			
Cheese Curds, 71 g	200	8	28
Cheese Fries, 113 g	310	12	45
Chili Cheese Fries, 156 g	430	17	61
• Extra Burger Patty, 70 g	180	8	20
Regular Breaded Onion Rings, 170 g	390	18	50
Regular Corn Dog Nuggets, 113 g	350	16	45
• Regular French Fries, 156 g	480	27	62
Sweets & Treats: Polar Swirls			
M&M's® Polar Swirl®, 340 g	710	25	107
• Oreo® Polar Swirl®,340 g	690	24	107
• Reese's® Polar Swirl®,340 g	740	31	97
Sweets & Treats: Sundaes (Medium)			
Chocolate Milkshake, 594 g	880	36	125
• Strawberry Milkshake, 594 g	840	36	113
• Vanilla Milkshake, 594 g	900	39	121
Sweets & Treats: Soft Serve Cones			
Vanilla Cone, 157 g	260	7	41
Sweets & Treats: Shakes			
Caramel Sundae, 189 g	340	9	57
Chocolate Sundae, 189 g	320	8	53
• Hot Fudge Sundae, 189 g	350	11	54
Strawberry Sundae, 189 g	300	8	47

AMAZON CAFÉ

	Cal	Fat	Cbs
Smoothie (Medium)			
Amazon Power Boost, 16 oz.	229	1	68
Bananarama, 16 oz.	239	1	65
Chocolate Nirvana, 16 oz.	225	1	76
Citrus Sunrise, 16 oz.	254	2	88
Coldblaster, 16 oz.	247	1	65

• MOST HEALTHY   • LEAST HEALTHY

AMAZON CAFÉ (cont.)

	Cal	Fat	Cbs
Orange Outrage, 16 oz.	215	1	65
Orange Sensation, 16 oz.	242	2	63
Paradise Lust, 16 oz.	265	3	60
• Piña Colada, 16 oz.	320	4	63
Raspberry Rage, 16 oz.	234	1	69
Raspberry Razzle, 16 oz.	207	1	62
• Skinny Delight, 16 oz.	186	1	44
Soy Smoothie, 16 oz.	191	0	50
Strawberry Supreme, 16 oz.	221	1	55
Tropical Passion, 16 oz.	236	1	71

Soup

	Cal	Fat	Cbs
Broccoli & Cheese, 8 oz.	110	6	10
Chicken & Sausage Gumbo, 8 oz.	100	3	12
Chicken & Wild Rice, 8 oz.	120	3	17
• Chili Con Carne, 8 oz.	250	7	29
Chipotle Black Bean, 8 oz.	130	1	21
Classic Chicken Noodle, 8 oz.	80	2	9
Corn Chowder, 8 oz.	110	4	19
Cream of Broccoli, 8 oz.	110	5	14
Cream of Potato with Bacon, 8 oz.	120	4	18
Hearty Vegetable, 8 oz.	70	1	15
Italian Wedding, 8 oz.	130	4	16
Mushroom Barley, 8 oz.	80	2	14
New England Clam Chowder, 8 oz.	90	2	15
Rosemary Chicken Dumpling, 8 oz.	80	1	12
Rustic Beef & Mushroom, 8 oz.	70	2	6
Split Pea with Ham, 8 oz.	160	5	22
Sweet Pepper & Beef, 8 oz.	90	2	14
Three Bean Chili, 8 oz.	130	0	47
• Tomato & Three Cheese, 8 oz.	60	2	7

APPLEBEE'S

Chicken

	Cal	Fat	Cbs
Chicken Fried Chicken	1250	N/A	114
Chicken Parmesan	1330	N/A	114
Chicken Tenders Basket	1000	N/A	81
Chicken Tenders Platter	1300	N/A	104
Fiesta Lime Chicken®	1230	N/A	97
Grilled Dijon Chicken & Portobellos	450	N/A	32
Margherita Chicken	750	N/A	67
Riblet and Chkn Tenders Basket	1240	N/A	92
• Riblet and Chkn Tenders Platter	1735	N/A	121
Roasted Garlic & Asiago Chicken	810	N/A	56
• Weight Watchers® Garlic Herb Chicken	370	N/A	37

Desserts

	Cal	Fat	Cbs
Blue Ribbon Brownie	1290	N/A	172

• MOST HEALTHY   • LEAST HEALTHY

APPLEBEE'S (cont.)

	Cal	Fat	Cbs
• Chocolate Chip Cookie Sundae	1660	N/A	224
Chocolate Mousse Shooter	450	N/A	44
• Hot Fudge Sundae Shooter	340	N/A	45
Maple Butter Blondie	990	N/A	116
Sizzling Apple Pie	900	N/A	144
Strawberry Cheesecake Shooter	380	N/A	41
Triple Chocolate Meltdown®	810	N/A	91

Pasta & Bowls

	Cal	Fat	Cbs
Cheddar-Jack Mac & Chz w/ Chicken	1030	N/A	66
Chicken Broccoli Pasta Alfredo	1200	N/A	104
• Crispy Orange Chicken Bowl	1900	N/A	231
Grilled Shrimp Pesto Alfredo Fettuccine	1610	N/A	109
Shrimp Fettuccine Alfredo Bowl	1220	N/A	105
• Spicy Shrimp Diavolo	500	N/A	79
Three-Cheese Chicken Penne	1310	N/A	120

Pick N Pair Lunch Combos

	Cal	Fat	Cbs
Applebee's Reuben	620	N/A	25
Asian Crunch Salad	220	N/A	21
Baked Potato Soup	380	N/A	24
Black Bean Soup	220	N/A	25
• Breadstick	80	N/A	14
Broccoli Cheddar Soup	320	N/A	17
Caesar Salad	220	N/A	8
California Turkey Club	460	N/A	30
Chicken Noodle Soup	140	N/A	15
Chicken Tortilla Soup	160	N/A	17
Chili	480	N/A	21
Clam Chowder	310	N/A	20
French Dip Sliders	580	N/A	50
French Onion Soup	280	N/A	18
Grilled Shrimp 'N Spinach Salad	270	N/A	21
Oriental Chicken Salad	390	N/A	25
• Three-Cheese Chicken Penne	690	N/A	54
Tomato Basil Soup	230	N/A	25

Realburgers

	Cal	Fat	Cbs
Bacon Cheddar Cheeseburger	940	N/A	48
Cheeseburger	850	N/A	47
Cowboy Burger	1120	N/A	74
Fire Pit Bacon Burger	1070	N/A	50
Hamburger	770	N/A	47
Philly Burger	1090	N/A	70
• Quesadilla Burger	1420	N/A	45
Southwest Jalapeño Burger	1110	N/A	65
Steakhouse Burger w/ A.1.® Steak Sauce	1190	N/A	63
The Original Brewtus Burger™	1140	N/A	48
Veggie Burger	530	N/A	61

• MOST HEALTHY   • LEAST HEALTHY

APPLEBEE'S (cont.)

	Cal	Fat	Cbs
Fresh Fruit, Side	70	N/A	17
Fries, Side	400	N/A	51
• Seasonal Vegetables, Side	40-60	N/A	9
Side	540	N/A	62
Small House Salad	230	N/A	12

Ribs & Fajitas

	Cal	Fat	Cbs
• Applebee's Riblets Basket	1075	N/A	75
Double-Glazed Baby Back Ribs	1350	N/A	109
Sizzling Fajitas - Chicken	1470	N/A	163
Sizzling Fajitas - Combo	1520	N/A	163
• Sizzling Fajitas - Steak	1560	N/A	164

Salads

	Cal	Fat	Cbs
Apple Walnut Chicken Salad, Regular	1000	N/A	53
Asian Crunch Salad	490	N/A	57
Crispy Shrimp Caesar, Regular	1060	N/A	57
Fried Chicken Salad, Regular	1060	N/A	49
Grilled Chicken Caesar, Regular	820	N/A	25
Grilled Shrimp 'N Spinach, Regular	1050	N/A	68
Grilled Steak Caesar, Regular	900	N/A	25
Oriental Chicken Salad, Regular	1310	N/A	88
Oriental Grilled Chicken Salad, Regular	1240	N/A	87
• Pecan-Crusted Chicken Salad, Regular	1340	N/A	108
Santa Fe Chicken Salad, Regular	1300	N/A	57
• Weight Watchers® Paradise Chkn Salad	340	N/A	35

Sandwiches

	Cal	Fat	Cbs
Applebee's Reuben	1130	N/A	49
Bacon Cheese Chicken Grill	720	N/A	47
Blackened Tilapia Sandwich	710	N/A	52
California Turkey Club	1050	N/A	62
Chicken Fajita Rollup	1040	N/A	61
Club House Grill	1140	N/A	66
Hand-Battered Fish Sandwich	820	N/A	60
Honey BBQ Chicken Sandwich	900	N/A	72
Knife & Fork Chkn Cordon Bleu Snd	730	N/A	35
Grilled Sirloin Sandwich (w/o fries)	690	N/A	49
Oriental Chicken Rollup	1060	N/A	110
• Weight Watchers® Itln Chkn & Portobello Snd w/fruit	360	N/A	49
• Zesty Ranch Chicken Sandwich	1140	N/A	74

Seafood

	Cal	Fat	Cbs
Double Crunch Shrimp	1280	N/A	129
Garlic Herb Salmon	750	N/A	59
Grilled Shrimp & Island Rice	380	N/A	59
Hand-Battered Fish & Chips	1560	N/A	106
• New England Fish & Chips	1910	N/A	121
Orange Glazed Salmon	790	N/A	98
• Weight Watchers® Cajun Lime Tilapia	310	N/A	39

• MOST HEALTHY   • LEAST HEALTHY

APPLEBEE'S (cont.)

	Cal	Fat	Cbs
Signature Steaks			
Asiago Peppercorn Steak w/sides	390	N/A	26
Bourbon Street Steak w/Mshr & onions	600	N/A	9
• Chkn Fried Steak (potato, gravy & veg)	1290	N/A	123
Chop Steak	740	N/A	11
Shrimp 'N Parmesan Sirloin	540	N/A	5
Steak & Fried Shrimp Combo	630	N/A	35
Steak & Grilled Shrimp Combo	390	N/A	2
Steak & Honey BBQ Chicken Combo	530	N/A	25
Steak & Riblets Combo	915	N/A	29
• Weight Watchers® Steak & Portobellos	330	N/A	38
Sliders			
BBQ Pulled Pork Sliders	1020	N/A	89
Cheeseburger Sliders	1240	N/A	81
• Cheeseburger Sliders add bacon	1310	N/A	82
• French Dip Sliders	830	N/A	74
Steaks & Toppers			
House Sirloin 9 oz.	310	N/A	0
• New York Strip 12 oz.	590	N/A	0
Ribeye 12 oz.	590	N/A	0
• Topper - Grilled Onions	60	N/A	7
Topper - Sautéed Garlic & Mshr	130	N/A	2
Topper - Shrimp 'N Parmesan	230	N/A	4
Ultimate Trios			
Boneless Buffalo Wings, Classic	580	N/A	33
Bnlss Buffalo Wings, Sweet & spicy sc	570	N/A	45
Buffalo Chicken Wings, Classic	360	N/A	4
Buffalo Chkn Wings, Sweet & spicy sc	350	N/A	16
Wings Bleu Chz Dipping Sauce	220	N/A	1
• Wings Ranch Dipping Sauce	210	N/A	1
• Cheeseburger Sliders	870	N/A	54
Dynamite Shrimp	730	N/A	40
Mozzarella Sticks	430	N/A	39
Spinach Artichoke Dip	580	N/A	42
Steak Quesadilla Towers	600	N/A	37
Others			
Asiago Peppercorn Steak	390	N/A	26
Asian Crunch Salad	490	N/A	57
Grilled Dijon Chicken & Portobellos	450	N/A	32
• Grilled Shrimp & Island Rice	380	N/A	59
• Spicy Shrimp Diavolo	500	N/A	79

ARBY'S

	Cal	Fat	Cbs
Beverages, Shakes & Desserts			
Apple Turnover (no icing), 89 g	270	15	32
Cherry Turnover (no icing), 89 g	270	15	31

• MOST HEALTHY   • LEAST HEALTHY

ARBY'S (cont.)

Sharable Appetizers	Cal	Fat	Cbs
• Appetizer Sampler	2475	N/A	171
Boneless Buffalo Wings, Classic	1170	N/A	66
Boneless Buffalo Wings, Sweet & Spicy	1150	N/A	90
Buffalo Chicken Wings, Classic	710	N/A	7
Buffalo Chkn Wings, Sweet & spicy	690	N/A	32
Wings Bleu Cheese Dipping Sauce	220	N/A	1
• Wings Ranch Dipping Sauce	210	N/A	1
Cheese Quesadilla Grande	1300	N/A	85
Cheeseburger Sliders	1240	N/A	81
Cheeseburger Sliders add bacon	1310	N/A	82
Chicken Quesadilla Grande	1460	N/A	90
Chicken Wonton Tacos	610	N/A	58
Chili Cheese Nachos	1680	N/A	133
Chips & Salsa	990	N/A	113
Crunchy Onion Rings	1230	N/A	161
Dynamite Shrimp	730	N/A	40
Mozzarella Sticks	940	N/A	84
Pork Wonton Tacos	940	N/A	71
Potato Skins	1380	N/A	70
Potato Twisters	840	N/A	64
Queso Blanco	1360	N/A	115
Queso Blanco with chili	1470	N/A	119
Spinach & Artichoke Dip	1535	N/A	123
Steak Quesadilla Towers	1190	N/A	76
Veggie Patch™ Pizza	950	N/A	51
Sides			
Add Fried Shrimp	390	N/A	35
Add Grilled Shrimp	220	N/A	2
Baked Potato	380	N/A	28
Baked Potato Soup (Bowl)	420	N/A	27
Broccoli Cheddar Soup (Bowl)	360	N/A	18
Chicken Noodle Soup (Bowl)	160	N/A	17
Chicken Tortilla Soup (Bowl)	180	N/A	18
• Chili (Bowl)	540	N/A	24
Clam Chowder (Bowl)	350	N/A	22
Dressing, Mexi-Ranch	150	N/A	2
French Onion Soup (Bowl)	280	N/A	19
Garlic Mashed Potatoes	330	N/A	38
Loaded Baked Potato	450	N/A	28
Loaded Mashed Potatoes	430	N/A	30
• Seasonal Vegetables	50	N/A	9
Small Caesar Salad	90	N/A	10
Small House Salad	230	N/A	12
Tomato Basil Soup (Bowl)	250	N/A	27

ARBY'S (cont.)

	Cal	Fat	Cbs
Icing Adds, 21 g	70	1	16
Chocolate Chunk Cookies (2), 91 g	420	21	54
• Chocolate Swirl Shake, 482 g	630	17	109
• Diet Blackberry FruiTea, 327 g	5	0	5
Diet Peach FruiTea, 327 g	5	0	5
Jamocha Swirl Shake, 482 g	610	17	106
Mandarin Peach FruiTea, 333 g	90	0	23
Passion Fruit FruiTea, 334 g	100	0	25
Vanilla Shake, 482 g	540	17	85
Chicken			
• Buffalo Dipping Sauce Adds, 28 g	10	1	2
Chicken Bacon & Swiss – Crispy, 205 g	590	27	54
Chicken Bacon & Swiss – Roast, 194 g	470	19	43
• Chicken Cordon Bleu – Crispy, 241 g	610	29	51
Chicken Cordon Bleu – Roast, 230 g	490	20	40
Chicken Sandwich – Crispy, 200 g	520	24	51
Chicken Sandwich – Roast, 189 g	400	16	40
Crispy Chicken Tenders – Regular, 131 g	360	17	28
Popcorn Chicken – Regular, 135 g	360	16	27
Roast Chicken Club Egg, Milk,, 258 g	460	19	39
Kids Meal			
• Applesauce, 113 g	90	0	21
Curly Fries – Kids, 77 g	240	13	29
Homestyle Fries – Kids, 85 g	230	10	33
• Junior Roast Beef, 125 g	300	9	37
Lowfat Chocolate Milk 1%, 249 g	160	3	27
Popcorn Chicken – Kids, 99 g	260	12	20
Potato Cakes (2), 100 g	260	14	16
Reduced Fat White Milk 2%, 244 g	130	5	13
Market Fresh® Chopped Salads			
• Chpd Farmhouse Chkn Salad – Crsp, 349 g	460	25	29
Chpd Farmhouse Chkn Salad – Grld, 307 g	260	14	10
Chpd Farmhouse Chkn Salad – Rst, 307 g	260	14	10
Chopped Italian Salad, 312 g	390	31	10
Balsamic Vinaigrette Dressing, 43 g	130	12	5
• Chopped Side Salad, 120 g	70	5	4
Chopped Turkey Club Salad, 307 g	250	14	9
Market Fresh® Sandwiches			
Pecan Chkn Salad Snd - Grilled, 322 g	870	44	88
Pecan Chkn Salad Snd - Roast, 322 g	860	44	89
Reuben Sandwich, 295 g	690	32	65
Roast Beef & Swiss Sandwich, 345 g	820	37	84
Roast Beef Gyro, 220 g	420	23	32
• Roast Chicken Ranch Sandwich, 211 g	340	9	41
Roast Ham & Swiss Sandwich, 345 g	750	30	85
Roast Turkey & Swiss Sandwich, 345 g	740	28	84

• MOST HEALTHY   • LEAST HEALTHY

ARBY'S (cont.)

	Cal	Fat	Cbs
Roast Turkey, Ranch & Bacon Snd, 363 g	850	37	84
• Ultimate BLT Sandwich, 295 g	880	46	84

Roast Beef Sandwiches

	Cal	Fat	Cbs
All-American Roastburger®, 245 g	390	16	40
Arby's Melt, 146 g	320	11	38
Bacon & Bleu Roastburger®, 235 g	450	21	39
• Dbl Meat Roastburger® Option Adds, 71 g	120	8	0
Bacon Cheddar Roastburger®, 235 g	430	18	39
Ham & Swiss Melt, 131 g	300	8	37
• Medium Beef 'n Cheddar, 251 g	530	25	42
Medium Roast Beef, 154 g	450	19	37

Sides & Sidekickers® (Medium)

	Cal	Fat	Cbs
• Curly Fries, 170 g	540	29	64
Homestyle Fries, 170 g	470	21	66
• Jalapeño Bites® (5), 110 g	300	17	32
Loaded Potato Bites® (5), 112 g	340	20	29
Mozzarella Sticks (4), 137 g	430	23	36
Onion Petals, 99 g	330	18	38
Potato Cakes (3), 150 g	380	20	25

Toasted Sandwiches

	Cal	Fat	Cbs
• Classic Italian Toasted Sub, 291 g	590	30	57
Frn Dip & Swiss Tst Sub w/Au Jus, 297 g	500	17	59
Philly Beef Toasted Subs, 254 g	570	27	55
• Roast Beef Patty Melt, 200 g	460	21	43
Turkey Bacon Club Toasted Sub, 292 g	570	24	56

ATLANTA BREAD COMPANY

Baked Goods: Bagels

	Cal	Fat	Cbs
Apple Spice, 4 oz.	360	3	73
• Asiago Cheese, 4 oz.	380	10	53
Blueberry, 4 oz.	270	1	55
Cinnamon Crisp, 4 oz.	330	3	68
Cinnamon Raisin, 4 oz.	270	1	56
Everything, 9 oz.	320	4	60
• Lower Carb Cranberry Walnut, 2 oz.	110	4	16
Onion, 4 oz.	290	1	59
Plain, 3 oz.	270	1	55
Poppy Seed, 4 oz.	320	5	57
Sesame, 4 oz.	360	9	57
Wheat, 4 oz.	270	2	54

Baked Goods: Breads

	Cal	Fat	Cbs
ABC Roll, 4 oz.	260	1	54
Asiago Loaf, 2 oz.	160	2	29
Asiago Strip, 2 oz.	160	2	28
Challah, 2 oz.	160	3	29
Cinnamon Raisin Loaf, 2 oz.	150	2	28

• MOST HEALTHY   • LEAST HEALTHY

ATLANTA BREAD COMPANY (cont.)

	Cal	Fat	Cbs
Cracked Wheat, 2 oz.	160	2	30
Foccacia Round, Asiago, 2 oz.	180	5	26
Foccacia Round, Basil Pesto, 2 oz.	190	8	26
Foccacia Round, Tomato Onion, 2 oz.	150	3	27
• Foccacia, Rosemary Tomato, 3 oz.	350	12	50
French Baguette, 2 oz.	140	1	30
French Loaf, 2 oz.	140	1	28
French Roll, 2 oz.	160	1	33
Honey Wheat, 2 oz.	150	2	28
• Lower Carb Multigrain Bread, 2 oz.	100	2	16
Nine Grain, 2 oz.	160	3	28
Pumpernickel, 2 oz.	140	2	26
Rye, 2 oz.	150	2	28
Sourdough Baguette, 2 oz.	140	0	29
Sourdough Loaf, 2 oz.	140	0	29
Sourdough Roll, 2 oz.	160	0	34

Baked Goods: Cream Cheese Spreads

	Cal	Fat	Cbs
Garden Vegetable Cream Cheese, 2 oz.	170	17	4
Onion & Chive Cream Cheese, 2 oz.	190	17	4
• Plain Cream Cheese, 2 oz.	190	19	1
• Plain Cream Cheese, Light, 2 oz.	120	10	6
Strawberry Cream Cheese, 2 oz.	190	15	12

Beverages: Cold

	Cal	Fat	Cbs
Caramel Latte Caffechillo, 19 oz.	250	10	32
• Frozen Spiced Chai Tea, 16 oz.	260	6	43
Kona Mocha Caffechillo, 19 oz.	250	10	32
Vanilla Caffechillo, 19 oz.	250	10	32

Beverages: Hot

	Cal	Fat	Cbs
Café Latte, tall, 16 oz.	170	6	18
Café Mocha, tall, 16 oz.	340	8	57
Cappuccino, tall, 16 oz.	130	5	14
Caramel Macchiato, tall, 16 oz.	390	8	69
• Espresso, single shot, 2 oz.	5	0	1
• Hot Chocolate, tall, 16 oz.	450	10	78
Hot Spiced Chai Tea, 15 oz.	260	6	43
House Latte, tall, 16 oz.	380	10	65

Beverages: Smoothies

	Cal	Fat	Cbs
• Pineapple Mango Banana, 16 oz.	290	0	72
Strawberry Banana, 16 oz.	290	0	71
• Strawberry Blueberry Banana, 16 oz.	280	0	69

Breakfast: Gourmet Breakfast

	Cal	Fat	Cbs
Belgian Waffle w/ syrup, 7 oz.	480	13	82
Belgian Waffle w/o syrup, 5 oz.	320	13	41
• French Toast w/ syrup, 9 oz.	560	9	103
French Toast w/o syrup, 7 oz.	400	9	61
• Scrambled eggs, 5 oz.	220	16	2

• MOST HEALTHY   • LEAST HEALTHY

ATLANTA BREAD COMPANY (cont.)

	Cal	Fat	Cbs
Breakfast: Hot Sandwiches			
Bacon, Egg & Cheese on Croissant, 5 oz.	530	34	39
• Egg & Cheese on Croissant, 5 oz.	480	30	39
Ham, Egg & Cheese on Croissant, 7 oz.	540	31	41
Sausage, Egg & Chz on Croissant, 7 oz.	690	48	39
Breakfast: Omelets			
Florentine, 8 oz.	350	24	6
• Greek, 8 oz.	290	20	5
• Ham and Swiss, 8 oz.	390	26	4
Spanish, 8 oz.	350	24	6
Tomato Bacon, 8 oz.	370	27	4
Breakfast: Side Orders			
Bacon (3 slices), 1 oz.	80	7	0
Breakfast Potatoes, 4 oz.	170	9	20
• Ham, 2 oz.	60	2	2
• Sausage (2 patties), 3 oz.	310	27	1
Pastas			
Asiago Cream, 14 oz.	860	51	63
• Basil Pesto, 14 oz.	940	53	69
Chicken Parmesan, 15 oz.	780	27	75
• Kid's Pasta, 9 oz.	410	12	56
Pasta Puttanesca, 14 oz.	590	21	63
Penne Pomodoro Pasta, 18 oz.	920	44	66
Pastries & Sweets: Cheesecakes			
• Carrot Cake Cheesecake, 1 slice	680	49	53
Chocolate Truffle Cheesecake, 1 slice	640	40	63
Oreo Cheesecake, 1 slice	630	39	60
Pecan Turtle Cheesecake, 1 slice	640	42	56
Plain Cheesecake, 1 slice	570	36	42
• Pumpkin Praline Cheesecake, 1 slice	510	31	50
Snickers Cheesecake, 1 slice	620	50	54
Pastries & Sweets: Cookies			
Chocolate Chunk, 3 oz.	400	19	51
• Chocolate Dipped Peanut, 4 oz.	530	30	52
Chocolate Dipped Shortbread, 4 oz.	440	23	55
Oatmeal Raisin, 3 oz.	360	15	50
Peanut Butter, 3 oz.	430	24	42
Shortbread, 3 oz.	370	18	47
Toffee Chocolate Chunk, 3 oz.	400	21	49
White Macadamia, 3 oz.	410	22	49
Pastries & Sweets: Croissants			
• Almond Croissant, 6 oz.	660	38	67
Apple Croissant, 5 oz.	430	17	65
Cheese Croissant, 6 oz.	510	29	56
Chocolate Croissant, 4 oz.	520	27	61
• Plain Croissant, 3 oz.	360	20	39

• MOST HEALTHY   • LEAST HEALTHY

ATLANTA BREAD COMPANY (cont.)	Cal	Fat	Cbs
Raspberry Cheese Croissant, 5 oz.	440	19	63
Pastries & Sweets: Danish			
Apple, 4 oz.	450	18	66
Cheese, 4 oz.	480	22	65
• Gooey Butter, 4 oz.	550	25	73
• Raspberry, 4 oz.	430	18	62
Pastries & Sweets: Muffins and Tops			
Banana Nut Muffin, 5 oz.	560	33	57
Blueberry Muffin, 4 oz.	430	21	54
Bran Raisin Muffin, 4 oz.	410	18	55
Chocolate Chip Muffin, 5 oz.	560	27	73
Cranberry Apple Muffin, 5 oz.	490	23	64
• Cranberry Orange Muffin, 5 oz.	560	34	55
Low Fat Apple Muffin, 4 oz.	340	5	66
• Low Fat Pumpkin Muffin, 4 oz.	320	5	65
Mocha Muffin, 5 oz.	560	27	73
Pumpkin Muffin, 5 oz.	470	18	73
Pastries & Sweets: Scones			
Cinnamon Scone, 4 oz.	350	11	57
Raspberry Scone, 4 oz.	360	13	56
Pastries & Sweets: Other			
Austrian Pretzel, 4 oz.	550	34	55
Banana Nut Bread, 2 oz.	230	14	24
Bear Claw, 6 oz.	540	24	73
• Boston Cream Pound Cake, 2 oz.	200	12	21
Cinnamon Roll, 5 oz.	630	26	91
Cranberry Orange Bread, 2 oz.	240	14	24
Key Lime Pie, 4 oz.	450	13	52
Lower Carb Chocolate Cake, 2 oz.	200	15	17
Marble Pound Cake, 2 oz.	230	15	22
• Pecan Roll, 6 oz.	860	60	72
Pumpkin Bread, 2 oz.	210	8	33
Sticky Bun, 5 oz.	560	30	66
Walnut Brownies, 4 oz.	490	24	63
Pizzas			
BBQ Chicken, 1/2 pizza	320	5	53
• Cheese (Kid's), 1/2 pizza	300	7	44
• Four Cheese, 1/2 pizza	530	23	46
Pepperoni, 1/2 pizza	340	10	44
White Pizza, 1/2 pizza	460	22	47
Salad Dressings			
• Fat-Free Raspberry Vinaigrette, 2 tbsp.	35	0	8
Greek Dressing, 2 tbsp.	100	10	1
Sesame Ginger Dressing, 2 tbsp.	130	11	8
Salads (w/o dressing)			
Add Grilled Chicken, 3 oz.	70	2	2

• MOST HEALTHY   • LEAST HEALTHY

ATLANTA BREAD COMPANY (cont.)	Cal	Fat	Cbs
Balsamic Bleu Salad, 10 oz.	330	18	35
Caesar Salad, 8 oz.	190	10	11
Chicken Salad on Lettuce, 4 oz.	280	21	2
Chopstix Chicken Salad, 13 oz.	280	13	24
Extra Croutons, 1 oz.	50	2	6
Fruit Salad, 10 oz.	130	0	34
Greek Salad, 12 oz.	200	13	13
• House, 10 oz.	50	0	11
• Tuna Salad on Lettuce, 4 oz.	360	32	4
Sandwiches			
• Chicken Salad (Scoop), 4 oz.	280	21	2
Chicken Salad on Sourdough, 10 oz.	540	19	62
Grilled Cheese on French Bread, 5 oz.	390	11	57
Honey Maple Ham, Honey Wheat, 10 oz.	410	5	63
w/ Cheese and Mayo, 11 oz.	620	26	64
w/ Mayo, 10 oz.	520	17	64
w/ Cheddar Cheese, 11 oz.	520	15	63
PB & Jelly on French Bread, 7 oz.	600	14	99
Roasted Turkey Breast on 9 Grain, 10 oz.	430	7	61
• w/ Cheese and Mayo, 11 oz.	630	26	62
w/ Cheese, 11 oz.	530	15	61
w/ Mayo, 10 oz.	530	18	62
Tuna Salad (Scoop), 4 oz.	360	32	4
Tuna Salad on French Bread, 10 oz.	610	29	62
Veggie Sandwich on Nine Grain, 9 oz.	340	5	63
w/ Cheese and Dill Sauce, 11 oz.	500	19	63
w/ Dill Sauce, 10 oz.	401	11	63
Sandwiches: Paninis (Full)			
• Chicken Pesto, 12 oz.	800	35	83
Cordon Bleu, 10 oz.	660	18	82
Cuban Pork Loin, 10 oz.	660	19	81
• Italian Vegetarian, 12 oz.	640	16	93
Turkey Club, 12 oz.	750	27	83
Soups			
Black Bean and Ham, 10 oz.	250	9	40
Chicken Tortilla, 10 oz.	190	9	20
Chunky Baked Potato, 10 oz.	290	16	30
Classic Chicken Noodle, 10 oz.	140	3	21
Cream of Broccoli, 10 oz.	200	11	19
Creamy Tomato, 10 oz.	130	9	10
French Onion with Toppings, 10 oz.	200	10	16
• French Onion, 10 oz.	80	3	10
Garden Vegetable, 10 oz.	100	2	19
• Homestyle Chkn and Dumpling, 10 oz.	290	18	25
New England Clam Chowder, 10 oz.	280	16	24
Pasta Fagioli, 10 oz.	170	6	24

• MOST HEALTHY   • LEAST HEALTHY

ATLANTA BREAD COMPANY (cont.)	Cal	Fat	Cbs
Spicy Chicken Gumbo, 10 oz.	120	3	16
Wisconsin Cheese, 10 oz.	240	14	21
Soups: Chili			
Frontier Chicken Chili, 10 oz.	270	10	26
Hearty Beef Chili, 10 oz.	350	15	33
Specialty Sandwiches			
ABC Special on French Roll, 12 oz.	420	5	61
w/ Cheese and Mayo, 14 oz.	680	28	62
w/ Cheese, 14 oz.	570	16	61
w/ Mayo, 13 oz.	530	16	62
Bella Basil on Tom & Rosemary Focaccia, 10 oz.	660	35	58
w/ Cheese, 11 oz.	760	44	58
Cali Avocado on Tom Onion Focaccia, 12 oz.	690	40	71
• w/ Cheese, 14 oz.	790	48	71
Hot Pastrami, 8 oz.	460	10	59
w/ Swiss Cheese, 9 oz.	570	18	59
• Tangy Roast Beef, 10 oz.	390	4	56
w/ Horseradish Cheddar & Mayo, 12 oz.	790	39	60
w/ Horseradish Cheddar, 12 oz.	690	28	59

AU BON PAIN			
Bagels			
Asiago Cheese Bagel, 4 oz.	370	8	57
• Cinnamon Crisp Bagel, 4 oz.	410	7	71
Cinnamon Raisin Bagel, 4 oz.	320	1	68
Everything Bagel, 4 oz.	320	4	60
Honey 9 Grain Bagel, 4 oz.	350	4	69
Honey Butter Pecan Bagel Braid, 4 oz.	360	9	59
Jalapeño Double Cheddar Bagel, 4 oz.	340	10	53
Onion Dill Bagel, 4 oz.	280	1	57
• Plain Bagel, 4 oz.	280	1	56
Poppy Bagel, 4 oz.	320	4	58
Sesame Seed Bagel, 4 oz.	330	5	59
White Choco Toffee Bagel Braid, 4 oz.	350	6	63
Blasts & Smoothies (Medium)			
• Caramel Blast, 16 fl.oz.	540	17	104
Mocha Blast, 16 fl.oz.	440	17	80
Peach Smoothie, 16 fl.oz.	310	1	69
• Strawberry Smoothie, 16 fl.oz.	310	1	66
Vanilla Blast, 16 fl.oz.	540	17	104
Breads			
Artisan Baguette Sandwich Size, 4 oz.	310	3	61
Artisan Honey Multigrain Baguette Snd Size, 5 oz.	340	5	66
Artisan Sundried Tomato Bread, 4 oz.	270	1	57
Asiago Breadstick, 2 oz.	190	4	28
• Bread Bowl, 9 oz.	620	3	123

• MOST HEALTHY   • LEAST HEALTHY

▶ AU BON PAIN (cont.)	Cal	Fat	Cbs
Caraway Rye Flatbread, 5 oz.	280	5	49
• Cheddar Jalapeño Breadstick, 2 oz.	130	2	26
Ciabatta Small, 3 oz.	180	1	38
Cinnamon Raisin Breadstick, 2 oz.	190	1	41
Country White Bread, 4 oz.	270	1	56
Everything Breadstick, 2 oz.	180	3	31
Farm House Rolls, 5 oz.	360	7	63
Focaccia, 5 oz.	360	7	62
Lahvash, 4 oz.	280	4	56
Rosemary Garlic Bread Stick, 2 oz.	190	5	31
Sesame Breadstick, 2 oz.	180	4	30
Whole Wheat Multigrain Bread, 4 oz.	260	3	53

Breakfast Sandwiches

	Cal	Fat	Cbs
• Bacon and Bagel, 4 oz.	340	6	58
Bacon and Egg Melt on Ciabatta, 7 oz.	470	23	39
Egg and Broccoli Baked Sandwich, 8 oz.	430	19	42
Egg on a Bagel, 7 oz.	430	12	58
Egg on a Bagel with Bacon, 7 oz.	490	16	58
Egg on a Bagel with Bacon and Chz, 8 oz.	570	23	59
Egg on a Bagel with Cheese, 8 oz.	510	18	59
Portobello, Egg and Cheddar, 8 oz.	460	23	40
Prosciutto and Egg on Asiago Bagel, 9 oz.	590	23	58
• Ssg, Egg and Cheddar on Asiago Bagel, 10 oz.	810	46	57
Smkd Salmon & Wasabi on Onion Dill Bagel, 7 oz.	430	11	64

Café Sandwiches

	Cal	Fat	Cbs
Arizona Chicken Sandwich, 12 oz.	710	29	62
Baja Turkey Sandwich, 13 oz.	700	27	71
Black Bean Burger, 10 oz.	560	18	76
Caprese Sandwich, 11 oz.	680	32	65
Chicken Pesto Sandwich, 13 oz.	660	24	66
Mozzarella Chicken Sandwich, 14 oz.	680	24	67
Pastrami Sandwich, 10 oz.	590	23	52
Portobello and Goat Chz Snd, 10 oz.	500	20	65
• Prosciutto Mozzarella Sandwich, 12 oz.	810	41	71
Roast Beef Caesar Sandwich, 10 oz.	680	27	68
• Spicy Tuna Sandwich, 10 oz.	470	16	60
Turkey Club Sandwich, 12 oz.	700	31	59

Coffee & Espresso (Medium)

	Cal	Fat	Cbs
• Caffe Americano, 16 fl.oz.	10	0	2
Caffe Latte, 16 fl.oz.	260	14	21
Caffeine Free Pepsi, 22 fl.oz.	280	0	77
Cappuccino, 16 fl.oz.	150	8	13
Caramel Macchiato, 16 fl.oz.	430	12	68
Chai Latte, 16 fl.oz.	380	14	51
Chocolate Milk, 12 fl.oz.	320	9	54
• Hot Chocolate, 16 fl.oz.	460	15	74

▶ AU BON PAIN (cont.)

	Cal	Fat	Cbs
Iced Caffe Latte, 16 fl.oz.	150	8	13
Iced Caramel Macchiato, 16 fl.oz.	390	10	65
Iced Chai Latte, 16 fl.oz.	260	7	42
Iced Decaf French Roast Coffee, 22 fl.oz.	10	0	2
Iced Mocha Latte, 16 fl.oz.	300	15	40
Iced Vanilla Latte, 16 fl.oz.	330	7	59
Iced White Chocolate Latte, 16 fl.oz.	330	13	51
Mocha Latte, 16 fl.oz.	390	20	48
Vanilla Latte Medium, 16 fl.oz.	410	12	66
White Chocolate Latte Medium, 16 fl.oz.	410	17	58
Cookies & Desserts			
Banana Nut Pound Cake, 4 oz.	480	26	56
Blondie, 4 oz.	460	33	59
Chocolate Cheesecake Brownie, 4 oz.	460	19	74
Chocolate Cherry Tulip, 4 oz.	410	21	54
Chocolate Chip Brownie, 4 oz.	510	19	74
Chocolate Chip Cookie, 2 oz.	280	13	40
Choco Dipped Cran Almond Macaroon, 2 oz.	300	15	36
Chocolate Dipped Shortbread, 3 oz.	380	22	42
Confetti Cookie with M&M's, 2 oz.	280	13	39
Crème de Fleur, 5 oz.	500	25	56
Crumb Cake, 6 oz.	750	40	97
English Toffee Cookie, 2 oz.	250	14	27
Hazelnut Mocha Brownie, 4 oz.	490	22	74
Iced Cinnamon Roll, 4 oz.	410	15	60
Lemon Drop Tulip, 4 oz.	410	19	55
Lemon Pound Cake, 5 oz.	520	25	67
Marble Pound Cake, 5 oz.	490	26	59
Mini Chocolate Chip Cookie, 5 oz.	70	3	10
• Mini Oatmeal Raisin Cookie, 5 oz.	60	3	10
Mint Chocolate Pound Cake, 5 oz.	530	29	64
Oatmeal Raisin Cookie, 2 oz.	250	9	40
Palmier, 4 oz.	440	23	53
• Pecan Roll, 6 oz.	810	41	99
Rocky Road Brownie, 4 oz.	490	22	74
Shortbread Cookie, 2 oz.	340	20	37
Wht Choco Chunk Mac. Nut Cookie, 2 oz.	300	16	36
Croissants			
• Almond Croissant, 5 oz.	600	38	55
Apple Almond Croissant, 5 oz.	460	23	59
• Apple Croissant, 4 oz.	280	11	44
Chocolate Croissant, 4 oz.	440	22	58
Ham and Cheese Croissant, 4 oz.	390	21	35
Plain Croissant, 3 oz.	310	17	31
Raspberry Cheese Croissant, 4 oz.	370	17	46
Spinach and Cheese Croissant, 4 oz.	290	16	28

● MOST HEALTHY   • LEAST HEALTHY

AU BON PAIN (cont.)	Cal	Fat	Cbs
Sweet Cheese Croissant, 4 oz.	400	19	49

Danish
	Cal	Fat	Cbs
• Cherry Danish, 4 oz.	420	20	54
Lemon Danish, 4 oz.	440	20	57
• Sweet Cheese Danish, 4 oz.	470	24	54

Dressings
	Cal	Fat	Cbs
• Fat Free Raspberry Vinaigrette, 2 oz.	50	0	12
FF Sun Dried Tomato Vinaigrette, 2 oz.	110	0	28
• Hazelnut Vinaigrette Dressing, 2 oz.	270	25	11
Lite Olive Oil Vinaigrette, 2 oz.	110	10	6
Pomegranate Vinaigrette Dressing, 2 oz.	250	22	12
Sesame Ginger Dressing, 2 oz.	230	20	12
Thai Peanut Dressing, 2 oz.	160	8	20

Grab n Go Sandwiches
	Cal	Fat	Cbs
Demi Chkn Sandwich on Baguette, 7 oz.	370	9	49
Demi Chkn Snd w/ Chdr Chz on Bag., 8 oz.	450	16	50
Demi Ham Sandwich on Baguette, 7 oz.	330	5	56
Demi Ham Snd w/ Swiss Chz on Bag., 8 oz.	400	10	56
Demi Roast Beef Snd on Baguette, 8 oz.	370	9	49
Demi Rst Beef Snd w/ Brie Chz on Bag., 9 oz.	480	19	50
Demi Tuna Snd on Baguette, 7 oz.	320	7	49
Demi Tuna Snd w/ Cheddar Chz on Bag., 8 oz.	400	14	50
Demi Turkey Sandwich on Baguette, 7 oz.	320	6	49
Demi Tkey Snd w/ Swiss Chz on Bag., 8 oz.	400	12	49
Half Snd Ham & Swiss on Farmhouse Roll, 6 oz.	320	13	34
Half Snd Rst Beef & Brie on Farmhouse Roll, 6 oz.	350	14	34
Half Snd Tuna & Chdr on Farmhouse Roll, 6 oz.	360	16	35
• Half Snd Turkey & Swiss on Farmhouse Roll, 6 oz.	320	11	34
Whl Snd Ham & Swiss on Cntry Wht Bread, 11 oz.	530	17	60
Whl Snd Rst Beef & Brie on Cntry White Bread, 11 oz.	600	21	59
• Whl Snd Tuna & Chdr on Cntry Wht Bread, 11 oz.	610	25	63
Whl Snd Tkey & Swiss on Cntry White Bread, 11 oz.	530	14	60

Harvest Rice Bowls
	Cal	Fat	Cbs
• Angus Steak Teriyaki, 19 oz.	660	18	101
Angus Steak Teriyaki w/ Brown Rice, 19 oz.	620	19	86
Mayan Chicken, 19 oz.	550	11	87
• Mayan Chicken w/ Brown Rice, 19 oz.	510	13	72

Hot & Cold Lunch Bar
	Cal	Fat	Cbs
• Aegean Pasta Salad, 1 oz.	90	4	10
Baked Potato, 1 oz.	25	0	5
BBQ Beef Salad, 1 oz.	35	1	4
Brown Rice, 1 oz.	30	0	6
Brown Rice Waldorf Nut Salad, 1 oz.	45	3	5
Burgundy Beef Penne, 1 oz.	30	1	4
Cajun Chicken Penne, 1 oz.	40	2	4
Chicken Broccoli Alfredo Penne, 1 oz.	60	4	3

AU BON PAIN (cont.)

	Cal	Fat	Cbs
Chicken Penne Pesto, 1 oz.	60	3	4
Chicken Provencal, 1 oz.	25	0	4
Creamed Spinach, 1 oz.	30	2	2
Egg and Cucumber Salad, 1 oz.	40	3	1
Eggplant Parmesan, 1 oz.	50	3	4
Fire Roasted Exotic Grains and Vegs, 1 oz.	40	1	7
Italian Sausage, Peppers and Onions, 1 oz.	25	1	1
Jambalaya, 1 oz.	25	1	2
Macaroni and Cheese, 1 oz.	40	3	3
Meat Lasagna, 1 oz.	45	2	4
Meatballs and Marinara Sauce, 1 oz.	50	4	2
Meatloaf with Wine Sauce, 1 oz.	50	3	2
Oriental Noodle Salad, 1 oz.	90	2	19
Orzo Toscano Salad, 1 oz.	35	1	6
Penne Marinara, 1 oz.	30	1	5
Polenta Marinara, 1 oz.	25	1	3
Potato Bacon Salad, 1 oz.	40	2	3
Quinoa, 1 oz.	25	0	4
Red Bliss Potato Salad, 1 oz.	30	2	5
Roasted Apple Cranberry Orzo, 1 oz.	45	1	9
Roasted Carrots, 1 oz.	15	0	3
Roasted Green Beans with Almonds, 1 oz.	20	1	1
• Roasted Zucchini & Summer Squash, 1 oz.	5	0	1
Sesame Brown Rice & Orange Salad, 1 oz.	45	3	6
Southwest Fusilli Pasta Salad, 1 oz.	45	3	4
Southwest Panzanella Salad, 1 oz.	50	3	7
Stuffed Peppers with Lentils, 1 oz.	20	0	3
Tomato Cucumber Salad, 1 oz.	10	0	2
Tom, Green Bean and Almond Salad, 1 oz.	20	2	2
Tsaziki, 1 oz.	15	0	2
Tuna Salad, 1 oz.	40	3	1
Vegetarian Lasagna, 1 oz.	45	3	3
Watermelon and Feta Salad, 1 oz.	15	1	3
White Rice, 1 oz.	35	0	8

Hot Breakfast Bar

	Cal	Fat	Cbs
• Apple Croissants Tart, 1 oz.	80	2	12
Cinnamon Walnut Quinoa, 1 oz.	45	0	4
French Pecan Toast, 1 oz.	70	2	8
Pineapple Blueberry Cobbler, 1 oz.	45	0	8
• Roasted Potatoes, 1 oz.	35	0	6
Sausage with Peppers and Onions, 1 oz.	50	2	1
Scrambled Eggs, 1 oz.	35	1	1
Southwest Corn Casserole, 1 oz.	60	2	4

Hot Entrees

	Cal	Fat	Cbs
Ancho Chicken Quesadilla, 12 oz.	700	28	62
Chicken Broccoli Alfredo Penne, 12 oz.	680	43	38

• MOST HEALTHY   • LEAST HEALTHY

AU BON PAIN (cont.)

	Cal	Fat	Cbs
• Meat Lasagna, 11 oz.	470	24	41
Rstd Angus Steak Teriyaki Bowl w/ Brown Rice, 18 oz.	680	24	91
• Rstd Angus Steak Teriyaki Bowl w/ White Rice, 18 oz.	730	23	107
Rst Mayan Chkn Bowl w/ Brown Rice, 18 oz.	580	17	78
Rst Mayan Chkn Bowl w/ White Rice, 18 oz.	630	16	92

Hot Sandwiches and Melts
	Cal	Fat	Cbs
Angus Steak Teriyaki Hot Wrap, 14 oz.	630	16	100
Baked BBQ Chicken Sandwich, 12 oz.	680	19	80
• Baked Turkey Sandwich, 12 oz.	720	26	79
Eggplant and Mozzarella Snd, 12 oz.	670	30	73
• Mayan Chicken Hot Wrap, 14 oz.	580	13	93
Meatball Sandwich, 11 oz.	670	26	77
Steakhouse on Ciabatta, 12 oz.	640	23	73
Tuna Melt, 13 oz.	690	30	71

Kid's
	Cal	Fat	Cbs
• Chz Sandwich on Farmhouse Roll, 4 oz.	360	22	32
• Grilled Chkn Snd on Multigrain Bread, 5 oz.	230	6	28
Rst Tkey Snd on Farmhouse Roll, 5 oz.	270	7	33
Macaroni and Cheese, 8 oz.	330	19	24

Muffins
	Cal	Fat	Cbs
Blueberry Muffin, 6 oz.	490	17	74
Carrot Walnut Muffin, 6 oz.	560	27	72
Chocolate Chip Muffin, 5 oz.	580	23	83
Corn Muffin, 6 oz.	490	17	75
Cranberry Walnut Muffin, 6 oz.	540	25	66
• Double Chocolate Chunk Muffin, 6 oz.	620	25	86
• Low-fat Triple Berry Muffin, 4 oz.	300	3	65
Raisin Bran Muffin, 6 oz.	480	11	85
Southwest Jalapeño Muffin, 5 oz.	560	30	64

New Items
	Cal	Fat	Cbs
• Apple Cinnamon Oatmeal Medium, 12 oz.	280	4	56
Honey Butter Pecan Bagel Braid, 4 oz.	360	9	59
Lobster Bisque Medium, 12 fl.oz.	390	28	23
• Meatball Sandwich, 11 oz.	670	26	77
Pastrami Sandwich, 10 oz.	590	23	52

Oatmeal
	Cal	Fat	Cbs
Apple Cinnamon Oatmeal Medium, 12 oz.	280	4	56
Oatmeal Medium, 12 oz.	260	5	47

Portions
	Cal	Fat	Cbs
Apples, Blue Chz and Cranberries, 5 oz.	200	10	27
Black Bean and Corn Salad, 6 oz.	130	0	25
Brie, Fruit and Crackers, 4 oz.	200	11	18
Brown Rice & Hazelnut Waldorf Salad, 5 oz.	180	9	22
• Brown Rice and Mushrooms, 5 oz.	200	13	18
Cheddar, Fruit and Crackers, 4 oz.	200	12	18
Chicken Pesto Salad, 4 oz.	160	8	1

• MOST HEALTHY   • LEAST HEALTHY

AU BON PAIN (cont.)

	Cal	Fat	Cbs
Chickpea and Tomato Salad, 6 oz.	100	1	19
Herb Cheese, Fruit and Crackers, 4 oz.	190	11	20
Hummus and Cucumber, 4 oz.	130	8	10
Mediterranean Tuna Salad, 4 oz.	120	8	4
Mozzarella and Tomato, 5 oz.	180	14	5
Smkd Salmon, Egg and Guacamole, 5 oz.	140	10	6
Thai Beef and Peanut, 4 oz.	120	5	5
Tkey, Asparagus, Cran Chutney & Gorgonzola, 5 oz.	140	5	10
• Watermelon, Feta and Almonds, 4 oz.	70	3	11

Salads

Apple Goat Cheese Salad, 10 oz.	290	13	39
Caesar Asiago Salad, 6 oz.	220	12	18
Chef's Salad, 9 oz.	250	15	7
Chicken BLT Salad, 11 oz.	300	16	7
Chkpea & Tomato Cucumber Salad, 11 oz.	230	12	23
• Garden Salad, 7 oz.	70	2	12
Grilled Chicken Caesar Asiago, 9 oz.	300	13	18
Mandarin Sesame Chicken Salad, 10 oz.	310	17	29
Mediterranean Chicken Salad, 10 oz.	290	16	12
Thai Peanut Chicken Salad, 11 oz.	240	8	19
Tuna Garden Salad, 11 oz.	240	12	15
• Turkey Cobb Salad, 11 oz.	330	19	14
White Bean and Asparagus Salad, 14 oz.	250	10	26

Scones

• Chocolate Orange Pecan Scone, 5 oz.	580	28	74
Cinnamon Scone, 4 oz.	520	27	60
• Orange Scone, 4 oz.	470	23	57

Snacks

Chocolate Covered Almonds, 1 oz.	230	15	20
Choco Covered Pretzels, 2 oz.	160	5	24
• Chocolate Covered Strawberry, 1 oz.	35	2	5
Dark Chocolate Covered Raisins, 1 oz.	180	8	26
Fresh Grapes, 8 oz.	160	0	41
Fresh Pineapple, 8 oz.	110	0	30
Fresh Watermelon, 8 oz.	70	0	17
Fruit Cup, Small, 6 oz.	70	0	18
Gelatin Dessert, Lemon, 8 oz.	120	0	29
Gelatin Dessert, Lime, 8 oz.	120	0	29
Gelatin Dessert, Orange, 8 oz.	130	0	30
Malted Milk Mini Eggs, 1 oz.	170	6	30
Mixed Nuts, 1 oz.	180	16	7
• Muesli, 8 oz.	390	8	76
Red Licorice, 1 oz.	140	1	30
Sugar Free Cinnamon Buttons, 6 oz.	70	0	15
The 19th Hole Snack Mix, 1 oz.	160	10	15
Turkish Apricots, 1 oz.	120	0	29

• MOST HEALTHY   • LEAST HEALTHY

> ### AU BON PAIN (cont.)

Soups - Medium

	Cal	Fat	Cbs
• Baked Stuffed Potato, 12 oz.	350	20	29
Black Bean Soup, 12 oz.	260	1	46
Broccoli Cheddar Soup, 12 oz.	300	21	20
Butternut Squash & Apple Soup, 12 fl.oz.	200	8	32
Carrot Ginger Soup, 12 oz.	140	5	22
Chicken And Dumpling Soup, 12 oz.	210	7	28
Chicken Florentine Soup, 12 oz.	250	13	25
Chicken Gumbo Soup, 12 oz.	180	8	21
Chicken Noodle Soup, 12 oz.	130	3	19
Clam Chowder, 12 oz.	320	18	27
Corn and Green Chili Bisque, 12 oz.	260	15	27
Corn Chowder, 12 oz.	350	18	40
Cream of Chkn and Wild Rice Soup, 12 oz.	240	14	22
Curried Rice and Lentil Soup, 12 oz.	170	2	30
Frn Moroccan Tomato Lentil Soup, 12 oz.	190	2	32
French Onion Soup, 12 oz.	130	5	19
• Garden Vegetable Soup, 12 oz.	80	2	13
Gazpacho, 12 oz.	90	5	11
Harvest Pumpkin Soup, 12 fl.oz.	240	13	27
Hearty Cabbage Soup, 12 oz.	110	5	14
Italian Wedding Soup, 12 oz.	170	7	19
Jamaican Black Bean Soup, 12 oz.	250	1	43
Mediterranean Pepper Soup, 12 oz.	170	5	26
Old Fashioned Tomato Soup, 12 oz.	200	7	27
Pasta E Fagioli Soup, 12 oz.	260	8	35
Portuguese Kale Soup, 12 oz.	130	5	15
Potato Cheese Soup, 12 oz.	260	14	24
Potato Leek Soup, 12 oz.	300	19	28
Red Beans, Itln Ssg & Rice Soup, 12 oz.	270	6	40
Scandinavian Fruit Soup, 12 fl.oz.	280	0	69
Southern Black-Eyed Pea Soup, 12 oz.	170	2	29
Southwest Tortilla Soup, 12 oz.	190	10	23
Southwest Vegetable Soup, 12 oz.	170	5	28
Split Pea with Ham Soup, 12 oz.	250	2	41
Thai Coconut Curry Soup, 12 oz.	160	7	21
Tomato Basil Bisque, 12 oz.	210	9	27
Tomato Cheddar Soup, 12 oz.	240	16	17
Tomato Florentine Soup, 12 oz.	130	3	19
Tomato Rice Soup, 12 oz.	120	1	24
Tuscan Vegetable Soup, 12 oz.	170	5	23
Vegetable Beef Barley Soup, 12 oz.	140	3	21
Vegetarian Chili, 12 oz.	220	2	39
Vegetarian Lentil Soup, 12 oz.	170	2	31
Vegetarian Minestrone Soup, 12 oz.	120	2	20
Wild Mushroom Bisque, 12 oz.	190	9	22

• MOST HEALTHY   • LEAST HEALTHY

AU BON PAIN (cont.)

	Cal	Fat	Cbs
Spreads			
Artichoke Aioli, 1 oz.	70	6	2
Basil Pesto, 1 oz.	120	12	1
Chili Dijon, 1 oz.	130	13	4
Herb Bagel Spread, 2 oz.	140	12	4
• Honey Pecan Cream Cheese, 2 oz.	200	16	10
Lite Cream Cheese Spread, 2 oz.	120	9	5
Mediterranean Spread, 1 oz.	120	11	2
Sundried Tomato Cream Cheese, 2 oz.	140	11	5
• Sun-Dried Tomato Spread, 1 oz.	45	4	1
Vegetable Cream Cheese, 2 oz.	170	16	3
Stews - Medium			
BBQ Chicken and Beef Stew, 12 fl.oz.	300	10	35
Beef and Vegetable Stew, 12 oz.	310	16	25
Beef Chili, 12 oz.	300	13	28
• Chicken and Vegetable Stew, 12 oz.	290	17	26
Lobster Bisque, 12 fl.oz.	390	28	23
• Macaroni and Cheese, 12 oz.	600	29	36
Strudel			
Apple Strudel, 4 oz.	440	24	50
Cherry Strudel, 5 oz.	460	26	50
Toppings			
All Natural Chicken Breast, 4 oz.	120	2	0
Bacon, 1 Portion, 1 oz.	60	5	0
Bagged Croutons, 2 oz.	190	6	29
Brie Cheese, 1 oz.	170	15	1
Cheddar Cheese, 2 oz.	160	13	1
Feta Cheese, 1 oz.	80	6	1
Goat Cheese, 1 oz.	45	4	1
Gorgonzola Cheese, 2 oz.	200	16	2
• Granola Topping, 2 oz.	230	8	37
Guacamole, 1 oz.	50	5	2
Ham, 4 oz.	100	4	0
Mozzarella Cheese, 2 oz.	120	9	0
Pastrami, 4 oz.	140	5	1
Prosciutto, 1 oz.	110	6	2
Roast Beef, 3. 7 oz.	150	6	0
Roasted Red Pepper Hummus, 2 oz.	80	5	6
• Roasted Red Peppers, 2 oz.	10	0	2
Sausage Patty, 2 oz.	210	20	0
Swiss Cheese, 1 oz.	150	12	2
Tuna Salad Mix, 4 oz.	170	10	3
Turkey Breast, 4 oz.	90	1	1
Wraps			
Chicken BLT Wrap, 13 oz.	690	33	61

AU BON PAIN (cont.)

	Cal	Fat	Cbs
Chicken Caesar Asiago Wrap, 11 oz.	610	28	61
Mediterranean Wrap, 13 oz.	610	29	73
• Southwest Tuna Wrap, 14 oz.	760	41	66
• Thai Peanut Chicken Wrap, 13 oz.	530	15	79

Yogurt - Small

	Cal	Fat	Cbs
• Blueberry Yogurt with Blueberries, 9 oz.	250	3	50
• Granola Topping, 2 oz.	230	8	37
Strawberry Yogurt with Blueberries, 9 oz.	250	2	50
• Vanilla Yogurt with Blueberries, 9 oz.	220	3	41

AUNTIE ANNE'S

Beverages

	Cal	Fat	Cbs
Blue Raspberry Dutch Ice®, 374 g	170	0	43
Blue Raspberry Dutch Smoothie, 298 g	280	10	45
Blue Raspberry ICEE®, 376 g	160	0	41
Caramel Dutch Latté™, 405 g	370	17	49
Chocolate Dutch Shake, 288 g	570	27	75
Kiwi-Banana Dutch Ice®, 374 g	150	0	37
Kiwi-Banana Dutch Smoothie, 298 g	270	10	41
Mocha Dutch Ice®, 374 g	270	8	50
Mocha Dutch Latté™, 405 g	360	17	47
Mocha Dutch Smoothie, 298 g	340	15	49
Orange Fanta®, 473 g	220	0	60
Piña Colada Dutch Ice®, 374 g	210	0	51
Piña Colada Dutch Smoothie, 298 g	300	10	49
• Poland Springs® Bottled Water, 501 g	0	0	0
Strawberry Dutch Ice®, 374 g	160	0	40
• Strawberry Dutch Shake, 288 g	600	27	79
Strawberry Dutch Smoothie, 298 g	280	10	43
Vanilla Dutch Shake, 258 g	510	27	57
Watermelon Dutch Ice®, 539 g	270	0	66
Wild Cherry Dutch Smoothie, 298 g	300	10	47
Wild Cherry ICEE®, 376 g	160	0	43

Dipping Sauces

	Cal	Fat	Cbs
• Caramel Dip, 40 g	130	3	23
Cheese Sauce, 31 g	90	7	3
Cream Cheese, 35 g	80	6	1
• Heated Marinara Sauce, 60 g	20	1	5
Hot Salsa Cheese, 31 g	90	7	4
Marinara Sauce, 57 g	45	1	7
Melted Cheese Dip, 60 g	80	6	7
Sweet Dip, 40 g	130	0	32

Pretzels & More

	Cal	Fat	Cbs
Almond Pretzel, 131 g	390	6	74
• Cinnamon Sugar Party Pretzels, 882 g	2940	72	519
Cinnamon Sugar Pretzel, 147 g	470	12	84

• MOST HEALTHY   • LEAST HEALTHY

AUNTIE ANNE'S (cont.)

	Cal	Fat	Cbs
Cinnamon Sugar Stix, 147 g	470	12	84
Garlic Pretzel, 123 g	350	5	65
Garlic Pretzel no Salt, 122 g	350	5	65
• Jalapeño Pretzel, 124 g	330	5	63
Jumbo Pretzel Dog, 212 g	610	29	67
Original Party Pretzels, 738 g	2140	32	405
Original Pretzel, 123 g	340	5	65
Original Stix, 123 g	340	5	65
Pepperoni Pretzel, 149 g	480	16	65
Pretzel Dog, 119 g	360	20	33
Pretzel Pocket – Bcn, Egg & Chz, 214 g	580	23	71
Pretzel Pocket – Pep & Mozz., 204 g	650	27	75
Pretzel Pocket – Tkey & Cheddar, 205 g	470	10	73
Raisin Pretzel, 127 g	360	5	69
Sesame Pretzel, 132 g	400	10	67
Sour Cream & Onion Pretzel, 127 g	360	5	68

BAJA FRESH

Americano Soft Taco

	Cal	Fat	Cbs
Breaded Fish, 129 g	240	11	23
Carnitas, 142 g	250	12	21
• Chicken, 142 g	230	10	20
Mahi Mahi, 150 g	240	10	20
Shrimp, 150 g	230	10	21
• Steak, 142 g	260	13	21

Baja Burrito

	Cal	Fat	Cbs
Breaded Fish, 426 g	850	44	78
Carnitas, 440 g	830	45	67
Chicken, 440 g	790	38	65
Mahi Mahi, 451 g	780	38	66
• Shrimp, 454 g	760	37	66
• Steak, 437 g	850	46	67

Baja Ensalada®

	Cal	Fat	Cbs
Charbroiled Chicken, 473 g	310	7	18
• Charbroiled Shrimp, 445 g	230	6	18
• Charbroiled Steak, 473 g	450	18	18
Savory Pork Carnitas, 473 g	370	18	20

Baja Fish Taco - Fried

	Cal	Fat	Cbs
Breaded Fish, 134 g	250	13	27

Bare Burrito®-Served

	Cal	Fat	Cbs
Carnitas, 590	680	14	99
• Chicken, 590	640	7	97
• Steak, 587	700	15	99

Bean and Cheese

	Cal	Fat	Cbs
Breaded Fish, 477 g	1030	41	108
Carnitas, 491 g	1010	42	98

• MOST HEALTHY   • LEAST HEALTHY

BAJA FRESH (cont.)	Cal	Fat	Cbs
Chicken, 491 g	970	35	96
Mahi Mahi, 502 g	960	35	96
• No Meat, 392 g	840	33	96
Shrimp, 505 g	950	34	96
• Steak, 488 g	1030	43	97
Burrito Mexicano			
Breaded Fish, 499 g	850	19	129
Carnitas, 514 g	830	20	119
Chicken, 514 g	790	13	117
Mahi Mahi, 525 g	791	13	117
• Shrimp, 528 g	770	13	117
• Steak, 511 g	860	21	118
Burrito Ultimo			
Breaded Fish, 465 g	940	42	96
Carnitas, 480 g	920	44	86
Chicken, 481 g	880	36	84
Mahi Mahi, 491 g	880	36	84
• Shrimp, 494 g	860	36	85
• Steak, 477 g	950	44	85
Chicken Tortilla Soup			
With Charbroiled Chicken, 388 g	320	14	29
Without Charbroiled Chicken, 354 g	270	14	29
Chicken Taquitos			
• Chicken Taquitos, 304 g	630	33	60
• Chicken Taquitos w/Beans, 518 g	780	40	68
Chicken Taquitos w/Rice, 449 g	740	40	66
"Enchilado" Style			
To Burrito add, 420 g	630	40	45
Fajitas			
Breaded Fish w/ Corn Tortillas, 817 g	1060	37	130
• Breaded Fish w/ Flour Tortillas, 876 g	1340	46	172
Breaded Fish w/ Mix Tortillas, 869 g	1260	43	162
Carnitas w/ Corn Tortillas, 788 g	920	34	108
Carnitas w/ Flour Tortillas, 847 g	1190	43	150
Carnitas w/ Mix Tortillas, 840 g	1120	40	140
Chicken w/ Corn Tortillas, 788 g	860	24	105
Chicken w/ Flour Tortillas, 847 g	1140	33	147
Chicken w/ Mix Tortillas, 840 g	1070	30	137
• Mahi Mahi w/ Corn Tortillas, 794 g	840	23	105
Mahi Mahi w/ Flour Tortillas, 853 g	1120	32	147
Mahi Mahi w/ Mix Tortillas, 846 g	1050	29	138
Shrimp w/ Corn Tortillas, 817 g	840	23	106
Shrimp w/ Flour Tortillas, 876 g	1120	32	148
Shrimp w/ Mix Tortillas, 869 g	1045	29	138
Steak w/ Corn Tortillas, 788 g	960	36	107
Steak w/ Flour Tortillas, 847 g	1240	45	149

▷ BAJA FRESH (cont.)

	Cal	Fat	Cbs
Steak w/ Mix Tortillas, 840 g	1170	42	139
Grilled Mahi Mahi			
Mahi Mahi, 177 g	230	9	26
Grilled Veggie			
Grilled Veggie, 506 g	800	33	94
Mini Bean & Cheese Burrito			
Mini Bean & Cheese Burrito, 348 g	540	14	14
Mini Bean & Chz Burrito w/ Chkn, 382	590	15	15
Mini Cheese Quesadilla			
3 oz. side Guacamole, 85 g	110	13	5
5 oz. side of Corn Tortilla Chips, 142 g	740	34	90
• 8 oz. side Pico de Gallo, 227 g	50	1	12
8 oz. side Salsa Baja, 227 g	70	3	7
8 oz. side Salsa Roja, 227 g	70	1	13
8 oz. side Salsa Verde, 227 g	50	0	11
Black Beans, 327 g	360	3	61
• Chips and Guacamole, 425 g	1340	83	141
Chips and Salsa Baja, 369 g	810	37	98
Mini Cheese Quesadilla, 283 g	610	26	72
Mini Cheese Quesadilla w/ Chkn, 317 g	650	27	72
Pinto Beans, 300 g	320	1	56
Pronto Guacamole™, 170 g	560	34	60
Rice, 181 g	280	4	55
Rice & Beans Plate, 325 g	420	5	72
Side Breaded Fish, 170 g	390	16	25
Side Carnitas, 170 g	300	16	4
Side Chicken, 170 g	230	4	0
Side Mahi Mahi, 184 g	210	3	1
Side Salad, 186 g	130	6	16
Side Shrimp, 156 g	150	2	1
Side Steak, 142 g	330	14	0
Tostada Shell, 91 g	490	28	44
Veggie Mix, 221 g	110	0	24
Nachos			
Breaded Fish, 867 g	2090	116	176
Charbroiled Chicken, 882 g	2020	110	164
Charbroiled Mahi Mahi, 893 g	2020	110	164
Charbroiled Shrimp, 893 g	2000	110	164
• Charbroiled Steak, 879 g	2120	118	163
• Cheese, 782 g	1890	108	163
Savory Pork Carnitas, 882 g	2060	117	166
Original Baja Taco			
Carnitas, 116 g	220	7	29
Chicken, 116 g	210	5	28
• Shrimp, 125 g	200	5	28
• Steak, 113 g	230	8	28

• MOST HEALTHY   • LEAST HEALTHY

BAJA FRESH (cont.)

	Cal	Fat	Cbs
Quesadilla			
Breaded Fish, 539 g	1400	86	96
Charbroiled Chicken, 553 g	1330	80	84
Charbroiled Mahi Mahi, 565 g	1330	79	84
Charbroiled Shrimp, 567 g	1310	79	84
• Charbroiled Steak, 550 g	1430	87	84
• Cheese, 454 g	1200	78	84
Savory Pork Carnitas, 553 g	1370	87	86
Veggie, 565 g	1260	78	96
Salad Burrito			
Cabo Style, 454 g	980	52	81
Caesar Style, 420 g	940	50	75
Salad Dressing			
Fat Free Salsa Verde, 71 g	15	0	3
Olive Oil Vinaigrette, 71 g	290	31	2
Torta			
With Chips, 57 g	880	35	96
Without Chips, 43 g	620	23	64
Tostada Salad			
Breaded Fish, 744 g	1200	61	111
Charbroiled Chicken, 758 g	1140	55	98
Charbroiled Fish, 769 g	1130	55	99
Charbroiled Shrimp, 772 g	1120	55	99
• Charbroiled Steak, 755 g	1230	63	98
• No Meat, 659 g	1010	53	98
Savory Pork Carnitas, 758 g	1180	62	100
Veggie & Cheese Bare Burrito -Served			
Veggie and Cheese, 563 g	580	10	101

BAKER'S DRIVE-THRU

	Cal	Fat	Cbs
American: Chicken Sandwiches			
Caribbean	450	4	50
• Grilled	480	5	48
• Monterey	410	7	43
Teriyaki	470	4	51
American: HamBurgers			
• Double Baker w/ Double Cheese	710	17	42
Grilled Boca Burger®	500	7	54
Grilled Cheese Sandwich	480	12	41
• Single Baker	420	5	41
Single Baker w/Cheese	500	10	41
Baker Breaks			
• Chili Cheese Fries	970	17	96
• Fiesta Salad	290	8	15
Guacamole & Chips	380	4	47
Not-So-Big Nachos	750	18	66

• MOST HEALTHY   • LEAST HEALTHY

► BAKER'S DRIVE-THRU (cont.)

	Cal	Fat	Cbs
Beverages			
• Baker's Bold Roast	0	0	0
Cappuccino Hot or Iced	120	4	9
• Hot Chocolate	300	2	54
Breakfast			
• All Beef Sausage & Egg Burrito	770	15	56
All Beef Sausage & Egg Sandwich	700	15	40
Chorizo & Egg Burrito	680	14	56
Chorizo Egg & Potato Taco	460	10	30
Egg Burrito	590	10	55
Egg Sandwich	520	10	38
Egg Soft Taco	240	4	17
• Hash Browns	200	3	24
Machaca Burrito	680	11	57
Monterey Egg Sandwich	400	8	39
Monterey Egg Taco	310	7	22
Breakfast: Meals			
• ? Chorizo Egg & Potato Tacos	1540	30	111
2 Egg Soft Tacos	1060	17	84
2 Monterey Egg Soft Tacos	1240	24	95
Chorizo & Egg Burrito	1390	24	107
Egg Burrito	1200	19	106
• Egg Sandwich	830	15	70
Egg Burrito w/ Meat & Beans	1375	19	147
Machaca Burrito	1325	20	111
Monterey Egg Sandwich	1125	17	91
Sausage & Egg Burrito	1380	24	111
Sausage & Egg Sandwich	1310	25	91
Budget Meals			
Bean and Cheese Burrito	770	8	116
Grilled Cheese	775	14	85
• Original Taco	465	6	55
Plain Hamburger	630	6	86
Quesadilla	745	12	94
Single Baker	740	8	86
• Spicy Rolled Quesadilla	805	15	95
Tostada	605	7	76
Drinks			
Powerade®	120	0	35
Mama Meals			
• 2 Tacos, Shrd Beef, Chkn, or Original	615	8	77
Combination Burrito	865	11	113
Single Baker w/Cheese	765	12	83
Taco Burger w/Ground Beef	640	12	65
• Veggie Wrap	905	8	143

► BAKER'S DRIVE-THRU (cont.)

	Cal	Fat	Cbs
Mex Meals			
Burrito	930	10	124
Mexican Salad	1100	20	111
• Nachos	1575	29	173
• Tacos	670	5	111
Mexican: Burritos			
• All Chicken	500	5	56
Bean & Cheese	500	5	70
Combination	600	8	72
Green	620	5	90
Ground Beef	670	13	55
Red	620	5	90
Rice & Bean	550	2	95
Shredded Beef	540	8	56
• Veggie Wrap	680	6	101
Mexican: Quesadillas			
• Cheese	470	10	52
• Chicken	600	10	54
Monterey	470	10	56
Shredded Beef	560	11	55
Spicy Rolled Quesadilla	530	13	53
Mexican: Tacos			
Chicken Texas Taco	250	5	23
Original Taco	170	4	10
Soft Taco w/Chicken	190	3	18
• Soft Taco w/Shredded Beef	170	3	19
• Taco Burger	360	7	38
Texas Taco w/Ground Beef	290	7	22
Tostada	280	5	29
Papa Meals			
2 Texas Tacos, Chkn or Grnd Beef w/flour tortilla	850	15	81
• Any Chicken Sandwich	750	8	98
Chicken Burrito	810	8	111
• Double Baker w/Double Cheese	1030	20	95
Grilled Boca Burger®	830	9	110
Ground Beef Burrito	940	15	105
Quesadilla, Chkn or Shredded Beef	900	14	107
Shredded Beef Burrito	830	10	104
Shakes			
Banana	600	16	82
• Butterfinger®	720	20	92
Cherry	630	16	89
Chocolate	600	16	81
Oreo®	720	18	91
Snickers®	720	19	88
• Strawberry	580	16	75

● MOST HEALTHY   ● LEAST HEALTHY

BAKER'S DRIVE-THRU (cont.)

	Cal	Fat	Cbs
Vanilla	630	16	88
Sides & More			
Bean Cup	310	5	37
Chili	230	3	27
• Large Fries	340	4	41
Mexican Rice Cup	290	3	46
• Side Salad	45	2	4
Smoothies			
• Cappuccino	500	15	59
• Chocolate Banana	670	14	113
Chocolate Raspberry	670	14	112
Mango	660	14	111
Strawberry Banana	650	14	107
Very Berry	670	14	113
Vegetarian			
• Vegetarian Combination Burrito	560	5	77
Vegetarian Soft Taco	170	2	26
• Vegetarian Taco	160	2	18
Vegetarian Taco Burger	350	5	49
Vegetarian Texas Taco	230	5	26

BAKERS SQUARE

	Cal	Fat	Cbs
Breakfast			
Rise & Shine Breakfast	510	19	66
Entrees			
Chicken and Vegetable Stir-Fry	465	14	61
Small Sirloin Steak	500	25	32
Pitas & Wraps			
Fajita Pita	610	22	65
Stir-Fry Pita	660	23	74
Salads			
Chicken Caesar Salad	315	15	14
Stir-Fry Salad	555	22	53

BASKIN ROBBINS

	Cal	Fat	Cbs
31 Below Pies			
Heath®, 1 Slice, 115 g	310	14	43
• OREO®, 1 Slice, 115 g	290	13	40
• Reese's® Peanut Butter Cup, 115 g	340	18	38
Cappuccino blast (Medium)			
Caramel, 24 fl.oz.	670	23	111
Mocha (w/ Whipped Cream), 24 fl.oz.	620	21	100
• Nonfat, 24 fl.oz.	340	0	78
OREO® 'n Cookies, 24 fl.oz.	740	29	113
Original, 24 fl.oz.	480	19	72
Soft Serve, 24 fl.oz.	410	13	65

• MOST HEALTHY   • LEAST HEALTHY

BASKIN ROBBINS (cont.)

	Cal	Fat	Cbs
• Turtle, 24 fl.oz.	780	22	137
Floats, Freezes & Ice Cream Sodas (Medium)			
• Freeze (with Orange Sherbet), 652 g	510	5	112
Ice Crm Float (w/ Vanilla Ice Crm & RtBeer), 675 g	680	30	99
• Ice Crm Soda (w/ Vanilla Ice Crm), 594 g	720	30	103
Fruit Blast (Medium)			
Peach Passion Fruit Blast, 24 fl.oz.	370	1	94
• Strawberry Citrus Fruit Blast, 24 fl.oz.	330	0	83
• Wild Mango Fruit Blast, 24 fl.oz.	470	2	116
Fruit Blast Smoothies (Medium)			
• Mango, 24fl.oz.	620	2	148
• Peach Passion Banana, 24fl.oz.	540	1	131
Strawberry Banana, 24fl.oz.	560	1	135
Grab N Go			
Choco Chip Cookie Dough Ice Crm Qt, 73 g	200	10	23
Chocolate Chip Ice Cream Quart, 73 g	170	10	18
Chocolate Ice Cream Quart, 73 g	170	9	21
Gold Medal Ribbon® Ice Cream Quart, 73 g	170	8	22
Jamoca® Almond Fudge Ice Crm Qt, 76 g	180	10	21
Mint Choco Chip Ice Cream Quart, 73 g	170	10	18
Old Fash Butter Pecan Ice Crm Qt, 73 g	180	12	16
OREO® Cookies 'n Crm Ice Crm Qt, 73 g	180	10	21
• Peanut Butter 'n Choco Ice Crm Qt, 73 g	200	13	20
Pralines 'n Cream Ice Cream Quart, 76 g	190	9	24
• Rainbow Sherbet Quart, 85 g	120	2	26
Rocky Road Ice Cream Quart, 73 g	190	10	23
Vanilla Ice Cream Quart, 73 g	170	10	17
Very Berry Strawberry Ice Crm Quart, 73 g	140	7	18
Novelties n treats			
Brownie a la Mode, 78 g	260	13	36
Raspberry Fudge Truffle, 78 g	280	15	36
Shakes (Medium)			
• Choco Chip Cookie Dough Shake, 24 fl.oz.	1030	42	137
Chocolate Chip Shake, 555 g	900	44	108
Choco Shake (w/ Choco Ice Crm), 24 fl.oz.	990	40	149
Mint Chocolate Chip Shake, 24 fl.oz.	930	44	116
Raspberry Chip Shake, 24 fl.oz.	760	21	125
Strwby Shake (w/Very Bry Strwby Ice Crm), 24 fl.oz.	770	31	105
Vanilla Shake, 24 fl.oz.	980	45	125
Fruit Cream (Medium)			
• Mango Fruit Cream, 16 oz.	640	18	110
• Peach Passion Fruit Cream, 16 oz.	630	17	109
Strawberry Fruit Cream, 16 oz.	630	19	102
Ice Cream: Classic Flavour			
Cherries Jubilee Ice Cream, 113 g	240	12	30
Choco Chip Cookie Dough Ice Crm, 113 g	310	15	36

▶ BASKIN ROBBINS (cont.)

	Cal	Fat	Cbs
Chocolate Chip Ice Cream, 113 g	270	16	28
Chocolate Ice Cream, 113 g	260	14	33
Gold Medal Ribbon® Ice Cream, 113 g	260	13	34
Jamoca® Almond Fudge Ice Crm, 113 g	270	15	31
Jamoca® Ice Cream, 113 g	240	13	26
Made with Snickers® Ice Cream, 71 g	180	10	22
Mint Chocolate Chip Ice Cream, 113 g	270	16	28
Nutty Coconut Ice Cream, 113 g	190	12	17
Old Fash Butter Pecan Ice Crm, 113 g	280	18	24
OREO® Cookies 'n Crm Ice Cream, 113 g	280	15	32
• Peanut Butter 'n Choco Ice Cream, 113 g	320	20	31
Pistachio Almond Ice Cream, 113 g	290	19	25
Pralines 'n Cream Ice Cream, 113 g	280	14	35
• Rainbow Sherbet, 71 g	100	2	21
Reese's® PB Cup Ice Crm, 113 g	300	18	31
Rocky Road Ice Cream, 113 g	290	15	36
Vanilla Ice Cream, 113 g	260	16	26
Very Berry Strawberry Ice Cream, 113 g	220	11	28
World Class® Choco Ice Cream, 113 g	280	16	31

Ice Cream: Regional Flavour

	Cal	Fat	Cbs
Banana Nut Ice Cream, 113 g	160	9	16
Bananas 'n Strawberries Ice Cream, 113 g	230	11	31
• Black Walnut Ice Cream, 113 g	280	19	25
Chocolate Almond Ice Cream, 71 g	190	12	20
Cotton Candy Ice Cream, 71 g	160	8	20
Creole Cream Cheese Ice Cream, 113 g	240	13	28
Fudge Brownie Ice Cream, 71 g	190	11	22
Lemon Blueberry Frozen Yogurt, 71 g	120	4	21
Lemon Custard Ice Cream, 113 g	260	13	30
Mississippi Mud Ice Cream, 113 g	270	13	38
Orange Sherbet, 113 g	160	2	34
Oregon Blackberry Ice Cream, 113 g	250	12	28
Rum Raisin Ice Cream, 113 g	250	11	34
• Splish Splash® Sherbet, 71 g	90	1	21
Wild 'n Reckless Sherbet, 113 g	160	2	33

Ice Cream: Seasonal Flavour

	Cal	Fat	Cbs
Chocolate Fudge, 113 g	270	15	35
• Chocolate Mousse Royale®, 113 g	310	18	35
• Daiquiri Ice, 71 g	80	0	21
German Chocolate Cake, 71 g	200	10	24
Icing on the Cake, 71 g	210	11	25
Love Potion #31®, 71 g	170	9	20
Pink Bubblegum, 113 g	260	12	36
Premium Churned Light Mint OREO®, 113 g	240	7	40
Strawberry Cheesecake, 71 g	170	9	20
Super Fudge Truffle, 71 g	190	10	24

• MOST HEALTHY   • LEAST HEALTHY

▶ BASKIN ROBBINS (cont.)

	Cal	Fat	Cbs
Watermelon Chip, 71 g	90	1	22
Winter White Chocolate®, 113 g	260	14	30

Soft Serve Sundaes

	Cal	Fat	Cbs
Strawberry Soft Serve Sundae, 10 oz.	450	18	59

Soft Serve: 31 below (Medium)

	Cal	Fat	Cbs
Butterfinger®, 16 oz.	860	31	132
Choco Chip Cookie Dough, 16 oz.	940	34	143
Choco OREO®, 16 oz.	1290	55	187
• Fudge Brownie, 16 oz.	1390	58	199
Heath®, 16 oz.	1160	54	151
Jamoca® Almond Fudge, 16 oz.	960	40	133
Jamoca® OREO®, 16 oz.	860	33	128
OREO®, 16 oz.	1000	41	143
Reese's® Peanut Butter Cup, 16 oz.	1220	67	134
• Strawberry Banana, 16 oz.	710	23	112

Soft Serve: Cups & Cones (Regular)

	Cal	Fat	Cbs
Vanilla Soft Serve, 6 oz.	280	11	37
w/ Berry Magic Sprinkles, 6 oz.	290	11	39

Classic Sundaes

	Cal	Fat	Cbs
Banana Royale Sundae, 321 g	620	28	87
Brownie Sundae, 303 g	920	47	119
• Classic Banana Split, 571 g	1010	34	173
• Strawberry Soft Serve Sundae, 10 oz.	450	18	59

Premium Sundaes

	Cal	Fat	Cbs
• Choco Chip Cookie Dough Sundae, 337 g	990	43	138
Made with Snickers® Sundae, 340 g	1000	46	138
• Reese's® PntBtr Cup Sundae, 344 g	1220	80	109

▶ BD'S MONGOLIAN BARBECUE

Desserts

	Cal	Fat	Cbs
• Cheesecake Mini, 1 oz.	220	13	23
Cookies and Cream Mini, 1 oz.	330	18	40
• Peanut Butter Cup Mini, 1 oz.	410	24	43

Meats

	Cal	Fat	Cbs
Chicken, 3 oz.	102	3	0
Lamb, 3 oz.	126	7	0
• Strip Steak, 3 oz.	79	1	1
Pork, 3 oz.	123	5	0
Ribeye, 3 oz.	123	4	0
• Sausage, 3 oz.	273	26	2
Turkey, 3 oz.	102	3	0

Noodles

	Cal	Fat	Cbs
• Pasta, 2 oz.	210	1	42
Rice Noodle, 2 oz.	161	1	33
• Tortillas, 1 ea	90	3	16

• MOST HEALTHY   • LEAST HEALTHY

▶ BD'S MONGOLIAN BARBECUE (cont.)	Cal	Fat	Cbs
Rice			
Brown Rice, 3/4 cup	150	1	32
Rice, 3/4 cup	160	0	35
Salad Dressings			
Greek Feta, 1 oz.	70	5	1
Raspberry Vinaigrette, 1 oz.	35	0	8
Sauces			
Asian Black Bean, 1 oz.	34	1	3
Chili Garlic, 1 oz.	40	3	3
Fajita, 1 oz.	10	0	2
Kung Pao, 1 oz.	35	1	7
Lemon, 1 oz.	30	0	7
• Lite Soy, 1 oz.	10	0	1
Mandarin Orange, 1 oz.	70	0	16
Mongo Marinara, 1 oz.	30	1	3
Mongolian Ginger, 1 oz.	42	1	5
Pad Thai, 1 oz.	15	0	2
• Peanut, 1 oz.	100	7	9
Ponzu, 1 oz.	00	0	11
Sesame Oil, 0.5 tsp	10	1	0
Shanghai Barbeque, 1 oz.	45	0	10
Shiitake Mushroom, 1 oz.	35	0	8
Spicy Buffalo, 1 oz.	40	5	0
Sweet & Sour, 1 oz.	45	0	12
Szechwan, 1 oz.	27	0	5
Teriyaki, 1 oz.	16	0	3
Seafood			
Calamari, 3 oz.	78	1	3
Crawfish, 3 oz.	80	2	0
Krab (Surimi), 3 oz.	85	1	9
• Salmon, 3 oz.	156	10	0
Scallops, 3 oz.	84	1	3
• Shrimp, 3 oz.	65	0	0
Soups			
Clam Chowder, 8 oz.	160	4	15
Golden Broccoli Cheese, 8 oz.	190	10	17
• Rosemary Chkn & Dumpl, 8 oz.	80	1	12
• Tomato Bisque, 8 oz.	320	20	29
Wisconsin Cheese, 8 oz.	200	12	16
Vegetables			
Bean Sprouts, 1 oz.	29	0	2
Beets, 1 oz.	10	0	2
Black Olives, 1 oz.	53	5	2
Bok Choy, 1 oz.	2	1	0
Broccoli, 1 oz.	8	1	2
Cabbage (Green), 1 oz.	7	1	2

• MOST HEALTHY   • LEAST HEALTHY

BD'S MONGOLIAN BARBECUE (cont.)

	Cal	Fat	Cbs
Cabbage (Red), 1 oz.	6	1	1
Carrots, 1 oz.	12	1	3
Celery, 1 oz.	5	0	1
• Cheddar Cheese, 1 oz.	120	10	1
• Cilantro, 1 tsp	0	0	0
Corn (Baby), 1 oz.	6	0	1
Crouton, 7 pieces	35	2	4
Cucumbers, 1 oz.	4	1	1
Head Lettuce, 1 leaf	1	0	0
Lemons, 1 wedge	2	0	1
Limes, 1 lime	20	1	7
Mushrooms, 1 oz.	7	1	1
Onions (Yellow), 1 oz.	11	1	2
Pea Pods, 1 oz.	11	1	3
Peppers (Green), 1 oz.	8	0	2
Peppers (Red), 1 oz.	9	1	2
Pineapple, 1 oz.	14	0	3
Romaine Lettuce, 1 oz.	1	0	0
Water Chestnuts, 1 oz.	9	0	2
Others: Limited Time Offerings			
Bistro French Onion Soup, 8 oz.	120	6	13
Ginger Soy Sauce, 1 oz.	60	0	13

BEN & JERRY'S

Ice Cream

	Cal	Fat	Cbs
Butter Pecan 86 g	260	20	17
Cake Batter 92 g	242	14	24
Cherry Garcia® 87 g	200	11	23
Chocolate 88 g	200	12	21
Chocolate Chip Cookie Dough 87 g	220	12	26
Chocolate Fudge Brownie 87 g	220	11	27
Chocolate Macadamia 92 g	253	17	23
Chocolate Peanut Butter Swirl 89 g	250	17	22
Chocolate Therapy™ 86 g	210	12	25
Chunky Monkey® 87 g	240	14	24
Cinnamon Buns 88 g	240	12	30
• Coconut Seven Layer Bar 92 g	276	17	25
Half Baked® 114 g	230	11	28
Imagine Whirled Peace™ 91 g	252	15	26
Mint Chocolate Chunk 88 g	230	14	23
New York Super Fudge Chunk® 87 g	250	17	24
Oatmeal Cookie Chunk, 87 g	240	13	28
One Cheesecake Brownie™, 92 g	234	14	23
• Orange and Cream, 92 g	152	6	23
Peanut Butter Cookie Dough, 92 g	268	17	25
Phish Food®, 88 g	230	11	32

• MOST HEALTHY   • LEAST HEALTHY

BEN & JERRY'S (cont.)	Cal	Fat	Cbs
Strawberry Cheesecake, 86 g	210	11	24
Strawberry, 84 g	170	9	18
Sweet Cream & Cookies, 88 g	240	13	24
Triple Caramel Chunk, 88 g	230	12	28
Vanilla HEATH® Bar Crunch, 82 g	240	14	24
Vanilla, 88 g	190	12	18
Low Fat Frozen Yogurt			
Black Raspberry Swirl, 93-94 g	140	2	28
Chocolate Fudge Brownie, 93-94 g	160	3	32
Half Baked®, 93-94 g	160	3	31
• Vanilla, 93-94 g	130	2	25
• Vanilla Fudge Chip, NSA 80 g	180	13	20
Sorbet			
Berry Berry Extraordinary®, 92 g	100	0	27
Mango Mango, 91 g	100	0	27
Strawberry Kiwi, 92 g	100	0	27

BIG APPLE BAGELS			
BAB's Choice Bagels			
Blueberry Cobbler, 70 g	196	4	35
• Cheddar Nacho, 70 g	176	3	30
Cinnamon Apple Pie, 70 g	193	4	34
• Cinnamon Bun, 70 g	200	4	35
Cinnamon Danish, 70 g	198	4	36
French Toast, 70 g	186	2	37
Quiche Lorraine, 70 g	177	4	27
Strawberry White Chocolate, 70 g	182	2	36
Swiss Melt, 70 g	184	4	29
White Chocolate Swirl, 70 g	198	4	35
Big Apple Bagels® Regular Bagels			
Apple Cinnamon, 70 g	166	1	35
Banana Nut, 70 g	170	1	34
Blueberry, 70 g	165	1	34
Cheddar Herb, 70 g	176	3	30
Chocolate Chip, 70 g	174	1	34
Cinnamon Raisin, 70 g	168	1	35
Cinnamon Sugar, 70 g	175	1	37
Cranberry Walnut, 70 g	176	1	36
Egg, 70 g	164	1	33
Everything, 70 g	168	1	34
Garlic, 70 g	165	1	34
Honey Oat, 70 g	160	1	34
Jalapeño, 70 g	175	3	30
Onion, 70 g	168	1	35
Plain, 70 g	167	1	34
Poppy, 70 g	172	1	34

● MOST HEALTHY   • LEAST HEALTHY

▶ BIG APPLE BAGELS (cont.)

	Cal	Fat	Cbs
Pumpernickel, 70 g	166	1	34
Salt, 70 g	162	1	33
• Sesame, 70 g	179	2	33
Spinach, 70 g	178	1	36
Strawberry, 70 g	171	1	36
Tomato Basil, 70 g	161	1	33
• Vegetable, 70 g	159	1	33
Wheat, 70 g	165	1	34

Classic Recipe Cream Cheese

	Cal	Fat	Cbs
Cheddar Jalapeño, 30 g	90	8	2
• Garden Vegetable, 30 g	90	9	2
Onion Chive, 30 g	80	8	2
• Plain Lite, 30 g	60	5	3
Plain, 30 g	90	9	2
Strawberry, 30 g	90	7	5

Icepresso Drinks

	Cal	Fat	Cbs
Caramel Decadence Icepresso, 16 oz.	300	12	42
• Classic Icepresso, 16 oz.	300	5	52
• Java Chip Icepresso, 16 oz.	360	18	48
Latte Icepresso, 16 oz.	300	12	42
Mocha Icepresso, 16 oz.	301	12	42
Strawberry Icepresso, 16 oz.	340	12	56

Knorr Soups

	Cal	Fat	Cbs
Beef Barley Mushroom, 8 oz.	100	3	12
Beef Pot Roast, 8 oz.	110	4	12
Boston Clam Chowder, 8 oz.	210	13	20
California Medley, 8 oz.	170	9	16
• Cheese & Bacon, 8 oz.	310	21	18
Chicken & Dumplings, 8 oz.	250	14	20
Chicken & Wild Rice, 8 oz.	190	9	22
Chicken Gumbo, 8 oz.	130	3	19
Chicken Noodle, 8 oz.	110	4	12
Country Bean, 8 oz.	140	2	24
Cream of Broccoli (w/Cheese), 8 oz.	170	11	15
Cream of Broccoli (w/o Cheese), 8 oz.	230	17	17
Cream of Potato, 8 oz.	240	14	24
• French Onion, 8 oz.	60	2	9
Garden Vegetable, 8 oz.	110	1	22
Hearty Vegetable Beef, 8 oz.	100	1	16
Minestrone, 8 oz.	150	3	26
Navy Bean w/Ham, 8 oz.	110	2	23
New England Clam Chowder, 8 oz.	220	13	21
Potato Chowder, 8 oz.	210	13	20
Sirloin Beef w/Pasta, 8 oz.	190	7	22
Split Pea w/Ham, 8 oz.	90	2	15
Turkey & Sausage Gumbo, 8 oz.	190	10	14

• MOST HEALTHY   • LEAST HEALTHY

▶ BIG APPLE BAGELS (cont.)	Cal	Fat	Cbs
Vegetable Beef, 8 oz.	110	3	16
Wisconsin Cheese, 8 oz.	210	11	20
Fat Free Muffins			
• Fat Free Blueberry, 55 g	108	0	26
Fat Free Cherry Pie, 55 g	109	0	26
Fat Free Chocolate Marble, 55 g	125	0	29
• Fat Free Cinnamon Bun, 55 g	168	0	42
Fat Free Raspberry Amaretto, 55 g	127	0	31
Regular Muffins			
Banana Nut, 55 g	195	11	21
Blueberry Cheesecake, 55 g	199	12	20
• Blueberry, 55 g	168	8	22
Boston Cream Pie, 55 g	176	7	26
Cherry Cheesecake, 55 g	170	10	19
Chocolate Cheesecake, 55 g	202	12	22
Chocolate Chip, 55 g	211	11	27
Cinnamon Crumb Cake, 55 g	212	13	21
• Cinnamon Swirl Cheesecake, 55 g	214	11	20
Deep Dish Apple Pie, 55 g	177	8	25
Double Chocolate, 55 g	201	9	28
Golden Corn Bread, 55 g	197	9	26
Lemon Poppyseed, 55 g	201	10	25
Pumpkin Spice, 55 g	181	8	26
My Favorite Muffin® Bagels			
• Blueberry, 113 g	320	2	66
Cinnamon Raisin, 113 g	310	1	66
Honey Grain, 113 g	310	3	61
• Plain, 113 g	310	1	64
Russian Black Bread, 113 g	320	1	67
Sour Dough, 113 g	310	1	64
Whole Wheat, 113 g	310	2	66
Breakfast Sandwiches			
• Breakfast B.L.T., 9 oz.	704	31	83
Lox & Cream Cheese, 11 oz.	602	21	78
• Morning Classic, 8 oz.	486	11	73
Northern Omelette, 10 oz.	699	31	73
So. Tradition (w/bacon), 8 oz.	566	18	73
So. Tradition (w/ham), 9 oz.	547	15	73
So. Tradition (w/sausage), 10 oz.	696	31	73
Build Your Own Sandwiches			
Ham, 10 oz.	495	9	77
Roast Beef, 10 oz.	480	6	77
• Tuna, 10 oz.	547	14	77
• Turkey, 10 oz.	465	3	77
Gourmet Sandwiches			
Classic Turkey, 10 oz.	552	14	74

● MOST HEALTHY　　● LEAST HEALTHY

▶ BIG APPLE BAGELS (cont.)

	Cal	Fat	Cbs
• Holey Guacamole, 11 oz.	476	5	76
• Kick-N Roast Beef, 11 oz.	579	15	79
Mediterranean Veg-Out, 11 oz.	506	9	90
Overstuffed Sandwiches			
Classic Reuben, 14 oz.	962	43	57
• Corned Beef, 11 oz.	661	19	77
Ham and Cheese, 14 oz.	889	36	79
• Manhattan Club, 16 oz.	1122	40	120
Pastrami, 11 oz.	661	19	77
TD California Club, 16 oz.	759	12	113
TD Classic Club, 19 oz.	1119	43	122
TD The Clubhouse, 15 oz.	1079	37	117
Pizzaah! Sandwiches (per piece)			
• Bruschetta Pizzaah, 13 oz.	162	12	7
Cheese Pizzaah, 14 oz.	189	7	23
Grilled Chkn Bruschetta Pizzaah, 14 oz.	343	21	24
• Pepperoni Pizzaah, 14 oz.	398	26	23
Sausage Pizzaah, 14 oz.	211	17	6
Veggie Pizzaah, 12 oz.	238	10	32
Specialty Sandwiches			
All-American Duo, 13 oz.	752	28	78
• Big Apple Club, 12 oz.	797	37	75
Chicken Caesar, 11 oz.	611	19	78
• Grilled Chicken, 10 oz.	571	17	77
Roma Italian, 13 oz.	764	34	76
Turkey Club, 12 oz.	782	34	75
Toasted Sandwiches			
• Cafe Chicken Melt, 14 oz.	815	32	80
Deli-Style Turkey, 12 oz.	732	25	76
• Roast Beef Parmesan Grinder, 11 oz.	583	15	76
Spicy Italian Sub, 14 oz.	770	34	77
Tuna Melt, 10 oz.	641	23	75
Gourmet Salads			
Calypso Chicken Salad, 14 oz.	637	49	34
Chicken Caesar Salad, 12 oz.	524	41	15
Classic Caesar Cafe Salad, 4 oz.	225	19	9
Classic Caesar Salad, 8 oz.	414	36	12
Garden Mix Cafe Salad (w/o egg), 7 oz.	63	2	9
Garden Mix Cafe Salad, 7 oz.	100	5	9
Garden Mix Salad (w/o egg), 12 oz.	123	4	18
Garden Mix Salad, 12 oz.	197	9	18
Grilled Chicken Club Salad, 18 oz.	820	69	16
• Mediterranean Bread Salad, 19 oz.	973	73	52
Snacks			
Enchilada Bagellata, 8 oz.	522	11	84
Pizza Bagel, 8 oz.	481	6	85

• MOST HEALTHY   • LEAST HEALTHY

▶ BIG APPLE BAGELS (cont.)

	Cal	Fat	Cbs
Specialty Drinks (prepared w/ fat free milk)			
Cappuccino, 16 oz.	133	1	18
Cinnamon Toast Latte, 16 oz.	240	1	44
Creme Caramel Latte, 16 oz.	244	1	45
• Italiano, 16 oz.	89	1	12
Jittery Monkey, 16 oz.	429	6	80
Latte, 16 oz.	145	1	20
Mocha w/whipped cream, 16 oz.	392	6	70
Oregon Chai® Tea Latte, 16 oz.	231	1	47
Raspberry Cheesecake Latte, 16 oz.	259	1	50
• Turtle Mocha, 16 oz.	522	12	90
Vanilla Creme Latte, 16 oz.	132	1	18

▶ BIG BOY

	Cal	Fat	Cbs
Breakfast			
Belgian Waffle w/Powdered Sugar, 1 waffle	526	25	65
w/ Apple Topping, 1 waffle	746	26	122
w/ Strawberry Topping, 1 waffle	836	26	145
Big Boy Fav No Meat No Grain Product, 1 serv	440	32	25
Biscuits Plain, 2 Biscuits	424	20	51
Canadian Bacon, 2 sl.	146	7	2
Cinnamon Roll, 2 oz.	218	8	34
Eggs Benedict	947	61	60
English Muffin Plain, 1 muffin	140	2	27
French Toast, 2 sl.	365	7	363
Hash Brown Potatoes, 4 oz.	254	18	23
Hot Cakes w/ Apple Top, no syrup, 3 hot cakes	1330	26	243
Hot Cakes w/ Blbry, no syrup, 3 hot cakes	1115	26	187
• Hot Cakes w/ Strwby Top, no syrup, 3 hot cakes	1420	26	266
Hot Cakes, No Syrup, 3 hot cakes	1110	25	186
Multi-Grain Hot cakes Plain, 1 order	698	25	105
Omelet Cheese w/Toast	866	53	61
w/ Biscuits	1092	70	79
Omelet Farmer's w/Toast	899	51	69
w/ Biscuits	1125	68	87
Omelet Ham &Cheese w/Toast	902	53	61
w/ Biscuits	1128	70	79
Omelet Plain w/ Toast	749	44	59
w/ Biscuits	975	61	77
Omelet Southern Country w/Toast	1102	70	72
w/ Biscuits	1328	87	90
Pecan Roll Plain, 1 Roll	419	30	35
Pork Sausage Links, 2 links	133	11	1
Pork Sausage Patties, 1 patty	134	11	3
Potato Pancakes Plain, 1 order	404	14	68
• Sliced Bacon, 2 sl.	75	1	0

• MOST HEALTHY   • LEAST HEALTHY

BIG BOY (cont.)

	Cal	Fat	Cbs
Sliced Breakfast Ham, 1/2 sl.	311	21	1
Dinner			
Chkn & Veg Stir Fry w/ Plain Bkd Potato	717	8	128
• Chkn Breast Tenders Only, 2 tenders	280	11	24
Chicken Parmesan Dinner	904	44	95
Country Fried Steak Dinner	990	66	68
• Fish & Chips	1252	84	87
Shrimp (7 Pieces) No Potato	512	20	55
Spaghetti Dinner	612	13	105
Spaghetti Marinara Dinner	364	4	71
Veal Parmesan	833	31	92
Salads			
Caesar Salad, Side	66	4	7
Cole Slaw	120	10	9
Sandwiches			
Big Chz & Bacon Chkn w/ am Chz (only)	847	50	40
w/ Mozz. Cheese (only)	849	50	40
w/ Swiss Cheese (only)	876	52	40
Big Shrooms & Onion's (only)	801	44	45
Brawny Lad (only)	471	25	36
• Patty Melt	900	54	36
Plain Big Topping Burger (only)	694	38	38
• Plain Chicken Burger Sandwich (only)	351	9	39
Slim Jim (only)	548	27	51
Super Big Boy (only)	853	55	35
Super Slim Jim Sandwich	858	44	77
Swiss Miss (only)	604	37	33
Sides			
French Fries (Combo & Side), 5 oz.	490	26	57
Onion Rings, 8 Rings	304	16	36

BLACKJACK PIZZA

Pizza			
14" Lg Chz Pep, 108 g	250	9	28
14" Lg Chz Sausage, 109 g	240	8	28
14 Large Cheese, 99 g	200	5	28
• Cheesebread, 163 g	410	15	52
• Cinnabread, 66 g	190	5	31
Mediterranean Chicken, 78 g	190	11	15
Santa Fe, 98 g	210	11	17

BLIMPIE

Breads/Wraps			
Bread, Cheddar Jalapeño, 6", 3 oz.	210	5	36
Bread, Ciabatta, serving, 4 oz.	230	5	43
Bread, Honey Oat 6", 4 oz.	260	8	41

BLIMPIE (cont.)

	Cal	Fat	Cbs
Bread, Marble Rye 6", 4 oz.	240	5	46
• Bread, Pretzel, 4 oz.	320	6	65
Bread, Wheat, 6", 3 oz.	210	4	38
• Bread, White, 6", 3 oz.	210	3	40
Bread, Zesty Parmesan, 6", 3 oz.	240	5	39
Wrap, Spinach Herb 12", 4 oz.	310	8	52
Wrap, Traditional 12", 4 oz.	310	8	52

Breakfast Items

	Cal	Fat	Cbs
Bagel, 112 g	290	1	58
Bagel, Cream Cheese, 141 g	390	11	59
Biscuit with Sausage Gravy, 214 g	460	27	43
Biscuit, Bacon Egg & Cheese, 176 g	520	30	38
Biscuit, Egg & Cheese, 151 g	380	20	37
Biscuit, Ham Egg & Cheese, 180 g	420	21	39
Biscuit, Sausage Egg & Cheese, 194 g	530	34	37
Bluffin, Bacon Egg & Cheese, 123 g	270	12	27
Bluffin, Egg & Cheese, 119 g	240	10	27
Bluffin, Ham Egg & Cheese, 147 g	280	10	29
• Bluffin, Plain, 57 g	130	1	25
Bluffin, Sausage Egg & Cheese, 162 g	390	24	27
Burrito, Bacon Egg & Cheese, 260 g	580	28	57
Burrito, Egg & Cheese, 246 g	500	23	57
Burrito, Ham Egg & Cheese, 302 g	580	24	60
• Burrito, Sausage Egg & Cheese, 331 g	800	50	57
Burrito, Turkey Egg & Cheese, 302 g	560	23	59
Cinnamon Roll, 142 g	450	20	60
Egg & Cheese on a Roll, 101 g	200	9	22
Grilled Breakfast Snd, Bacon, 216 g	480	23	44
Grilled Breakfast Snd, Ham, 258 g	480	19	47
Grilled Breakfast Snd, Sausage, 286 g	710	45	44
Grilled Breakfast Snd, Turkey, 258 g	460	18	46

Cheese

	Cal	Fat	Cbs
American, 1 oz.	100	9	1
• Cheddar Shredded, serving, 1 oz.	110	9	0
• Parmesan Shredded, serving, 1 oz.	50	4	1
Pepper Jack, serving, 1 oz.	80	7	0
Provolone, serving, 1 oz.	80	6	0
Smoked Cheddar, serving, 1 oz.	80	6	1
Swiss, serving, 1 oz.	80	6	0

Chips/Snacks

	Cal	Fat	Cbs
Baked BBQ, 1 oz.	130	4	25
Cheddar Sour Cream, 2 oz.	240	15	21
Cheetos Crunchy, 1 oz.	160	10	15
Doritos Cooler Ranch, 2 oz.	240	12	31
Doritos Nacho Cheese, 2 oz.	240	12	30
• Fritos, 2 oz.	320	20	30

• MOST HEALTHY   • LEAST HEALTHY

▶ BLIMPIE (cont.)

	Cal	Fat	Cbs
KC Master BBQ, 2 oz.	240	15	22
• Potato Baked, 1 oz.	120	1	26
Potato Regular, 2 oz.	220	15	22
Pretzels Classic Thin Style, 2 oz.	220	2	47
SunChips Multigrain Harvest Chdr, 2 oz.	210	9	28
SunChips Multigrain Original, 2 oz.	210	9	29

Desserts, Snacks and Sides

	Cal	Fat	Cbs
Brownie, 2 oz.	230	10	28
Chocolate Chunk Cookie, 2 oz.	200	10	25
• Oatmeal Raisin Cookie, 2 oz.	180	7	27
Peanut Butter Cookie, 2 oz.	210	13	21
• Sugar Cookie, 3 oz.	320	16	42
White Choco Mac Nut Cookie, 2 oz.	200	11	25

Dressings/Sauces

	Cal	Fat	Cbs
Blimpie Special Sauce, 1 oz.	40	5	0
Oil, Blend, 1 oz.	130	14	0
• Peppercorn, 1 oz.	240	26	1
• Red Wine Vinegar, 1 oz.	5	0	1
Sauce, Red Hot Original, 1 oz.	10	0	2

Kids Meals

	Cal	Fat	Cbs
3" Ham, 165 g	260	8	32
3" Tuna, 160 g	280	11	30
• 3" Turkey, 152 g	190	3	31

Meats/Protein

	Cal	Fat	Cbs
Bacon, 1 oz.	110	8	0
Cappacola, 1 oz.	20	1	0
Chicken (Grilled) Strips, 3 1 oz.	110	4	0
Corned Beef, 1 oz.	35	1	1
Ham, 1 oz.	35	1	2
Meatballs, 3 oz.	220	16	8
Pastrami, 1 oz.	45	3	1
Pepperoni, 1 oz.	70	6	1
Philly Steak & Onion, 4 oz.	210	15	5
• Prosciuttini, 1 oz.	15	0	1
Roast Beef, 1 oz.	30	1	0
Salami, 1 oz.	35	3	0
Seafood Salad, 3 oz.	90	4	10
• Tuna, 3 oz.	240	18	0
Turkey, 1 oz.	30	0	1

Salads

	Cal	Fat	Cbs
Antipasto, 330 g	250	14	12
Buffalo Chicken, 220 g	220	9	10
Chicken Caesar, 269 g	190	8	6
Cole Slaw Salad, side, 110 g	160	9	20
• Garden, 184 g	30	0	6
• Macaroni Salad, side, 145 g	330	22	28

• MOST HEALTHY   • LEAST HEALTHY

▶ BLIMPIE (cont.)

	Cal	Fat	Cbs
Northwest Potato Salad, side, 140 g	260	17	22
Potato Salad, side, 135 g	230	12	28
Tuna, 269 g	270	19	6
Ultimate Club, 289 g	260	14	10
Sandwiches/Wraps			
Blimpie Best, 6", 296 g	450	17	49
Blimpie Best, 6" Super Stacked, 364 g	550	22	52
Blimpie Burger, 173 g	460	24	42
Blimpie Dog, 179 g	510	29	45
Blimpie Trio, 6" Super Stacked, 384 g	510	15	51
BLT, 6", 204 g	430	22	43
BLT, 6" Super Stacked, 238 g	640	41	43
Chicken Cheddar Bacon Ranch, 6", 346 g	600	29	48
Chicken Teriyaki, 6", 249 g	450	12	52
Chicken Teriyaki, 6" Wheat, 260 g	450	14	50
Ciabatta, Buffalo Chicken, 322 g	540	23	49
Ciabatta, French Dip, 394 g	430	11	49
Ciabatta, Grilled Chicken Caesar, 289 g	580	20	62
Ciabatta, Mediterranean, 289 g	450	8	65
Ciabatta, Rst Beef, Tkey & Chdr, 286 g	520	24	51
Ciabatta, Sicilian, 285 g	590	22	66
• Ciabatta, Spicy Chkn & Pepperoni, 288 g	710	34	65
Ciabatta, Tuscan, 282 g	570	20	65
Ciabatta, Ultimate Club, 210 g	520	24	47
Club, 6", 290 g	410	13	49
Club, 6" Wheat, 301 g	410	14	47
Cuban, 6", 233 g	410	11	43
French Dip, 6", 382 g	410	11	46
Ham & Swiss, 6", 285 g	420	14	49
Ham & Swiss, 6" Wheat, 295 g	420	15	47
Ham, Salami & Provolone, 6", 287 g	470	20	49
Hot Pastrami, 6", 204 g	430	16	42
Hot Pastrami, 6" Super Stacked, 289 g	570	23	43
Meatball 6", 286 g	580	31	50
Philly Steak & Onion, 6", 223 g	600	35	46
Pretzel, Ham and Swiss, 310 g	520	15	75
Pretzel, Turkey Bacon, 264 g	560	18	70
Reuben, 6", 261 g	530	20	52
Roast Beef & Provolone, 6", 307 g	430	14	46
Rst Beef & Provolone, 6" Wheat, 323 g	430	16	44
Special Veg (Doritos Sub), 6", 335 g	590	30	66
Tuna, 6", 255 g	470	21	43
Turkey & Provolone, 6", 307 g	410	13	49
Turkey & Provolone, 6" Wheat, 323 g	420	14	47
Turkey and Avocado 6", 319 g	360	7	51
Tkey and Bacon, 6" Super Stacked, 367 g	640	29	49

• MOST HEALTHY   • LEAST HEALTHY

BLIMPIE (cont.)

	Cal	Fat	Cbs
• Turkey and Cranberry 6", 279 g	350	4	58
Veggie & Cheese, 6", 319 g	460	21	50
Veggie Supreme, 6", 343 g	550	27	50
VegiMax, 6", 291 g	520	20	56
VegiMax, Wheat 6", 301 g	520	21	54
Wrap, Chicken Caesar, 277 g	560	24	56
Wrap, Southwestern, 287 g	530	22	61

Soups

	Cal	Fat	Cbs
Bean with Ham, 9 oz.	140	1	23
Beef Steak & Noodle, 9 oz.	120	4	14
Beef Stew, 9 oz.	170	4	18
Captain's Corn Chowder, 9 oz.	210	7	29
Chicken & Dumpling, 9 oz.	170	7	19
Chicken Gumbo, 9 oz.	90	2	13
Chicken Noodle, 9 oz.	130	4	18
Chicken with White & Wild Rice, 9 oz.	250	10	15
Cream of Broccoli with Cheese, 9 oz.	250	19	13
Cream of Potato, 9 oz.	190	9	24
French Onion, 9 oz.	80	4	11
• Garden Vegetable, 9 oz.	80	1	14
• Grande Chili with Bean & Beef, 9 oz.	310	9	31
Harvest Vegetable, 9 oz.	100	1	19
Italian Style Wedding, 9 oz.	130	4	17
Minestrone, 9 oz.	90	3	14
New England Clam Chowder, 9 oz.	170	3	28
Pasta Fagioli with Sausage, 9 oz.	150	5	22
Split Pea with Ham, 9 oz.	130	2	21
Tomato Basil with Raviolini, 9 oz.	110	1	22
Vegetable Beef, 9 oz.	80	2	13
Yankee Pot Roast, 9 oz.	80	2	12

Toppings

	Cal	Fat	Cbs
• Guacamole, 1 oz.	45	4	2
Lettuce, serving, 2 oz.	5	0	1
Olives, serving, 1 oz.	15	2	1
Onion, serving, 3 ea	10	0	3
• Peppers, Hot Ring, 12pcs, 1 oz.	0	0	1
Peppers, Jalapeño, 18pcs, 1 oz.	10	0	1
Peppers, Red Roasted, serving, 2 oz.	10	0	2
Peppers, Sweet Strips, 6pcs, 1 oz.	20	0	5
Tomato, serving, 2 ea	5	0	2

BOB EVANS RESTAURANTS

Appetizers

	Cal	Fat	Cbs
Blue Ribbon Apple Pie, 213, g	503	12	96
County Fair Cheese Bites, 323, g	942	66	47
• Itsy Bitsy Sandwich Trio, 454, g	1134	54	110

● MOST HEALTHY • LEAST HEALTHY

BOB EVANS RESTAURANTS (cont.)	Cal	Fat	Cbs
• Itsy Bitsy Trio, Mini Pot Roast Snd, 99, g	243	11	23
Itsy Bitsy Trio, Mini Pld Pork Snd, 102, g	281	14	20
Itsy Bitsy Trio, Mini Sausage Snd, 105, g	298	17	20
Loaded Potato Bites, 397, g	1008	63	93
Wildfire Chicken Quesadilla, 431, g	765	34	55
Beverages			
• Arnold Palmer, 269 g	47	0	11
• Caramel Mocha, 283 g	268	9	45
Cherry Hot Chocolate, 247 g	246	7	46
Breads			
Banana Nut Bread (1), 85 g	215	8	34
Biscuit (1), 86 g	260	13	32
Cherry Bread (1), 85 g	279	12	39
• Cinnamon Swirl (unfrosted), 139 g	532	28	67
Dinner Rolls (1), 64 g	201	5	34
English Muffin (1), 62 g	146	3	25
• Kaiser Bun (1), 62 g	195	5	31
Mini Bun (1), 40 g	126	3	20
Parmesan Crusted Garlic Bread (1), 80 g	195	9	23
Pumpkin Bread (1), 82 g	222	7	37
Rye Bread (1), 43 g	109	1	21
Sourdough Bread (1), 43 g	130	3	21
Texas Toast (1), 45 g	122	3	10
• Wheat Bread (1), 31 g	77	1	14
White Bread (1), 31 g	83	1	15
Breakfast			
Bacon (1) (a la carte), 7 g	36	4	0
Biscuit Sandwich, 207 g	581	39	33
Blueberry & Banana Yogurt Parfait, 190 g	177	1	39
Blueberry Crepe (1), 162 g	306	14	40
Blueberry Hotcake, No Topping (1), 176 g	343	10	58
Blueberry Stuffed French Toast, 434 g	730	19	90
Border Scramble Biscuit Bowl, 524 g	1029	57	75
Border Scrmbl Burrito w/ Bob Evans Egg Lites, 530 g	661	32	54
Border Scramble Burrito w/ Egg, 539 g	850	51	54
w/ Egg Whites, 530 g	654	32	54
Border Scramble Omelet, 428 g	637	46	14
w/ Bob Evans Egg Lites, 422 g	418	24	13
w/ Egg Whites, 422 g	408	24	13
Bowl of Grits, 295 g	265	10	40
Bowl of Oatmeal, 303 g	168	3	31
Bowl of Sausage Gravy, 332 g	294	19	23
Buttermilk Hotcake, No Topping (1), 164 g	337	10	56
Cinnamon Hotcake, No Topping (1), 173 g	382	12	62
Country Biscuit Breakfast, 287 g	652	45	39
Cup of Grits, 164 g	148	6	22

BOB EVANS RESTAURANTS (cont.)

	Cal	Fat	Cbs
Cup of Oatmeal, 164 g	91	2	17
Cup of Sausage Gravy, 193 g	171	11	14
Eggs (1) (a la carte), 60 g	131	11	1
Farmer's Market Omelet, 403 g	631	45	14
w/ Bob Evans Egg Lites, 397 g	413	23	13
w/ Egg Whites, 397 g	403	23	13
French Toast (1) (a la carte), 96 g	164	3	18
Fruit & Yogurt Plate, 524 g	347	2	82
Garden Harvest Omelet, 374 g	542	38	14
w/ Bob Evans Egg Lites, 369 g	323	16	13
w/ Egg Whites, 369 g	313	16	13
Ham & Cheddar Omelet, 289 g	515	36	4
w/ Bob Evans Egg Lites, 283 g	296	14	3
w/ Egg Whites, 283 g	286	14	3
Hardcooked Egg (1) (a la carte), 43 g	57	4	1
Meat Lover's BoBurrito, 380 g	805	52	40
w/ Bob Evans Egg Lites, 371 g	615	32	40
w/ Egg Whites, 371 g	609	32	40
Multigrain Hotcake, No Topping (1), 184 g	374	11	61
Mush (1) (a la carte), 94 g	171	7	25
Omelet Shell (a la carte), 116 g	194	14	2
Omelet Shell, Bob Evans Egg Lites, 170 g	85	0	2
Omelet Shell, Egg Whites, 170 g	75	0	2
Plain Crepe (1) (a la carte), 119 g	255	14	27
Pot Roast Hash, 374 g	681	45	30
Roasted Caramel Apple Crepe (1), 142 g	279	14	33
Rst Caramel Apple Stuffed French Toast, 448 g	731	19	91
Sausage & Cheddar Omelet, 283 g	552	43	4
w/ Bob Evans Egg Lites, 278 g	334	20	3
w/ Egg Whites, 278 g	324	20	3
Sausage Biscuit Bowl, 552 g	1024	63	78
Sausage Breakfast Patty (1), 48 g	140	11	0
Sausage Link (1) (a la carte), 34 g	133	12	0
Scrmbld Bob Evans Egg Lites (1 egg equiv), 57 g	28	0	1
Scrambled Egg (1 egg equiv), 57 g	84	5	1
• Scrambled Egg Whites (1 egg equiv), 57 g	25	0	1
Smoked Ham (1) (a la carte), 113 g	99	3	3
Spinach, Bcn & Tom Biscuit Bowl, 522 g	1039	62	81
• Stkd & Stfd Blbry Crm Hotcakes, 644 g	1490	70	204
Stkd & Stfd Caramel Banana Pecan Hotcakes, 479 g	1070	43	155
Stkd & Stfd Cinnamon Crm Hotcakes, 683 g	1377	53	211
Stkd & Stfd Rst Caramel Apple Crm Hotcakes, 550 g	1047	36	165
Stkd & Stfd Strwbry Banana Crm Hotcakes, 757 g	1168	36	197
Strawberry Banana Crepes (1), 198 g	314	14	44
Strwby Banana Mini Fruit & Yogurt Parfait, 188 g	151	1	33
Strwbry Blbry Mini Fruit & Yogurt Parfait, 190 g	158	1	34

• MOST HEALTHY   • LEAST HEALTHY

▶ BOB EVANS RESTAURANTS (cont.)	Cal	Fat	Cbs
Stuffed French Toast, No Topping, 349 g	627	19	65
Sunshine Skillet, 400 g	557	36	32
Sweet Cream Waffle, No topping, 179 g	394	8	66
Three Cheese Omelet, 235 g	528	40	5
w/ Bob Evans Egg Lites, 230 g	309	18	3
w/ Egg Whites, 230 g	299	18	3
Turkey & Spinach Omelet, 400 g	618	40	9
w/ Bob Evans Egg Lites, 394 g	399	18	8
w/ Egg Whites, 394 g	389	18	8
Turkey Sausage (1) (a la carte), 45 g	72	4	1
Turkey Sausage Breakfast, 329 g	362	7	48
Western BoBurrito, 414 g	738	44	42
w/ Bob Evans Egg Lites, 405 g	548	24	42
w/ Egg Whites, 405 g	542	24	42
Western Omelet, 335 g	529	36	8
w/ Bob Evans Egg Lites, 329 g	310	14	6
w/ Egg Whites, 329 g	300	14	6
Condiments			
Apple Butter (1), 14 g	34	0	8
Captain Wafers Crackers (1), 6 g	28	1	4
• Diet Blackberry Jam (1), 11 g	5	0	2
Grape Jelly (1), 14 g	36	0	9
Half and Half Cups (1), 15 g	40	3	1
Honey, 14 g	43	0	12
Margarine Buttery Taste Spread Cup (1), 5 g	27	3	0
Non-Dairy Creamer Cups (1), 14 g	19	1	1
Orange Marmalade (1), 14 g	36	0	9
• Pancake Syrup, 85 g	213	0	55
Saltine Crackers (1), 11 g	47	1	8
Strawberry Jam (1), 14 g	36	0	9
Sugar Free Pancake Syrup, 85 g	39	0	10
Desserts			
Apple Dumpling Pie, 247 g	568	28	77
Blackberry Cobbler, 227 g	566	26	79
• Cherry Deep Dish Cobbler, 232 g	667	29	101
Coconut Cream Pie, 198 g	514	29	59
French Silk Pie, 156 g	655	44	59
Lemon Supreme Pie, 206 g	642	38	71
NSA Apple Pie, 191 g	499	30	56
Strawberry Shortcake, 361 g	555	22	86
Strawberry Sundae, 315 g	419	20	56
Strawberry Supreme Pie, 246 g	651	47	58
• Vanilla Ice Cream, 79 g	111	6	13
Dinner			
Chicken-N-Noodles Deep-Dish, 564 g	701	29	66
Chkn Parmesan w/ Meat Sauce, 541 g	845	44	57

BOB EVANS RESTAURANTS (cont.)

	Cal	Fat	Cbs
Chicken Salad Plate, 590 g	710	43	69
Chicken & Broccoli Alfredo, 471 g	470	24	35
Country Fried Steak w/ Gravy (1), 232 g	550	37	37
Country Fried Steak (1), 150 g	496	33	31
Cranberry Apple Pork Loin (1), 201 g	241	12	25
Fried Buttermilk Shrimp, 221 g	685	48	36
Fried Btrmlk Shrimp & Flounder Combo, 258 g	521	31	27
Fried Btrmlk Shrimp & Haddock Combo, 306 g	707	42	45
Fried Chkn Breast, 142 g	285	13	13
Fried Chkn Strips, 43 g	137	8	10
Fried Haddock (a la carte), 184 g	363	18	27
Garlic Butter Grld Chkn Breast (1), 128 g	180	6	1
Garlic Butter Salmon, 224 g	256	9	1
Grilled Chkn Breast, 113 g	165	5	0
• Grilled Chkn Tenders, 31 g	36	1	0
Meatloaf, 252 g	435	22	22
Open-Faced Roast Beef, 272 g	476	24	22
Pot Roast Beef Stew Deep-Dish, 571 g	713	34	67
Pot Roast Stroganoff, 672 g	813	43	65
Potato-Crusted Flounder, 136 g	177	7	9
Salmon, 210 g	243	8	0
Sirloin Steak, 142 g	421	29	3
Slow-Roasted Chicken-N-Noodles, 309 g	186	4	25
• Slow-Roasted Chicken Pot Pie, 510 g	884	60	66
Slow-Roasted Turkey, 113 g	136	5	3
Spaghetti with Meat Sauce, 380 g	489	25	44
Turkey and Dressing, 493 g	690	30	56
Wildfire Grilled Chicken Breast (1), 147 g	236	6	15
Wildfire Salmon, 244 g	312	9	15

'Fit from the Farm' Menu Items

	Cal	Fat	Cbs
AppleCran Spinach Salad w/RF Rspbry Dressing, 235 g	381	15	47
Applesauce, 94 g	69	0	18
Beef Veg Soup w/ Saltine Crackers, 190 g	137	3	21
Blueberry-Banana French Toast, 232 g	323	6	36
Blbry-Banana Mini Fruit & Yogurt Parfait, 190 g	177	1	39
Bob Evans Egg Lites w/ a Sl. of Tomato, 139 g	62	0	2
Chkn-N-Noodles w/ Saltine Crackers, 238 g	184	4	26
Chicken, Spinach & Tomato Pasta, 346 g	526	16	67
Classic Bean Soup w/ Saltine Crackers, 164 g	157	4	23
Cup of Quaker Oatmeal w/ Brown Sugar & Milk, 255 g	218	3	44
Dry English Muffin w/ Smucker's Jelly, 71 g	156	1	33
Dry Wheat Toast w/ Smucker's Jelly, 45 g	113	1	23
Fresh Fruit Cup, 218 g	148	1	38
Fresh Fruit Plate w/ LowFat Cottage Chz, 513 g	347	4	69
Fresh Fruit Plate w/ Low Fat Strwby Yogurt, 519 g	353	2	84
• Fresh Garden Salad w/o Croutons or Dress, 79 g	15	0	3

• MOST HEALTHY   • LEAST HEALTHY

▶ BOB EVANS RESTAURANTS (cont.)	Cal	Fat	Cbs
• Fruit & Yogurt Crepe w/ Quaker Oatmeal, 516 g	616	17	104
Grilled Chicken Breast, 558 g	403	6	58
Grilled Salmon Fillet, 655 g	481	9	58
Low-Fat Strawberry Yogurt, 91 g	93	1	18
Plain Baked Potato, 286 g	193	0	50
Potato Crusted Flounder, 581 g	415	8	67
Steamed Broccoli Florets, 159 g	44	1	8
Veggie Omelet, 383 g	272	2	43
Kids Menu			
Applesauce, 94 g	69	0	18
Baked Potato, 286 g	193	0	50
Broccoli Florets, 159 g	44	1	8
Chocolate Milk 1%, Kids, 312 g	212	3	37
Corn, 101 g	166	11	17
Cottage Cheese, 108 g	92	4	4
French Fries, 128 g	319	13	46
Fresh Garden Salad, 43 g	49	4	1
Fried Chicken Strips, 43 g	137	8	10
Fruit & Yogurt Dippers, 303 g	222	1	51
Fudge Blast Sundae, 113 g	216	9	31
Glazed Carrots, 102 g	101	5	14
Green Beans, 108 g	47	2	6
Grilled Cheese Triangles, 96 g	313	15	32
• Grilled Chkn Tenders, 31 g	36	1	0
Home Fries, 145 g	164	6	24
Macaroni and Cheese, 184 g	318	8	41
Mashed Potatoes, 159 g	192	7	16
Mini Cheeseburgers (1), 85 g	284	15	22
Plenty-o-Pancakes, 156 g	337	12	52
Reese's I'm Smiling Sundae, 122 g	274	13	35
Smiley Face Potatoes, 88 g	271	16	29
• Spaghetti with Meat Sauce, 374 g	467	24	44
Strawberry Sundae, Kids, 125 g	177	8	24
Strawberry Yogurt, 91 g	93	1	18
Turkey Lurkey, 142 g	163	7	4
Salads			
Caesar Dressing (Dinner), 79 g	432	47	2
Cobb Salad, 408 g	517	31	10
Colonial Dressing (Dinner), 79 g	433	38	22
• Country Caesar Salad, 473 g	744	53	20
Country Spinach Salad, 303 g	428	25	12
Cranberry Pecan Chicken Salad, 400 g	672	45	38
French Dressing (Dinner), 79 g	410	38	18
Garden Salad, 91 g	58	1	9
Heritage Chef Salad, 352 g	398	25	11
Hot Bacon Dressing (Dinner), 79 g	198	6	33

BOB EVANS RESTAURANTS (cont.)	Cal	Fat	Cbs
Rspbry RF Dressing (Dinner), 79 g	199	10	27
Specialty Garden Salad, 105 g	124	7	10
Sweet Italian Dressing (Dinner), 62 g	253	23	12
Swiss Bacon Dressing (Dinner), 79 g	423	48	3
• Vinegar & Oil Dressing (Dinner), 85 g	54	6	0
Wildfire Fried Chicken Salad, 425 g	711	34	70
Wildfire Grilled Chicken Salad, 383 g	389	13	37
Sandwiches			
Bacon Cheeseburger, 307 g	719	38	35
Biscuit Sandwich, 207 g	581	39	33
Bob-B-Q Pulled Pork Sandwich, 224 g	596	24	65
Bob's BLT & E, 282 g	639	41	26
Cheeseburger, 292 g	648	31	35
Chicken Salad Sandwich, 272 g	637	37	54
Fried Chicken Club Sandwich, 288 g	637	31	47
Fried Chicken Sandwich, 252 g	489	18	47
Fried Haddock Sandwich, 320 g	732	33	71
Grilled Cheese Sandwich, 119 g	350	15	22
Grilled Chicken Club Sandwich, 259 g	512	23	34
Grilled Chicken Sandwich, 224 g	370	10	33
Hamburger, 264 g	542	22	34
• Hamburger Patty (a la carte), 128 g	336	17	0
• Knife & Fork Bob-B-Q Pulled Pork Snd, 425 g	856	30	89
Knife & Fork Meatloaf Sandwich, 539 g	845	39	52
Knife & Fork Pork Loin Sandwich, 454 g	771	46	51
Knife & Fork Turkey Sandwich, 439 g	718	37	48
Pot Roast Sandwich, 241 g	574	28	50
Turkey Bacon Melt, 294 g	588	28	49
Sauces			
Bacon Bits, 28 g	145	11	1
• Beef Gravy, 62 g	25	1	3
Blueberry Topping, 85 g	103	0	25
Brown Sugar, 26 g	95	0	24
Caramel Topping, 28 g	74	0	18
Chicken-Roasted Gravy, 57 g	54	4	3
Chocolate Fudge Topping, 28 g	86	2	16
Cocktail Sauce, 35 g	31	0	7
Country Gravy, 85 g	56	4	6
Cranberries, 20 g	68	0	17
Cranberry Apple Topping, 74 g	92	1	20
Honey Roasted Pecans, 20 g	132	13	5
Marinara Sauce, 85 g	35	1	5
Pork-Roasted Gravy, 57 g	64	5	3
• Queso Sauce, 113 g	159	9	8
Raisins, 26 g	84	0	20
Ranchero Picante, 37 g	37	0	0

BOB EVANS RESTAURANTS (cont.)	Cal	Fat	Cbs
Roasted Caramel Apple Topping, 85 g	89	1	21
Shredded Cheddar Cheese, 28 g	112	9	1
Strawberry Topping, 85 g	55	0	14
Tarter Sauce, 20 g	116	12	1
Whipped Topping, 11 g	37	3	3
Seniors			
Bowl of Sausage Gravy, 332 g	294	19	23
Chicken & Broccoli Alfredo, 471 g	470	24	35
Chkn Parmesan w/ Meat Sauce, 541 g	845	44	57
Country Fried Steak (1) (a la carte), 150 g	496	33	31
Cup of Sausage Gravy, 193 g	171	11	14
Fried Chicken Breast (1) (a la carte), 142 g	285	13	13
Fried Haddock (a la carte), 184 g	363	18	27
Garlic Butter Grilled Chkn Breast (1), 128 g	180	6	1
• Grilled Chicken Breast (1), 113 g	165	5	0
Meatloaf (1) (a la carte), 252 g	435	22	22
Open-Faced Roast Beef, 272 g	476	24	22
Pot Roast Stroganoff, Savor Size, 346 g	425	23	33
• Slow-Roasted Chkn Pot Pie, 510 g	884	60	66
Slow-Roasted Chkn-N-Noodles, 309 g	186	4	25
Spaghetti with Meat Sauce, 380 g	489	25	44
Turkey and Dressing, Senior, 380 g	554	26	53
Turkey Sausage Breakfast, 329 g	362	7	48
Wildfire Grilled Chkn Breast (1), 147 g	236	6	15
Sides			
American Cheese (1), 14 g	53	4	1
Applesauce, 94 g	69	0	18
Baked Potato, 286 g	193	0	50
Blue Cheese, 28 g	97	8	0
Bread and Celery Dressing, 176 g	296	16	31
Broccoli Florets, 159 g	44	1	8
Coleslaw, 102 g	208	14	19
Corn, 101 g	166	11	17
Cottage Cheese, 108 g	92	4	4
Cranberry Relish, 34 g	68	0	16
• Dill Pickle Slices, 26 g	2	0	0
French Fries, 128 g	319	13	46
Fruit Dish, 108 g	58	0	14
Garden Vegetables, 170 g	119	8	11
Glazed Carrots, 102 g	101	5	14
Green Beans, 108 g	47	2	6
Grilled Mushrooms, 198 g	87	5	10
Home Fries, 145 g	164	6	24
Lettuce & Tomato, 48 g	9	0	2
Lettuce, Tomato and Pickle, 74 g	12	0	2
• Loaded Baked Potato, 329 g	395	16	53

• MOST HEALTHY   • LEAST HEALTHY

BOB EVANS RESTAURANTS (cont.)	Cal	Fat	Cbs
Mashed Potatoes, 159 g	192	7	16
Monterey Jack Cheese (1), 20 g	71	6	0
Onion Petals, 136 g	288	14	35
Strawberry Yogurt, 91 g	93	1	18
Tomato Slices (2), 51 g	11	0	2
Soups			
Cup of Bean Soup, 153 g	110	2	15
Cup of Chdr Baked Potato Soup, 175 g	172	9	15
• Cup of Sausage Chili, 170 g	215	14	15
• Cup of Vegetable Beef Soup, 179 g	90	2	13

BOJANGLES			
Biscuit Sandwiches			
Bacon	290	17	26
Bacon, Egg & Cheese	550	42	27
• Biscuit (plain)	243	12	29
Cajun Filet	454	21	46
Country Ham	270	15	26
Egg	400	30	26
Sausage	350	23	26
Smoked Sausage	380	26	27
• Steak	649	49	37
Cajun Spiced Chicken			
Breast	278	17	12
• Leg	122	16	11
• Thigh	310	23	11
Wing	160	25	11
Individual Fixin'			
Botato Rounds	235	11	31
Cajun Pintos	110	0	18
Dirty Rice	166	6	24
• Green Beans	25	0	5
Macaroni & Cheese	198	14	12
Marinated Cole Slaw	136	3	26
Potatoes w/o gravy	80	1	16
• Seasoned Fries	344	19	39
Sandwiches			
Cajun Filet	337	11	41
Grilled Filet	235	5	25
Snacks			
Buffalo Bites	180	5	5
Chicken Supremes	337	16	26
Sweet Biscuits			
Bo Berry™	220	10	29
Cinnamon	320	18	37

• MOST HEALTHY   • LEAST HEALTHY

BOSTON MARKET

	Cal	Fat	Cbs
Desserts			
• Apple Pie (slice), 6 oz.	580	30	74
Chocolate Cake, 5 oz.	580	34	67
Chocolate Chip Fudge Brownie, 3 oz.	320	13	49
Chocolate Chunk Cookie, 3 oz.	370	18	50
• Cornbread, 2 oz.	180	5	31
Family Meals			
Beef Brisket, 113	280	20	1
• Meatloaf, 218	480	36	21
• Roasted Turkey, 142	180	3	0
Rotisserie Chicken, 170	310	15	0
Individual Meals			
1 Thigh & 1 Drumstick, 145 g	290	17	0
1/4 White Rotisserie Chicken, 187 g	320	12	0
1/4 White Rotisserie Chkn, No Skin, 181 g	240	4	1
3 Pc Dark (2 Thighs & Drumstick), 253 g	490	29	0
3 Piece Dark Individual Meal, 208	390	22	1
3 Pc Dark Sknlss (2 Thighs & Drumstick), 202 g	350	18	0
3 Pc Dark Sknlss (Thigh & 2 Drumsticks), 171 g	290	11	0
Baked Whitefish, 269	470	28	21
Beef Brisket, 113 g	230	13	0
Half Rotisserie Chicken, 341 g	610	29	1
Meatloaf, 215 g	480	30	25
• Pastry Top Chicken Pot Pie, 425 g	810	48	60
• Roasted Turkey, 113 g	150	3	0
Salads			
Beef Brisket, 6 oz.	280	20	1
Caesar Salad Entree w/o dressing, 3 oz.	140	8	7
• Market Chopped Salad, 3 oz.	480	40	24
Market Chopped Salad Dressing, 4 oz.	360	39	2
• Roasted Turkey, 14 oz.	110	2	0
Rotisserie Chicken, 5 oz.	180	3	0
Sandwiches			
Boston Chicken Carver, 321 g	750	29	64
• Boston Meatloaf Carver, 449 g	940	40	96
Boston Turkey Carver, 344 g	700	26	65
Brisket Dip Carver, 304 g	840	45	62
Classic Chicken Salad Sandwich, 363 g	800	41	65
Half Boston Chicken Carver, 199 g	375	15	32
Half Boston Turkey Carver, 172 g	350	13	32
Meatloaf Open-faced Sandwich, 374 g	670	38	48
Roasted Tkey Open-faced Snd, 300 g	330	6	43
• Rotisserie Chkn Open-faced Snd, 289 g	320	8	34
Soups & Sides			
• Beef Gravy, 3 oz.	35	2	4
Chicken Noodle Soup, 14 oz.	250	8	23

BOSTON MARKET (cont.)

	Cal	Fat	Cbs
Chkn Tortilla Soup w/ Toppings, 13 oz.	410	26	30
Chkn Tortilla Soup w/o toppings, 11 oz.	160	8	13
Cinnamon Apples, 5 oz.	210	3	47
Creamed Spinach, 7 oz.	280	23	12
Fresh Steamed Vegetables LF, 5 oz.	60	2	8
Fresh Vegetable Stuffing, 5 oz.	190	8	25
Garlic Dill New Potatoes LF, 6 oz.	140	3	24
Green Beans, 3 oz.	60	4	7
Macaroni and Cheese, 8 oz.	300	11	35
Mashed Potatoes, 8 oz.	270	11	36
Poultry Gravy, 4 oz.	50	2	7
Sweet Corn, 6 oz.	170	4	37
• Sweet Potato Casserole, 7 oz.	460	16	77

BROWN'S CHICKEN & PASTA

Main Chicken Items

	Cal	Fat	Cbs
• Chicken Breast	284	N/A	12
Chicken Legs	287	N/A	9
Chicken Thigh	355	N/A	13
• Chicken Wing	385	N/A	17

Miscellaneous Items

	Cal	Fat	Cbs
• Chicken Gizzards	387	N/A	26
Chicken Livers	341	N/A	20
• Mushrooms	289	N/A	30

Pasta Items

	Cal	Fat	Cbs
Mostaccioli (in Marinara)	792	10	74
Spaghetti (in Marinara)	792	10	146

Premium Side Items

	Cal	Fat	Cbs
• Cheezy Potatoes, 12 oz.	188	11	16
Mostaccioli (in Marinara)	792	10	74
• Spaghetti (in Marinara)	792	10	146

Regular Side Items

	Cal	Fat	Cbs
Cole slaw	131	N/A	9
• Corn Fritters	415	N/A	42
• Potato salad	95	N/A	13

BRUEGGER'S

Bagels

	Cal	Fat	Cbs
Asiago Parmesan, 4 oz.	330	4	61
Blueberry, 4 oz.	310	2	62
Chocolate Chip, 4 oz.	330	4	65
Cinnamon Raisin, 4 oz.	310	2	65
Cinnamon Sugar, 4 oz.	320	2	63
Cranberry Orange, 4 oz.	310	2	64
Egg, 4 oz.	310	3	63
Everything, 4 oz.	310	3	62

• MOST HEALTHY   • LEAST HEALTHY

▶ BRUEGGER'S (cont.)

	Cal	Fat	Cbs
• Fortified Multi-Grain, 4 oz.	340	3	66
Garlic, 4 oz.	300	2	61
Honey Grain, 4 oz.	310	3	61
Jalapeño, 4 oz.	310	2	62
LTO - Baked Apple Bagel, 4 oz.	320	2	67
Onion, 4 oz.	300	2	61
Plain, 4 oz.	300	2	60
Poppy, 4 oz.	310	3	61
Pumpernickel, 4 oz.	300	2	62
Rosemary Olive Oil, 4 oz.	330	6	59
Rye, 4 oz.	330	2	59
Salt, 4 oz.	300	2	61
Sesame, 4 oz.	310	3	60
Sourdough, 4 oz.	290	2	56
• Sundried Tomato, 4 oz.	280	2	57
Whole Wheat, 4 oz.	300	4	56

Beverages: Other (Medium)

	Cal	Fat	Cbs
Hot Chocolate, 8 oz.	140	2	31

Syrup Flavors

	Cal	Fat	Cbs
Almond Flavored Syrup, 1 oz.	90	0	23
Caramel Flavored Syrup, 1 oz.	100	0	24
• Chocolate Syrup, 1 oz.	88	1	20
Hazelnut Flavored Syrup, 1 oz.	90	0	22
• Vanilla Flavored Syrup, 1 oz.	100	0	25

Breads & Wraps

	Cal	Fat	Cbs
• Bagel Bowl, 10 oz.	720	9	136
Ciabatta, 4 oz.	250	3	48
Hearty White, 4 oz.	260	1	54
Honey Wheat, 4 oz.	280	3	54
• White Wrap, 2 oz.	180	2	32

Cream Cheese

	Cal	Fat	Cbs
Bacon Scallion, 2 oz.	140	12	5
Garden Veggie, 2 oz.	130	11	5
Honey Walnut, 2 oz.	150	12	8
Jalapeño, 2 oz.	140	13	4
• Light Garden Veggie, 2 oz.	90	6	3
Light Herb Garlic, 2 oz.	100	6	4
Light Plain, 2 oz.	100	6	4
• LTO - Cucumber Dill (seasonal), 2 oz.	150	14	3
LTO - Pumpkin (seasonal), 2 oz.	120	11	4
Olive Pimiento, 2 oz.	140	13	3
Onion and Chive, 2 oz.	140	13	3
Plain, 2 oz.	130	11	6
Smoked Salmon, 2 oz.	150	13	3
Strawberry, 2 oz.	140	13	4
Vermont Maple, 2 oz.	120	11	4

● MOST HEALTHY   • LEAST HEALTHY

BRUEGGER'S (cont.)

	Cal	Fat	Cbs
Dessert Bars			
Chocolate Chunk Brownies, 3 oz.	310	18	38
• Marshmallow Chew, 2 oz.	280	6	55
• Seven Layer Bar, 5 oz.	650	43	58
Toffee Almond Bar, 3 oz.	400	19	53
Kids & Prepared			
• Kids' Grilled Cheese Sandwich, 3 oz.	300	14	27
Plain Bagel/L Plain Cream Cheese, 6 oz.	400	8	64
Plain Bagel w/Hummus, 6 oz.	410	8	70
Plain Bagel w/Peanut Butter, 6 oz.	550	23	70
• Plain Bagel w/Peanut Butter & Jelly, 7 oz.	650	23	69
Plain Bagel w/Plain Cream Cheese, 6 oz.	430	13	66
Salad Dressings			
• Asian Sesame Ginger, 2 oz.	260	21	17
• Balsamic Vinaigrette, 2 oz.	110	9	8
Caesar, 2 oz.	110	9	8
Ranch, 2 oz.	190	21	2
Salads & Dressings			
• Build Your Own Base, 5 oz.	30	1	5
Caesar No Dressing, 6 oz.	160	8	14
Caesar Caesar Dressing, 8 oz.	270	17	22
Caesar w/Chkn/Caesar Dressing, 11 oz.	380	20	23
Mandarin Medley No Dressing, 8 oz.	220	8	29
Mandarin Medley Balsamic Vinaigrette, 10 oz.	340	17	36
Mandarin Medley w/Chkn Balsamic Vinaigrette, 13 oz.	450	21	37
Sesame Salad No Dressing, 6 oz.	120	5	12
Sesame Salad Asian Sesame Drss, 8 oz.	380	26	29
• Sesame Salad w/Chkn Asian Sesame Drss, 11 oz.	490	29	30
Breakfast Sandwiches			
Bagel - Egg / Cheese, 7 oz.	470	14	63
Bagel - Egg / Cheese / Bacon, 7 oz.	480	21	63
• Bagel - Egg / Cheese / Ham, 8 oz.	440	9	65
Bagel - Egg / Cheese /Sausage, 8 oz.	560	23	63
Classic Wrap w/Bacon, 9 oz.	730	44	39
Classic Wrap w/Ham, 10 oz.	570	27	38
Classic Wrap w/Sausage, 9 oz.	690	41	37
Rio Grande w/Bacon / Wrap, 9 oz.	640	38	41
Rio Grande w/Ham / Wrap, 9 oz.	480	21	41
Rio Grande w/Sausage / Wrap, 9 oz.	600	35	39
Smoked Salmon / Plain Bagel, 8 oz.	460	10	66
Spinach & Chdr Omelet/Plain Bagel, 7 oz.	500	16	64
w/ Bcn / Plain Bagel, 8 oz.	570	22	64
w/ Ham / Plain Bagel, 9 oz.	550	17	66
Spinach, Chdr & Ssg Omelet /Plain Bagel, 9 oz.	670	31	64
• Western / Plain Bagel, 7 oz.	760	56	66

• MOST HEALTHY • LEAST HEALTHY

BRUEGGER'S (cont.)

	Cal	Fat	Cbs
Deli Sandwiches			
BLT / Plain Bagel, 8 oz.	530	23	64
BLT / Hearty White, 11 oz.	720	42	62
Chicken Breast / Plain Bagel, 11 oz.	550	6	81
Chicken Breast / Hearty White, 15 oz.	610	4	94
• Garden Veggie / Plain Bagel, 12 oz.	360	2	72
Garden Veggie / Wheat Bread, 15 oz.	360	3	67
Ham / Plain Bagel, 9 oz.	430	8	64
Ham / Honey Wheat, 15 oz.	540	16	64
Roast Beef / Plain Bagel, 10 oz.	450	11	63
Roast Beef / Hearty White, 16 oz.	560	18	59
Tuna Salad / Plain Bagel, 9 oz.	570	25	63
• Tuna Salad / Hearty White, 14 oz.	810	46	58
Turkey / Plain Bagel, 9 oz.	440	8	64
Turkey / Honey Wheat, 15 oz.	560	15	60
Hot Panini			
Four Chz & Tomato / Hearty White, 10 oz.	700	34	56
• Ham & Swiss / Honey Wheat, 10 oz.	600	17	72
Primo Pesto Chkn / Hearty White, 11 oz.	700	32	56
• Tuna & Chdr Melt / Honey Wheat, 12 oz.	970	61	57
Turkey Toscana / Hearty White, 12 oz.	650	28	58
Signature & Classic Sandwiches			
• Herby Turkey Sesame Bagel, 10 oz.	530	14	73
Leonardo da Veg Plain Softwich, 12 oz.	560	15	76
Roma Roast Beef Hearty White, 13 oz.	770	44	62
Tarragon Chkn Salad Hearty White, 14 oz.	750	37	75
Thai Peanut Chkn Plain Bagel, 11 oz.	580	11	91
• Tkey Chipotle Club Honey Wheat, 12 oz.	800	51	57
Cookies			
Chocolate Chip, 3 oz.	390	17	52
• Double Chocolate, 3 oz.	390	19	51
• Everything, 3 oz.	380	18	49
Muffins			
Banana Nut, 5 oz.	450	26	50
Blueberry (Bake N Joy), 5 oz.	430	22	53
• Blueberry (Main Street Gourmet), 5 oz.	355	10	59
Cappuccino, 5 oz.	490	26	60
• Cinna. Coffee Cake (Bake N Joy), 5 oz.	510	27	61
Corn (Bake N Joy), 5 oz.	490	23	63
Cranberry (Main Street Gourmet), 5 oz.	355	10	59
Cranberry Nut (Bake N Joy), 5 oz.	430	23	53
Soups			
Beef Chili, 8 oz.	190	8	18
Butternut Squash, 8 oz.	240	17	21
Chicken Spaetzle, 8 oz.	140	5	15
• Chicken Wild Rice, 8 oz.	280	22	12

• MOST HEALTHY   • LEAST HEALTHY

BRUEGGER'S (cont.)

	Cal	Fat	Cbs
Fire Roasted Tomato, 8 oz.	130	6	17
Four Cheese Broccoli, 8 oz.	260	20	12
New England Clam Chowder, 8 oz.	230	14	16
• Spinach & Lentil, 8 oz.	110	4	16
White Chicken Chili, 8 oz.	240	9	26
Square Bagels			
Asiago Parmesan, 5 oz.	360	5	68
Everything, 5 oz.	350	2	64
• Plain, 5 oz.	330	3	67
• Sesame, 5 oz.	370	4	70
Cheese			
• American Cheese, 2 oz.	160	14	0
• Asiago Cheese, Shredded, 1 oz.	50	4	0
Blue Cheese, 1 oz.	80	5	0
Cheddar Cheese, 1 oz.	160	12	0
Muenster Cheese, 2 oz.	120	9	0
Provolone Cheese, 1 oz.	100	8	0
Swiss Cheese, 1 oz.	100	8	0
Condiments			
Chipotle Sauce, 1 oz.	100	11	0
• Cranberry Horseradish Relish, 1 oz.	35	1	8
Cranberry Sauce, 3 oz.	110	0	27
Horseradish Mayo, 1 oz.	140	13	6
Hummus, 2 oz.	110	6	10
Jelly/Jam - Grape, 1 oz.	50	0	13
Jelly/Jam - Strawberry, 1 oz.	50	0	13
• Peanut Butter, 1 oz.	190	16	7
Pesto, 1 oz.	100	10	0
Sundried Tomato Mayo, 1 oz.	140	15	1
Sundried Tomato Spread, 1 oz.	79	6	5
Thai Peanut Sauce, 1 oz.	45	3	4
Egg Patties & Omelets			
• Egg White Patty, 2 oz.	30	0	1
• Spinach & Cheddar Omelet, 3 oz.	120	8	3
Whole Egg Patty, 2 oz.	90	6	2
Meat			
• Bacon, 1 oz.	70	6	1
Chicken Breast, 4 oz.	140	4	1
Ham, 4 oz.	100	2	5
Roast Beef, 4 oz.	110	5	2
Salmon, 2 oz.	80	3	0
Sausage, 2 oz.	220	20	1
Tarragon Chicken Salad, 5 oz.	460	37	19
• Tuna Salad, 5 oz.	520	46	2
Turkey, 4 oz.	100	1	3

BRUEGGER'S (cont.)

	Cal	Fat	Cbs
Nuts/Other			
• Almonds (Sliced)	25	3	1
Chow Mein Noodles	40	2	6
• Croutons, 1 oz.	70	3	8
Sesame Seeds	40	4	2
Vegetables & Fruit			
• Cranberries (Dried), 1 oz.	60	0	15
Cucumbers, 1 oz.	5	0	0
Green Peppers, 1 oz.	6	0	1
Jalapeños, 1 oz.	5	0	1
Lettuce	1	0	0
Mandarin Oranges, 1 oz.	20	0	5
Roasted Red Peppers, 2 oz.	15	0	3
Sprouts	1	0	0
• Tomatoes	0	0	2

BUCA DI BEPPO

	Cal	Fat	Cbs
Insalate (Small)			
• Mixed Green Salad	159	2	6
Mxd Grn Salad w/ Prosciutto & Gorgonzola	317	8	7
Caesar Salad	160	2	8
Chopped Antipasto Salad	341	9	8
Apple Gorgonzola Salad	451	10	25
• Lunch Soup & Caesar Salad	648	6	39
Lunch Soup & Mixed Green Salad	634	6	36
Zuppa Di Giorno, Bowl	378	5	26
Pizza (Small)			
• Margherita	250	3	34
Chicken Pesto	512	11	43
• Supremo Italiano	744	16	58
Four Cheese	448	10	36
Pepperoni	567	18	34
Veggie	613	9	64
Baked Pasta Specialties (Small)			
Cheese Manicotti	370	12	27
Chicken Cannelloni	367	11	15
• Baked Ravioli	323	7	36
Stuffed Shells	398	9	20
Lasagna	347	7	35
• Baked Rigatoni	518	7	59
Pasta (Small)			
Spaghetti Marinara	394	0	71
Spaghetti w/ Meatballs	398	2	63
Spaghetti w/ Meat sauce	916	11	100
Penne Basilica	669	16	59
Shrimp fra Diavolo	687	12	58

• MOST HEALTHY   • LEAST HEALTHY

BUCA DI BEPPO (cont.)

	Cal	Fat	Cbs
Linguini Frutti di Mare	827	3	73
• Raviolo al Pomodoro	318	7	3
Raviolo w/ Meat Sauce	349	8	36
Penne San Remo	655	12	67
Gnocchi al Telefono	392	6	58
Spicy Chicken Rigatoni	719	12	62
Penne Arrabbiata	640	14	60
Fettuccine Alfredo	839	28	83
Fettuccine Supremo	734	22	62
• Chicken Carbonara	1008	25	70

Entrées (Small)

	Cal	Fat	Cbs
Chicken Limone	408	16	7
Chicken Saltimbocca	450	17	10
Chicken Marsala	406	5	10
Prosciutto stuffed Chicken	439	5	14
Chicken Parmigiana	312	1	22
Eggplant Parmigiana	482	4	46
Veal Parmigiana	287	2	25
• Chianti Braised Short Ribs	566	22	5
Oven Roasted Salmon	436	7	11
Veal Saltimbocca	491	18	9
Chicken Cacciatore	512	3	13

Side Dishes (Small)

	Cal	Fat	Cbs
Garlic Mashed Potatoes	411	17	33
• Green Beans	91	1	9
Italian Broccoli Romano	92	1	6
Italian Sausage, 2 links	684	19	10
• Italian Sausage & Peppers	1918	26	133
Meatball, 1/2 lb.	818	17	49

Kids Menu

	Cal	Fat	Cbs
• Macaroni & Cheese	1058	24	132
Spaghetti & Meatball	463	9	83
Fettuccine Alfredo	593	19	62
• Cheese Pizza	253	1	49
Pepperoni Pizza	359	5	49

Beverages

	Cal	Fat	Cbs
Wild Raspberry Italian Soda, 11 oz.	180	0	46
Wild Raspberry Cream Soda, 11 oz.	473	18	51
Sassy Strawberry Italian Soda, 11 oz.	204	0	50
• Sassy Strawberry Cream Soda, 11 oz.	497	18	55
Purple Pear Italian Soda, 11 oz.	188	0	46
Purple Pear Cream Soda, 11 oz.	481	18	51
Wild Raspberry Lemonade, 11 oz.	40	0	63
Sassy Strawberry Lemonade, 11 oz.	258	0	66
Purple Pear Lemonade, 11 oz.	246	0	63
• Espresso, 5 oz.	1	0	0

● MOST HEALTHY   • LEAST HEALTHY

BUCA DI BEPPO (cont.)	Cal	Fat	Cbs
Latte, 5 oz.	144	10	11

BUCK'S PIZZA

	Cal	Fat	Cbs
14 Canadian Bacon Pizza, 1 sl.	313	9	47
• 14 Cheese Pizza, 1 sl.	296	8	47
14 Pepperoni Pizza, 1 sl.	361	14	47
• 14 Sausage Pizza, 1 sl.	362	14	47

BURGER KING

Beverage

	Cal	Fat	Cbs
Regular Cappuccino, 46 g	64	2	7

Breakfast

	Cal	Fat	Cbs
Bacon, Egg & Cheese Biscuit, 146 g	410	25	31
Cini-minis, 108 g	490	7	74
Croissan'wich Bacon, Egg & Chz 122 g	340	7	26
• Croissan'wich Egg & Cheese 115 g	300	7	26
Croissan'wich Ham, Egg & Chz, 149 g	350	7	27
Croissan'wich Sausage & Chz, 106 g	380	10	26
Double Croissan'wich Ham, Bacon, 206 g	420	11	28
• Double Croissan'wich Ssg, Bacon, 210 g	550	15	28
French Toast Sticks (3 piece), 65 g	310	11	50
Hash Browns, 140 g	420	6	40

Burger

	Cal	Fat	Cbs
Angus Burger, 239 g	555	28	44
Bacon Double Cheeseburger, 160 g	479	25	30
Cheeseburger, 123 g	320	13	31
Double Angus, 323 g	796	45	44
Double Cheeseburger, 173 g	465	23	32
Double WHOPPER®, 355 g	876	53	49
• Double WHOPPER® w/ Chz, 380 g	963	60	50
• Hamburger, 110 g	275	9	31
Smoked Bacon & Cheddar Angus, 270 g	679	37	45
Smkd Bcn & Chdr Double Angus, 354 g	920	54	45
WHOPPER JR.®, 148 g	343	16	31
WHOPPER JR.® with Cheese, 161 g	388	20	31
WHOPPER®, 274 g	634	35	48
WHOPPER® with Cheese, 299 g	721	42	49
XL Bacon Double Cheeseburger, 302 g	928	55	46

Desserts

	Cal	Fat	Cbs
• BK Fusions® Strawberry Chzcake, 170 g	345	12	55
• Regular BK® Shake (Chocolate), 401 g	467	11	79
Regular BK® Shake (Strawberry), 401 g	452	11	76
Regular BK® Shake (Vanilla), 401 g	421	12	65

Kids

	Cal	Fat	Cbs
BK® Angus Mini Burgers, 97 g	272	11	30
• BK® Angus Mini Burgers w/ Chz, 110 g	321	15	30

• MOST HEALTHY   • LEAST HEALTHY

▶ BURGER KING (cont.)

	Cal	Fat	Cbs
• BK® Fresh Apple Fries (UK only), 60 g	28	0	7
BK® Veggie Bean Burger - Kids, 116 g	278	7	49
Char Grilled Chicken Mini Burger, 109 g	214	3	30
Char-Grilled Chicken Fillet Strips x3, 75 g	95	2	0
Chicken Bites x7, 56 g	158	7	14
KIDS Cheeseburger, 113 g	317	13	31
KIDS Hamburger, 100 g	272	9	31

Salad

	Cal	Fat	Cbs
Flame-Grilled Chicken Salad, 240 g	128	3	6
Garden Salad, 165 g	33	1	6

Sauces

	Cal	Fat	Cbs
Sweet Chilli Sauce Dip Pot, 40 g	96	0	24

Sides (Regular)

	Cal	Fat	Cbs
Fries, 111 g	300	15	43
Onion Rings, 126 g	462	24	54

Veggie, Fish, Chicken

	Cal	Fat	Cbs
BK® Veggie Bean Burger, 280 g	590	20	85
• Chicken Bites x14, 112 g	317	15	28
• Chicken Royale with Cheese, 263 g	698	39	55
Chicken Royale, 210 g	606	32	53
Ocean Catch, 188 g	495	27	43
Piri Piri Chicken Sandwich, 196 g	336	6	42
Sweet Chilli Chicken Royale, 210 g	542	23	58

▶ BURGERVILLE, USA

Beverages

	Cal	Fat	Cbs
• Hot Chocolate - Regular, 12 fl.oz.	230	8	38
Odwalla® Lemonade, Regular, 16 fl.oz.	170	0	43
• Odwalla® Orange, 10 fl.oz.	138	0	31

Breakfast

	Cal	Fat	Cbs
American cheese 2 slices, 25 g	90	7	0
Bacon 2 slices, 11 g	60	5	1
Bagel w/Egg and bacon, 156 g	400	15	47
Bagel w/Egg and ham, 202 g	400	12	48
Bagel w/Egg and sausage, 202 g	570	32	47
Breakfast Platter Egg only, 278 g	550	33	49
Breakfast Platter/Bacon, 241 g	540	34	49
Breakfast Platter/Ham, 335 g	600	35	51
• Breakfast Platter/Sausage, 335 g	770	55	49
Egg, one, fried, 55 g	110	10	1
English Muffin w/Egg and sausage, 183 g	530	42	27
English Muffin w/Egg and bacon, 133 g	330	23	27
English Muffin w/Egg and ham, 183 g	350	22	28
Hash Browns (2), 102 g	230	14	24
Plain Bagel, 90 g	230	1	46
Plain English Muffin, toasted, 66 g	140	6	26

● MOST HEALTHY • LEAST HEALTHY

BURGERVILLE, USA (cont.)

	Cal	Fat	Cbs
Sausage patty, 2 oz., 57 g	227	22	0
Scrambled eggs, 2 eggs, 108 g	200	17	2
• Sliced Canadian-style Bacon, 2 oz., 57 g	53	2	1
Tillamook Cheese 1 slice, 28 g	110	9	0
Condiments/Dressings			
Burgerville Spread Cup	300	32	4
Cream Cheese	100	10	1
• Garlic Aioli Dip	330	36	0
Green Garden Sweet & Sour Sauce	90	4	12
• Litehouse Fat Free Raspberry Vinaigrette	60	0	14
Cones			
Vanilla Ice cream cone, 118 g	250	11	32
Vanilla YoCream cone, 147 g	190	0	39
Entrees			
Burgerville Classic Hamburger, 224 g	530	30	42
w/out mayo, 196 g	430	19	41
Cheeseburger, 130 g	380	20	30
Chicken Strips-5 piece, 142 g	040	17	27
Colossal Cheeseburger, 236 g	540	30	43
Crispy Chicken Sandwich, 223 g	460	19	54
Deluxe Crispy Chicken Sandwich, 257 g	600	30	54
Double Beef Cheeseburger, 151 g	450	27	30
Halibut Fillet Sandwich, 192 g	490	27	43
w/out tartar sauce, 163 g	350	13	42
Halibut Fish piece, 133 g	310	16	25
Hamburger, 110 g	320	17	30
Low Fat Grilled Chicken Sandwich, 223 g	330	5	45
Nine Grain Turkey Club Sandwich, 229 g	610	37	37
w/out mayo, 201 g	410	15	37
• w/out mayo cheese, 173 g	300	7	37
Parmesan Sole Fillet Sandwich, 175 g	440	26	38
w/out tartar sauce, 146 g	310	12	37
Parmesan Sole Fish 3 pieces, 136 g	330	18	24
• Pepper Bacon Cheeseburger, 259 g	680	43	39
w/out mayo, 245 g	580	32	39
Seasoned Turkey Burger, 266 g	520	22	47
w/out mayo, 252 g	420	11	47
Spicy Anasazi Bean Burger, 274 g	680	34	72
w/out mayo, 245 g	500	14	70
w/out mayo & cheese, 224 g	420	8	70
The Oregon Harvest Burger, 252 g	550	19	85
w/out mayo, 238 g	450	8	85
Tillamook Cheeseburger, 252 g	640	39	42
w/out mayo, 238 g	540	28	42
Individual Menu Ingredients			
5 inch bun, 74 g	200	4	36

BURGERVILLE, USA (cont.)

	Cal	Fat	Cbs
9 Grain Bun, 86 g	180	2	35
American cheese (1 slice), 13 g	45	4	0
Anasazi bean patty, 95 g	200	4	39
Blue Cheese, 28 g	113	9	0
Breads, Plain Bagel, 90 g	230	1	46
BV Spread, 14 g	71	8	1
• Chicken Strips 5 pieces, 140 g	340	17	27
Chipotle Mayo, 28 g	182	20	2
Crispy Chicken patty, 84 g	185	9	13
Croutons, 7 g	35	2	4
Fried Bacon (2 piece), 13 g	65	5	0
Grilled Chicken breast, 84 g	100	3	0
Halibut 1 piece, 44 g	108	5	8
Halibut fillet for sandwich, 88 g	210	11	17
Hamburger Small patty-cooked, 36 g	103	7	0
Hazelnuts, 28 g	183	18	5
• Kosher Dill Chips (3), 9 g	0	0	0
Lettuce (1 piece), 24 g	2	0	0
Meat, Eggs and NutsEgg, one, fried, 55 g	110	10	1
Onion, chopped (1 Tbsp), 10 g	4	0	1
OregonHarvest patty, 95 g	223	5	44
Plain English Muffin, toasted, 66 g	140	6	26
Sausage patty, 2 oz., 57 g	227	22	0
Sides, Hash Brown 1 triangle, 57 g	115	7	12
Sliced Canadian Ham, 56 g	53	2	1
Smoked Salmon, 56 g	117	2	2
Sole 1 piece, 45 g	110	6	8
Sole Fillet for sandwich, 72 g	180	9	13
Tartar Sauce, 28 g	132	14	1
Tillamook cheese (1 slice), 28 g	110	9	0
Tillamook Pepper Jack chz (1 slice), 21 g	80	6	0
Tillamook Shredded, 28 g	110	9	0
Tillamook Swiss cheese (1 slice), 28 g	110	8	1
Tomatoes (2 slices), 40 g	6	0	1
Turkey Breast, 56 g	81	3	0
Turkey Burger -cooked, 101 g	195	8	5
Vegetables Tomatoes (1 piece), 20 g	4	0	1
Whole Wheat Hot Dog Bun, 50 g	120	2	22
Kids Meals			
• Apple Slices, 60 g	35	0	9
• Cheeseburger, 130 g	380	20	30
Hamburger, 110 g	320	17	30
Kid's French Fries 2 -3/4 oz., 78 g	200	8	28
Kid's Hot Dog, 114 g	290	16	26
Parmesan Fish 2 pieces, 91 g	220	12	16

▍ BURGERVILLE, USA (cont.)

	Cal	Fat	Cbs
Milkshakes			
Chocolate Monkey - Regular, 16 g	870	33	133
Chocolate-Regular, 16 g	790	36	105
• Mocha Perk - Regular, 16 g	780	37	100
• NW Cherry Chocolate - Regular, 16 g	1030	47	138
Strawberry Splash - Regular, 16 g	840	35	124
Strawberry-Regular, 16 g	810	33	115
Triple Berry Blast - Regular, 16 g	880	36	126
Vanilla-Regular, 16 g	810	33	117
Salads/no dressing			
• Grilled Chicken Salad, 366 g	420	27	15
w/out hazelnuts, 344 g	280	14	11
Rogue River Smokey Blue Salad, 214 g	290	11	38
• Side Salad, 119 g	50	3	4
Wild Smkd Salmon & Hazelnut Salad, 326 g	370	26	15
w/out hazelnuts, 322 g	240	13	12
Sides (Regular)			
Apple Slices, 60 g	35	0	9
French Fries/No Added Salt, 142 g	360	15	52
Smoothies (Regular)			
Chocolate, 16 g	450	0	93
Chocolate Monkey, 16 g	460	0	100
Mocha Perk, 16 g	460	0	95
• NW Cherry Chocolate, 16 g	550	0	118
Strawberry, 16 g	440	0	92
• Strawberry Splash, 16 g	380	1	83
Triple Berry Blast, 16 g	430	0	91
Vanilla, 16 g	440	0	92
Sundaes/Ice Cream			
Caramel, 170 g	380	15	56
• Hot Fudge, 170 g	380	18	51
• Triple Berry, 182 g	340	14	46
Yocream Sundaes			
Caramel, 170 g	260	1	56
• Hot Fudge, 170 g	260	4	51
• Triple Berry, 170 g	200	1	43

▶ CAPTAIN D'S SEAFOOD

	Cal	Fat	Cbs
Add-a-Piece			
• Batter Dipped Fish Filet (1), 65 g	182	12	8
Breaded Chicken Tender (1), 58 g	170	10	11
Premium Shrimp (3), 57 g	154	6	0
• Stuffed Crab Shell, 57 g	100	5	9
D's Classics			
Bite Size Shrimp Dinner, 428 g	1140	61	120
Catfish Feast, 400 g	995	57	88

• MOST HEALTHY   • LEAST HEALTHY

CAPTAIN D'S SEAFOOD (cont.)	Cal	Fat	Cbs
Chicken Dinner 3 Pc, 432 g	1190	70	102
Country Style Fish Dinner, 435 g	1069	59	97
Fish & Fries, 307 g	1034	64	83
Fish Dinner 2 Pc, 416 g	1204	76	96
• Fried Flounder Dinner, 580 g	1530	93	115
LB Clam Platter 1/2, 486 g	1450	87	133
Oyster Dinner, 413 g	1000	58	100
• Seasoned Tilapia Dinner, 457 g	540	10	76
Shrimp Lover's Trio, 684 g	863	25	80
Shrimp Skewers Dinner, 583 g	610	7	75
Ultimate Premium Shrimp Platter, 485 g	1290	65	69
Wild Alaskan Salmon Dinner, 628 g	550	8	76
Dressings & Sauces			
• Ginger Teriyaki Sauce, 68 g	60	0	13
• Scampi Butter Sauce (2 oz.), 57 g	120	10	5
Sweet Chili Sauce, 68 g	100	0	25
Family & Kids Meals			
Family Value Pack 10 Pc, 539 g	590	54	72
Fish & Chicken Family Pack, 482 g	600	32	53
Fish & Shrimp Family Pack, 500 g	635	30	42
• Fish or Chicken Only 10 Pc, 213 g	400	47	45
Kids Chicken, 567 g	684	31	86
Kids Fish, 574 g	696	33	83
Kid's Mac & Cheese, 516 g	414	12	66
Kids Shrimp, 594 g	744	31	101
• Seafood Feast, 625 g	1147	65	289
Salads			
• Bite Size Shrimp Salad, 317 g	267	10	33
Fried Chicken Salad, 290 g	207	10	18
• Side Salad, 232 g	19	0	3
Wild Alaskan Salmon Salad, 403 g	177	1	8
Sandwiches			
Chicken Ranch Sandwich, 234 g	710	36	69
• Classic Fish Sandwich, 253 g	744	41	63
Great Little Fish Sandwich, 136 g	672	41	56
• Wild Alaskan Salmon Sandwich, 294 g	520	18	48
Seafood Selections			
Classic Fish & Chicken Dinner, 474 g	1374	86	107
Classic Fish & Shrimp Dinner, 492 g	1409	84	96
• Deluxe Seafood Platter, 606 g	1609	94	114
Fish & Blue Bay Crab Cake Dinner 2 Pc, 459 g	1218	75	97
Fish & Coconut Shrimp 2 Pc, 528 g	1525	95	123
• Seafood Scampi Platter, 519 g	600	10	76
Side Choices			
Baked Potato, 255 g	240	0	54
Breadsticks, 85 g	300	11	42

● MOST HEALTHY • LEAST HEALTHY

CAPTAIN D'S SEAFOOD (cont.)

	Cal	Fat	Cbs
• Broccoli, 100 g	40	1	5
Corn on the Cob, 163 g	190	2	37
French Fries, 99 g	310	15	38
Fried Okra, 113 g	230	14	23
Green Beans, 113 g	60	2	10
Home-style Cole Slaw, 109 g	170	12	13
• Hush Puppies, 99 g	400	26	36
Macaroni & Cheese, 113 g	160	7	17
Roasted Red Potatoes, 124 g	170	7	25
Seasoned Rice, 113 g	160	1	35
Side Salad, 201 g	60	0	14
Starters & Desserts			
Cheesecake with Strawberries, 142 g	430	26	45
Cheesesticks (4 pc), 66 g	220	12	16
Chocolate Cake, 85 g	300	11	49
Jalapeño Poppers (5 pc), 76 g	155	7	20
Pecan Pie, 113 g	470	26	56
Pineapple Cream Cheese Pie, 106 g	720	14	43

CARIBOU COFFEE

	Cal	Fat	Cbs
Amy's Blend Pink Ribbon Bagel, 113 g	310	4	61
Blackberry & White Choco Scone, 128 g	490	22	70
Blueberry Muffin, 135 g	410	18	55
Caprese Salad, 287 g	378	32	8
Caribou Coffee Snack Bars, 35 g	140	4	26
Cheddar Cheese Bagel, 113 g	290	4	53
Chocolate Chocolate Chip Muffin, 135 g	480	24	62
Chocolate Chunk Cookie, 94 g	441	22	58
Cinnamon Chip Scone, 120 g	500	22	68
• Cinnamon Hoof Mints, 1 g	0	0	1
Cinnamon Raisin Bagel, 113 g	300	2	63
Cinnamon Roll Popover, 159 g	580	30	70
Cinn. Streusel Muff w/Wh Choco Chp, 135 g	530	25	71
Dark Chocolate Graham, 28 g	140	8	18
Double Chocolate Biscotti, 57 g	250	10	36
Fruit Salad, 250 g	105	0	27
Italian Beef Sandwich, 272 g	626	30	56
Lemon Poppy Seed Loaf Cake, 128 g	470	26	56
Milk Chocolate Graham, 28 g	140	8	18
Multi Grain Bagel, 113 g	360	7	63
Orange Walnut Wht Choco Biscotti, 57 g	250	11	34
Original Almond Biscotti, 57 g	230	8	34
Peanut Butter Cookie, 94 g	450	23	55
Peppermint Hoof Mints, 1 g	0	0	1
Pumpkin Bread, 124 g	430	22	54
Reduced Fat Banana Bread, 129 g	380	11	72

• MOST HEALTHY　• LEAST HEALTHY

CARIBOU COFFEE (cont.)

	Cal	Fat	Cbs
RedFat Cranberry Orange Scone, 128 g	450	14	78
Reduced Fat Mountain Brry Muffin, 135 g	300	6	54
Roasted Chicken Sandwich, 238 g	540	19	53
Roasted Vegetable Sandwich, 296 g	622	36	61
Rosemary Romano Chkn Salad Snd, 258 g	637	65	49
Smoked Turkey Sandwich, 245 g	590	29	53
Tomato Gorgonzola Pasta Salad, 258 g	397	19	45
• Tortellini Salad, 278 g	820	48	72
Turkey and Pesto Sandwich, 239 g	431	16	42
Turkey Cherry Pasta Salad, 247 g	571	33	44
Wht Choco Macadamia Nut Cookie, 94 g	420	20	55
White Chocolate Pretzel, 24 g	110	5	17
Wintergreen Hoof Mints, 1 g	0	0	1
Beverages (Small)			
Açaí Smoothie, 16 fl.oz.	290	3	65
• Americano, 12 fl.oz.	5	0	1
Blended Chai w/ 2% Milk, 16 fl.oz.	180	4	31
Blended Chai w/ Skim Milk, 16 fl.oz.	150	0	31
Breve, 12 fl.oz.	310	26	11
• Campfire Mocha, 12 fl.oz.	460	16	71
Cappuccino, 12 fl.oz.	140	5	14
Caramel Cooler, 16 fl.oz.	340	12	56

CARL'S JR.

Breakfast	Cal	Fat	Cbs
Bacon & Egg Burrito, 208 g	550	32	37
Breakfast Burger™, 295 g	780	41	64
French Toast Dips® - No Syrup, 130 g	460	21	60
• Hash Brown Nuggets, 108 g	350	23	32
• Loaded Breakfast Burrito, 312 g	780	49	51
Sourdough Breakfast Snd, 174 g	470	25	37
Steak & Egg Burrito, 311 g	650	36	43
Sunrise Croissant®, 175 g	590	44	27
Charbroiled Burgers			
Big Hamburger, 209 g	460	17	54
Double Wstrn Bacon Chzburger™, 319 g	960	52	70
Famous Star™ with Cheese, 278 g	660	39	53
Jalapeño Burger™, 287 g	720	46	50
Kid's Cheeseburger, 118 g	290	15	24
• Kid's Hamburger, 102 g	230	10	24
Super Star® with Cheese, 383 g	920	58	54
Teriyaki Burger™, 309 g	610	29	60
The Big Carl™, 315 g	920	59	51
• The Guac. Bacon 6 Dollar Burger®, 411 g	1040	70	53
The Jalapeño Six Dollar Burger™, 384 g	930	61	52
The Low Carb Six Dollar Burger®, 300 g	570	43	7

• MOST HEALTHY   • LEAST HEALTHY

CARL'S JR. (cont.)

	Cal	Fat	Cbs
The Original Six Dollar Burger®, 384 g	890	54	58
The Portobello Mshr $6 Burger™, 393 g	870	53	52
The Six Dollar Cheeseburger™, 311 g	790	43	53
The Wstrn Bacon $6 Burger®, 340 g	1020	53	81
Western Bacon Cheeseburger®, 236 g	710	33	69

Chicken & Other Choices

	Cal	Fat	Cbs
• Bacon Swiss Crispy Chkn® Snd, 310 g	750	40	62
Carl's Catch Fish Sandwich®, 291 g	710	37	74
Charbroiled BBQ Chkn™ Snd, 239 g	380	7	49
Charbroiled Chkn Club™ Snd, 262 g	560	27	44
Charbroiled Santa Fe Chkn™ Snd, 266 g	630	35	44
• Chicken Strips (3 pieces), 108 g	370	26	19
Spicy Chicken Sandwich, 156 g	420	27	33

Desserts

	Cal	Fat	Cbs
Chocolate Cake, 85 g	300	12	48
• Chocolate Chip Cookie, 71 g	370	19	48
Strawberry Swirl Cheesecake, 99 g	290	16	32

Hand-Scooped Ice Cream Shakes & Malts™

	Cal	Fat	Cbs
Chocolate Malt, 414 n	780	34	100
Chocolate Shake, 397 g	710	33	86
• OREO® Cookie Malt, 414 g	790	38	95
OREO® Cookie Shake, 397 g	730	38	81
Strawberry Malt, 414 g	770	34	99
• Strawberry Shake, 397 g	700	33	85
Vanilla Malt, 414 g	780	34	101
Vanilla Shake, 397 g	710	33	86

Salad Dressings

	Cal	Fat	Cbs
• Chipotle Caesar Dressing, 57 g	270	27	5
House Dressing, 57 g	220	22	3
• Raspberry Vinaigrette, 43 g	160	12	12

Salads - Without Dressings

	Cal	Fat	Cbs
Cran Apple Walnut Grilled Chkn Salad, 300 g	300	11	25
Original Grilled Chicken Salad, 354 g	200	6	13
• Side Salad, 121 g	50	3	5
• Southwest Grilled Chkn Salad, 322 g	440	23	24

Sides

	Cal	Fat	Cbs
• Chicken Stars™ (4 pieces), 56 g	210	16	10
• Chili Cheese Fries, 344 g	980	56	88
CrissCut® Fries, 139 g	450	29	42
Fish & Chips, 284 g	730	39	72
Fried Zucchini, 139 g	330	18	36
Natural-Cut Fries, 169 g	460	22	60
Onion Rings, 128 g	530	28	61

CARVEL ICE CREAM

	Cal	Fat	Cbs
Blended Drinks			
Arctic Blender® - Cookie Dough, 16 oz.	920	40	126
Arctic Blender® - Fried Ice Cream, 16 oz.	670	31	85
Arctic Blender® - Peanut Butter, 16 oz.	870	33	88
• Banana Barge®, 16 oz.	970	46	128
Carvelanche® - Butterfinger®, 16 oz.	730	38	92
Carvelanche® - Cake Mix, 16 oz.	770	31	110
Carvelanche® - Cookies & Cream, 16 oz.	610	33	70
Carvelanche® - M&M'S®, 16 oz.	760	39	88
Carvelanche® - Reese's®, 16 oz.	750	39	85
Carvelatte® - Caramel Macchiato, 16 oz.	680	27	97
Carvelatte® - Mocha, 16 oz.	610	25	88
• Float Choco Ice Cream & Coke®, 16 oz.	360	14	54
Float Choco Ice Crm & Soda Water, 16 oz.	420	15	69
Float Vanilla Ice Cream &Coke®, 16 oz.	380	17	53
Float Vanilla Ice Crm & Soda Water, 16 oz.	440	18	68
Thick Chocolate Shake, 16 oz.	650	27	93
Thick Shake Float - Chocolate, 16 oz.	790	34	109
Thick Shake Float - Strawberry, 16 oz.	750	39	85
Thick Shake Float - Vanilla, 16 oz.	810	39	102
Thick Strawberry Shake, 16 oz.	600	31	70
Thick Vanilla Shake, 16 oz.	660	31	86
Classic Sundaes (small)			
• Caramel	700	36	84
• Hot Fudge	540	30	60
Strawberry	610	34	67
Cones - Small			
Cake Cone with Chocolate	440	21	51
Cake Cone with Vanilla	470	26	50
• Slice of Carvel Ice Cream Cake	250	13	29
Sugar Cone with Chocolate	460	21	59
Sugar Cone with Vanilla	490	26	57
Waffle Cone with Chocolate	490	23	63
• Waffle Cone with Vanilla	510	24	61
Dashers®			
Banana's Foster, 12 oz.	660	23	105
Fudge Brownie, 12 oz.	850	45	102
Mint Chocolate Chip, 12 oz.	770	42	95
• Peanut Butter Cup, 12 oz.	1060	60	95
• Strawberry Shortcake, 12 oz.	580	29	74
Ice Cream (Small Cup)			
Chocolate, 8 oz.	410	21	48
• No Sugar Added Vanilla, 8 oz.	260	7	51
Sherbet, 8 oz.	290	3	67
• Vanilla, 8 oz.	450	26	47

• MOST HEALTHY   • LEAST HEALTHY

CARVEL ICE CREAM (cont.)

	Cal	Fat	Cbs
Low Fat			
• Arctic Blender® - Cookie Dough	720	18	129
Arctic Blender® - Fried Ice Cream	500	10	95
Arctic Blender® - Peanut Butter	710	14	93
Cake Cone with Low Fat Chocolate	300	6	53
Cake Cone with Low Fat Vanilla	320	6	57
Carvelatte® - Caramel Macchiato	500	7	100
Carvelatte® - Mocha	440	6	91
Flying Saucer® (Low Fat Chocolate)	190	5	34
• Flying Saucer® (Low Fat Vanilla)	190	5	35
Small Cup (8 wt oz) Low Fat Choco	280	6	49
Small Cup (8 wt oz) Low Fat Vanilla	290	6	54
Sugar Cone with Low Fat Chocolate	320	6	59
Sugar Cone with Low Fat Vanilla	340	6	64
Waffle Cone with Low Fat Chocolate	360	8	64
Waffle Cone with Low Fat Vanilla	370	8	68
Smoothies			
• Raspberry - Strawberry, 16 oz.	300	0	75
• Strawberry, 16 oz.	330	0	80
Strawberry - Banana, 16 oz.	320	0	78
Take Home Treats			
Brown Bonnet®	390	23	43
• Carvel Sinful Love Bar®	470	30	48
Chipster®	350	17	45
Cupcake	270	12	36
Deluxe Flying Saucer® - Sprinkles	350	16	49
Flying Saucer® - Chocolate	230	10	33
Flying Saucer® - Vanilla	250	11	33
Lil' Rounder® - Chocolate Chip	180	9	23
Lil' Rounder® - Double Chocolate Chip	180	9	23
• Lil' Rounder® - Oreo®	160	7	25
Lil' Rounder® - Sugar Cookie	190	9	22
Mini Sundae (Chocolate Syrup)	220	10	29
Olde Fashion Sundae	340	15	47
Sprinkle Cup	260	14	31

CHARLEY'S GRILLED SUBS

	Cal	Fat	Cbs
Breakfast			
• 2 pieces of Toast	160	4	30
Bacon Omelet	410	32	8
Bacon, Egg & Cheese Sandwich	540	26	54
Egg & Cheese Sandwich	310	5	54
Ham Omelet	410	26	10
Ham, Egg & Cheese Sandwich	540	20	55
Hash Browns, 4 oz.	200	9	27
Sausage Omelet	474	35	8

• MOST HEALTHY   • LEAST HEALTHY

CHARLEY'S GRILLED SUBS (cont.)	Cal	Fat	Cbs
Sausage, Egg & Cheese Sandwich	604	29	54
• Steak, Egg & Cheese Sandwich	620	25	55
Two Eggs Scrambled	160	12	2
Veggie Omelet	359	24	13
Western Omelet	521	25	13
Fresh Grilled Subs			
Bacon 3 Cheese	635	32	54
Chicken Bacon Club	570	25	53
Chicken Buffalo	531	16	60
Chicken Caledonia	500	16	52
Chicken Cordon Blue	570	18	54
Chicken Teriyaki	522	16	58
Italian Deli	585	25	53
Mushroom Swiss Steak	519	19	57
Philly Cheesesteak	521	19	55
Philly Chicken	517	16	57
Philly Ham & Swiss	517	16	59
Philly Steak and Bleu	521	19	55
Philly Steak Deluxe	527	19	58
• Philly Veggie	449	15	62
• Sicilian Steak	640	31	53
Turkey Cheddar Melt	470	12	53
Ultimate Club	560	23	54
Fries & Kid's Meal			
5 Chicken Fingers	334	20	17
• Cheddar Bacon Fries	553	30	47
Cheddar Fries	523	30	47
• Kid's (3 Chicken Fingers)	200	12	10
Ranch Bacon Fries	530	25	51
Reg.Fries	453	25	41
Salads (Cheese & Dressing Not Included)			
Buffalo Chicken Salad	208	8	14
• Chicken Teriyaki Salad	213	7	12
• Fresh Garden	58	2	9
Grilled Chicken Salad	198	7	10
Grilled Steak Salad	208	10	10
Toppings			
12 Rings Banana Peppers	5	0	0
• Black Olives, 1 oz.	36	3	2
• Lettuce, 1 oz.	4	0	1
Tomatoes, 1 oz.	7	0	2

CHEVY'S FRESH MEX			
A La Carte			
Beans a la Charra Setup	210	4	32
Black Bean Setup	190	2	32

• MOST HEALTHY • LEAST HEALTHY

CHEVY'S FRESH MEX (cont.)

	Cal	Fat	Cbs
Carnitas Crispy Taco	270	12	27
Carnitas Enchilada	300	21	15
Carnitas Soft Taco	360	23	27
Cheddar Cheese Enchilada	390	27	17
Chile Relleno	260	30	7
Crispy Chicken Flautas	430	23	36
Crispy Picadillo Beef Taco	240	15	18
Crispy Salsa Chicken Taco	230	13	17
El Machino® Tortilla	140	4	22
Fresh Mex® Rice Setup	180	5	29
• Guacamole	130	12	7
Homemade Black Beans	190	2	32
• Mini Chimichanga*	600	35	47
Picadillo Beef Enchilada	260	14	18
Refried Beans	280	14	28
Salsa Chicken Enchilada	240	12	19
Salsa Chicken Tamale	330	10	49
Slow-Roasted Pork Tamale	370	10	54
Soft Picadillo Beef Taco	290	15	27
Soft Salsa Chicken Taco	280	14	26
Sour Cream	180	18	4
Sweet Corn Tamalito	190	7	29
Appetizers & Quesadillas			
Carnitas Quesadilla	1650	107	112
Chile Con Queso	1510	85	131
Crab & Shrimp Quesadilla	1790	126	86
Crispy Chicken Flautas	970	56	82
Dilla Duo Dinner	865	47	65
Farmers' Market Quesadilla	1590	104	105
• Fresh Mex® Sampler	2560	139	179
Grilled Steak Quesadilla	1380	88	78
Guac-My-Way	730	53	62
Nachos Grande	1890	105	163
Original Chicken Quesadilla	1260	80	77
Original Fajita Nachos	1595	97	83
• Red Chile Pork Taquitos	610	37	44
San Antonio Chicken Quesadilla	1170	65	72
Shrimp & Sweet Corn Cake Tamalito	690	42	55
Spicy Wings	1520	99	37
Dessert			
Chevys Flan	740	23	116
Chiquita Sundae	575	30	70
• Deep Fried Ice Cream	1100	60	131
Ooey Gooey Chewy Sundae	1020	48	145
• Sopapillas	550	24	78

• MOST HEALTHY   • LEAST HEALTHY

CHEVY'S FRESH MEX (cont.)	Cal	Fat	Cbs
Fajitas			
Mix & Match: Chicken & Shrimp	410	17	18
• Mix & Match: Chicken & Steak	410	18	13
Original Chicken	360	11	14
Fresh Mex® Burritos			
Cheeseburger*	1550	79	139
Fajita Burrito Steak	1370	59	152
• Grande Chimi Beef	1725	89	152
Smothered Burrito	1515	71	158
• Smothered Chile Verde Burrito	1360	71	134
Veggie Burrito	1440	62	177
Fresh Mex® Specialties			
• Chile Verde	1030	44	113
• Crispy Chicken Flautas	1510	76	156
Red Chile Pork Taquitos	1350	69	136
Grande Salads & Soup			
Grilled Fajita Salad	1515	119	67
BBQ Chicken Salad	1140	69	72
Bowl of Homemade Tortilla Soup	390	17	35
Grilled Chicken Caesar	860	69	32
• Kickin' Chicken Corn Chowder	280	16	28
Santa Fe Chopped	670	39	30
• Tostada Salad	1615	105	103
Kids Menu			
Bean & Cheese Burrito	1020	45	131
Cheese Quesadilla	1020	47	125
• Flour Flautas	1175	65	123
Fresh Mex® Chicken Bites	810	36	97
Kiddie Cheeseburger	1060	50	112
• Taco	795	34	102
Lunch Bowls			
Chicken Mole Enchilada Bowl	860	47	70
• Chile Verde Bowl	510	25	39
Grilled Fresh Salmon Bowl	540	26	45
Red Chile Pork Taquitos	770	48	55
• Smothered Chile Verde Burrito	1130	57	109
Lunch Duos			
• Baby Greens (side)	80	3	13
Caesar Salad (side)	360	32	16
Chicken Quesadilla	490	27	35
• Grilled Steak Quesadilla	550	31	35
Santa Fe Chopped Salad	370	23	15
Mesquite Grilled Tacos			
• 2 Grilled Chicken Tacos Plates	590	24	50
Grilled Chicken Tacos	1050	35	125
Grilled Fresh Fish Tacos	1060	39	125

● MOST HEALTHY   • LEAST HEALTHY

CHEVY'S FRESH MEX (cont.)

	Cal	Fat	Cbs
• Grilled Steak Tacos	1110	44	124
Grilled Tacos Combo	1080	40	125
Misc			
Guacamole, 1 Tbs.	20	2	1
• Pico de Gallo, 1 Tbs.	5	0	1
• Sweet Corn Tamalito, 1 Tbs.	30	1	5
Salads And Soup			
Cilantro Lime Chicken Salad	510	24	38
Mixed Baby Green Salad - w/o dressing	130	4	22
Signature Enchiladas			
• Chicken Mole Enchiladas	950	51	84
Chipotle Chicken Enchiladas	1070	64	87
Fresh Mex® Artichoke/Mushroom	1120	75	94
• Shrimp & Crab Enchiladas	1360	97	87
Sizzling Fajitas			
Carnitas	1291	77	103
Fresh Salmon	1127	51	96
Juicy Achiote Shrimp	1200	64	102
Mix & Match	1346	71	117
• Mixed Grill	1533	87	103
• Original Famous Chicken	932	32	95
Sizzling Steak	1030	46	94
Veggie Fajitas & Chile Relleno	1080	53	119

CHICK-FIL-A

Breakfast	Cal	Fat	Cbs
Bacon, Egg & Cheese Biscuit, 172 g	520	29	44
Biscuit, 86 g	310	13	41
Biscuit & Gravy, 199 g	420	20	51
Chicken Biscuit, 150 g	450	20	48
Chicken Breakfast Burrito, 199 g	450	20	43
Chicken, Egg & Cheese Bagel, 213 g	530	23	50
Chick-n-Minis: 3-count, 94 g	260	10	30
Cinnamon Cluster, 105 g	400	15	61
Hash Browns, 77 g	280	19	25
• Sausage Biscuit, 149 g	590	41	42
Sausage Breakfast Burrito, 199 g	510	29	40
• Yogurt Parfait, 184 g	180	3	37
Yogurt Parfait with Granola, 198 g	240	5	47
Yogurt Parfait with Oreo, 193 g	200	5	40
Classics			
Chargrilled Chicken Club Snd, 258 g	410	12	39
• Chargrilled Chicken Sandwich, 228 g	300	4	38
Chicken Salad Sandwich, 233 g	500	20	52
Chicken Sandwich, 179 g	430	17	39
• Chick-n-Strips: 4-count, 218 g	500	24	24

• MOST HEALTHY   • LEAST HEALTHY

CHICK-FIL-A (cont.)

	Cal	Fat	Cbs
Nuggets: 12-count, 170 g	400	17	18
Desserts			
Cheesecake, 91 g	310	23	22
Chocolate Milkshake, 515 g	750	28	113
Cookies & Cream Milkshake, 508 g	700	33	100
Fudge Nut Brownie, 79 g	370	19	45
• Icedream: cone, 135 g	170	4	31
Lemon Pie, 120 g	360	13	58
• Peach Milkshake, 595 g	850	21	153
Strawberry Milkshake, 565 g	770	28	118
Vanilla Milkshake, 480 g	660	27	91
Dressings & Sauces			
• Buffalo Sauce, 21 g	10	0	1
Chick-fil-A Sauce, 28 g	140	13	6
Polynesian Sauce, 28 g	110	6	14
RedFat Berry Balsamic Vinaigrette, 37 g	70	2	12
• Spicy Dressing, 29 g	140	14	2
Salads			
Chargrilled & Fruit Salad, 347 g	230	6	23
Chargrilled Chicken Garden Salad, 298 g	180	6	11
• Chick-n-Strips Salad, 390 g	470	23	27
• Garlic and Butter Croutons, 14 g	60	2	9
Harvest Nut Granola, 14 g	60	2	10
Honey Roasted Sunflower Kernels, 14 g	90	7	4
Southwest Chargrilled Salad, 326 g	240	9	18
Tortilla Strips, 14 g	80	4	8
Side Items			
Carrot & Raisin Salad: large, 255 g	390	18	59
Chicken Salad Cup, 170 g	350	24	6
• Cole Slaw: large, 298 g	580	50	31
Fruit Cup: large, 194 g	100	0	27
Hearty Breast of Chkn Soup: large, 439 g	220	6	30
• Side Salad, 113 g	70	5	5
Waffle Potato Fries: large, 128 g	430	23	50
Wraps			
Chargrilled Chicken Cool Wrap, 291 g	410	12	50
• Chicken Caesar Cool Wrap, 232 g	460	15	47
• Spicy Chicken Cool Wrap, 277 g	410	12	48

CHILI'S RESTAURANT

	Cal	Fat	Cbs
Appetizers			
Baby Back Rib Snackers	570	31	50
Boneless Buffalo Wings w/ Bleu Chz	1200	81	44
Bottomless Tostada Chips w/ Salsa	480	39	26
Crsp Onion String & Jalapeño Stk w/ Jalapeño Ranch	1020	86	49
Hot Spinach & Artichoke Dip w/ Chips	1130	90	41

• MOST HEALTHY   • LEAST HEALTHY

CHILI'S RESTAURANT (cont.)

	Cal	Fat	Cbs
Loaded Nachos - Beef (8)	1150	82	42
Loaded Nachos - Chicken (8)	1060	66	44
Skillet Queso w/ Chips	920	73	46
SW Eggrolls w/ Avocado Ranch	910	57	72
• Texas Cheese Fries w/ Jalapeño Ranch	1930	135	97
Triple Dipper™ Big Mouth® Bites w/ Jalapeño Ranch	740	48	46
Triple Dipper™ Bnlss Buffalo Wings w/ Bleu Chz	740	60	27
Triple Dipper™ Chkn Crispers® No Drss	570	39	29
• Triple Dipper™ Crispy Onion String & Jalapeño Stk	410	37	16
Triple Dipper™ Hot Spinach & Artichoke Dip w/ Chips	570	45	20
Triple Dipper™ SW Eggrolls w/ Avocado Ranch	640	42	48
Triple Dipper™ Wings Over Buffalo® w/ Bleu Chz	790	69	4
Wings Over Buffalo® w/ Bleu Cheese	1320	110	4

Burgers

	Cal	Fat	Cbs
Big Mouth® Bites w/ Jalapeño Ranch	1810	110	140
Classic Bacon Burger	1520	88	115
Ground Peppercorn Burger w/ Bleu Chz	1520	88	120
• Jalapeño Smkhs Burger w/ Jalapeño Ranch	2130	139	127
Mushroom-Swiss Burger	1460	84	116
• Oldtimer®	1260	62	118
Shiner Bock® BBQ Burger	1510	78	136
Sthrn Smkhs Burger w/ Ancho Chile BBQ	2080	127	141

Create Your Own Combo

	Cal	Fat	Cbs
Classic Sirloin	310	19	4
Fried Shrimp w/ Tequila Lime Sauce	400	28	18
Grilled Salmon w/ Garlic & Herbs	370	23	1
• Half Rack of Baby Back Ribs	560	41	17
• Margarita Grilled Chicken	110	6	14
Monterey Chicken®	470	25	13
Spicy Garlic & Lime Grilled Shrimp	120	8	3

Everything's Better On The Grill

	Cal	Fat	Cbs
Beef Fajitas w/o Tortillas & Condiments	480	25	26
Buffalo Chkn Fajitas w/o Tortillas & Condiments	240	8	9
Cajun Pasta w/ Grilled Chicken	530	26	28
Cajun Pasta w/ Grilled Shrimp	1350	70	104
Chkn Fajitas - w/o Tortillas & Condiments	1030	76	43
Chili's Classic Sirloin - w/o Sides	1310	75	105
• Fajita Condiments, 1 Each	230	19	7
Fajita TRIO - w/o Tortillas & Condiments	360	12	23
Flame-Grilled Ribeye - w/o Sides	450	26	19
Flour Tortillas, 3 Each	380	10	62
GG Classic Sirloin	900	68	18
GG Salmon w/ Garlic & Herbs	620	29	44
Grilled Salmon w/ Garlic & Herbs	530	19	43
Margarita Grilled Chicken	380	8	67
Monterey Chicken®	870	47	53

● MOST HEALTHY   ● LEAST HEALTHY

CHILI'S RESTAURANT (cont.)

	Cal	Fat	Cbs
Quesadilla Bacon Ranch Chkn w/ Salsa Ranch	1520	102	99
• Quesadilla Jalapeño Steak w/ Ancho Chile Ranch	1550	94	93

Hand-Battered Wins Everytime

	Cal	Fat	Cbs
Country-Fried Steak	1440	83	123
Crispy Chicken Crispers® - w/o Sauce	1510	86	132
• Crispy Honey-Chipotle Chkn Crispers® w/ Ranch	1950	104	202
• Fried Shrimp w/ Tequila Lime Sauce	1050	60	94

Kid's Menu

	Cal	Fat	Cbs
Cheese Pizza	570	24	67
Cheese Quesadilla	460	24	42
Chocolate Shake	490	24	67
Corn Dog	280	17	25
Country Fried Chicken Crispers	560	38	27
Grilled Cheese Sandwich	520	41	28
Grilled Chicken Platter	150	3	1
Grilled Chicken Sandwich	220	4	25
• Little Chicken Crispers	570	39	29
Little Mouth Burger	350	17	24
Little Mouth Cheeseburger	420	23	25
Macaroni & Cheese	400	10	68
Side Black Beans	90	1	17
Side Cinnamon Apples	200	8	36
Side Homestyle Fries	150	2	32
Side Kernel Corn	250	10	36
Side Mandarin Oranges	130	2	23
Side Rice	70	0	17
Side Seasonal Veggies	170	1	36
• Side Corn Cob w/o Butter	35	1	6

Not "Just" Sides

	Cal	Fat	Cbs
Add Fried Shrimp to any Entrée	200	8	36
Add Rice and Black Beans, 3 Each	120	7	8
Add Spicy Garlic & Lime Shrimp	240	25	1
Applewood Smoked Bacon	170	17	3
Avocado Slices, 6 Each	270	15	16
Black Bean Pattie Only, 3 Each	60	4	2
Black Beans	270	2	53
Cheese, American, 6 Each	130	8	3
Cheese, Cheddar, 3 Strips	100	8	0
Cheese, Provolone	70	7	4
Cheese, Swiss	60	0	14
Cinnamon Apples	100	1	17
Dressing, Ancho Chile Ranch	200	2	25
Dressing, Asian Vinaigrette	70	6	1
Dressing, Avocado Ranch	80	7	0
Dressing, Caribbean	50	4	0
Dressing, Citrus Balsamic Vinaigrette	250	25	6

• MOST HEALTHY • LEAST HEALTHY

▶ CHILI'S RESTAURANT (cont.)

	Cal	Fat	Cbs
Dressing, Honey Lime	200	17	13
Dressing, Jalapeño Ranch	140	15	2
Gravy, Black Pepper	35	2	4
Guacamole	40	4	2
Homestyle Fries	380	16	55
Honey Chipotle Sauce	130	0	34
• Loaded Mashed Potatoes	390	25	29
Mashed Potatoes w/ Black Pepper Gravy	280	15	33
Rice	170	1	36
• Salsa Only as served w/ Chips	30	0	6
Salsa Ranch Only as served w/ Chips	250	24	5
Seasonal Veggies	80	6	7
Spicy Cole Slaw	180	12	16
Sweet Corn on the Cob w/ Butter	200	7	32
Wheat Bun	360	3	62
Ribs, Slow-smoked In-house			
Memphis Dry Rub Ribs	1180	87	34
• Original Ribs	1110	81	33
• Shiner Bock® BBQ Ribs	1230	81	58
Salads			
Asian Salad w/ Grilled Chicken, Small	540	33	40
Asian Salad w/ Salmon, Small	650	42	40
Asian Salad w/ Steak, Small	610	39	41
Boneless Buffalo Chicken Salad	1150	84	52
Caribbean Salad w/ Grilled Chicken, Sm	490	24	64
Caribbean Salad w/ Grilled Shrimp, Small	550	28	64
Chicken Caesar Salad	710	42	25
GG Asian Salad	360	22	22
GG Caribbean Salad	450	24	4
GG House Salad w/ Lo Fat Ranch	140	6	0
Grilled BBQ Smoked Chicken Salad	1060	63	19
• House Salad No Dressing	100	3	0
• Quesadilla Explosion Salad	1400	88	26
Sandwiches			
BBQ Pulled Pork Sandwich	1250	53	147
• Buffalo Chicken Ranch Sandwich	1560	86	140
Chili's Cheesesteak Sandwich	1240	55	116
• GG Grilled Chicken Sandwich w/ Veggies	610	12	78
GG Santa Fe Chicken Wrap w/ Veggies	610	22	75
Grilled Chicken Sandwich	1240	62	114
Santa Fe Chkn Wrap w/ Ancho-Chile Ranch	1270	69	121
Smoked Turkey on Chile-Pepper Roll	1230	58	118
Smkd Tkey on Chile-Pepper Roll Combo	810	37	90
Steakhouse Sandwich	1080	51	115
Soups & Chili			
Baked Potato Soup, 1 Bowl	280	15	28

CHILI'S RESTAURANT (cont.)

	Cal	Fat	Cbs
Blackbean, 1 Bowl	290	8	40
Broccoli Cheese, 1 Bowl	250	15	17
• Chicken & Green Chili, 1 Bowl	190	5	21
Chicken Enchilada, 1 Bowl	430	26	22
• Chili's Terlingua Chili w/Toppings, 1 Bowl	460	30	24
Southwestern Vegetable, 1 Bowl	210	10	21
Sweet Corn, 1 Bowl	450	36	31

Stupendously Sweet Endings

	Cal	Fat	Cbs
• Brownie Sundae	1340	68	188
Cheesecake	710	42	68
Chocolate Chip Cookie Molten Cake	1140	56	150
Chocolate Chip Paradise Pie	1290	68	163
Frosty Chocolate Shake	740	35	100
Molten Chocolate Cake	1070	51	143
• Sweet Shot Key Lime Pie	240	12	30
Sweet Shot Red Velvet Cake	250	9	39
Sweet Shot Warm Cinnamon Roll	280	13	38
Sweet Shot Warm Double Choco Fudge Brownie	420	24	51
White Chocolate Molten Cake	1250	65	150

Tacos Wrapped In Flavor

	Cal	Fat	Cbs
Crispy Chicken Tacos w/ Corn Tortillas	1360	69	125
• Crispy Chicken Tacos w/ Flour Tortillas	1480	74	140
Crispy Shrimp Tacos w/ Corn Tortillas	830	28	111
Crispy Shrimp Tacos w/ Flour Tortillas	950	33	126
Pulled Pork Tacos w/ Corn Tortillas	800	22	99
Pulled Pork Tacos w/ Flour Tortillas	920	27	114
Seasoned Ground Beef Tacos w/ Corn Tortillas	1000	46	90
Seasoned Ground Beef Tacos w/ Flour Tortillas	1120	51	104
• Smoked Chicken Tacos w/ Corn Tortillas	700	15	98
Smoked Chicken Tacos w/ Flour Tortillas	820	20	113

CHIPOTLE

	Cal	Fat	Cbs
Flour Tortilla (burrito), 1 ea.	290	9	44
Flour Tortilla (taco), 1 ea.	90	3	13
Crispy Taco Shell, 1 ea.	60	2	9
Cilantro-Lime Rice, 3 oz.	130	3	23
Black Beans, 4 oz.	120	1	23
Pinto Beans, 4 oz.	120	1	22
Fajita Vegetables, 2.5 oz.	20	1	4
Barbacoa, 4 oz.	170	7	2
Chicken, 4 oz.	190	7	1
Carnitas, 4 oz.	190	8	1
Steak, 4 oz.	190	7	2
Tomato Salsa, 3.5 oz.	20	0	4
Corn Salsa, 3.5 oz.	80	2	15
Red Tomatillo Salsa, 2 fl.oz.	40	1	8

● MOST HEALTHY   ● LEAST HEALTHY

CHIPOTLE (cont.)

	Cal	Fat	Cbs
Green Tomatillo Salsa, 2 fl.oz.	15	0	3
Cheese, 1 oz.	100	9	0
Sour Cream, 2 oz.	120	10	2
Guacamole, 3.5 oz.	150	13	8
Romaine Lettuce (salad), 2.5 oz.	10	0	2
• Romaine Lettuce (tacos), 1 oz.	5	0	1
• Chips, 4 oz.	570	27	73
Vinaigrette, 2 fl, oz.	260	25	12

CHUCK E. CHEESE

Complements

	Cal	Fat	Cbs
Breadsticks, 1 stick	175	9	18
1/4 Sheet Cake, Chocolate, Slice	310	14	41
Apple Dessert Pizza, Slice	192	5	33
Buffalo Wings, 1 wing	75	5	4
Chocolate Cake, Slice	290	13	41
Cinnamon Sticks, 1 stick	70	2	11
• French Fries, 4 oz.	420	20	55
Hot Dogs, 1 oz.	310	19	35
Mozzarella Sticks, 1 stick	93	6	6
Sampler Platter, 1/7th	329	19	25
Sandwich Platter, 1/12th (1 piece)	183	8	20
Side Carrot Sticks with Ranch, 4 oz.	183	15	12
Side Celery & Bleu Cheese, 4 sticks	269	26	6
Side French Fries, 4 oz.	420	20	55
• Side Mandarin Oranges, 3¼ oz.	56	0	15
Vanilla Buttercream Cake, Slice	310	18	35
Veggie Platter, 1/8th	129	11	7

Oven-Baked Sandwiches

	Cal	Fat	Cbs
• Chicken Ciabatta, 6 oz.	65	0	9
Ham & Cheese, 6 oz.	150	4	24
Italian Sub, 1 oz.	715	28	80
Side Fruit Garnish, 1 oz.	685	27	79
Side Pasta Salad, 1 oz.	790	39	78

Pizza (Medium)

	Cal	Fat	Cbs
All Meat Combo, Slice	180	9	19
BBQ Chicken, Slice	185	6	24
• Cheese, Pizza	540	19	69
Super Combo, Slice	185	8	22
• Veggie Combo, Slice	135	5	20

CHURCH'S CHICKEN

Condiments

	Cal	Fat	Cbs
• Creamy Jalapeño Sauce, 1 pkg.	80	9	1
• Hot Sauce, 1 pkg.	18	0	0
Purple Pepper Sauce, 1 pkg.	45	0	12

• MOST HEALTHY   • LEAST HEALTHY

CHURCH'S CHICKEN (cont.)

	Cal	Fat	Cbs
Sweet & Sour Sauce, 1 pkg.	24	0	6
Main Courses			
BBQ Chicken Sandwich	516	17	36
Boneless Wings w/ BBQ Sauce, 6 pieces	550	21	60
Boneless Wings w/ Hot Sauce, 6 pieces	460	21	36
Chicken Sandwich w/ Chz, Snd	503	26	48
Country Fried Steak, 1 piece	470	28	36
Double Chkn N Chz Snd	738	38	63
Nuggets, 5 pieces	162	7	13
Original Breast, 1 piece	200	11	3
Original Chicken Sandwich	458	22	48
• Original Leg, 1 piece	110	6	3
Original Thigh, 1 piece	330	23	8
Original Wing, 1 piece	300	19	7
Premium Homestyle Fillet, 1 fillet	349	17	17
w/ 3 oz., Brown Gravy, 1 fillet	630	21	71
w/ 3 oz. White Gravy, 1 fillet	409	20	25
Premium Homestyle Sandwich	623	32	51
• Shrimp & Fries Basket, 1 basket	750	36	86
Spicy Breast, 1 piece	320	20	12
Spicy Chicken Sandwich, sandwich	456	21	47
Spicy Leg, 1 piece	180	11	8
Spicy Tender Strips™, 1 piece	135	7	7
Spicy Thigh, 1 piece	480	35	20
Spicy Wing, 1 piece	430	27	17
Steak Fingers, 3 pieces	494	36	23
Tender Strips™, 1 piece	120	6	6
Sides			
Apple Pie, 1 pie	260	11	39
Cajun Rice (Reg.), 6 oz.	130	7	16
Churro - Caramel, 1 piece	140	7	18
Cole Slaw (Reg.), 6 oz.	150	10	15
Corn-on-the-cob, 1 piece	140	3	24
French Fries (Reg.), 4 oz.	290	14	38
Honey-Butter Biscuit, 1 biscuit	190	10	22
Jalapeño Chz Bombers® (Reg.), 4 pieces	240	10	29
• Jalapeño Pepper, 1 pepper	5	0	1
Macaroni & Cheese (Reg.), 6 oz.	221	10	24
Mashed Potatoes & Gravy (Reg.), 6 oz.	70	2	12
• Okra (Reg.), 3.41 oz.	350	22	36

CICI'S PIZZA

12" Buffet Pizzas

Alfredo, 1 slice	120	4	18
• Bacon Cheddar, 1 slice	110	5	19
BBQ, 1 slice	150	3	25

• MOST HEALTHY   • LEAST HEALTHY

CICI'S PIZZA (cont.)

	Cal	Fat	Cbs
Beef, 1 slice	150	4	20
Buffalo Chicken	140	5	19
Cheese, 1 slice	150	4	19
Classic Chicken	140	5	19
• Deep Dish	170	6	19
Ham	150	4	19
Ham & Pineapple, 1 slice	150	4	21
Macaroni & Cheese	170	3	29
Ole, 1 slice	120	3	20
Pepperoni & Jalapeño, 1 slice	150	5	20
Pepperoni Flip	120	6	13
Pepperoni, 1 slice	160	5	20
Sausage, 1 slice	140	5	20
Spinach Alfredo, 1 slice	120	4	19
Tomato Alfredo	120	3	19
Zesty Ham & Cheddar, 1 slice	120	4	19
Zesty Pepperoni, 1 slice	150	6	19
Zesty Veggie, 1 slice	130	4	20

Extras & Desserts

	Cal	Fat	Cbs
• Apple Pizza, 1 slice	150	4	26
Brownies, 1 slice	140	6	22
Cinnamon Rolls, 1 slice	140	5	20
• Garlic Bread, 1 slice	100	5	10

CINNABON

	Cal	Fat	Cbs
Apple Minibon	285	5	53
• Caramel Pecanbon	1100	56	141
Cinnabites, 6 count	520	140	78
CinnaPretzel	750	6	156
CinnaStixs	379	21	41
Classic Cinnabon	813	32	117
• Frosting, 1 oz.	180	11	20
Minibon	339	13	49
Strawberry Minibon	250	5	46

COLD STONE CREAMERY

Cakes and Pies

	Cal	Fat	Cbs
A Cheesecake Named Desire™, 162 g	420	22	55
Birthday Cake, 119 g	310	18	34
Cake Batter Confetti™, 141 g	440	21	58
Chocolate Chipper™, 142 g	470	28	53
• Coffeehouse Crunch™, 155 g	540	31	61
Cookie Dough Delirium™, 147 g	460	23	55
Cookies & Creamery™, 129 g	370	19	45
Dark Peppermint Pleasure™, 140 g	450	25	52
Midnight Delight™, 146 g	470	27	54

• MOST HEALTHY   • LEAST HEALTHY

COLD STONE CREAMERY (cont.)	Cal	Fat	Cbs
MMMMMM Chip™, 130 g	380	20	44
Peanut Butter Playground™, 148 g	490	30	53
• Pumpkin Pie, 98 g	270	15	33
Strawberry Passion™, 151 g	410	21	53
Candy			
Butterfinger® Candy, 30 g	140	6	22
Almond Joy® Candy, 35 g	170	9	21
Chocolate Chips, 25 g	130	7	16
Chocolate Shavings, 17 g	90	5	9
• Ghirardelli Caramel Square, 15 g	70	4	9
Gumballs, 35 g	90	0	23
Gummi Bears, 30 g	120	0	30
Heath® Candy Bar, 20 g	110	7	12
Kit Kat® Candy Bar, 20 g	110	5	13
M & M's® Candy, 35 g	170	7	25
Nestle® Crunch Bar, 25 g	130	7	16
Peanut M & M's®, 30 g	150	8	18
• Reese's® Peanut Butter Cup, 35 g	190	11	19
Reese's® Pieces, 35 g	180	9	21
Snickers® Candy, 35 g	170	9	21
Twix® Candy, 30 g	150	7	20
White Chocolate Chips, 30 g	160	9	18
Whoppers® Candy, 25 g	120	4	19
York® Peppermint Patties, 30 g	120	2	24
Cupcakes			
Cake Batter Delux, 120 g	380	19	50
• Double Chocolate, 120 g	360	19	45
• Sweet Cream, 120 g	390	21	48
Fruit			
Apple Pie Filling, 60 g	60	0	16
Bananas, 60 g	50	0	14
Blackberries, 30 g	10	0	2
• Black Cherries, 35 g	80	0	18
Blueberries, 15 g	10	0	2
Cherry Pie Filling, 45 g	50	0	13
• Maraschino Cherries, 5 g	5	0	1
Pineapple Chunks, 25 g	15	0	4
Raspberries, 35 g	25	0	5
Strawberries, 45 g	20	0	7
Peach Pie Filling, 60 g	60	0	16
Raisins, 25 g	70	0	20
Ice Cream			
Amaretto Ice Cream, 227 g	530	31	53
Banana Ice Cream, 227 g	500	29	53
Black Cherry Ice Cream, 227 g	530	30	58
Blueberry Muffin Ice Cream, 227 g	530	30	61

COLD STONE CREAMERY (cont.)	Cal	Fat	Cbs
Butter Pecan Ice Cream, 227 g	520	31	53
Cake Batter Ice Cream™, 227 g	550	30	66
Cheesecake Ice Cream, 227 g	520	29	59
Choco Cake Batter Ice Cream™, 227 g	550	30	68
Chocolate Devotion™, 74 g	200	11	26
Chocolate Ice Cream, 227 g	520	32	53
Choco Raspberry Truffle Ice Cream, 227 g	510	28	63
Cinnamon Bun Ice Cream, 227 g	600	33	68
Cinnamon Ice Cream, 227 g	530	32	55
Coconut Ice Cream, 227 g	520	31	52
Coffee Ice Cream, 227 g	530	31	54
Coffee Lovers Only®, 74 g	210	13	22
Cookie Batter Ice Cream, 227 g	600	32	71
Cotton Candy Ice Cream, 227 g	530	31	55
Crème De La Berry™, 74 g	180	9	23
Dark Chocolate Ice Cream, 227 g	540	32	51
Dark Choco Peppermint Ice Cream, 227 g	540	32	54
Egg Nog Ice Cream, 227 g	410	24	42
Founder's Favorite®, 74 g	210	12	24
French Toast Ice Cream, 227 g	530	31	56
French Vanilla Ice Cream, 227 g	540	30	60
Ghirardelli Chocolate Ice Cream, 227 g	520	31	59
Gingerbread Ice Cream, 227 g	510	30	58
Irish Cream Ice Cream, 227 g	530	32	54
JELL-O® Banana Pudding Ice Crm, 227 g	550	28	74
JELL-O® Btrsctch Pnddng Ice Crm, 227 g	550	28	73
JELL-O® Choco Pudding Ice Crm, 227 g	550	28	73
JELL-O® Vanilla Pudding Ice Crm, 227 g	550	28	74
Macadamia Nut Ice Cream, 227 g	530	31	54
Mango Ice Cream, 227 g	490	29	53
Marshmallow Ice Cream, 227 g	530	28	66
Mint Ice Cream, 227 g	530	30	57
Mocha Ice Cream, 227 g	520	31	53
• Nutter Butter Ice Cream, 227 g	630	39	65
Oatmeal Cookie Batter Ice, 227 g	540	31	58
Orange Dreamsicle Ice Cream, 227 g	510	30	55
Peanut Butter Cup Perfection™, 74 g	220	13	24
Peanut Butter Ice Cream, 227 g	590	39	53
Pecan Praline Ice Cream, 227 g	530	30	58
Pistachio Ice Cream, 227 g	520	31	54
Pumpkin Ice Cream, 227 g	460	24	53
Raspberry Ice Cream, 227 g	520	30	57
Rocky Off Road™, 74 g	230	14	25
Shock-A-Cone®, 74 g	220	13	26
Sinless Cake Batter Ice Cream, 227 g	300	2	65
Sinless Sans Fat™ Sweet Cream, 227 g	220	0	55

• MOST HEALTHY   • LEAST HEALTHY

COLD STONE CREAMERY (cont.)

	Cal	Fat	Cbs
Strawberry Ice Cream, 227 g	510	30	55
Sweet Cream Ice Cream, 227 g	530	32	53
Vanilla Bean Ice Cream, 227 g	530	31	52
White Chocolate Ice Cream, 227 g	520	31	53
• Zenilla™, 74 g	170	11	17
Lifestyle			
Banana Banana, 655 g	510	5	117
Banana Strawberry, 672 g	450	6	102
Blueberry Banana, 582 g	430	5	95
• Blueberry Pineapple, 539 g	360	5	78
Mango Pineapple, 627 g	510	5	115
• Mango Strawberry, 687 g	520	6	118
Pineapple Coconut Orange, 617 g	490	14	90
Raspberry Banana, 642 g	460	5	104
Strawberry Raspberry, 669 g	400	6	89
Mix-ins: Other			
Brownies, 40 g	170	4	32
Coconut, 15 g	80	5	7
• Cookie Dough, 40 g	180	8	26
Graham Cracker Pie Crust, 25 g	130	6	17
Granola, 30 g	120	2	23
Marshmallows, 30 g	100	0	24
• Nilla Wafers, 15 g	70	3	11
OREO® Cookies, 25 g	120	5	18
OREO® Pie Crust, 30 g	180	8	19
Peanut Butter, 25 g	150	13	5
Toasted Coconut, 15 g	90	7	7
Yellow Cake, 25 g	80	3	13
Nuts			
Cashews, 30 g	170	14	9
Macadamia Nuts, 25 g	180	19	3
Peanuts, 35 g	210	18	5
• Pecan Pralines, 30 g	210	21	5
Pecans, 20 g	140	15	3
Pistachio Nuts, 35 g	200	16	10
Roasted Almonds, 25 g	150	14	4
Sliced Almonds, 35 g	210	20	6
• Walnuts, 20 g	130	13	3
Shakes			
Cake 'n Shake™, 602 g	1400	73	172
Cherry Cheeseshake™, 636 g	1290	66	157
Cream de Menthe™, 571 g	1280	74	138
Lotta Caramel Latte™, 660 g	1530	72	200
Milk and Cookies™, 598 g	1400	80	154
Oh Fudge!™, 773 g	1660	91	191
• PB&C™, 687 g	1690	111	149

• MOST HEALTHY   • LEAST HEALTHY

► COLD STONE CREAMERY (cont.)	Cal	Fat	Cbs
• Savory Strawberry™, 636 g	1200	67	138
Very Vanilla™, 607 g	1390	69	173
Shakes made with Sinless			
• Sinless Cake n Shake, 607 g	840	9	175
Sinless Milk and Cookies, 587 g	710	9	147
Sinless Oh Fudge, 599 g	670	4	149
Sinless Very Vanilla, 570 g	590	1	135
Sinless			
2 to Mango™, 652 g	250	0	63
Berry Lemony™, 691 g	200	1	50
• Berry Trinity™, 749 g	160	2	41
Citrus Sunsation™, 718 g	220	0	57
• Man-Go Bananas™, 670 g	300	0	75
On The YoGo™, 687 g	240	2	60
Strawberry Bananza™, 783 g	220	2	57
Sorbet and Yogurt			
• Countrytime Pink Lmnade Sorbet, 227 g	380	0	95
Lemon Sorbet, 227 g	250	0	64
Raspberry Sorbet, 227 g	260	0	67
Tart and Tangy Berry Yogurt, 227 g	240	0	59
• Tart and Tangy Yogurt, 227 g	230	0	53
Watermelon Sorbet, 227 g	260	0	66
Supplements			
• Nrgize Antioxidant/Immune Supplement, 4 g	4	0	2
Nrgize Anti-Stress, 4 g	4	0	2
Nrgize Energy Supplement, 4 g	4	0	2
• Nrgize Whey Protein Supplement, 15 g	60	1	4
Toppings			
Butterscotch Fat Free, 30 g	80	0	19
Caramel, 30 g	90	1	21
Caramel Fat Free, 30 g	80	0	19
Chocolate Sprinkles, 25 g	25	0	6
• Cinnamon, 1 g	0	0	0
Fudge, 30 g	90	2	18
Fudge Fat Free, 30 g	80	0	20
Honey, 30 g	90	0	25
• Marshmallow Crème, 30 g	100	0	24
Rainbow Sprinkles, 25 g	25	0	6
Reddi Wip® Original, 20 g	45	3	5
Waffle Products			
• Dipped Waffle, 68 g	310	15	46
• Sugar Cone, 13 g	50	0	11
Waffle Cone or Bowl, 38 g	160	4	29

● MOST HEALTHY   • LEAST HEALTHY

CORNER BAKERY CAFÉ

	Cal	Fat	Cbs
Add On for Breakfast Panini Combo			
Breakfast Potatoes	140	5	21
Seasonal Fruit Salad Medley - LF, LS	70	0	17
Additional Bakery Breads			
Asiago Cheese Bread	390	10	53
Ciabatta Ficelle	370	5	70
• Croissant	340	16	39
• Poblano Cheese Batard	410	13	60
Pretzel Demi	410	5	77
Asian Wonton Salads (Dressing Included)			
Asian Wonton Salad - cafe size	260	9	29
Baby Bundt Cakes			
Banana Baby Bundt Cake	620	30	81
Chocolate Baby Bundt Cake	580	30	70
Bagel Spreads			
Green Onion Cream Cheese	130	12	2
• Peanut Butter	240	21	2
• Strawberry Cream Cheese	110	10	3
Vegetable Cream Cheese	110	11	2
Whipped Plain Cream Cheese	130	13	2
Bagels (without Cream Cheese)			
• 8-Grain Bagel - LF	330	2	72
Blueberry Bagel - LF	340	2	73
Cinnamon Raisin Bagel - LF	330	2	72
Everything Bagel - LF	330	3	69
Plain Bagel - LF	330	2	70
• Sesame Seed Bagel - LF	340	4	69
Bakery Rolls			
Focaccia Roll - LF	110	2	19
Harvest Roll	180	3	32
Bars & Brownies			
Cream Cheese Brownie	590	37	53
Fudge Brownie	590	28	86
Lemon Bar	590	24	90
• Maple Pecan Bar	730	44	80
• Raspberry Bar	530	24	72
Bowl of Soup			
Big Al's Chili w/ Cheddar Cheese	590	27	44
Topping - Cheddar Cheese	70	6	0
Cheddar Broccoli	550	41	28
• Ld Baked Potato	630	43	36
Topping - Cheddar Cheese	70	6	0
• Topping - Green Onions	0	0	0
Mom's Chicken Noodle - LF	210	6	28
Roasted Poblano Corn Chowder	420	25	43
Roasted Tomato Basil	320	11	49

• MOST HEALTHY   • LEAST HEALTHY

CORNER BAKERY CAFÉ (cont.)

	Cal	Fat	Cbs
Topping - Croutons	100	6	10
Three Lentil Vegetable - LF	210	4	36
Zesty Chicken Tortilla	360	16	41
Topping - Tortilla Strips	40	2	5
Bread			
Focaccia Roll - LF	110	2	19
Garlic Bread	110	3	17
Bread & Garnish			
Focaccia Roll - LF	110	2	19
Mixed Greens w/ Drss, garnish service	30	3	1
Breakfast Pastries			
• Cinnamon Creme Cake - Slice	770	34	108
Cinnamon Roll	660	24	95
Croissant	340	16	39
Breakfast Sandwiches			
• Anaheim Panini	740	37	71
Anaheim Panini w/ Egg Whites	660	29	70
Commuter	690	45	43
Commuter w/ Egg Whites	610	36	42
Ham & Swiss Panini	630	23	68
• Ham & Swiss Panini w/ Egg Whites	550	14	67
Smoked Bacon & Cheddar Panini	690	33	66
Smkd Bacon & Chdr Panini w/ Egg Wht	610	25	66
Breakfast Scramblers			
All American Scrambler	350	27	3
• w/ Egg Whites (w/ bacon)	200	11	2
• Anaheim Scrambler	570	45	9
Anaheim Scrambler w/ Egg Whites	410	28	8
Farmer's Scrambler	420	28	13
Farmer's Scrambler w/ Egg Whites	270	11	12
By The Slice			
Cinnamon Raisin	220	7	32
Country Small Oblong	170	1	34
Harvest	160	1	31
Mom's White	160	5	24
• Raisin Pecan	140	4	23
Steakhouse Rye	160	1	30
• Traditional Sesame Baguette (1/6 loaf)	270	5	48
White Rye	160	3	27
Caesar Salads (Dressing Included)			
Caesar Salad - cafe size	360	31	12
Caesar Salad w/ Chicken - cafe size	420	35	12
Chopped Salads (Dressing Included)			
Chopped Salad - cafe size	400	29	17

• MOST HEALTHY   • LEAST HEALTHY

CORNER BAKERY CAFÉ (cont.)

	Cal	Fat	Cbs
Cookies			
Chocolate Chip Cookie	300	13	46
• Monster Cookie	340	14	51
• Oatmeal Raisin Cookie	290	10	47
Snickerdoodle Cookie	290	10	47
Sugar Cookie	290	10	47
Cream Cakes			
Cinnamon Cream Cake, Slice	770	34	108
Crisps			
Harvest Crisp, each	60	1	10
Sweet Crisp, each	150	4	25
Cup of Soup			
Big Al's Chili	380	17	29
Topping - Cheddar Cheese	40	3	0
Cheddar Broccoli	370	28	19
• Loaded Baked Potato	410	27	24
Topping - Cheddar Cheese	40	3	0
• Topping - Green Onions	0	0	0
Mom's Chicken Noodle - LF	140	4	19
Roasted Poblano Corn Chowder	280	16	29
Roasted Tomato Basil - LF	200	7	31
Topping - Croutons	50	3	5
Three Lentil Vegetable - LF	140	3	24
Zesty Chicken Tortilla	230	11	26
Topping - Tortilla Strips	20	1	2
Current Offerings			
Asian Edamame Salad	90	5	8
Caesar Salad - trio & side portion	230	20	8
DC Chicken Salad	240	16	14
• Greek Marinated Vegetable Salad	60	3	6
Mixed Greens Salad - trio & side portion	120	8	9
Pasta Caprese Salad	140	7	12
Roasted Potato Bacon Salad	150	5	21
Seasonal Fruit Salad Medley - LF, LS	70	0	17
• Tuna Salad	280	20	2
Entrees			
• Macaroni & Cheese	350	11	48
Pasta Marinara - LF	340	8	53
• Parmesan Chz - Subtract to Customize	40	3	0
French Toast (with Vanilla Syrup)			
Baked French Toast	1250	52	187
w/ Bacon & Fresh Fruit	1340	62	192
Greek Salad (Dressing Included)			
Greek Salad - cafe size	260	16	20
Grits			
Buckhead Cheese Grits	350	22	20

• MOST HEALTHY   • LEAST HEALTHY

CORNER BAKERY CAFÉ (cont.)

	Cal	Fat	Cbs
Harvest Salads (dressing included)			
Harvest Salad - cafe size	410	25	37
Harvest Salad w/ Chicken - cafe size	470	28	37
Medium Bundt Cakes (8-10 Slices/Cake)			
Banana Bundt Cake	3500	170	460
Chocolate Bundt Cake	3200	170	380
Mixed Greens Salads (Dressing Included)			
Mixed Greens Salad - cafe size	220	17	14
Mom's Cheeses			
Provolone Cheese	80	6	0
• Swiss Cheese	90	6	0
• White Cheddar Cheese	70	7	0
Yellow Cheddar Cheese	70	7	0
Mom's Snd			
Mom's Corned Beef on Rye Bread - LF	480	4	76
• Mom's Rst Beef on Sourdough Bread - LF	510	7	71
Mom's Roast Chkn on Harvest Bread - LF	420	6	55
Mom's Slicd Ham on White Bread - LF	490	15	57
• Mom's Turkey on Harvest Bread - LF	410	2	59
Muffins			
Banana Muffin	530	20	67
Blueberry Muffin	510	22	70
Chocolate Muffin	530	28	60
• Cinnamon Crumb Muffin	660	30	90
• Pumpkin Muffin	460	18	69
Oatmeal			
• Honey Banana Crunch Oatmeal w/ top - LF	480	10	83
Loaded Oatmeal w/ toppings - LF	340	9	49
Brown Sugar - LF	45	0	12
Currants - LF	35	0	8
• Dried Cranberries - LF	25	0	6
Toasted Almonds	35	3	1
Toasted Walnuts	50	5	1
Oatmeal w/out toppings - LF	140	2	21
Spiced Cranberry Apple Oatmeal - LF	330	6	57
Swiss Oatmeal - LF	360	3	78
Paninis			
• California Grille	700	28	82
Chicken Pomodori	780	35	73
Club	760	37	70
• Corned Beef Reuben	880	43	80
Grilled Ham & Swiss	700	26	73
Pasta Entrees			
Chicken Carbonara	1110	61	85
Half Moon Cheese Ravioli	640	25	73
• Penne Marinara - LF	600	18	89

• MOST HEALTHY   • LEAST HEALTHY

CORNER BAKERY CAFÉ (cont.)

	Cal	Fat	Cbs
• Pesto Cavatappi	1100	63	82
Pasta Toppings			
Parmesan Cheese	90	6	0
Pound Cakes			
Banana Walnut Bread - Slice	420	18	63
Lemon Pound Cake - Slice	480	22	64
Rugalach			
Apricot Walnut Rugalach	240	15	23
Cinnamon Pecan Rugalach	250	16	24
Salad Dressings			
Asian Dressing - cafe portion	80	5	10
White Balsamic Vinaigrette - cafe portion	70	5	0
Salad Toppings			
• Avocado - cafe portion	30	3	2
Bacon - cafe portion	40	4	0
Bacon - entree portion	70	7	0
Blue Cheese - cafe portion	80	7	0
Cheddar Cheese - cafe portion	70	6	0
Croutons - cafe portion	50	3	5
Feta Cheese - cafe portion	80	6	1
Harvest Crisp Pieces - cafe portion	60	1	10
Roast Chicken - entree portion	120	5	0
• Toasted Walnuts - cafe portion	120	11	2
Wonton Strips - cafe portion	40	0	8
Sandwiches			
Grilled Cheese Sandwich	610	35	52
Ham Sandwich - LF	410	13	52
• Peanut Butter & Jelly Sandwich	810	38	103
• Turkey Sandwich - LF	410	11	53
Sante Fe Salads (dressing included)			
Sante Fe Ranch Salad - cafe size	480	28	39
Sides			
Baby Carrots - LS, LF	30	0	7
Bakery Chips	190	12	22
Chocolate Chip Cookie	300	13	46
• Monster Cookie	340	14	51
• Pickle Spear	10	0	1
Seasonal Fruit Salad Medley - LF, LS	70	0	17
Sides			
Bacon, 3-slice	110	11	0
Breakfast Potatoes	140	5	21
• Buckhead Cheese Grits	180	11	10
Harvest Toast - LF	160	1	31
• Seasonal Fruit Salad Medley - LF, LS	70	0	17
Sweet Crisp, each	150	4	25

• MOST HEALTHY   • LEAST HEALTHY

▶ CORNER BAKERY CAFÉ (cont.)

	Cal	Fat	Cbs
Signature Sandwiches			
Bavarian Ham on Pretzel Bread - LF	680	19	84
Bavarian Turkey on Pretzel Bread - LF	670	15	87
Chicken Pesto on Ciabatta Ficelle Bread	760	27	87
D.C. Chkn Salad on Steakhouse Rye Bread	630	18	91
Poblano Fresco Chkn on Poblano Chz Bread	820	40	70
• Poblano Pesto Rst Beef on Poblano Chz Bread	830	40	71
Poblano Fresco Veg on Poblano Chz Bread	770	42	71
Tomato Mozz. on Ciabatta Ficelle Bread	700	26	81
• Tuna Salad on Harvest Bread	570	22	59
Turkey Frisco on Asiago Cheese Bread	730	26	67
Uptown Turkey on Harvest Bread	580	19	63
Toast per Slice			
• Cinnamon Raisin	220	7	32
Country Small Oblong - LF	170	1	34
Mom's White - LF	160	5	24
• Raisin Pecan	140	4	23
Steakhouse Rye - LF	160	1	30
White Rye - LF	180	0	27
Whole Loafs			
Cinnamon Raisin	2540	87	389
• Country Boule	1040	3	213
Country Small Oblong	3150	14	640
Focaccia Loaf	1110	15	190
Harvest	2080	15	401
Mom's White	2090	67	314
Raisin Pecan Miche	2050	61	340
Steakhouse Rye	1990	15	393
Traditional Sesame Baguette	1620	30	287
• White Rye Oblong	3540	59	649
Whoopee Pies			
• Peanut Butter Whoopee Pie	440	29	38
• Pumpkin Whoopee Pie	400	22	45
Vanilla Cream Whoopee Pie	430	26	43
Yogurt			
Fresh Berry Parfait - LF, LS	380	12	64

▶ COSI

	Cal	Fat	Cbs
Baked Omelette Sandwiches			
• Club Omelette, 9 oz.	683	28	64
• Pesto Garden Omelette Croissant, 1 oz.	740	45	56
Western Croissant, 1 oz.	713	40	56
Beverages (Grande)			
Arctic Latte, 16 oz.	264	7	48
Arctic Mocha, 16 oz.	343	5	70
• Café Americano, 16 oz.	8	0	1

• MOST HEALTHY   • LEAST HEALTHY

COSI (cont.)

	Cal	Fat	Cbs
Café Au Lait, 16 oz.	145	8	12
Cappuccino, 16 oz.	155	8	13
Chai Tea Latte, 16 oz.	214	8	29
• Così Sangria, 16 oz.	553	0	134
Country Club Tea, 24 oz.	98	0	26
Double Oh! Arctic Mocha, 16 oz.	549	23	82
Green Tea Smoothie, 16 oz.	326	7	63
Iced Tea, 16 oz.	22	0	6
Mango Smoothie, 16 oz.	280	0	74
Mocha, 16 oz.	411	10	68
Slim Vanilla Latte, 16 oz.	135	0	20
Strawberry Smoothie, 16 oz.	332	0	82
Watermelon Habanero Lemonade, 14 oz.	284	0	93
Breakfast			
Bananas Foster Parfait, 11 oz.	389	5	77
Cosi Oatmeal, 8 oz.	101	0	16
• Fruit Salad Breakfast, 8 oz.	84	1	21
Strawberry Parfait, 12 oz.	331	5	62
• Veggie Quiche, 1 oz.	522	36	30
Breakfast Wraps			
Italian Sausage Bolognese, 11 oz.	446	28	21
Santa Fe, 11 oz.	437	27	24
• Spinach Florentine, 11 oz.	334	21	21
Desserts			
• Cinnamon Apple Pie, 14 oz.	964	41	145
Così Bread Pudding, 7 oz.	621	36	66
Cream Brulee Cheesecake, 1 oz.	644	46	48
Double Trouble Brownie, 8 oz.	690	75	86
Mississippi Mud Pie, 9 oz.	566	35	61
S'mores, 3 oz.	361	10	61
• S'mores (with Oreo®), 3 oz.	351	11	59
Kids Sandwiches			
Kids Gooey Grilled Chz Snd, 3 oz.	269	15	22
Kids Gooey Grilled Ham and Chz, 4 oz.	320	18	22
• Kids Peanut Butter & Jelly, 4 oz.	343	15	45
• Pesto Turkey Sandwich, 3 oz.	151	1	22
Melt			
• Bacon Turkey Cheddar Melt, 12 oz.	572	24	48
Chicken TBM Melt, 12 oz.	693	31	49
Italian Roast Beef Melt, 14 oz.	658	30	47
Pesto Chicken Melt, 11 oz.	671	31	52
Steakhouse Gorgonzola Melt, 12 oz.	752	47	49
TBM Melt, 12 oz.	636	32	49
• Tuna Melt, 14 oz.	874	40	51
Muffins, Scones & Pastries			
Blueberry Muffin, 150 g	440	19	60

● MOST HEALTHY   ● LEAST HEALTHY

COSI (cont.)

	Cal	Fat	Cbs
Blueberry Scone, 120 g	410	17	60
Break Bar, 3 oz.	359	18	44
Carrot Muffin, 150 g	470	22	62
• Chocolate Chip Muffin, 147 g	506	27	67
Cranberry Orange Scone, 120 g	400	15	61
• Stawberry Parfait, 12 oz.	331	5	62

Our Lighter Side

	Cal	Fat	Cbs
• Bombay Chicken Salad Low Cal, 13 oz.	188	2	21
• Hummus & Veggie Sandwich, 10 oz.	397	7	72
Lighter Side Cosi Cobb Salad, 11 oz.	519	34	17
Lighter Side Cosi Signature Salad, 11 oz.	371	19	45
• Lighter Side Grilled Chicken TBM, 12 oz.	531	17	50
Lighter Side TBM Sandwich, 9 oz.	372	11	50
Sesame Ginger Chicken, 10 oz.	480	7	69

Pizza

	Cal	Fat	Cbs
• Cheese Flatbread Pizza, 14 oz.	887	21	123
Margherita Chicken Flatbread Pizza, 13 oz.	703	31	96
Margherita Flatbread Pizza, 14 oz.	790	32	92
Pepperoni Flatbread Pizza, 14 oz.	874	44	95
Smky BBQ Chkn Flatbread Cosi Org Crust, 14 oz.	874	44	95
• Trifecta Flatbread Pizza, 12 oz.	683	29	95

Salad

	Cal	Fat	Cbs
Bombay Chicken Salad, 13 oz.	481	32	17
Buffalo Chicken Salad, 12 oz.	592	44	18
Caesar Salad, 9 oz.	488	40	20
Chicken Caesar Salad, 11 oz.	621	44	20
• Cosi Cobb Salad, 13 oz.	708	55	16
Cosi Signature Salad, 11 oz.	611	45	44
Greek Salad, 14 oz.	517	47	19
Grilled Wild Alaskan Salmon Salad, 15 oz.	457	27	24
Salad Bruschetta, 15 oz.	645	14	79
• Shanghai Chicken Salad, 10 oz.	313	13	26
Steakhs Salad w/ Bleu Chz Drss, 14 oz.	614	49	14
Tuscan Steak Salad, 15 oz.	532	34	26

Sandwiches

	Cal	Fat	Cbs
Buffalo Bleu Sandwich, 10 oz.	565	25	47
Chicken TBM Sandwich, 11 oz.	691	36	47
Cosi Club Sandwich, 9 oz.	497	10	47
Cosi Market with Turkey Sandwich, 9 oz.	687	32	62
• Fire-Roasted Veggie Sandwich, 9 oz.	324	8	44
Hummus & Veggie Sandwich, 10 oz.	397	7	72
Italiano Sandwich, 10 oz.	747	42	49
Meatball Aurora Sandwich, 10 oz.	558	25	53
Sesame Ginger Chicken, 10 oz.	480	7	69
Shrimp Remoulade, 10 oz.	456	20	48
• Steak TBM Sandwich, 11 oz.	829	55	46

• MOST HEALTHY   • LEAST HEALTHY

▶ COSI (cont.)

	Cal	Fat	Cbs
Tandoori Chicken Sandwich, 9 oz.	541	23	48
TBM Sandwich, 9 oz.	532	30	46
Tuna Sandwich, 10 oz.	539	6	52
Turkey Light Sandwich, 9 oz.	390	5	62
Tuscan Pesto Chicken Sandwich, 10 oz.	510	6	49
Wasabi Roast Beef Sandwich, 10 oz.	556	27	49

Shareables

	Cal	Fat	Cbs
• Brie & Fruit, 8 oz.	616	41	36
• Chicken Queso Tortilla, Side, 5 oz.	100	4	9
Hummus Shareable, 6 oz.	339	5	62
Spinach & Artichoke Dip, 6 oz.	299	13	47

Soups

	Cal	Fat	Cbs
Beef w/ Winter Garden Vegs Soup, 5 oz.	75	4	7
• Cheese Flatbread Pizza, 12 oz.	683	29	95
Lentil Soup, 5 oz.	99	2	16
New England Clam Chowder, 5 oz.	220	14	12
• Three Bean Chili, 5 oz.	75	0	18
Tomato & Basil Soup, 5 oz.	112	8	9

Squagals

	Cal	Fat	Cbs
• Asiago Cheese, 6 oz.	453	8	75
Cinnamon Raisin, 7 oz.	447	2	95
Cranberry Orange, 6 oz.	418	1	87
• Low-Fat Cream Cheese, 2 oz.	106	8	4
Low-Fat Vegetable Cream Cheese, 2 oz.	113	9	2
Plain, 5 oz.	309	1	61
Plain Cream Cheese, 2 oz.	189	19	0
Poppyseed, 5 oz.	361	3	69
Sesame, 6 oz.	363	3	69
Whole Grain, 5 oz.	339	3	65

▶ COUNTRY BUFFET

Beverages

	Cal	Fat	Cbs
• Cappuccino, all flavors, 8 fl.oz.	150	4	30
Hot Chocolate, 8 fl.oz.	130	1	32
• Icee,® all flavors, 12 fl.oz.	110	0	27

Breads

	Cal	Fat	Cbs
Biscuits, 41 g	130	6	16
Buns, Hot Dog, 43 g	120	2	22
Caramel Rolls, 43 g	140	5	22
Cinnamon Bread, 50 g	160	3	32
Cinnamon Rolls, 40 g	140	5	23
Corn Bread, 50 g	160	6	25
Dinner Rolls, 38 g	130	5	18
Dinner Rolls, White-Pull-A-Part, 39 g	130	5	18
• English Muffins, dry, 26 g	60	1	13
Flour Tortilla, 38 g	120	3	20

● MOST HEALTHY   • LEAST HEALTHY

▶ COUNTRY BUFFET (cont.)

	Cal	Fat	Cbs
Garlic Bread, 18 g	70	3	9
• Garlic Cheese Biscuit, 60 g	230	15	20
Honey Corn Bread, 50 g	170	7	26
Jalapeño Cornbread, 50 g	160	6	25

Breakfast

	Cal	Fat	Cbs
Bacon, 8 g	40	4	0
Brown Sugar, 9 g	35	0	9
Buttermilk Pancakes, 60 g	120	2	19
• Diced Bacon, 46 g	240	19	0
Diced Ham, 28 g	35	1	0
French Toast, 85 g	220	9	29
Grits, 121 g	60	0	13
Hashbrown Patties, 50 g	110	7	13
Maple Flavored Syrup, 68 g	180	0	47
Oatmeal, 117 g	60	2	12
Omelet-plain, 88 g	140	11	2
Peach Topping, 42 g	45	0	11
Poached Eggs, 36 g	70	5	0
Potatoes O' Brien, 110 g	150	0	20
Sausage Gravy, 55 g	40	2	5
Sausage Links, 21 g	100	10	0
• Sautéed Bell Peppers, 28 g	15	1	2
Sautéed Onions, 28 g)	15	1	3
Scrambled Eggs, 62 g	120	10	0
Sliced Ham, 43 g	80	5	1
Strawberry Topping, 42 g	60	0	16
Waffles, 41 g	120	6	15

Dessert

	Cal	Fat	Cbs
Apple Crisp, 94 g	150	3	32
Apple Spice Cake, 63 g	180	7	26
Banana Nut Cake, 74 g	270	12	37
Banana Pudding, 90 g	150	5	24
• Banana Split, 175 g	340	6	58
Black Forest Cake, 60 g	150	6	20
Bread Pudding, 100 g	190	8	27
Butterfinger® Pieces, 15 g	70	3	11
Butterscotch Brownie, 38 g	170	9	20
Butterscotch Topping, 41 g	130	0	31
Cappuccino Cake, 65 g	180	10	18
Caramel Apple Crisp, 95 g	170	5	32
Carrot Cake, 64 g	240	12	29
Cheesecake, 80 g	230	12	28
Cheesecake, Cherry, 90 g	240	12	30
Cherry Cobbler, 100 g	210	9	32
Cherry Crisp, 94 g	160	3	32
Chewy Bears, 20 g	60	0	15

• MOST HEALTHY　• LEAST HEALTHY

COUNTRY BUFFET (cont.)

	Cal	Fat	Cbs
Chocolate Cake, 60 g	180	8	25
Chocolate Chip Cookie Bars, 65 g	290	13	39
Chocolate Chip Cookie Pizza, 35 g	160	8	21
Chocolate Chip Cookie, 26 g	130	6	18
Chocolate Chips, 15 g	90	5	10
Chocolate Cookie Pieces, Crushed, 8 g	35	2	6
Chocolate Cream Pie, 64 g	180	9	24
Chocolate Decadence Cake, 64 g	220	10	30
Chocolate Haystacks, 31 g	160	8	19
Chocolate Marble Cake, 60 g	190	8	26
Chocolate Pudding, 90 g	120	5	19
Chocolate Syrup, 39 g	100	0	25
Coconut Cream Pie, 64 g	240	12	24
• Cone, Ice Cream, 4 g	15	0	3
Cookies and Cream, 70 g	290	16	35
Crispy Rice Bar, 32 g	120	2	24
Crispy Rice Bar-Chocolate Drizzle, 33 g	130	3	25
Crispy Rice Bar-Fun E Chips, 32 g	120	2	25
Crispy Rice Bar-Sprinkles, 32 g	120	2	25
Crushed Pineapple, 32 g	25	0	6
Cupcakes: Black Forest Cupcake, 90 g	230	9	36
Cupcakes: Caramel Topped Cupcake, 90 g	310	16	38
Cupcakes: Chocolate Cupcake, 90 g	280	12	41
Cupcakes: Peach Cupcake, 90 g	260	13	33
Cupcakes: Rocky Road Cupcake, 90 g	310	16	38
Cupcakes: Wht Cupcake, decorated, 90 g	310	16	38
Decorated Cookies, 27 g	120	5	17
Dessert Pizza, 47 g	110	4	17
Dutch Apple Cake, 80 g	230	9	36
Flurries, vanilla soft serve, 174 g	260	10	40
Fudge Brownies, 56 g	200	6	34
Fudge, 10 g	40	2	7
Fun E Chips, 15 g	80	3	12
German Chocolate Cake, 80 g	270	13	35
Heath® Bar Bits, 15 g	80	5	9
Honey Nut Topping, 28 g	170	12	9
Hot Fudge Sundae Cake, 86 g	160	3	33
Hot Fudge Topping, 37 g	120	3	22
Iced Decorated Cookies, 42 g	190	9	25
Key Lime, 60 g	170	11	16
Ko Ko Bits, 15 g	70	4	10
Lemon Bars, 68 g	190	5	35
Lemon Cake, 60 g	190	10	24
Lemon Cream Pie, 64 g	170	4	32
Lemon Meringue Pie, 60 g	130	5	23
Malted Milk Balls, Ground, 15 g	70	3	11

• MOST HEALTHY   • LEAST HEALTHY

COUNTRY BUFFET (cont.)

	Cal	Fat	Cbs
Maple Walnut Cake, 63 g	240	15	24
Nestle® Crunch Pieces, 15 g	80	4	10
Oatmeal Raisin Cookies, 26 g	120	6	16
Orange Dreamsicle, 89 g	240	11	33
Peach Cobbler, 100 g	210	8	33
Peanut Butter Cookies, 26 g	120	6	14
Peanut Butter Mocha, 52 g	230	16	21
Pecan Pie, 74 g	310	19	33
Pumpkin Pie, 92 g	200	11	23
Reduced Sugar Apple Pie, 116 g	230	13	28
Reduced Sugar Banana Cream Pie, 91 g	180	11	20
Reduced Sugar Choco Cream Pie, 79 g	190	12	19
Reduced Sugar Pie-Cherry, 95 g	170	10	18
Reduced Sugar Pie-Lemon, 95 g	170	10	18
Reduced Sugar Pie-Lime, 95 g	170	10	18
Reduced Sugar Pie-Orange, 95 g	170	10	18
Reduced Sugar Pie-Raspberry, 95 g	170	10	18
Reduced Sugar Pie-Strawberry, 95 g	170	10	18
Red. Sugar/Calorie Choc Pudding, 86 g	70	1	12
Red. Sugar/Calorie Vanilla Pudding, 86 g	40	1	5
Rocky Road Pudding, 90 g	160	6	27
Scotcheroos, 39 g	180	7	27
Seven Layer Bar, 58 g	220	9	32
Snickerdoodle Cookie Pizza, 48 g	180	9	22
Snickerdoodle Cookies, 26 g	120	5	17
Soft Serve, Chocolate, 87 g	120	3	21
Soft Serve, Vanilla, 87 g	130	5	20
Sprinkles, 15 g	70	2	13
SS FroYo, Nonfat Orange Sorbet, 89 g	90	0	22
SS FroYo, Nonfat, NutraSweet,® Vanilla, 89 g	80	0	16
Strawberry Marble Cake, 63 g	200	10	26
Strawberry Mousse Cake, 74 g	190	11	22
Strawberry Topping, 39 g	60	0	15
Sugar Free Ranger Cookies, 20 g	90	5	10
Supreme Cake, 70 g	190	8	26
Sweet Potato Pie, 71 g	280	18	26
Tres Leches, 90 g	250	15	25
Turtle Brownies, 40 g	130	4	23
Vanilla Pudding, 90 g	130	5	20
Whipped Topping, 21 g	60	5	3
Dressings			
• Greek Vinaigrette, 30 g	130	13	1
Oriental Sesame, 30 g	90	5	12
• Raspberry Vinaigrette, fat free, 30 g	35	0	8
Entrées			
BBQ Beef, 57 g	70	3	8

• MOST HEALTHY   • LEAST HEALTHY

▶ COUNTRY BUFFET (cont.)

	Cal	Fat	Cbs
BBQ Beef Ribs, 143 g	300	23	7
BBQ Pork Ribs, 41 g	140	9	5
Beef Stroganoff, 140 g	190	8	19
Butter Crumb Alaskan Pollack, 50 g	110	5	2
Butterfly Shrimp, 11 g	35	2	4
Carved Ham, 85 g	100	5	0
Carved Grilled Pork Loin, 85 g	140	10	0
Carved Roast Beef, 85 g	230	15	0
Carved Rope Sausage, 85 g	270	24	3
Carved Salmon Filet, 85 g	190	11	0
Carved Sirloin Steak, 85 g	180	9	0
Chicken & Dumplings, 140 g	160	5	17
Chicken Strips, 56 g	170	10	10
Chinese Chicken Livers, 85 g	200	11	14
Clam Strips, 85 g	320	20	28
Country BBQ Chicken-breast, 165 g	310	16	6
Country BBQ Chicken-drumstick, 75 g	100	6	2
Country BBQ Chicken -wing, 58 g	80	5	3
Country BBQ Chicken-thigh, 122 g	180	11	5
Country Fried Steak-w/o Gravy, 62 g	210	13	15
Country Pasta Gratine, 140 g	160	4	24
Creamy Penne Carbonara, 140 g	250	15	20
Fire Grilled Chicken Alfredo, 140 g	220	14	14
Fried Catfish, 46 g	100	5	4
Fried Fish, 30 g	80	4	9
Fried Shrimp, 44 g	120	6	12
Grilled BBQ Pork Steak, 60 g	150	9	3
Grilled BBQ Smoked Sausage, 80 g	170	13	8
Grilled Cheese, 93 g	310	18	28
Grilled Italian Sausage Penne, 140 g	180	11	14
Grilled Pork Steak, 57 g	140	9	0
Grilled Smoked Sausage, 56 g	190	17	2
Grilled Teriyaki Pineapple Chicken, 85 g	130	6	6
• Hand Breaded Fried Chkn-breast, 154 g	360	22	0
Hand Breaded Fried Chkn-drumstick, 45 g	100	7	0
Hand Breaded Fried Chkn-thigh, 122 g	200	13	0
Hand Breaded Fried Chkn-wing, 58 g	90	6	0
Honey BBQ Pork Riblets, 34 g	120	9	3
Honey Glazed Baked Ham, 85 g	120	5	3
Italian Sausage, 80 g	150	13	3
Macaroni & Cheese, 100 g	110	3	18
Meatloaf, 85 g	180	11	7
New Orleans Bourbon Street Chkn, 85 g	180	8	9
Orange Chicken, 85 g	340	22	26
Oven Roasted Rotisserie Style Tkey, 85 g	100	4	1
Pepperoni & Sausage Calzone, 69 g	150	6	15

► COUNTRY BUFFET (cont.)

	Cal	Fat	Cbs
Perfect Pot Roast, 140 g	160	7	9
Pizza, Cheese, 76 g	150	4	22
Roasted Jerk Chicken-breast, 154 g	320	18	0
Roasted Jerk Chicken-drumstick, 45 g	100	7	0
Roasted Jerk Chicken-thigh, 122 g	180	11	0
Roasted Jerk Chicken-wing, 58 g	80	5	0
Rotisserie Chicken-breast, 154 g	310	17	1
Rotisserie Chicken-drumstick, 45 g	90	6	0
Rotisserie Chicken-thigh, 122 g	140	11	1
Rotisserie Chicken-wing, 58 g	80	5	0
Salisbury Steak, 100 g	150	9	8
• Sauerkraut, 28 g	5	0	1
Seafood Patties, 57 g	120	6	13
Shrimp Scampi, 140 g	280	15	20
Sizzling BBQ Beef Brisket, 85 g	170	6	6
Traditional Baked Chicken-breast, 154 g	310	17	1
Traditional Baked Chicken-drumstick, 45 g	80	6	1
Traditional Baked Chicken-thigh, 122 g	180	11	1
Traditional Baked Chicken-wing, 58 g	80	5	0
Turkey Hot Dogs, 56 g	130	11	2
Wood Seared Salmon, 85 g	220	16	0

Fruits

	Cal	Fat	Cbs
• Bananas, 70 g	60	0	16
• Cantaloupe, 85 g	25	0	6
Grapes, 80 g	60	0	15
Honeydew, 88 g	30	0	8
Orange Wedges, 70 g	30	0	8
Pineapple, 78 g	35	0	10
Strawberries, 72 g	25	0	6
Watermelon, 76 g	25	0	6

Gravies and Sauces

	Cal	Fat	Cbs
• Au Jus, 55 g	0	0	0
Beef Gravy, 55 g	25	1	4
Cheese Sauce, 62 g	45	2	7
Chicken Gravy, 55 g	30	0	5
Country Gravy, 55 g	50	2	7
Marinara Sauce, 70 g	30	1	5
Meat Sauce, 71 g	45	2	3
• Queso Dip, 62 g	50	2	8
Thick Cheese Sauce, 62 g	50	2	7
Turkey Gravy, 55 g	20	1	4
White Gravy, 55 g	50	2	7

Loaf Bread

	Cal	Fat	Cbs
• French, 25 g	70	1	14
• Pumpernickel, 25 g	60	1	12
Wheat, 25 g	70	1	12

▶ COUNTRY BUFFET (cont.)

	Cal	Fat	Cbs
Muffins			
• Apple Walnut, 73 g	220	8	34
Banana Walnut, 83 g	270	13	35
Blueberry, 80 g	230	9	34
Cherry, 77 g	240	9	35
Coconut Almond, 68 g	230	10	32
• Corn Muffin, 105 g	320	12	49
Cranberry Walnut, 79 g	250	11	34
Hot Fudge Chocolate Chip, 83 g	280	12	42
Hot Fudge Sundae, 91 g	290	12	43
Oatmeal Raisin, 81 g	270	10	43
Peach, 89 g	250	9	38
Pina Colada, 90 g	220	9	33
Poppy Seed. 66 g	220	10	29
Pumpkin w/ Raisins, 85 g	240	9	38
Rum Raisin, 76 g	240	8	40
Strawberry, 89 g	260	9	41
Zucchini, 72 g	220	9	32
Salad			
Ambrosia, 89 g	160	9	23
BLT Salad, 70 g	120	12	2
Broccoli Apple Salad, 100 g	160	11	13
Broccoli Bacon Salad, 100 g	180	13	14
Bruschetta Tomato Salad, 100 g	90	7	4
Caesar Salad, 65 g	70	6	4
California Coleslaw, 100 g	100	0	24
Carrot & Raisin Salad, 100 g	140	9	17
Chicken Caesar Salad, 72 g	90	7	3
Chicken Pasta Salad, 100 g	240	18	13
Corn Salsa, 85 g	60	1	14
Creamy Pea Salad, 100 g	180	15	10
Cucumber Tomato Salad, 100 g	30	1	4
Dilled Potato Salad, 83 g	110	8	10
Gelatin, 70 g	40	0	10
Gelatin Whip, 68 g	80	3	13
Greek Salad, 75 g	120	8	10
Italian Chopped Salad, 75 g	90	7	4
Italian Pasta Salad, 100 g	190	13	14
Macaroni Vegetable Salad, 100 g	240	16	21
Marinated Vegetables, 100 g	50	4	5
Oriental Chicken-without dressing, 72 g	50	2	6
Oriental Pasta, 100 g	150	8	14
Pickled Beets, 100 g	60	0	18
Potato Salad, 85 g	120	7	15
Prunes, Stewed, 71 g	100	0	27
Raisin Fluff, 80 g	120	4	21

• MOST HEALTHY   • LEAST HEALTHY

COUNTRY BUFFET (cont.)

	Cal	Fat	Cbs
• Seafood Salad, 117 g	310	26	15
Seven Layer Salad, 75 g	190	17	4
Sicilian Pasta Salad, 100 g	140	7	16
Spinach Salad, 57 g	90	7	3
• Spring Mix, 45 g	5	0	1
Strawberry Walnut Salad, 66 g	90	7	6
Strawberry Whip, 76 g	230	18	17
Strawberry-Banana Salad, 85 g	80	1	20
Tarragon Potato Salad, 82 g	120	7	13
Three Bean Salad, 100 g	90	5	12
Tossed Green Salad, 45 g	5	0	1
Waldorf Salad, 60 g	110	7	12

Salad Toppers

	Cal	Fat	Cbs
Bacon Bits, imitation, 7 g	30	1	2
Bacon Bits, real, 7 g	25	2	0
Broccoli, 10 g	5	0	1
Carrots, Matchsticks, 8 g	5	5	1
Cauliflower, 10 g	5	0	1
Cherry Peppers, 11 g	4	0	1
Cherry Tomatoes, 17 g	5	0	1
Chow Mein Noodles, 7 g	35	2	4
Cottage Cheese, 28 g	20	1	1
Crispy Noodles, 7 g	30	1	5
Croutons, 7 g	35	1	4
• Cucumbers, sliced, 15 g	2	0	1
Diced Eggs, 15 g	20	2	0
• Feta Cheese, 40 g	110	9	2
Garbanzo Beans, 15 g	10	0	2
Imitation Shredded Cheese, 10 g	20	1	2
Kidney Beans, 15 g	10	0	2
Mushrooms, 10 g	2	0	1
Olives, 15 g	15	2	1
Parmesan Cheese, 7 g	30	2	0
Peaches, sliced, 15 g	10	0	2
Peas, 15 g	10	0	2
Peel & Eat Shrimp, 9 g	5	0	0
Pepperoncini, 11 g	2	0	1
Radishes, 10 g	2	0	1
Raisins, 12 g	40	0	10
Red Onions, sliced, 6 g	2	0	1
Spinach Leaves, 32 g	5	0	1
Sunflower Seeds, 11 g	70	5	2

Sides

	Cal	Fat	Cbs
AuGratin Potatoes, 110 g	120	7	10
Baked Potatoes, 130 g	150	0	36
BBQ Baked Beans, 85 g	130	3	26

• MOST HEALTHY   • LEAST HEALTHY

COUNTRY BUFFET (cont.)

	Cal	Fat	Cbs
Broccoli Florets (fresh), 85 g	25	0	6
Broccoli Florets and Cheese Sauce, 85 g	50	2	8
Broccoli/Cauliflower Medley, 85 g	25	0	6
Cajun Dirty Rice, 70 g	90	2	16
Candied Yams, 118 g	140	2	33
Cauliflower AuGratin, 85 g	50	2	8
Cheesy Hashbrowns, 100 g	140	9	10
Collard Greens w/Bacon, 110 g	40	3	3
• Corn Bread Dressing, 100 g	220	13	22
Corn on the Cob, 130 g	80	3	13
French Fries, 60 g	170	9	23
Fried Okra, 85 g	220	12	28
Fried Rice w/Ham, 100 g	130	6	14
German Boiled Cabbage, 85 g	40	3	4
Green Bean Casserole, 110 g	100	7	9
• Green Beans, 85 g	15	0	3
Green Beans El Greco, 85 g	20	0	6
Green Cabbage, 85 g	70	5	6
Grilled Cowboy Potatoes, 100 g	180	9	23
Grilled Vegetables, 85 g	40	3	4
Jo Jo Potatoes, 82 g	160	8	22
Joe's Cracked Ppr Green Beans w/Bacon, 85 g	70	5	6
Mashed Potatoes, 110 g	70	1	13
Montreal Vegetable Medley, 85 g	50	5	3
Potato Skins, 14 g	80	5	7
Ranch Red Potatoes, 100 g	100	5	16
Risotto Style Rice, 70 g	100	4	15
Sautéed Zucchini, 85 g	50	4	4
Seasoned Green Beans, 85 g	40	2	6
Spaghetti, 100 g	150	3	27
Spanish Rice, 70 g	140	7	9
Spinach Marie, 110 g	190	14	8
Squash, 85 g	150	9	18
Steamed Carrots, 85 g	40	3	7
Steamed Corn, 85 g	90	3	17
Steamed Red Potatoes, 100 g	90	5	15
Vegetable Rice Pilaf, 70 g	60	0	14
White Rice, 70 g	90	0	20

Soup

	Cal	Fat	Cbs
Chicken Noodle Soup, 123 g	80	2	8
Chicken Rice Soup, 123 g	60	2	5
• Chicken Tortilla Soup, 123 g	40	1	5
Chili Bean Soup, 123 g	80	4	9
Corn Chowder, 123 g	80	4	12
Cream of Broccoli Soup, 123 g	80	6	6
Creamy Tomato Basil Soup, 123 g	60	1	11

• MOST HEALTHY   • LEAST HEALTHY

COUNTRY BUFFET (cont.)

	Cal	Fat	Cbs
French Onion Soup, 123 g	40	2	5
Italian Sausage & Bean Soup, 123 g	50	3	6
Minestrone Soup, 123 g	60	1	11
Navy Bean Soup w/Ham, 123 g	50	1	9
• New England Clam Chowder, 123 g	150	11	12
Potato Cheese Soup, 123 g	120	9	9
Vegetable Beef Soup, 123 g	50	2	7

Taco Bar

	Cal	Fat	Cbs
Beef Taco Meat, 57 g	50	3	2
Chicken Chilaquiles, 100 g	240	13	9
Chicken Fajita, 85 g	150	12	3
Chicken Quesadillas, 49 g	110	7	6
Chicken Taco Meat, 57 g	70	3	1
Diced Onions, 15 g	5	0	2
Diced Tomatoes, 15 g	5	0	1
• Enchiladas, all, 148 g	250	18	12
Fried Jalapeños, 14 g	10	1	1
Jalapeños, 11 g	2	0	1
King's Ranch Chicken, 100 g	200	10	21
• Lettuce, shredded, 14 g	0	0	0
Mexican Rice, 70 g	60	0	13
Nacho Chips, 14 g	70	4	9
Pico de Gallo, 30 g	10	0	3
Pinto Beans w/Bacon, 85 g	70	2	13
Potato Con Queso, 100 g	120	6	17
Red Beans w/Ham, 85 g	50	2	8
Refried Beans, 85 g	80	3	12
Salsa, 30 g	10	0	2
Shredded Cheddar Cheese, 10 g	40	4	0
Sliced Tomatoes, 15 g	2	0	1
Steak Fajita, 85 g	120	6	2
Taco Shell Baskets, 32 g	160	8	20
Taco Shells, 11 g	50	3	7
Tostadas, 32 g	110	6	14

COUSINS SUBS

7 1/2" Subs

	Cal	Fat	Cbs
BLT, 225 g	591	38	47
Cheese Steak, 290 g	503	19	49
Chicken Breast, 314 g	569	27	50
Chicken Cheddar Deluxe, 330 g	669	39	51
Club, 306 g	646	35	51
Double Cheese Steak, 393 g	747	36	49
• Garden Veggie, 253 g	390	12	51
Gyro, 344 g	710	41	61
Ham & Provolone, 256 g	604	34	50

• MOST HEALTHY   • LEAST HEALTHY

COUSINS SUBS (cont.)

	Cal	Fat	Cbs
Hot Veggie, 277 g	472	17	55
• Italian Special, 343 g	817	51	50
Meatball & Provolone, 280 g	723	38	54
Pepperoni Melt, 279 g	722	45	50
Philly Cheese Steak, 326 g	531	19	55
Pizza Sub, 324 g	709	39	55
Roast Beef, 301 g	607	30	50
Seafood with Crab, 314 g	642	38	60
Three Cheese, 276 g	685	44	50
Tuna, 263 g	643	38	49
Turkey Breast, 249 g	531	28	50
Better Bunch Salads			
Chef Salad, 198 g	125	3	9
Garden Salad, 113 g	34	0	7
• Garden Salad w/ Chkn Breast, 227 g	148	1	9
• Side Salad, 96 g	19	0	4
Better Bunch Subs (7½")			
Chicken Breast, 286 g	366	2	50
Club, 256 g	370	5	51
• Garden Veggie, 218 g	266	2	50
Ham, 206 g	328	4	50
Hot Veggie, 223 g	287	2	55
• Roast Beef, 272 g	405	6	50
Turkey Breast, 220 g	329	3	50
Breads			
7½" Garlic Herb Bread, 97 g	240	2	44
7½" Italian Bread, 96 g	240	2	44
• 7½" Parmesan-Asiago Bread, 98 g	248	2	45
7½" Wheat Bread, 96 g	240	3	44
• Flour Tortilla Wraps, 71 g	210	5	36
Limited Time Specials (7½")			
Chicken Salad, 314 g	556	23	62
• Deli Classic, 293 g	642	28	56
Ham & Salami Italiano, 231 g	497	21	51
• Horseradish Dijon Ham, 211 g	451	18	51
Hot Ham & Jack, 218 g	471	20	48
Hot Pepperoni Jack, 204 g	554	29	50
Steak Reuben, 276 g	619	30	50
Turkey Jalapeño Ranch, 229 g	468	20	49
Wisconsin Ham & Cheddar, 225 g	477	16	57
Salads			
Chef Salad, 248 g	327	14	25
Garden Salad, 163 g	235	11	23
Garden Salad w/ Chicken Breast, 276 g	349	12	25
Italian Salad, 255 g	403	24	24
Seafood Salad, 248 g	315	11	34

▶ COUSINS SUBS (cont.)

	Cal	Fat	Cbs
• Side Salad, 124 g	135	6	14
• Tuna Salad, 284 g	623	46	23

Sides & Other

	Cal	Fat	Cbs
Chocolate Chip Cookie, 43 g	210	11	26
Chocolate Chip with M&M's, 43 g	190	9	26
Coconut Toffee Chip Cookie, 43 g	200	9	23
Double Chocolate Chip Cookie, 43 g	190	9	25
• French Fries (Medium), 113 g	367	19	43
Oatmeal Cranberry Walnut Cookie, 43 g	170	7	25
• Oatmeal Raisin Cookie, 43 g	170	7	25
PntBtr w/ Reese's Pieces Cookie, 43 g	210	11	22
Snickerdoodle Cookie, 43 g	190	9	25
Sugar Cookie, 43 g	180	8	26
Wht Chunk Macadamia Nut Cookie, 43 g	200	11	24

Soups (Regular)

	Cal	Fat	Cbs
Beef Steak & Noodle Soup, 198 g	105	3	12
Cheddar Cauliflower Soup, 198 g	114	5	13
Cheddar Cheese Soup, 198 g	201	11	18
Chicken & Dumplings Soup, 198 g	149	4	17
Chicken Noodle Soup, 198 g	114	4	16
• Chicken with Wild Rice Soup, 198 g	219	9	13
Chili, 198 g	219	8	26
Cream of Broccoli with Chz Soup, 198 g	166	7	13
Cream of Mushroom Soup, 198 g	193	11	13
Cream of Potato Soup, 198 g	166	8	21
Eight Bean Soup with Ham, 198 g	105	1	18
Fiesta Tortilla Soup with Chicken, 198 g	114	5	11
New England Clam Chowder, 198 g	149	3	25
Tomato Basil with Raviolini, 198 g	96	1	19
• Vegetable Beef, 198 g	70	2	11

▶ CULVER'S

ButterBurgers

	Cal	Fat	Cbs
• ButterBurger "The Original," Single, 5 oz.	346	12	35
ButterBurger Cheese, Single, 6 oz.	398	16	36
• Culver's Bacon Deluxe, Single, 8 oz.	573	34	34
Culver's Deluxe, Single, 8 oz.	494	27	34
Cheddar ButterBurger, Single, 5 oz.	421	19	31
Chdr ButterBurger w/ Bacon, Single, 6 oz.	541	29	31
Mushroom & Swiss, Single, 6 oz.	431	20	33
Sourdough Cheddar Melt, Single, 6 oz.	413	20	33
Wisconsin Swiss Melt, Single, 6 oz.	403	20	33

Classic Sundaes

	Cal	Fat	Cbs
• Banana Split, 2 Scoop, 18 oz.	1084	64	115
• Bananas Foster Sundae, 1 Scoop, 8 oz.	421	20	53
Caramel Apple Pecan Sundae, 1 Sc, 7 oz.	517	30	55

• MOST HEALTHY   • LEAST HEALTHY

CULVER'S (cont.)	Cal	Fat	Cbs
Caramel Cashew, 1 Scoop, 7 oz.	586	33	58
Fudge Pecan Sundae, 1 Scoop, 7 oz.	606	42	51
Turtle Sundae, 1 Scoop, 7 oz.	606	41	53
Concrete Mixers (Medium)			
Chocolate Concrete Mixer, 16 oz.	996	49	122
• Turtle Concrete, 15 oz.	1156	71	114
• Vanilla Concrete Mixer, 13 oz.	836	49	82
Condiments			
American Cheese, Slice	50	5	0
Bacon, Slice	40	4	0
• Dill Pickles, Sliced	1	0	0
Horseradish Sauce, 1 oz.	150	14	6
Picante Sauce, Mild & Medium, 1 oz.	10	0	2
Shrimp Cocktail Sauce, 2 oz.	50	0	12
Steak Sauce	10	0	2
Sweet & Sour Dipping Sauce, 2 oz.	90	0	23
• Tartar Sauce, 1 oz.	188	18	1
Cones and Frozen Custard			
Chocolate Cake Cone, 1 Scoop, 5 oz.	319	14	40
Choco Dipped Waffle Cone, 1 Scp, 7 oz.	533	24	72
Chocolate Frozen Custard, 1 Pint, 14 oz.	819	39	98
Chocolate, Dish, 1 Scoop, 5 oz.	294	14	35
Chocolate, Waffle Cone, 1 Scoop, 6 oz.	384	15	55
Mini Scoop Chocolate Cake Cone, 3 oz.	193	8	25
Mini Scoop Vanilla Cake Cone, 3 oz.	201	10	22
NSA Caramel Fudge Swirl, 3 oz.	205	11	30
Oreo Frozen Custard Snd, Choco, 4 oz.	277	12	40
Oreo Frozen Custard Snd, Mint, 4 oz.	284	14	37
Oreo Frozen Custard Snd, Vanilla, 4 oz.	284	14	37
• Plain Cake Cone	25	0	5
Plain Waffle Cone, 1 oz.	90	1	20
Vanilla Cake Cone, 1 Scoop, 5 oz.	333	13	35
• Vanilla Frozen Custard, 1 Pint, 14 oz.	858	51	84
Vanilla, Choco Dipped Waffle Cone, 1 Scp, 7 oz.	547	28	67
Vanilla, Dish, 1 Scoop, 5 oz.	308	18	30
Vanilla, Waffle Cone, 1 Scoop, 6 oz.	398	19	50
Dinners			
Angus Chicken Fried Steak Dinner, 20 oz.	880	42	87
• Beef Pot Roast Dinner, 22 oz.	769	39	73
Butterfly Crispy Shrimp, 6 piece, 18 oz.	1285	62	151
Chopped Steak Dinner, 23 oz.	873	52	64
Fresh Fried Chicken, 2 piece, 25 oz.	1755	94	140
• North Atlantic Cod Filet, 2 piece, 23 oz.	1831	116	135
Favorites			
Angus Philly Steak Sandwich, 9 oz.	468	21	35
Beef Pot Roast Sandwich, 6 oz.	363	12	33

• MOST HEALTHY   • LEAST HEALTHY

▶ CULVER'S (cont.)

	Cal	Fat	Cbs
Cheese Hot Dog, 5 oz.	407	26	26
Chicken Tenders, Breaded, 4 piece, 6 oz.	440	20	32
Chili Dog with Bun, 6 oz.	379	24	28
Crispy Chicken Filet Sandwich, 8 oz.	578	35	50
• Flame Roasted Chicken Sandwich, 7 oz.	308	9	36
Grilled Ham 'N' Swiss on Rye, 8 oz.	497	25	33
Grilled Reuben Melt, 11 oz.	588	31	41
Hot Dog, 7 oz.	392	22	38
• North Atlantic Cod Filet Sandwich, 9 oz.	663	40	47
Pork Tenderloin Sandwich, 9 oz.	593	26	62
Shaved Prime Rib, 9 oz.	570	33	35
Turkey BLT, 9 oz.	562	31	36
Turkey, Stacked, Sandwich, 8 oz.	450	19	47

Garden Fresh Salads

	Cal	Fat	Cbs
Caesar w/ Flame Roasted Chkn, 10 oz.	340	16	14
• Chkn Cashew w/ Flame Roasted Chkn, 12 oz.	443	24	19
Garden Fresco, 9 oz.	229	10	19
• Side Caesar, 3 oz.	54	2	5
Side Salad, 3 oz.	60	2	6

Malts • Shakes • Floats (Medium)

	Cal	Fat	Cbs
• Chocolate Malt, 16 oz.	968	45	122
Chocolate Shake, 16 oz.	912	44	114
Culver's Root Beer Float, 20 oz.	548	18	90
• Old Fashioned Cherry Soda, 16 oz.	516	25	63
Vanilla Malt, 14 oz.	872	45	98
Vanilla Shake, 13 oz.	752	44	74

Salad Dressings

	Cal	Fat	Cbs
Raspberry Vinaigrette Reduced Calorie, 2 oz.	45	0	11
Sesame Ginger Dressing, 2 oz.	70	0	16

Scoopie Kid's Meals

	Cal	Fat	Cbs
ButterBurger, 5 oz.	346	12	35
• ButterBurger, Cheese, 6 oz.	396	16	36
• Chicken Tenders, Breaded, 2 piece, 3 oz.	220	10	16
Corn Dog, 3 oz.	260	14	26
Crinkle Cut Fries, 4 oz.	275	12	38
Grilled Cheese, 4 oz.	290	14	33
Hot Dog with Bun, 5 oz.	366	22	30

Sides

	Cal	Fat	Cbs
Chili Cheddar Fries, 9 oz.	607	29	72
Cole Slaw, 5 oz.	350	21	37
Crinkle Cut Fries, Regular, 5 oz.	385	17	53
Dairyland Cheese Curds, 7 oz.	670	38	54
Dinner Roll, 2 oz.	140	6	19
Green Beans, 5 oz.	150	13	8
• Mashed Potatoes, 6 oz.	120	1	24
Onion Rings, Breaded, 7 oz.	630	36	70

• MOST HEALTHY   • LEAST HEALTHY

CULVER'S (cont.)

	Cal	Fat	Cbs
Soups			
Baja Chicken Enchilada, 11 oz.	352	23	21
Bean with Ham, 11 oz.	190	3	33
Boston Clam Chowder, 11 oz.	252	11	25
Broccoli Cheese with Florets, 11 oz.	240	14	16
Cauliflower Cheese, 11 oz.	252	14	23
Cheddar Brat Soup, 11 oz.	380	25	26
Cheesy Chicken Tortilla, 11 oz.	180	7	16
Chicken & Dumpling, 11 oz.	300	22	19
Chicken Gumbo, 11 oz.	120	6	13
Chicken Noodle, 11 oz.	112	2	14
Corn Chowder, 11 oz.	276	13	35
Cream of Broccoli, 11 oz.	185	10	16
French Onion, 11 oz.	129	7	11
George's Chili, 11 oz.	336	18	27
Italian Style Wedding, 11 oz.	275	6	44
Lumberjack Mixed Vegetable, 11 oz.	150	6	21
• Minestrone, 11 oz.	100	1	19
Mushroom Medley, 11 oz.	252	16	20
Oven Roasted Turkey Noodle, 11 oz.	175	5	21
Potato Au Gratin, 11 oz.	350	22	28
Potato with Bacon, 11 oz.	225	9	28
Split Pea with Ham, 11 oz.	262	9	32
Stuffed Green Pepper with Beef, 11 oz.	150	3	25
Tomato Basil Ravioletti, 11 oz.	112	3	18
Tomato Florentine, 11 oz.	112	1	21
Vegetable Beef & Barley, 11 oz.	112	4	14
• Wild & Brown Rice with Chicken, 11 oz.	452	22	27
Wisconsin Cheese, 11 oz.	375	24	29
Special Treats			
Cookie Dough Craving Concrete Cake, 4 oz.	273	15	32
Cookies & Cream Concrete Cake, 4 oz.	245	14	26
Cooler, 392 g	168	0	42
• Lemon Ice Smoothie, 228 g	360	16	50
• Lemon Ice, 1 Scoop, 196 g	84	0	21
Turtle Concrete Cake, 4 oz.	280	17	30
Toppings			
Almond	84	8	3
Andes Creme De Menthe Thins, 1 oz.	151	10	16
Blackberry	14	0	4
Blueberry	17	0	4
• Brownie Pieces, 3 oz.	361	16	52
Butterfinger®, 1 oz.	110	5	18
Butterscotch	43	0	10
Cashew	90	7	4
Cheesecake Pieces, 3 oz.	300	18	30

CULVER'S (cont.)

	Cal	Fat	Cbs
Cherry, Red	20	0	5
Chocolate Chip Cookie Dough, 1 oz.	120	5	17
Chocolate Flake, 1 oz.	142	9	17
Culver's Chocolate Syrup, 1 oz.	64	0	16
Culver's Hot Caramel	44	1	9
Culver's Hot Fudge	44	1	8
Flat Pie Chips, 1 oz.	144	8	16
Heath® Toffee Chunks, 1 oz.	155	9	17
M&M Minis, 1 oz.	140	7	18
Marshmallow Creme	39	0	10
Mint	45	1	10
Nestle Crunch, 1 oz.	140	7	19
Novelty Coating	87	7	6
Oreo® Cookie Crumbs	62	2	9
Peach	15	0	4
Peanut Butter, 1 oz.	179	15	6
Pecan Halves	100	11	2
Pineapple	20	0	5
Raspberry	18	0	4
Reese's Pieces® Minis, 1 oz.	142	7	16
Reese's® Peanut Butter Cups, 1 oz.	150	9	16
Snickers® Candy Bar Pieces	67	4	8
Spanish Peanuts, 1 oz.	160	14	5
Sprinkles, Blue and White, 1 oz.	140	7	21
• Strawberry, Sliced	13	0	3

D'ANGELO

Dressing

	Cal	Fat	Cbs
• Balsamic, 85 g	180	18	9
• Creamy Italian, 85 g	350	36	7
Greek, 85 g	230	26	6

Kids

	Cal	Fat	Cbs
Cheeseburger Sub, 128 g	300	13	32
• Cookie Chocolate Chip, 43 g	170	6	26
Ham & Cheese Sub, 103 g	230	5	32
• Kidz Tuna Sub, 113 g	390	24	30
Meatball Sub, 153 g	340	16	37

Pokket Bread

	Cal	Fat	Cbs
Plain, 79 g	190	1	37

Pokkets

	Cal	Fat	Cbs
BLT & Cheese, 283 g	440	22	39
Caesar Salad, 298 g	560	37	47
Capicola & Cheese, 152 g	330	12	32
Cheese, 176 g	510	27	38
Cheeseburger, 237 g	460	23	35
Chicken Caesar Salad, 390 g	680	39	48

• MOST HEALTHY   • LEAST HEALTHY

▶ D'ANGELO (cont.)

	Cal	Fat	Cbs
Chicken Club, 275 g	550	30	34
Chicken Honey Dijon, 301 g	460	14	42
Chicken Salad, 184 g	600	41	31
Chicken Stir Fry, 283 g	400	10	39
Classic Vegetable, 288 g	360	13	43
Classic Veggie No Cheese, 241 g	200	1	40
• Greek, 450 g	750	55	46
Grilled Chicken, 261 g	300	5	35
Ham, 123 g	220	2	33
Ham & Cheese, 151 g	310	8	35
Ham & Salami, 148 g	380	18	32
Hamburger, 218 g	390	18	34
Italian, 152 g	440	24	32
Lobster, 255 g	490	26	34
Meatball, 346 g	600	32	52
Mortadella & Cheese, 151 g	530	32	33
Number 9, 329 g	530	22	39
Pastrami & Cheese, 213 g	540	33	33
Pepperoni, 131 g	400	21	32
Roast Beef, 149 g	250	4	32
• Salad, 298 g	190	1	39
Salami & Cheese, 162 g	500	31	31
Steak, 272 g	510	22	32
Steak & Cheese, 244 g	500	22	34
Steak Bomb, 343 g	590	28	43
Tuna, 184 g	630	46	31
Turkey, 149 g	260	1	31
Turkey Club, 283 g	360	8	32
Quesadillas			
Chicken Stir Fry, 223 g	360	15	31
• Number 9, 223 g	380	19	31
• Salsa, 57 g	20	0	0
Sour Cream, 57 g	110	9	2
Veggie, 223 g	290	13	33
Salad Entree			
Antipasto, 442 g	270	17	18
Caesar, 354 g	620	54	28
Chicken Caesar, 432 g	670	53	21
Chicken Stir Fry, 366 g	170	4	11
Cobb, 408 g	330	18	14
• Greek, 530 g	780	70	23
Greek no dressing, 445 g	320	22	20
Lobster, 415 g	380	25	12
Roast Beef, 352 g	140	4	11
• Tossed, 308 g	60	0	13
Turkey, 366 g	170	1	10

• MOST HEALTHY   • LEAST HEALTHY

D'ANGELO (cont.)

	Cal	Fat	Cbs
Soup (Small)			
Beef Stew, 227 g	220	8	23
Broccoli & Cheddar, 227 g	250	19	12
Chicken Noodle, 227 g	110	3	14
• Hearty Vegetable, 227 g	40	0	7
Italian Wedding, 227 g	120	6	11
• Lobster Bisque, 227 g	360	29	16
NE Clam Chowder, 227 g	320	18	31
Portuguese Kale, 227 g	130	5	16
Subs (Medium)			
Honey Wheat Roll, 139 g	340	6	62
Traditional Sub Roll, 139 g	370	4	73
Subs: One Pounder			
Number 9, 843 g	1460	64	105
• Steak, 595 g	1180	52	74
Steak and Cheese, 633 g	1300	61	78
• Steak Bomb, 896 g	1590	76	101
Subs (Small)			
Baked Stuffed Lobster, 243 g	640	33	54
BLT & Cheese, 258 g	500	23	51
Capicola & Cheese, 166 g	400	14	46
Cheese, 190 g	580	29	52
Cheeseburger, 251 g	530	25	49
Chicken Club, 289 g	620	32	48
Chicken Honey Dijon, 316 g	530	15	56
Chicken Salad, 198 g	670	43	45
Chicken Stir Fry, 297 g	470	12	53
Classic Veggie, 310 g	450	15	60
Grilled Chicken, 254 g	370	7	48
Ham, 208 g	300	4	49
Ham & Cheese, 165 g	380	10	49
Ham & Salami, 163 g	450	19	46
Hamburger, 232 g	460	20	48
Italian, 173 g	530	26	50
Lobster, 255 g	560	27	47
Lobster Roll, 184 g	390	22	24
Meatball, 360 g	670	34	66
Meatball & Cheese, 391 g	780	42	67
Mortadella & Cheese, 165 g	590	33	47
Number 9, 343 g	600	24	53
Pastrami & Cheese, 227 g	610	34	47
Pepperoni, 172 g	600	34	47
Roast Beef, 163 g	320	5	46
• Salad, 397 g	280	3	56
Salami & Cheese, 176 g	570	33	45

▶ D'ANGELO (cont.)	Cal	Fat	Cbs
Steak, 237 g	500	17	49
Steak & Cheese, 265 g	590	24	52
Steak Bomb, 343 g	630	29	51
Surf n' Turf, 373 g	800	40	55
Toasted Pastrami, 298 g	750	47	54
Toasted RB & Cheddar, 308 g	600	27	55
• Toasted Spicy MB, 453 g	860	49	68
Toasted Tuna & Swiss, 283 g	810	56	48
Toasted Turkey & Ham, 280 g	570	26	49
Toasted Turkey Thanksgiving, 234 g	620	17	81
Tuna, 198 g	700	48	45
Turkey, 163 g	330	3	45
Turkey Club, 266 g	420	10	48
Toppings			
American Cheese, 28 g	90	7	3
Bacon, 14 g	80	7	0
Buffalo Sauce, 28 g	10	0	0
Cheese Cheddar White, 28 g	110	9	1
Cucumber, 28 g	5	0	1
Hot Peppers, 21 g	0	0	1
Lettuce, 28 g	5	0	1
Mushrooms, 28 g	5	0	1
Olive Oil Blend, 36 g	70	2	17
Onions, 30 g	20	1	2
• Pickles, 27 g	240	27	0
Provolone Cheese, 14 g	5	0	1
• Sweet Peppers, 14 g	0	0	0
Swiss Cheese, 28 g	100	9	0
Tomato, 28 g	10	0	2
Turkey Gravy, 28 g	110	8	1
Vinegar, 60 g	10	0	2
Wraps			
BLT & Cheese, 266 g	590	30	55
Buffalo Chicken Salad, 415 g	810	45	65
Caesar Salad, 284 g	710	45	64
Capicola & Cheese, 191 g	480	21	50
Cheese, 215 g	670	36	56
Cheeseburger, 222 g	600	31	52
Chicken Caesar Salad, 401 g	830	48	65
Chicken Club, 328 g	710	39	53
Chicken Cobb, 464 g	910	54	72
Chicken Filet & Bacon, 335 g	710	39	53
Chicken Honey Dijon, 355 g	620	22	61
Chicken Salad, 223 g	760	49	49
Chicken Stir Fry, 322 g	550	19	57
Classic Veggie, 328 g	520	22	61

• MOST HEALTHY   • LEAST HEALTHY

D'ANGELO (cont.)

	Cal	Fat	Cbs
• Greek, 489 g	910	64	65
Grilled Chicken, 215 g	440	13	50
Ham & Cheese, 190 g	470	17	54
Ham & Salami, 199 g	550	26	50
Hamburger, 226 g	600	31	50
• Honey Wheat, 110 g	310	8	55
Italian, 191 g	600	33	50
Lobster, 294 g	650	34	52
Meatball, 385 g	760	41	70
Mortadella & Cheese, 190 g	680	40	52
Number 9, 368 g	680	31	58
Pastrami, 252 g	700	41	52
Pepperoni, 170 g	560	30	50
Plain, 110 g	310	9	49
Roast Beef, 188 g	410	12	50
Salad, 422 g	360	9	60
Salami & Cheese, 197 g	640	38	49
Steak, 311 g	670	30	50
Steak & Cheese, 283 g	660	31	53
Steak Bomb, 368 g	720	36	55
Tuna, 223 g	780	55	49
Turkey, 188 g	410	10	49
Turkey Club, 310 g	510	17	53

DAIRY QUEEN

Arctic Rush®

	Cal	Fat	Cbs
Arctic Rush, All Flavors - Medium, 595 g	310	0	63

Baskets

	Cal	Fat	Cbs
• Chkn Strip Basket™ w/ Country Gravy, 432 g	1360	63	103
Iron Grld Chkn Quesadilla Basket, 425 g	1070	50	117
Iron Grld Veg Quesadilla Basket, 396 g	1020	49	114
• Popcorn Shrimp Basket, 425 g	990	49	115

Blizzard® Treats (Medium)

	Cal	Fat	Cbs
Banana Cream Pie Blizzard, 385 g	780	30	115
• Banana Split Blizzard, 382 g	570	16	93
Butterfinger Blizzard, 383 g	740	26	114
Cappuccino Heath Blizzard, 411 g	870	38	122
Cherry CheeseQuake Blizzard, 361 g	690	28	92
Choco Cherry Love Blizzard, 382 g	730	33	94
Chocolate Chip Blizzard, 383 g	880	50	96
Chocolate Xtreme Blizzard, 392 g	980	44	130
Cookie Dough Blizzard, 446 g	1010	40	148
French Silk Pie Blizzard, 378 g	920	44	117
Georgia Mud Fudge Blizzard, 390 g	1010	54	114
Hawaiian Blizzard, 383 g	600	21	92
Heath Blizzard, 411 g	920	41	126

• MOST HEALTHY • LEAST HEALTHY

▶ DAIRY QUEEN (cont.)

	Cal	Fat	Cbs
M&M's Chocolate Candy Blizzard, 397 g	840	29	127
Mint Oreo Blizzard, 362 g	740	25	116
Mocha Chip Blizzard, 390 g	810	37	107
Oreo CheeseQuake Blizzard, 369 g	820	35	108
Oreo Cookies Blizzard, 334 g	680	25	100
PntBtr Butterfinger Blizzard, 399 g	1050	54	122
Reese's PntBtr Cups Blizzard, 371 g	760	31	101
Snickers Blizzard, 397 g	850	33	123
Strawberry CheeseQuake Blizzard, 371 g	690	28	92
Tropical Blizzard, 376 g	750	40	87
• Turtle Pecan Cluster Blizzard, 425 g	1050	54	127

Breakfast

	Cal	Fat	Cbs
Biscuits and Gravy, 369 g	820	47	87
Bacon Biscuit Sandwich, 146 g	480	31	37
Country Platter w/ Bacon, 350 g	1070	66	92
Country Platter w/ Ham, 404 g	1100	64	97
• Country Platter w/ Sausage, 432 g	1360	91	95
Ham Biscuit Sandwich, 163 g	460	28	38
Pancake Platter w/ Bacon, 148 g	400	13	57
• Pancake Platter w/ Ham, 187 g	380	8	59
Pancake Platter w/ Sausage, 187 g	530	25	57
Sausage Biscuit Sandwich, 163 g	540	37	37
Sausage Biscuit Twin Pack, 213 g	940	64	71
Ultimate Breakfast Burrito, 282 g	660	36	59
Ultimate Hash Browns w/ Bacon, 372 g	750	49	45
Ultimate Hash Browns w/ Ham, 412 g	740	45	47
Ult Hash Browns w/ Sausage, 411 g	880	62	45

Burgers

	Cal	Fat	Cbs
1/4 lb Bacon Cheddar GrillBurger™, 222 g	650	35	41
1/2 lb GrillBurger, 290 g	720	40	42
• 1/2 lb GrillBurger w/ Cheese, 323 g	870	51	42
1/4 lb Classic GrillBurger w/ Chz, 224 g	560	28	42
1/4 lb FlameThrower GrillBurger, 238 g	780	52	41
Classic GrillBurger, 205 g	470	21	42
Original Bacon Double Chzburger, 245 g	730	41	35
Original Cheeseburger, 156 g	400	18	34
Original Double Cheeseburger, 226 g	640	34	34
Original Double Hamburger, 198 g	540	26	33
• Original Hamburger, 142 g	350	14	33

DQ Cones (Medium)

	Cal	Fat	Cbs
Chocolate Cone, 199 g	340	10	54
• Dipped Cone, Butterscotch, 220 g	490	23	59
Dipped Cone, Cherry, 220 g	480	24	59
Dipped Cone, Chocolate, 220 g	470	22	60
• Vanilla Cone, 199 g	330	10	53

▶ DAIRY QUEEN (cont.)

	Cal	Fat	Cbs
DQ® Cakes			
• Choco Xtreme Blizzard Cake, 1/10 sl., 312 g	820	33	97
Cookie Dough Blizzard Cake, 1/10 sl., 311 g	760	34	103
DQ Cake, 10", 1/10 slice, 255 g	500	19	72
• DQ Heart Cake, 1/10 slice, 143 g	290	11	42
DQ Log Cake, 1/8 slice, 142 g	310	12	44
DQ Sheet Cake, 1/24 slice, 154 g	320	12	47
Oreo Blizzard Cake, 1/10 slice, 297 g	720	31	97
Reese's PntBtr Cups Blizzard Cake, 1/10 sl., 299 g	730	34	93
Strwbry ChzQuake Blizzard Cake, 1/10 sl., 314 g	630	27	84
DQ® Sundaes			
Sundae, Banana, 234 g	330	10	53
Sundae, Caramel, 234 g	430	11	75
Sundae, Cherry, 234 g	350	10	58
Sundae, Chocolate, 234 g	400	10	70
• Sundae, Hot Fudge, 234 g	440	14	66
Sundae, Marshmallow, 234 g	410	10	72
Sundae, Pineapple, 234 g	340	10	54
Sundae, Strawberry, 248 g	350	10	55
Hot Dogs			
All-Beef Cheese Dog, 94 g	290	19	19
• All-Beef Chili Cheese Dog, 158 g	430	22	39
All-Beef Chili Dog, 125 g	290	17	24
• All-Beef Hot Dog, 96 g	250	14	21
Iron Grilled Sandwiches			
Iron Grilled Classic Club Snd, 239 g	580	29	43
• Iron Grilled Supreme BLT Snd, 172 g	590	33	42
• Iron Grilled Turkey Sandwich, 233 g	530	25	42
Kids' Meals			
All-Beef Hot Dog Kids' Meal w/ Applesauce, 236 g	380	18	47
All-Beef Hot Dog Kids' Meal w/ Fries, 177 g	470	25	48
Chzburger Kids' Meal w/ Applesauce, 284 g	500	18	59
• Chzburger Kids' Meal w/ Fries, 227 g	590	27	61
• Chkn Strip Kids' Meal w/ Applesauce, 194 g	350	10	39
Chicken Strip Kids' Meal w/ Fries, 155 g	470	18	44
Hamburger Kids' Meal w/ Applesauce, 270 g	450	14	59
Hamburger Kids' Meal w/ Fries, 213 g	540	23	60
Iron Grld Chz Kids' Meal w/ Fries, 174 g	510	21	57
Iron Grid Chz Kids' Meal w/ Applesauce, 231 g	420	13	56
Local Menu Food			
Barbecue Beef Sandwich, 142 g	270	5	43
Barbecue Pork Sandwich, 142 g	340	12	41
• Breaded Mushrooms, 114 g	250	9	36
California GrillBurger, 198 g	620	39	39
• Chili Cheese Fries, 504 g	1240	71	119
Corn Dog, 175 g	460	19	56

• MOST HEALTHY   • LEAST HEALTHY

DAIRY QUEEN (cont.)

	Cal	Fat	Cbs
Crispy Fish Sandwich, 184 g	430	18	51
Crispy Fish Sandwich w/ Cheese, 198 g	480	22	52
Deluxe Cheeseburger, 177 g	400	18	35
Deluxe Double Cheeseburger, 247 g	640	34	35
Deluxe Double Hamburger, 219 g	540	26	34
Deluxe Hamburger, 163 g	350	14	34
DQ Ultimate® Burger, 259 g	780	48	33
Iron Grilled Cheese Sandwich, 103 g	320	13	30
Mushroom Swiss GrillBurger, 203 g	620	37	39
Pork Tenderloin Sandwich, 191 g	610	35	58
Shredded Chicken Sandwich, 170 g	290	7	30
Spicy Chili - Cup, 224 g	470	16	54

Local Menu Treats

	Cal	Fat	Cbs
Arctic Rush Float, All Flavors - Medium, 538 g	470	9	80
Arctic Rush Freeze, All Flavors - Medium, 518 g	560	14	89
• Diet Coke Float - Medium, 618 g	280	9	42
Frozen Lemonade - Medium, 583 g	290	0	61
Frozen Limeade - Medium, 597 g	300	0	64
Minute Maid Orange Float - Medium, 639 g	500	9	100
Pecan Mudslide® Treat, 198 g	300	10	45
Root Beer Float - Medium, 638 g	480	9	96
Strawberry Shortcake, 255 g	480	17	75
• Triple Chocolate Utopia, 283 g	750	36	93

MooLatte®

	Cal	Fat	Cbs
• Cappuccino MooLatte - 16 oz, 413 g	500	18	71
• Caramel MooLatte - 16 oz, 448 g	630	19	101
French Vanilla MooLatte - 16 oz, 433 g	560	18	88
Mocha MooLatte - 16 oz, 427 g	590	23	82

More Food

	Cal	Fat	Cbs
Crispy Chicken Sandwich, 198 g	560	28	48
Crispy Chicken Salad, 424 g	460	19	31
Crispy Chicken Sandwich w/ Chz, 212 g	610	32	48
Crispy Chicken Wrap, 85 g	290	16	17
• Crispy FlameThrower Chkn Snd, 260 g	860	55	51
Crispy FlameThrower Chkn Wrap, 85 g	310	19	17
Grilled Chicken Salad, 424 g	280	11	14
Grilled Chicken Sandwich, 180 g	370	16	32
• Grilled Chicken Wrap, 85 g	200	12	9
Grilled FlameThrower Chkn Snd, 233 g	590	36	34

More Treats

	Cal	Fat	Cbs
• Banana Split, 374 g	520	13	94
• Oreo Brownie Earthquake®, 304 g	760	27	117
Peanut Buster® Parfait, 304 g	700	30	94

Novelties

	Cal	Fat	Cbs
• Buster Bar® Treat, 148 g	480	31	45
Butterscotch Dilly Bar, 87 g	210	11	24

● MOST HEALTHY   • LEAST HEALTHY

▶ DAIRY QUEEN (cont.)

	Cal	Fat	Cbs
Cherry Dilly Bar, 88 g	210	12	24
Cherry StarKiss Bar, 85 g	80	0	21
Chocolate Dilly Bar, 87 g	240	15	24
Chocolate Mint Dilly® Bar, 87 g	240	15	24
• DQ Fudge Bar - no sugar added, 66 g	50	0	13
DQ Sandwich, 85 g	190	5	31
DQ Vanilla Orange Bar - NSA, 66 g	60	0	18
DQ Vanilla Take Home-Pak™ - 1/2 cup, 94 g	140	5	21
Heath Dilly Bar, 87 g	220	13	25
No Sugar Added Dilly Bar, 88 g	190	13	24
Stars & Stripes™ StarKiss® Bar, 85 g	80	0	21

Shakes and Malts (Medium)

	Cal	Fat	Cbs
Malt, Banana, 571 g	740	20	120
Malt, Caramel, 578 g	960	24	163
Malt, Cherry, 578 g	800	22	130
Malt, Chocolate, 578 g	900	22	154
• Malt, Hot Fudge, 578 g	970	31	146
Malt, Marshmallow, 578 g	900	22	157
Malt, Pineapple, 578 g	750	20	123
Malt, Strawberry, 578 g	770	20	128
• Shake, Banana, 543 g	620	19	96
Shake, Caramel, 550 g	850	23	140
Shake, Cherry, 550 g	690	21	106
Shake, Chocolate, 550 g	790	21	130
Shake, Hot Fudge, 550 g	850	30	123
Shake, Marshmallow, 550 g	780	21	133
Shake, Pineapple, 550 g	650	21	99
Shake, Strawberry, 550 g	650	21	97

Side Items

	Cal	Fat	Cbs
Bacon - 3 slices, 17 g	80	6	0
French Fries - Regular, 114 g	310	13	43
• Ham - 1 slice, 28 g	35	1	1
Hashbrowns, 71 g	190	12	18
Onion Rings, 113 g	360	16	47
Sausage - 1 patty, 28 g	110	10	0
Side Salad, 182 g	45	0	11

Waffle Treats

	Cal	Fat	Cbs
Choco Coated Waffle Cone w/ Soft Serve, 247 g	540	21	77
Choco Covered Strwbry Waffle Bowl Sundae, 318 g	790	40	99
Fab Fudge Waffle Bowl Sundae, 297 g	750	30	108
• Fudge Brownie Tempt. Waffle Bowl Sundae, 319 g	970	49	120
Nut & Fudge Waffle Bowl Sundae, 304 g	880	47	99
• Plain Waffle Cone w/ Soft Serve, 226 g	420	13	67
Turtle Waffle Bowl Sundae, 304 g	810	34	116

Xtra Stuff

	Cal	Fat	Cbs
Almond Pieces, 14 g	90	8	2

• MOST HEALTHY   • LEAST HEALTHY

DAIRY QUEEN (cont.)

	Cal	Fat	Cbs
• Banana Slices, 28 g	25	0	6
Blackberry Topping, 28 g	60	0	14
Blueberry Topping, 28 g	60	0	15
Butterfinger Pieces, 28 g	110	5	18
Butterscotch Topping, 28 g	90	0	20
Caramel Topping, 28 g	90	1	20
Cheesecake Pieces, 28 g	100	6	10
Cherry Topping, 28 g	40	0	9
Chewy Baked Brownie Pieces, 28 g	130	6	17
Choco Chunks, 28 g	150	10	17
Chocolate Topping, 28 g	70	0	17
Cocoa Fudge, 28 g	160	10	17
Coconut Flakes, 14 g	80	7	7
Cookie Dough Pieces, 28 g	130	6	18
Heath Pieces, 28 g	150	9	17
Hot Fudge Topping, 28 g	90	3	15
M&M's Chocolate Candies, 28 g	140	6	20
Maple Walnut Topping, 28 g	130	8	14
Marshmallow Topping, 28 g	70	0	18
Oreo Cookie Pieces, 28 g	140	6	20
• Peanut Butter Topping, 28 g	180	15	8
Peanuts, 14 g	80	7	3
Pecan Pieces, 14 g	100	11	2
Pineapple Topping, 28 g	30	0	7
Rainbow Sprinkles, 14 g	70	3	10
Red Raspberry Topping, 28 g	50	0	14
Reese's Peanut Butter Cups Pieces, 28 g	150	9	16
Snickers Pieces, 28 g	130	7	17
Strawberry Topping, 28 g	25	0	6
Whipped Topping, 28 g	90	7	7

DAMON'S GRILL

	Cal	Fat	Cbs
Aloha Chicken	516	12	45
BBQ Chicken Breast	420	16	27
Chimi Chicken	453	9	37
• Flame-Grilled Veggie Burger	660	27	75
Grilled Mediterranean Shrimp Skewers	380	11	26
Half Grilled Caesar Salad with Chicken	320	17	7
Maui Salmon, 8 oz.	537	21	40
Napa Valley Spinach Salad	600	25	79
• Specialty House Salad	80	0	19

DEL TACO

Breakfast

	Cal	Fat	Cbs
5-Piece Hash Brown Sticks, 71 g	210	15	18
Bacon & Egg Quesadilla, 163 g	430	20	37

• MOST HEALTHY   • LEAST HEALTHY

DEL TACO (cont.)

	Cal	Fat	Cbs
Big Fat Breakfast Taco, 169 g	400	19	34
Breakfast Burrito, 123 g	280	13	26
• Breakfast Del Carbon Taco, 98 g	140	5	18
Egg & Cheese Burrito, 214 g	400	18	35
• Steak & Hashbrown Brkfst Burrito, 192 g	470	24	34
Burgers			
Bacon Double Del® Cheeseburger, 276 g	770	52	40
Cheeseburger, 162 g	430	22	40
• Hamburger, 143 g	360	16	39
• Triple Del™ Cheeseburger, 342 g	950	66	40
Burritos			
Chkn Fajita Burrito (chkn & veggies only), 242 g	320	10	37
Del Beef Burrito™, 227 g	470	20	37
Del Classic Chicken Burrito™, 227 g	510	33	37
Del Combo Burrito, 269 g	510	16	61
Deluxe Combo Burrito™, 340 g	570	25	64
Deluxe Del Beef Burrito™, 298 g	510	23	39
Half Pound Green Burrito, 241 g	430	10	67
Half Pound Red Burrito, 241 g	450	10	66
• Kid's Burrito (Green Sauce), 142 g	300	9	43
• Kid's Burrito (Red Sauce), 142 g	310	9	42
Macho Chicken Burrito, 539 g	920	30	111
• Macho Combo Burrito™, 553 g	990	34	112
Shredded Beef Combo Burrito, 270 g	500	20	55
Spicy Chicken Burrito, 291 g	610	15	95
Veggie Works Burrito, 319 g	620	16	96
Dessert			
Chocolate Fudge Cake, 99 g	350	14	51
Caramel Chzcake Bites (2 Bites), 122 g	430	23	42
Drinks & Shakes			
• Caramel Mocha Hot Coffee, 443 g	280	4	56
Caramel Mocha Iced Coffee, 358 g	290	3	64
• Premium Caramel Mocha Shake, 443 g	720	13	138
Premium Chocolate Shake, 381 g	630	13	117
Premium Orange Shake, 429 g	590	13	106
Premium Strawberry Shake, 381 g	600	13	108
Premium Vanilla Shake, 375 g	560	13	100
Fries & Sides			
Chili Cheese Fries, 298 g	570	33	46
Chips and Salsa, 85 g	160	8	20
• Deluxe Chili Cheese Fries™, 340 g	610	36	48
Jalapeño Rings, 131 g	260	15	31
Macho Chips and Salsa, 255 g	480	23	61
Medium Fries, 198 g	380	22	44
Side of Cheddar Cheese, 14 g	50	4	0
Side of Guacamole, 14 g	25	2	1

• MOST HEALTHY   • LEAST HEALTHY

DEL TACO (cont.)

	Cal	Fat	Cbs
• Side of Salsa, 28 g	5	0	1
Side of Sour Cream, 14 g	30	2	0
Nachos & Salads			
Del Nachos, 206 g	480	21	56
• Macho Nachos®, 482 g	1090	53	116
• Nachos, 113 g	370	21	39
Quesadillas			
Cheddar Quesadilla, 151 g	480	25	36
• Kid's Quesadilla (2 Pack), 84 g	280	13	28
• Spicy Jack Chicken Quesadilla, 215 g	570	30	41
Spicy Jack Quesadilla, 151 g	480	25	38
Taco			
Big Fat Chicken Taco™, 153 g	330	14	34
• Big Fat Steak Taco™, 153 g	390	18	33
Chicken Soft Taco, 106 g	220	12	16
Chicken Taco Del Carbon, 98 g	150	5	19
Classic Taco, 92 g	200	12	10
Crispy Fish Taco™, 145 g	300	17	29
Crispy Shrimp Taco, 141 g	290	17	27
Del Carbon Shredded Beef Taco, 98 g	200	10	18
Soft Taco, 78 g	150	6	15
Steak Taco Del Carbon, 98 g	210	8	18
• Taco, 64 g	130	7	9
Value Menu			
Bean & Cheese Cup, 220 g	320	4	52
Cheeseburger, 162 g	430	22	40
• Chicken Soft Taco, 106 g	220	12	16
Half Pound Green Burrito, 241 g	430	10	67
• Half Pound Red Burrito, 241 g	450	10	66
Nachos, 113 g	370	21	39
Tostada, 128 g	260	13	26

DENNY'S

American Dinner Classics	Cal	Fat	Cbs
Chicken Strips, 8 oz.	560	24	41
Country-Fried Steak & Eggs, 11 oz.	660	43	29
• Country-Fried Steak w/gravy, 13 oz.	1000	65	54
Fit Fare Grilled Chicken, 15 oz.	380	10	12
Grilled Chkn Sizzlin' Skillet Dinner, 18 oz.	770	34	72
• Grilled Chicken, 10 oz.	280	4	4
Homestyle Meatloaf w/gravy, 7 oz.	600	46	14
Mushroom Swiss Chopped Steak, 13 oz.	940	66	13
Prime Rib Sizzlin' Skillet Dinner, 19 oz.	900	42	77
Sweet & Tangy BBQ Chicken, 20 oz.	650	11	108
Appetizers			
Chicken Strips w/ Buffalo Sauce, 13 oz.	730	32	53

• MOST HEALTHY   • LEAST HEALTHY

DENNY'S (cont.)

	Cal	Fat	Cbs
• Chicken Wings w/ Buffalo Sauce, 8 oz.	300	21	5
Fried Shrimp w/ Buffalo Sauce, 8 oz.	380	17	37
Mozzarella Cheese Sticks, 8 oz.	750	40	195
• Sampler, 17 oz.	1380	71	139
Smothered Cheese Fries, 10 oz.	840	50	74
Sweet & Tangy BBQ Chkn Strips, 13 oz.	820	30	83
Sweet & Tangy BBQ Chkn Wings, 8 oz.	420	19	41
Sweet & Tangy BBQ Shrimp, 8 oz.	460	14	66
Tsing Tsing Chicken, 15 oz.	890	31	92
Zesty Nachos, 22 oz.	1150	49	138

Better Burgers

	Cal	Fat	Cbs
• Baco Burger no fries, 11 oz.	420	11	57
Bacon Cheddar Burger, 15 oz.	940	52	49
Cheesy Three Pack, 25 oz.	1930	111	164
Classic Cheeseburger w/o cheese, 14 oz.	790	40	51
Classic Cheeseburger, 15 oz.	870	46	51
Double Cheeseburger, 23 oz.	1480	88	52
Fit Fare Baco Burger w/ fruit, 15 oz.	470	11	71
Mushroom Swiss Burger, 18 oz.	910	49	55
Slamburger, 15 oz.	990	54	59
• Smokin'Q Three Pack, 24 oz.	2020	110	185
Western Burger, 17 oz.	1160	65	79

Beverages

	Cal	Fat	Cbs
Blueberry Pomegranate Splash, 15 oz.	150	0	38
Blueberry Pomegranate Tea Chiller, 15 oz.	120	0	30
Cherry Cherry Limeade, 15 oz.	180	0	45
Cherry Lime Tea Chiller, 15 oz.	120	0	31
Flavored Cappuccino, 8 oz.	100	2	28
Four berry Fizz, 15 oz.	170	0	44
Four Berry Tea Chiller, 15 oz.	140	0	37
Hot Chocolate, 8 oz.	100	2	28
Milk Shake (van/choc/strawberry), 12 oz.	560	26	76
OJ Strawberry Mango, 15 oz.	250	0	61
Peach Tea Chiller, 15 oz.	150	0	38
• Straight Up Lemon Tea Chiller, 15 oz.	90	0	26
Strawberry Mango Pucker, 15 oz.	220	0	56
Strawberry mango Tea Chiller, 15 oz.	140	0	36
Very Double Berry, 15 oz.	280	1	69
White Peach Breeze, 15 oz.	180	0	46

Condiments

	Cal	Fat	Cbs
BBQ Sweet & Spicy, 2 oz.	110	0	30
Butter Roti, 2 oz.	91	9	2
Cherry Topping, 3 oz.	86	0	21
Croutons (for Salad), 0.25 oz.	90	3	15
• Garlic Dinner Bread, 2 pc	170	9	21
Maple-Flavored Syrup (3 Tbsp.), 2 oz.	143	0	36

• MOST HEALTHY   • LEAST HEALTHY

DENNY'S (cont.)

	Cal	Fat	Cbs
• Pico de Gallo, 3 oz.	21	0	5
Sugar-Free Maple-Flavored Syrup, 2 oz.	23	0	9
Whipped Margarine, 1 Tbsp	50	6	0
Desserts			
Apple Crisp a la mode, 13 oz.	750	21	134
Apple Pie, 7 oz.	510	23	72
Carrot Cake, 8 oz.	820	45	100
Cheesecake, 7 oz.	640	41	58
Cheesecake (No Sugar Added), 3 oz.	290	23	23
• Cherry Topping, 2 oz.	57	0	14
Chocolate Topping, 2 oz.	133	1	34
Chocolate Vanilla Pudding, 5 oz.	110	2	32
Coconut Cream Pie, 7 oz.	630	39	65
Double Scoop/Sundae, 5 oz.	325	15	44
Floats (Root Beer or Cola), 16 oz.	430	17	69
French Silk Pie, 7 oz.	770	57	59
Fudge Topping, 2 oz.	201	10	30
Hershey's Chocolate Cake, 5 oz.	580	28	75
Hot Fudge Brownie a la mode, 7 oz.	830	37	122
Milkshake (Van/Choc/Strawberry), 12 oz.	560	26	76
• Oreo Blender Blaster, 14 oz.	890	44	113
Oreo Sundae, 9 oz.	760	37	103
Strawberry Topping, 2 oz.	77	1	17
Dinner Sides			
Breaded Shrimp (6 ct.), 3 oz.	190	8	20
Coleslaw, 5 oz.	260	22	15
Corn, 4 oz.	130	3	26
Cottage Cheese, 3 oz.	70	2	5
• Country-Fried Potatoes, 5 oz.	390	28	30
Dinner Rolls, 2 pc	260	9	38
Dippable Veggies /no dressing, 3 oz.	30	0	5
Fiesta Corn, 4 oz.	135	3	26
Garlic Bread, 2 pc	170	9	21
Green Beans (canned), 4 oz.	45	1	7
Green Beans (frozen), 3 oz.	45	2	4
Grilled Shrimp Skewer, 1	90	4	0
Hash Browns, 1 Serv.	210	12	26
Mashed Potatoes, plain, 5 oz.	170	7	76
Ranchero Mashed Potatoes, 4 oz.	140	6	50
Smoked Cheddar Mashed Potatoes, 4 oz.	120	5	49
• Tomato Slice (3 slices), 2 sl.	10	0	2
Vegetable Rice Pilaf, 5 oz.	200	3	37
Favorites			
• Bacon Avocado Burrito, 17 oz.	1010	59	91
Country-Fried Steak & Eggs, 11 oz.	660	42	29
Moons Over My Hammy, 13 oz.	780	42	50

• MOST HEALTHY   • LEAST HEALTHY

DENNY'S (cont.)

	Cal	Fat	Cbs
Southwestern Steak Burrito, 13 oz.	910	52	76
T-Bone Steak & Eggs, 16 oz.	780	36	4
• Two-Egg Breakfast, 4 oz.	200	15	1
Kid's Meals Desserts			
Sundae Sundae Sundae!, 4 oz.	300	16	36
Breakaway Brownie, 2 oz.	310	16	42
• Kids OREO Blender Blaster, 12 oz.	680	33	88
Power Play Pudding, 5 oz.	110	2	32
mini chocolate chips, 13 g	53	3	7
• OREO cookie pieces, 9 g	42	2	6
white chocolate chips, 15 g	79	4	10
Soccer Shake-all flavors, 11 oz.	490	25	59
Kid's Meals Entrees			
Cheesy @ the Plate, 4 oz.	380	21	32
Chocolate Chip-In Pancakes, 7 oz.	450	18	61
Jr. Grand Slam, 5 oz.	380	19	39
Slam Dribblers, 6 oz.	410	11	74
• Slap Shot Slider (one), 8 oz.	620	30	43
• Softball Pancake w/ meat, 4 oz.	250	11	30
Spaghetti, Set, Go!, 6 oz.	260	7	40
Track & Cheese, 7 oz.	340	11	48
Triple Play Nuggets w/BBQ sauce, 4 oz.	340	13	43
Kids Meals Sides			
Apple Dunkers w/ caramel sauce, 3 oz.	130	0	30
• Finish Line Fries, 5 oz.	450	23	57
Fishing Goldfish Crackers, 2 oz.	260	9	38
• Game on Grapes, 3 oz.	55	0	29
High Diving Veggies w/ dip, 4 oz.	280	25	11
Home Plate Mash Potatoes w/ gravy, 5 oz.	140	6	52
Jump-Shot JELL-0, 3 oz.	70	0	22
Pit Stop Pizza, 4 oz.	320	14	38
Tumbling Vanilla Yogurt, 6 oz.	160	2	30
Omelettes			
Ham & Cheddar Omelette, 10 oz.	590	44	4
• Ultimate Omelette, 12 oz.	670	54	8
• Veggie-Cheese Omelette, 13 oz.	500	37	10
Rock Star Menu			
All Nighter Sampler, 19 oz.	1120	47	131
• Basket of Puppies, 10 pcs	490	5	98
Grand Slamwich w/o hash browns, 16 oz.	1320	90	71
• Hooburrito, 17 oz.	1430	67	164
Jewel's Smoked Chkn Quesadilla, 9 oz.	720	46	60
Los Lonely Boys Texican Burger, 15 oz.	1020	57	64
Nachitos, 10 oz.	570	24	47
Rascal Flatts Unstoppable Brkfst, 17 oz.	1130	73	68
Southwestern Steak Burrito, 13 oz.	910	52	76

• MOST HEALTHY   • LEAST HEALTHY

DENNY'S (cont.)

	Cal	Fat	Cbs
Tsing Tsing Chicken, 15 oz.	890	31	92
Sandwiches			
Bacon, Lettuce & Tomato, 7 oz.	520	35	35
Chicken Ranch Melt, 12 oz.	800	30	80
Chicken Snd-Breaded w/dress, 15 oz.	1150	64	98
Chicken Snd-Grilled w/dress, 15 oz.	880	51	64
Club Sandwich, 11 oz.	640	33	55
• Fit Fare Chicken Snd w/fruit, 15 oz.	450	6	62
• Grand Slamwich w/o side choice, 16 oz.	1320	90	71
Prime Rib Philly Melt, 13 oz.	730	43	53
Smoked Chicken Melt, 12 oz.	950	55	72
Spicy Buffalo Chicken Melt, 15 oz.	870	41	82
The Super Bird, 12 oz.	700	37	53
Scrambles			
Heartland Scramble, 20 oz.	1150	66	97
Meat Lover's Scramble, 19 oz.	1130	66	80
Seniors			
Bacon Cheddar Mini Burgers, 11 oz.	750	40	47
Belgian Waffle Slam w/Egg, 8 oz.	450	31	29
Club Sandwich, 10 oz.	570	34	37
Country-Fried Steak, 8 oz.	530	34	30
French Toast Slam w/Egg, 5 oz.	300	14	31
• Grilled Chicken, 5 oz.	140	2	2
Grilled Chz Deluxe Sndwch, 7 oz.	520	28	49
Grilled Shrimp Skewer, 8 oz.	290	6	39
Homestyle Meatloaf, 4 oz.	280	23	5
Lemon Pepper Grilled Tilapia, 9 oz.	450	24	5
Omelette, 9 oz.	480	37	6
• Scrambled Eggs & Cheddar, 13 oz.	800	47	58
Starter, 3 oz.	210	19	1
Sides			
Bacon Strips (4), 4 sl.	180	13	2
Bagel & Cream Cheese, 6 oz.	428	12	48
Biscuit, 2 pc	210	11	25
Biscuits & Sausage Gravy, 8 oz.	580	34	57
Cheddar Cheese Hash Browns, 5 oz.	310	19	26
Chicken Sausage Patties (2), 1.5 oz.	110	9	0
Country-Fried Potatoes, 5 oz.	550	37	48
Eggs (each) 2 oz. = 1 egg, 2 oz.	120	10	0
• Eggs, Whites, 4 oz.	50	0	1
English Muffin w/ margarine, 1 pc	180	3	25
Everything HshBrwn w/onions, chz & gravy, 8 oz.	480	22	60
Fruit – Banana, 1 ea	110	0	29
Fruit – Grapes, 3 oz.	55	0	29
• Granola 4 oz. w/ 8 oz. milk, 1 serv	690	12	131
Grilled Honey Ham Slice, 3 oz.	110	5	1

• MOST HEALTHY   • LEAST HEALTHY

DENNY'S (cont.)

	Cal	Fat	Cbs
Grits, 12 oz.	260	5	47
Hash Browns, 5 oz.	210	12	26
Oatmeal w/ 8 oz. milk, 16 oz.	270	7	37
Pancake Puppies (6), 6 oz.	390	12	67
Pancakes, Buttermilk (2), 6 oz.	510	6	102
Pancakes, Hearty Wheat (2), 2 ea	310	2	64
Sausage Links (4), 3 pcs	370	34	4
Seasonal Fruit, 4 oz.	70	0	18
Toast w/ margarine, 1 sl.	130	7	16
Turkey Bacon (4), 4 sl.	76	4	0
Yogurt, LF, 6 oz.	160	2	30

Skillets

	Cal	Fat	Cbs
Prime Rib Prem Sizzlin Brkfst Skillet, 21 oz.	850	40	77
Southwestern Sizzlin' Skillet, 17 oz.	990	61	71

Slams

	Cal	Fat	Cbs
All-American Slam, 10 oz.	820	69	5
Bacon Strips, 2 sl	90	7	1
Belgian Waffle Slam, 12 oz.	820	64	32
Buttermilk Biscuit, 1 pc	105	6	13
Buttermilk Pancakes (2), 2/serv	340	4	68
Chicken Sausage Patty (1 Patty), 1.5 oz.	110	9	0
Eggs. Scrambled (2), 4 oz.	250	21	1
• Eggs. Whites (2), 4 oz.	50	0	1
English Muffin, 1 pc	180	3	25
French Toast Slam, 15 oz.	940	53	68
• Grand Slamwich w/o hash browns, 16 oz.	1320	90	71
Granola 4 oz. w/8 oz. milk, 1 serv	690	12	131
Grits, 12 oz.	260	5	47
Hash Browns, 1 serv	210	12	26
Hearty Wheat Pancakes (2), 2/serv	310	2	64
Lumberjack Slam, 15 oz.	850	46	60
Oatmeal w/ 8 oz. milk, 16 oz.	270	7	37
Sausage Links, 2 links	182	18	2
Seasonal Fruit, 4 oz.	70	0	18
Toast Slices, 2 sl	260	14	32
Turkey Bacon Strips, 2 sl	76	4	0
Yogurt, LF, 6 oz.	160	2	30

Soups, Salads and Sides

	Cal	Fat	Cbs
Broccoli & Cheddar Soup, 12 oz.	374	29	16
Butter Roll, 2 oz.	260	9	38
• Chicken Dix Salad – Chkn Strips, 18 oz.	590	29	44
Chicken Dix Salad-Grilled Chkn, 17 oz.	290	10	15
Chicken Noodle Soup, 12 oz.	166	4	19
Clam Chowder, 12 oz.	266	17	24
Cran-Pecan Chicken Sld no/dress, 7 oz.	210	5	11
Dippable Veggies w/ranch dressing, 4 oz.	280	25	11

DENNY'S (cont.)

	Cal	Fat	Cbs
Fit-Fare Grilled Chicken Breast, 17 oz.	290	10	26
French Fries, salted, 5 oz.	425	23	50
• Garden Salad w/o dressing, 7 oz.	113	7	7
Garlic Dinner Bread, 2 oz.	170	9	21
Hash Browns, 5 oz.	210	12	26
Onion Rings, 5 oz.	520	36	48
Prime Rib & Bleu Salad/no dressing, 5 oz.	160	9	4
Seasoned Fries, 5 oz.	510	33	48
Vegetable Beef Soup, 12 oz.	124	1	18

Steak & Seafood

	Cal	Fat	Cbs
Fit Fare Grilled Tilapia, 17 oz.	600	11	66
• Grilled Shrimp Skewers, 10 oz.	370	10	39
Lemon Pepper Tilapia, 13 oz.	640	27	41
• T-Bone Steak & Breaded Shrimp, 13 oz.	920	34	20
T-Bone Steak & Eggs, 16 oz.	780	36	4
T-Bone Steak & Shrimp Skewer, 12 oz.	830	60	0
T-Bone Steak, 12 oz.	740	56	0
Tilapia Ranchero, 19 oz.	470	17	57

Sweets

	Cal	Fat	Cbs
Chocolate Chip Pancakes (3), 13 oz.	720	18	129
• Fabulous French Toast Platter, 15 oz.	1010	52	93
• Hearty Wheat Pancakes (3), 3/serv	460	2	96
Pancakes, Buttermilk (3), 3/serv	510	6	102

DIPPIN' DOTS

Chillz (Cups)

	Cal	Fat	Cbs
• Chocolate, 85 g	100	0	19
• Sour Razz Blue Raspberry Ice, 85 g	60	0	15
Wango Rainbo, 85 g	60	0	15

Dots N Cream

	Cal	Fat	Cbs
Banana Split, 100 g	220	14	22
Caramel Cappuccino, 100 g	190	12	18
Mint Chocolate, 100 g	230	14	25
• Orange Creme De La Creme, 100 g	180	12	17
Vanilla Over The Rainbow, 100 g	210	12	23
• Wild About Chocolate, 100 g	240	14	26

Flavored Ice (Cups)

	Cal	Fat	Cbs
• Liberty Ice, 75 g	90	0	23
• Rainbow Ice, 10 g	10	10	10
Watermelon Ice, 75 g	90	0	23

Ice Cream (Cups)

	Cal	Fat	Cbs
Banana Split, 85 g	170	10	16
• Bubble Gum, 85 g	165	10	15
Candy Bar Crunch, 85 g	208	13	34
Caramel Brownie Sundae, 85 g	170	10	16
Chocolate Chip Cookie Dough, 85 g	213	11	26

• MOST HEALTHY • LEAST HEALTHY

DIPPIN' DOTS (cont.)

	Cal	Fat	Cbs
Chocolate Cups, 85 g	165	10	15
Cookies 'n Cream w/ Oreo, 85 g	203	11	22
Cotton Candy, 85 g	170	10	16
Horchata, 85 g	170	10	16
Mint Chocolate, 85 g	165	10	15
• Moose Tracks, 85 g	218	13	21
Peanut Butter Chip, 85 g	165	10	15
Strawberry, 85 g	170	10	16
Tropical Tie Dye, 85 g	170	10	16
Vanilla, 85 g	170	10	16

Ice Cream Packs

	Cal	Fat	Cbs
Banana Split, 85 g	170	10	16
Chillz - Chocolate, 75 g	80	0	15
Chillz - Sour Blue Razz, 75 g	50	0	13
Chillz - Wango Rainbo, 75 g	50	0	13
Choc'um, 85 g	70	10	16
• Chocolate Chip Cookie Dough, 85 g	213	11	26
Cookies 'n Cream w/ Oreo, 85 g	203	11	22
Mint Chocolate, 85 g	165	10	15
• Rainbow Ice, 75 g	0	0	23
Strawberry, 85 g	170	10	16
Strawberry Cheesecake, 85 g	100	0	21
Vanilla, 85 g	170	10	16

No Sugar Added (Cups)

	Cal	Fat	Cbs
NSA Fat Free Fudge, 85 g	92	0	18
NSA Reduced Fat Vanilla, 85 g	123	6	13

Sherbet (Cups)

	Cal	Fat	Cbs
Lemon Lime Sherbet, 85 g	97	1	22
Orange Sherbet, 85 g	97	1	22
Raspberry Sherbet, 85 g	97	1	22

Yogurt (Cups)

	Cal	Fat	Cbs
Strawberry Cheesecake, 85 g	100	0	21

DOMINO'S PIZZA

Pizza Basics: Crust

	Cal	Fat	Cbs
• Deep Dish, 460 g	1290	43	199
Hand Tossed, 411 g	1060	23	181
• Thin Crust, 177 g	670	26	93

Pizza Basics: Cheese

	Cal	Fat	Cbs
• Cheese only pizza, 213 g	560	42	12
Extra Cheese (w/ toppings), 213 g	560	42	12
• Regular cheese, 142 g	380	28	8

Pizza Basics: Sauce

	Cal	Fat	Cbs
BBQ Sauce, 71 g	130	0	29
• Garlic Parm, 85 g	390	40	4
Hearty Marinara, 128 g	80	3	12

• MOST HEALTHY   • LEAST HEALTHY

DOMINO'S PIZZA (cont.)

	Cal	Fat	Cbs
• New Pizza Sauce, 120 g	70	0	13
Sides			
• Amazin' Greens: Croutons (1 pkg), 18 g	90	4	11
Amazin' Greens: Drss (1 pkg), 43 g	125	12	3
Amazin' Greens: Garden Fresh, 241 g	140	7	9
Amazin' Greens: Grld Chkn Caesar, 269 g	170	7	9
Breadsticks 1 order = 8 servings, 244 g	870	50	89
Buffalo Chkn Kickers, 253 g	510	21	36
• Buffalo Wings Hot or BBQ Sauce, 420 g	1060	69	23
Cheesy Bread, 286 g	930	51	91
Chocolate Lava Crunch Cakes, 171 g	690	34	93
Cinna Stix 1 order = 8 servings, 262 g	940	49	109
Dipping Cups, 28–71 g	160	16	27
Toppings			
American Cheese, 85 g	310	26	3
Anchovies, 57 g	110	8	63
Bacon, 71 g	340	26	6
Banana Peppers, 57 g	15	0	3
Beef, 99 g	300	26	0
Cheddar Cheese, 57 g	230	19	1
Chicken, 99 g	140	5	3
Chorizo, 99 g	90	4	1
Feta Cheese, 43 g	90	6	1
Garlic, 28 g	40	0	9
Green Chile Pepper, 57 g	10	0	3
Green Pepper, 57 g	10	0	3
Ham, 71 g	90	5	0
Jalapeños, 57 g	15	0	3
Mushroom, 99 g	20	0	2
Olive, Black, 57 g	100	10	2
Olive, Green, 57 g	100	10	2
Onion, 57 g	15	0	4
Parmesan, Shredded, 43 g	170	12	1
Pepperoni, 53 g	240	21	0
Pepperoni, Extra Large, 57 g	270	25	1
Philly Steak, 71 g	90	3	2
Pineapple, 99 g	60	0	16
Provolone Cheese, 57 g	200	16	1
• Red Pepper, Roasted, 57 g	10	0	2
Salami, 57 g	220	18	1
• Sausage, Italian, 99 g	350	30	9
Sausage, Sliced Italian, 89 g	290	26	0
Spinach, 43 g	10	0	2
Tomato, 99 g	20	0	5
Wing Sauce, 28 g	10	0	2

• MOST HEALTHY • LEAST HEALTHY

DON PABLO'S

	Cal	Fat	Cbs
Appetizers			
• Beef Taquitos, 6 taquitos	561	34	36
Chicken Flautas, 6 flautas	507	31	39
Single Flauta, 1 flauta	65	4	6
• Single Taquito, 1 each	63	3	5
Burritos			
Chicken Burrito, 1 burrito	878	48	70
Spicy Ground Beef & Bean Burrito, 1 burrito	1389	73	123
Caesar Salads			
• Caesar Salad (Plain), 1 salad	1388	21	79
Chicken Caesar Salad, 1 salad	1563	49	85
Steak Caesar Salad, 1 salad	1792	37	97
Carnitas			
Carnitas Cold Set, 1 order	187	14	19
Traditional Pork Carnitas, 1 order	1050	38	118
Chimichangas			
Chicken, 1 burrito	1099	42	114
Spicy Ground Beef Chimi De Oro, 1 burrito	1349	68	131
Classic Fajitas			
• Chicken, 1 order	851	29	90
• Steak, 1 order	1174	68	106
Steak and Chicken Combo, 1 order	1013	48	98
Classic Quesadillas (Large)			
Cheese, 8 slices	1597	99	105
• Mesquite Grilled Chicken, 8 slices	1332	65	110
Mesquite Grilled Steak, 8 slices	1561	91	122
• The Don's Sampler, 1 order	2002	118	129
Cool Amigos			
Chicken Nachos, 1 order	745	46	42
Chicken Sandwich, 1 order	1068	52	108
Cool Amigo Chicken Quesadilla, 1 order	1507	85	137
Cool Amigo Fajitas - Beef, 1 order	1272	63	134
Cool Amigo Fajitas - Chicken, 1 order	1099	44	125
• Cool Amigo Steak Quesadilla, 1 order	1622	98	143
• Fried Ice Cream (Small), 1 order	424	18	58
Hamburger, 1 order	1145	57	106
Steak Nachos, 1 order	859	59	48
Desserts			
Chocolate Volcano Cake, 1 order	1380	77	161
• Fried Ice Cream (Adult Serving), 1 order	827	35	116
• Sopapillas, 1 order	1402	78	160
Dos Tacos			
Don Diego, 1 order	758	38	58
• Dos Beef Tacos - Soft, 1 order	851	37	92
Dos Beef Tacos - Crispy, 1 order	820	41	81

• MOST HEALTHY   • LEAST HEALTHY

DON PABLO'S (cont.)

	Cal	Fat	Cbs
Dos Chicken Tacos - Crispy, 1 order	766	34	83
Dos Chicken Tacos - Soft, 1 order	780	29	94
• Mamma's Skinny Enchiladas, 1 order	476	14	51
Rico's Lunch, 1 order	794	39	70

Enchiladas

	Cal	Fat	Cbs
• Beef, 1 enchilada	263	18	4
Cheese, 1 enchilada	232	16	5
• Chicken, 1 enchilada	210	13	9
Spinach & Poblano, 1 enchilada	258	13	30

Fajita Cold Set

	Cal	Fat	Cbs
• Combo Cheese Topping, 1 oz.	108	8	0
Guacamole (optional), 1 oz.	52	5	2
Pico de Gallo, 1 oz.	8	0	2
• Shredded Lettuce, 1 oz.	0	0	0
Sour Cream, 1 oz.	77	7	2

Fajita Enchiladas

	Cal	Fat	Cbs
Chicken, 3 enchiladas	872	51	21
• Mama's Skinny Enchiladas, 3 enchiladas	368	14	18
• Steak, 3 enchiladas	1101	77	33
Three Amigos, 3 enchiladas	697	46	18

Fajita Nachos

	Cal	Fat	Cbs
Chicken Nacho, 1 order	1396	87	73
Steak Nacho, 1 order	1430	99	71

Little Amigos

	Cal	Fat	Cbs
• Beef Taco Dinner, 1 order	483	24	50
Cheese Enchilada Dinner, 1 order	515	29	33
Chicken Stix, 1 order	739	46	75
Corn Dog, 1 order	724	40	80
• Dogs in a Blanket, 1 order	1248	78	98
Grilled Cheese Crisp, 1 order	883	48	92

Lunch

	Cal	Fat	Cbs
Don Pablo's Lunch, 1 order	755	39	54
Dos Beef Enchiladas, 1 order	754	39	53
Dos Cheese Enchiladas, 1 order	755	39	55
• Dos Chicken Enchiladas, 1 order	729	35	63
• El Favorito, 1 order	982	52	81

Lunch-Sized Fajitas

	Cal	Fat	Cbs
• Classic Chicken, 1 order	600	20	74
• Classic Steak, 1 order	772	39	83
Combo Fajita, 1 order	685	29	78

Nachos

	Cal	Fat	Cbs
Cheese, 1 order	1317	98	48
Taco Beef, 1 order	1625	113	85

Numero Uno Favorito

	Cal	Fat	Cbs
• Chicken, 1 order	1168	56	93
• Conquistador, 1 order	1893	88	156

• MOST HEALTHY   • LEAST HEALTHY

▶ DON PABLO'S (cont.)	Cal	Fat	Cbs
El Matador, 1 order	1409	76	110
Steak and Chicken, 1 order	1200	63	90
Other			
Flour Tortilla Taco Shell, 1 shell	486	8	50
Tortilla Salad, 1 salad	549	14	59
Other Fajita Components			
7" Flour Tortilla, each	124	4	20
• Lettuce Wraps, 3-4 wraps	0	0	1
• Onions and Peppers, 7 oz.	186	13	17
Quesadillas & Salads			
• Cheese, 1 order	903	55	61
• Mesquite-Grilled Chicken, 1 order	773	39	63
Mesquite-Grilled Steak, 1 order	888	52	69
Rellenos			
Beef Relleno, 1 relleno	299	17	20
• Cheese Relleno, 1 relleno	396	26	19
• Chicken Rolleno, 1 relleno	235	11	21
Salad Dressing			
Cilantro Ranch Dressing, 3 oz.	494	3	20
Don's House Vinaigrette, 3 oz.	357	6	10
Sides, Sauces & Garnishes			
Black Beans, 4 oz.	119	2	20
Charro Beans, 5 oz.	96	2	16
Chile-mashed potatoes, 2.75 oz.	108	6	12
• Chips and Salsa, 1 order	338	17	43
Combo Cheese, 1 oz.	109	9	0
Combo Cheese Topping, 1/4-oz.	27	2	0
Guacamole, 1.25 oz.	52	5	2
Mexican Rice, 3 oz.	107	1	21
Pico de Gallo, 1.25 oz.	8	0	2
Ranchero Sauce, 5 oz.	44	0	9
Red Sauce, 2 oz.	17	0	4
Refritos, 5 oz.	262	10	31
• Salsa, 1 oz.	6	0	1
Salsa - Spicy Chili Macho, 2 oz.	14	0	3
Seasoned Vegetables, 6 oz.	98	5	13
Seasoned Vegetables, 6 oz.	98	5	13
Side Salad, 1 salad	108	7	8
Sour Cream Sauce, 2 oz.	66	4	5
Sour Crema, 1 oz.	57	5	1
Spoon Bread, 4 oz.	250	12	32
Sizzling Fajitas and Enchilada Combos			
Chkn Fajitas & Chicken Enchilada, 1 order	986	34	105
• Shrimp Fajitas & Shrimp Enchilada, 1 order	981	63	65
• Steak Fajitas & Steak Enchilada, 1 order	1255	66	119

DON PABLO'S (cont.)

	Cal	Fat	Cbs
Soup			
Tortilla Soup - Bottomless Bowl, 12 oz.	258	13	26
White Chkn Chili - Btmlss Bowl, 12 oz.	541	23	48
Tacos			
Crispy Beef Taco, 1 taco	291	18	21
• Crispy Chicken Taco, 1 taco	257	14	22
• Soft Beef Taco, 1 taco	327	18	29
Soft Chicken Taco, 1 taco	293	14	30
Tamales			
Chicken, 1 tamale	222	10	25
Pork, 1 tamale	270	14	24
The Don's Dips			
• Dip Sampler, 4, 2 oz. dips	519	39	27
• Dip Sampler - Guacamole, 2 oz.	83	8	4
Dip Sampler - Prairie Fire Bean Dip, 2 oz.	126	8	8
Dip Sampler - Queso, 2 oz.	105	8	3
Dip Sampler - Queso Blanco, 2 oz.	113	9	4
Prairie Fire Bean Dip Cup, 6 oz.	378	25	23
Queso Blanco Cup, 6 oz.	339	27	13
Queso Cup, 6 oz.	315	23	10

DONATOS PIZZA

	Cal	Fat	Cbs
Desserts			
Apple Timpano, 2 slices	406	9	3
Chocolate Chunk Cookie, 1 Cookie	430	21	2
• Cinnamon Timpano, 2 slices	523	22	2
• Cinnamon Twists, 2 pieces	260	5	2
Dressings			
Apple Cider Vinaigrette, 2 oz.	140	12	0
• Chicken Bacon Ranch Pizza Dip, 3 oz.	450	47	0
• Roasted Red Pepper Croutons, 1 oz.	50	3	0
Tuscan Caesar, 2 oz.	180	18	0
Oven Baked Subs - White (Whole Sub)			
Big Don™ Italian	717	34	3
Big Don™ Sausage Italian	998	56	3
Big Don™ Sausage w/Pizza Sauce	936	48	4
Big Don™ w/Pizza Sauce	656	26	4
Big Steak Hoagie	801	39	3
Big Steak Hoagie w/Mshr Gravy	801	39	3
Big Steak Hoagie w/Pizza Sauce	806	39	3
Chicken Bacon Cheddar	818	37	3
• Fresh Vegy™	540	19	5
• Meatball	1119	63	8
Roast Beef and Provolone	803	39	5
Turkey Club	743	30	3

• MOST HEALTHY   • LEAST HEALTHY

DONATOS PIZZA (cont.)

	Cal	Fat	Cbs
Pizza Bakery			
BBQ Chicken, 2 slices	361	13	2
Chicken Spinach Mozzarella, 2 slices	368	18	2
• Chicken Vegy Medley, 2 slices	281	10	3
Classic Trio, 2 slices	381	18	3
Founder's Favorite, 2 slices	381	18	3
Fresh Mozzarella Trio, 2 slices	350	17	3
Hawaiian, 2 slices	337	13	3
Margherita, 2 slices	352	18	2
Mariachi Beef, 2 slices	370	17	3
Mariachi Chicken, 2 slices	373	16	3
Pepperoni, 2 slices	347	16	3
Pepperoni Zinger, 2 slices	353	17	2
Serious Cheese, 2 slices	347	16	3
• Serious Meat, 2 slices	429	22	3
Vegy, 2 slices	325	13	4
Works, 2 slices	377	17	3
Pizza Hand Tossed			
BBQ Chicken, 2 slices	630	22	4
Chicken Spinach Mozzarella, 2 slices	587	25	4
Chicken Vegy Medley, 2 slices	517	17	5
Classic Trio, 2 slices	658	31	5
Founder's Favorite, 2 slices	678	31	5
• Fresh Mozzarella Trio, 2 slices	350	17	3
Hawaiian, 2 slices	578	22	6
Margherita, 2 slices	583	27	4
Mariachi Beef, 2 slices	591	24	5
Mariachi Chicken, 2 slices	617	24	5
Pepperoni, 2 slices	499	27	5
Pepperoni Zinger, 2 slices	645	30	5
Serious Cheese, 2 slices	597	25	5
• Serious Meat, 2 slices	735	37	5
Vegy, 2 slices	550	19	6
Works, 2 slices	669	31	6
Pizza No Dough (Whole Pizza)			
Chkn Veg Medley™ No Dough pizza	495	29	3
Classic Trio® No Dough pizza	532	37	3
Founder's Fav® No Dough pizza	558	38	3
Fresh Mozzarella Meatball	502	33	3
• Hawaiian™ No Dough pizza	436	26	4
Mariachi™ Beef No Dough pizza	528	34	4
Mariachi™ Chkn No Dough pizza	495	30	4
Pepperoni Zinger	584	42	3
Pepp No Dough pizza	499	35	2
Serious Chz™ No Dough pizza	457	31	2
• Serious Meat™ No Dough pizza	653	46	3

• MOST HEALTHY   • LEAST HEALTHY

DONATOS PIZZA (cont.)

	Cal	Fat	Cbs
The Works™ No Dough pizza	547	37	4
Pizza Thick Crust (1/4 Pizza)			
Chkn Spinach Mozzarella	803	39	3
• Chkn Vegy Medley™ thicker crust pizza	657	24	3
Classic Trio™ thicker crust pizza	832	41	5
Founder's Favorite™ thicker crust pizza	858	42	4
Fresh Mozzarella Trio	860	42	5
Hawaiian™ thicker crust pizza	758	32	5
Margherita	782	41	3
Mariachi Beef™ thicker crust pizza	796	36	5
Mariachi Chkn™ thicker crust pizza	806	35	4
Pepperoni thicker crust pizza	798	39	4
Pepperoni Zinger	827	41	4
Serious Chz™ thicker crust pizza	798	38	4
• Serious Meat™ thicker crust pizza	907	47	4
The Works™ thicker crust pizza	847	41	6
Vegy™ thicker crust pizza	715	29	6
Pizza Thin Crust (1/4 Pizza)			
• BBQ Chkn thin crust pizza	792	26	2
Chkn Spinach Mozzarella	643	34	2
• Chkn Vegy Medley™ thin crust pizza	497	20	3
Classic Trio® thin crust pizza	674	37	3
Founder's Favorite® thin crust pizza	702	38	2
Fresh Mozzarella Trio	740	42	3
Hawaiian™ thin crust pizza	588	27	4
Margherita	622	36	3
Mariachi™ Beef thin crust pizza	630	32	3
Mariachi™ Chkn thin crust pizza	639	30	3
Pepperoni thin crust pizza	627	34	2
Pepperoni Zinger	656	36	2
Serious Chz™ thin crust pizza	627	34	2
Serious Meat™ thin crust pizza	736	42	3
Spinach thin crust pizza	611	34	2
The Works™ thin crust pizza	689	37	4
Vegy thin crust pizza	544	24	4
White thin crust pizza	690	42	1
Salads (Whole Salad)			
• Entree Chkn Harvest Salad	410	23	6
Entree Italian Chef Salad	268	19	3
• Side Harvest Salad	81	3	2
Side Italian Salad	104	8	1
Starters			
3 Chz Garlic Bread, about 2 pieces	174	9	1
Breadsticks w/Nacho Chz Sauce, 2 sticks	398	22	2
Breadsticks w/Pizza Sauce, 2 sticks	261	9	3
Buffalo Wings - BBQ, 5 Wings	595	43	0

• MOST HEALTHY • LEAST HEALTHY

▶ DONATOS PIZZA (cont.)

	Cal	Fat	Cbs
Buffalo Wings - Garlic, 5 Wings	669	56	0
Buffalo Wings - Hot, 5 Wings	597	48	0
Buffalo Wings - Mild, 5 Wings	618	48	0
Buffalo Wings - Plain, 5 Wings	552	43	0
• Buffalo Wings - Spicy Garlic, 5 Wings	713	60	0
• Chicken Breast Strips, 2 Strips	125	4	0
Wedge Fries, Side Portion	261	13	6

Stromboli

	Cal	Fat	Cbs
3 Meat Stromboli, Whole Stromboli	689	31	5
Cheese Stromboli, Whole Stromboli	693	31	5
Deluxe Stromboli, Whole Stromboli	613	25	5
• Pepperoni Stromboli, Whole Stromboli	716	34	5
• Vegy Stromboli, Whole Stromboli	606	24	5

▶ DUNKIN' DONUTS

Bagels

	Cal	Fat	Cbs
Blueberry Bagel, 1 Bagel	330	3	65
Cinnamon Raisin Bagel, 1 Bagel	330	4	65
Everything Bagel, 1 Bagel	350	5	66
Garlic Bagel, 1 Bagel	340	3	68
• Multigrain Bagel, 1 Bagel	390	8	65
• Onion Bagel, 1 Bagel	310	2	63
Plain Bagel, 1 Bagel	320	3	63
Poppy Seed Bagel, 1 Bagel	350	6	64
Salt Bagel, 1 Bagel	320	3	63
Sesame Bagel, 1 Bagel	360	6	63
Wheat Bagel, 1 Bagel	320	4	61

Cookies

	Cal	Fat	Cbs
Chocolate Chunk Cookie, 1 Cookie	540	23	80
Oatmeal Raisin Cookie, 1 Cookie	480	14	83

Coolatta® (Medium)

	Cal	Fat	Cbs
Coffee Coolatta® with Cream, 24 fl.oz.	600	35	73
Coffee Coolatta® with Milk, 24 fl.oz.	360	6	75
• Coffee Coolatta® with Skim Milk, 24 fl.oz.	310	0	76
Strawberry Fruit Coolatta®, 24 fl.oz.	440	0	108
Tropicana Orange Coolatta®, 24 fl.oz.	330	0	79
• Vanilla Bean Coolatta®, 24 fl.oz.	650	9	136
Watermelon Coolatta®, 24 fl.oz.	370	0	91

Cravings Sandwiches

	Cal	Fat	Cbs
• Chicken Bruschetta Sandwich, 1 Snd	580	26	49
Chipotle Chicken Sandwich, 1 Snd	600	25	50
• Pastrami Supreme Sandwich, 1 Snd	750	39	51
Pressed Cuban Sandwich, 1 Snd	680	33	50

Cream Cheese

	Cal	Fat	Cbs
• Plain Cream Cheese, 50 g	150	15	3
Red. Fat Blbry Cream Chz, 50 g	150	9	15

• MOST HEALTHY   • LEAST HEALTHY

▶ DUNKIN' DONUTS (cont.)

	Cal	Fat	Cbs
• Red. Fat Cream Cheese, 50 g	100	8	5
Red. Fat Onion & Chive Cream Chz, 50 g	130	11	6
Red. Fat Smkd Salmon Cream Chz, 50 g	140	11	6
Red. Fat Strwbry Cream Chz, 50 g	150	10	15
Red. Fat Veggie Cream Chz, 50 g	120	10	6
Danish			
Apple Cheese Danish, 1 Danish	330	16	41
• Cheese Danish, 1 Danish	330	17	39
• Strawberry Cheese Danish, 1 Danish	320	16	40
Deli Classics Sandwiches			
Tuna (Albacore) Sandwich, 1 Snd	660	19	56
Turkey and Cheese Sandwich, 1 Snd	450	13	52
Donuts			
Apple Crumb Donut, 1 Donut	460	14	80
Apple 'n Spice Donut, 1 Donut	240	11	32
Bavarian Kreme Donut, 1 Donut	250	12	31
Blueberry Cake Donut, 1 Donut	330	18	38
• Blueberry Crumb Donut, 1 Donut	470	14	84
Boston Kreme Donut, 1 Donut	280	12	38
Chocolate Coconut Cake Donut, 1 Donut	340	18	42
Chocolate Frosted Cake Donut, 1 Donut	340	19	38
Chocolate Frosted Donut, 1 Donut	230	10	32
Chocolate Glazed Cake Donut, 1 Donut	280	15	33
Chocolate Kreme Filled Donut, 1 Donut	310	16	37
Cinnamon Cake Donut, 1 Donut	290	18	30
Double Chocolate Cake Donut, 1 Donut	290	16	34
French Cruller, 1 Donut	250	20	18
Glazed Cake Donut, 1 Donut	320	18	37
Glazed Donut, 1 Donut	220	9	31
Jelly Filled Donut, 1 Donut	260	11	36
Maple Frosted Donut, 1 Donut	230	10	33
Marble Frosted Donut, 1 Donut	230	10	32
Old Fashioned Cake Donut, 1 Donut	280	18	27
Powdered Cake Donut, 1 Donut	300	18	30
Strawberry Frosted Donut, 1 Donut	230	10	33
• Sugar Raised Donut, 1 Donut	190	9	22
Vanilla Kreme Filled Donut, 1 Donut	320	17	37
Fancies			
• Apple Fritter, 1 Fritter	400	15	63
• Bow Tie Donut, 1 Donut	310	15	39
Choco Frosted Coffee Roll, 1 Coffee Roll	380	19	50
Chocolate Iced Bismark, 1 Bismark	350	16	53
Coffee Roll, 1 Coffee Roll	370	18	49
Eclair, 1 Eclair	350	14	53
Glazed Fritter, 1 Fritter	400	15	63
Maple Frosted Coffee Roll, 1 Coffee Roll	380	18	50

• MOST HEALTHY • LEAST HEALTHY

▷ DUNKIN' DONUTS (cont.)

	Cal	Fat	Cbs
Vanilla Frosted Coffee Roll, 1 Coffee Roll	380	18	50
Favorites Sandwiches			
Steak and Cheese Sandwich, 1 Snd	470	16	50
Toasted Italian Sandwich, 1 Snd	560	25	52
• Tuna Melt Sandwich, 1 Snd	770	30	57
• Turkey and Bacon Club Sandwich, 1 Snd	440	13	51
Flavored Coffee (Small)			
Blueberry Coffee, 10 fl.oz.	15	0	2
Caramel Coffee, 10 fl.oz.	10	0	2
Cinnamon Coffee, 10 fl.oz.	15	0	2
• Hazelnut Coffee, 10 fl.oz.	10	0	1
Raspberry Coffee, 10 fl.oz.	15	0	2
Toasted Almond Coffee, 10 fl.oz.	10	0	1
French Vanilla Coffee, 10 fl.oz.	10	0	1
Coconut Coffee, 10 fl.oz.	10	0	1
• Mocha Coffee, 14 fl.oz.	170	1	39
Hot Espresso Drinks			
• Cappuccino Small, 10 fl.oz	80	4	7
Caramel Swirl Latte Small, 10 fl.oz.	220	0	26
Latte Lite Medium, 16 fl.oz.	120	0	19
Latte Small, 10 fl.oz.	120	6	10
• Mocha Raspberry Latte Medium, 16 fl.oz.	340	9	54
Mocha Spice Latte Medium, 16 fl.oz.	330	9	53
Mocha Swirl Latte Small, 10 fl.oz.	220	6	35
Vanilla Latte Lite Medium, 16 fl.oz.	130	0	20
White Chocolate Latte Medium, 16 fl.oz.	320	9	50
Iced Coffee (Medium)			
• Iced Coffee, 24 fl.oz.	15	0	2
Iced Coffee w/ Skim Milk & Splenda, 24 fl.oz.	40	0	8
• Iced Mocha Coffee with Cream, 24 fl.oz.	260	9	42
Iced Espresso Drinks			
Iced Caramel Swirl Latte Small, 16 fl.oz.	220	6	35
Iced Latte Lite Medium, 24 fl.oz.	120	0	19
Iced Latte Small, 16 fl.oz.	120	6	10
• Iced Mocha Rspbry Latte Med, 24 fl.oz.	340	9	54
Iced Mocha Spice Latte Medium, 24 fl.oz.	330	9	53
Iced Mocha Swirl Latte Small, 16 fl.oz.	220	6	35
• Iced Vanilla Latte Lite Small, 16 fl.oz.	90	0	14
Iced White Choco Latte Med, 24 fl.oz.	320	9	50
Muffins			
Blueberry Muffin, 1 Muffin	510	16	87
Chocolate Chip Muffin, 1 Muffin	630	23	98
• Coffee Cake Muffin, 1 Muffin	660	26	98
Corn Muffin, 1 Muffin	510	17	84
Honey Bran Raisin Muffin, 1 Muffin	500	14	86
• Red. Fat Blueberry Muffin, 1 Muffin	450	10	86

• MOST HEALTHY   • LEAST HEALTHY

▶ DUNKIN' DONUTS (cont.)

	Cal	Fat	Cbs
Munchkins			
Cinnamon Cake Munchkin, 1 Munchkin	60	3	6
Glazed Cake Munchkin, 1 Munchkin	60	3	8
Glazed Choco Cake Munchkin, 1 Munchkin	60	3	8
Glazed Munchkin, 1 Munchkin	50	3	7
Jelly Filled Munchkin, 1 Munchkin	60	3	8
Plain Cake Munchkin, 1 Munchkin	50	3	5
• Powdered Cake Munchkin, 1 Munchkin	60	4	6
• Sugar Raised Munchkin, 1 Munchkin	40	3	5
Other			
Biscuit, 1 Biscuit	280	14	32
Blbry White Hot Choco Medium, 14 fl.oz.	350	12	58
• Brownie, 1 Brownie	430	23	56
Caramel Hot Chocolate Medium, 14 fl.oz.	330	11	59
Coconut Hot Chocolate Medium, 14 fl.oz.	330	11	58
Dunkaccino® Small, 10 fl.oz.	230	11	35
English Muffin, 1 Muffin	160	2	31
Hot Chocolate Small, 10 fl.oz.	210	7	39
Plain Croissant, 1 Croissant	310	16	35
• Turbo Shot™ Medium, 2.5 fl.oz.	5	0	1
Vanilla Chai, 14 fl.oz.	330	9	53
White Hot Chocolate Medium, 14 fl.oz.	340	13	56
Other Oven Toasted Items			
Hash Browns, 9 Pieces	200	11	22
Oven Toasted Breakfast Sandwiches			
Bacon, Egg & Chz on Bagel, 1 Snd	510	17	66
Bacon, Egg & Chz on Biscuit, 1 Snd	470	29	36
Bacon, Egg & Chz on Croissant, 1 Snd	510	31	39
Bacon, Egg & Chz on English Muffin, 1 Snd	360	16	34
Bacon, Egg White & Chz on Eng Muffin, 1 Snd	310	8	34
Bacon, Egg White & Chz on Wheat Eng Muff, 1 Snd	300	9	33
Chicken Biscuit, 1 Snd	500	25	48
Egg & Chz on Bagel, 1 Snd	470	14	66
Egg & Chz on Biscuit, 1 Snd	430	26	36
Egg & Chz on Croissant, 1 Snd	470	28	39
Egg & Chz on English Muffin, 1 Snd	320	13	34
Egg White & Chz on English Muffin, 1 Snd	270	5	34
• Egg White & Chz on Wheat Eng Muffin, 1 Snd	260	6	33
Ham, Egg & Chz on Bagel, 1 Snd	510	16	67
Ham, Egg & Chz on Biscuit, 1 Snd	470	28	36
Ham, Egg & Chz on Croissant, 1 Snd	510	30	39
Ham, Egg & Chz on English Muffin, 1 Snd	360	15	35
Ham, Egg White & Chz on Eng Muffin, 1 Snd	310	7	34
Ham, Egg White & Chz on Wheat Eng Muff, 1 Snd	300	8	33
Sausage Biscuit, 1 Snd	450	28	33
Sausage, Egg & Chz on Bagel, 1 Snd	640	29	67

● MOST HEALTHY   ● LEAST HEALTHY

DUNKIN' DONUTS (cont.)

	Cal	Fat	Cbs
Sausage, Egg & Chz on Biscuit, 1 Snd	610	40	36
• Sausage, Egg & Chz on Croissant, 1 Snd	640	43	39
Ssge, Egg & Chz on English Muffin, 1 Snd	490	28	35
Ssge, Egg White & Chz on Eng Muffin, 1 Snd	440	20	35
Ssge, Egg White & Chz on Wheat Eng Muff, 1 Snd	430	20	33
Waffle Breakfast Snd w/ Sausage, 1 Snd	550	37	28

Oven Toasted Flats, Sandwiches & Wraps

	Cal	Fat	Cbs
• Bacon Jack Chkn Croissant Snd, 1 Snd	680	38	53
Bacon Jack Chicken Wrap, 1 Wrap	260	13	21
Bacon, Egg & Chz Wake-Up Wrap, 1 Wrap	200	12	14
Bacon, Egg White & Chz Wake-Up Wrap, 1 Wrap	180	8	14
Chicken Parmesan Flatbread, 1 Snd	500	24	49
Egg & Cheese Wake-Up Wrap, 1 Wrap	180	10	14
• Egg White & Chz Wake-Up Wrap, 1 Wrap	150	6	14
Egg White Tkey Ssge Flatbread, 1 Snd	280	6	37
Egg White Veggie Flatbread, 1 Snd	290	9	39
Grilled Cheese Flatbread, 1 Snd	380	18	35
Ham & Cheese Flatbread, 1 Snd	320	11	34
Original Chkn Croissant Snd, 1 Snd	640	35	53
Original Chicken Wrap, 1 Wrap	240	11	20
Tuna Salad Snd on a Plain Bagel, 1 Snd	540	20	69
Tkey Cheddar & Bacon Flatbread, 1 Snd	410	20	36

Salads

	Cal	Fat	Cbs
Caesar Salad, 7 oz.	320	29	11
• Chicken Caesar Salad, 10 oz.	440	33	11
• Garden Salad, 12 oz.	180	6	21

Soups

	Cal	Fat	Cbs
Broccoli Cheddar Soup, 8 oz.	190	11	14
Chicken Noodle Soup, 8 oz.	130	3	19

Sticks

	Cal	Fat	Cbs
Cinnamon Cake Stick, 1 Stick	310	20	30
Glazed Cake Stick, 1 Stick	340	20	38
Glazed Chocolate Cake Stick, 1 Stick	390	25	40
• Jelly Stick, 1 Stick	400	20	54
• Plain Cake Stick, 1 Stick	300	20	26
Powdered Cake Stick, 1 Stick	320	20	31

Tea

	Cal	Fat	Cbs
• Decaffeinated Tea, 10 fl.oz.	0	0	0
Earl Grey Tea, 10 fl.oz.	0	0	0
English Breakfast Tea, 10 fl.oz.	0	0	0
Freshly Brewed Unsweetened Iced Tea, 16 fl.oz.	5	0	1
Freshly Brewed Unsweetened Tea, 10 fl.oz.	0	0	0
Green Tea, 10 fl.oz.	0	0	0
Peach Flavored Iced Tea, 16 fl.oz.	15	0	2
Raspberry Flavored Iced Tea, 16 fl.oz.	15	0	2
• Sweet Tea, 16 fl.oz.	120	0	29

▶ DUNN BROS COFFEE	Cal	Fat	Cbs
A Seasonal Specialty			
Hot Spiced Apple Cider, 16 oz.	215	0	51
Brewed Coffee w/ Double Espresso			
• Chocolate Steamed Nirvana, 16 oz.	325	5	63
• Skim Chocolate Steamed Nirvana, 16 oz.	290	3	61
Soy Chocolate Steamed Nirvana, 16 oz.	300	5	60
Brewed from Fresh Roasted Coffee Beans			
• Brewed Coffee, 16 oz.	10	0	2
• Coffee with Steamed 2% milk, 16 oz.	70	3	8
Coffee with Steamed Skim milk, 16 oz.	55	0	8
Coffee with Steamed Soy Milk, 16 oz.	60	2	7
Depth Charge, 16 oz.	10	0	2
Espresso Drinks			
• Americano, 16 oz.	0	0	0
Caffe Latte, 16 oz.	142	5	14
Cappuccino, 16 oz.	70	3	7
Caramel Latte Macchiato, 16 oz.	230	5	38
Caramel Mocha Latte, 16 oz.	275	5	50
Mocha Latte, 16 oz.	275	5	50
Skim Milk Caffe Latte, 16 oz.	110	0	17
Skim Milk Cappuccino, 16 oz.	80	0	13
Skim Milk Caramel Latte Macchiato, 16 oz.	240	1	48
Skim Milk Caramel Mocha Latte, 16 oz.	240	1	50
Skim Milk Mocha Latte, 16 oz.	260	3	50
Skim Milk Vanilla Latte, 16 oz.	170	0	31
Skim Milk White Mocha Latte, 16 oz.	260	5	46
Soy Cappuccino, 16 oz.	90	2	12
Soy Milk Caffe Latte, 16 oz.	140	4	16
Soy Milk Caramel Latte Macchiato, 16 oz.	260	5	47
Soy Milk Mocha Latte, 16 oz.	280	6	49
Soy Milk Vanilla Latte, 16 oz.	180	4	28
• Soy Milk White Mocha Latte, 16 oz.	290	8	45
Vanilla Latte, 16 oz.	210	5	30
White Mocha Latte, 16 oz.	270	9	52
Fruit Smoothies			
• Mango, 16 oz.	250	0	58
Strawberry, 16 oz.	250	0	58
Wildberry, 16 oz.	250	0	58
• Strawberry Pink Freeze, 16 oz.	360	7	70
Ice Cremas			
Caramel IceCrema, 16 oz.	350	11	65
Caramel Mocha IceCrema, 16 oz.	400	11	74
Chai IceCrema, 16 oz.	410	11	74
Coffee IceCrema, 16 oz.	260	10	41
• Mocha IceCrema, 16 oz.	420	10	79
Skim Milk Caramel IceCrema, 16 oz.	300	4	65

● MOST HEALTHY • LEAST HEALTHY

DUNN BROS COFFEE (cont.)

	Cal	Fat	Cbs
Skim Milk Caramel Mocha IceCrema, 16 oz.	370	5	77
Skim Milk Chai IceCrema, 16 oz.	350	4	75
• Skim Milk Coffee IceCrema, 16 oz.	210	3	41
Skim Milk Mocha IceCrema, 16 oz.	370	3	80
Soy Milk Chai IceCrema, 16 oz.	360	5	75

Iced Drinks

	Cal	Fat	Cbs
• Cold Press Coffee, 16 oz.	10	0	2
Iced Caramel Latte Macchiato, 16 oz.	200	4	35
Iced Chai, 16 oz.	130	6	23
Iced Latte, 16 oz.	90	4	9
Iced Mocha, 16 oz.	230	3	45
Iced White Mocha, 16 oz.	230	7	47
Italian Cream Soda, 16 oz.	190	2	42
Italian Soda, 16 oz.	170	0	42
Skim Milk Iced Chai, 16 oz.	140	0	30
Skim Milk Iced Latte, 16 oz.	80	0	12
Skim Milk Iced Latte Macchiato, 16 oz.	170	1	35
Skim Milk Iced Mocha, 16 oz.	220	3	45
Skim Milk Iced White Mocha, 16 oz.	210	5	47
Soy Milk Iced Chai, 16 oz.	150	2	30
Soy Milk Iced Latte, 16 oz.	100	3	11
• Soy Milk Iced Mocha, 16 oz.	240	5	45
Soy Milk Iced White Mocha, 16 oz.	270	6	46
Vanilla Iced Nirvana, 16 oz.	210	16	17

Steamed Milk and Chocolate

	Cal	Fat	Cbs
Hot Chocolate, 16 oz.	380	6	71
Skim Hot Chocolate, 16 oz.	340	3	68

Sweetened Spiced Tea w/ Steamed Milk

	Cal	Fat	Cbs
• Chai Tea Latte, 16 oz.	165	4	27
• Skim Milk Chai Tea Latte, 16 oz.	140	0	27
Soy Milk Chai Tea Latte, 16 oz.	140	0	27

EAT N' PARK

Appetizers

	Cal	Fat	Cbs
• Appetizer Platter	1338	88	76
Basket of Loaded Fries	902	53	91
Buffalo Chicken Tenders	635	42	27
Fried Cheese Sticks	537	36	26
Grilled Chicken Quesadilla	907	55	51
Hand-Breaded Zucchini	478	26	50
• Onion Rings	244	16	23

Bakery

	Cal	Fat	Cbs
Apple Raisin Muffin	248	8	40
Banana Nut Muffin	284	14	36
Bearclaw	516	24	66
Blueberry Muffin	240	9	36

• MOST HEALTHY   • LEAST HEALTHY

EAT N' PARK (cont.)

	Cal	Fat	Cbs
Boston Brown Bread	281	9	43
Buttermilk Biscuit	202	12	23
Cheese Biscuit	119	6	16
Chocolate Chip Cookie	413	18	57
Chocolate Chip Muffin	275	11	40
Chocolate Nut Muffin	319	15	42
Cinnamon Buns	269	10	42
Corn Muffin	228	8	35
Cornbread	116	4	18
Cranberry Nut Muffin	265	11	38
Croissant	258	15	27
Crumby Buns	193	9	24
English Muffin	129	1	25
Garlic Toast	497	23	62
• Grilled Stickies	585	31	64
Hoagie Bun	178	2	34
Honey Bun (1)	172	8	22
Hot Dog Bun	128	3	21
• Italian Bread	54	1	10
Kaiser Roll	179	3	32
Mocha Java Muffin	216	9	31
Oat Bran Apple Raisin Muffin	306	11	47
Oat Bran Muffin	346	13	49
Plain Bagel	291	2	57
Pumpkin Muffin	279	9	45
Raisin Bread	71	1	14
Rye Bread	83	1	15
Six Grain Bread	79	1	15
Smiley Cookie	250	9	40
Sno-top roll (1)	111	4	16
Sourdough Bread	173	2	32
Strawberry Crème Muffin	272	10	40
Strawberry-Filled Muffin	279	10	42
Superburger Bun	179	3	31
Three-Cheese Hoagie	489	29	44
White Bread	67	1	13
Whole Wheat Bread	79	1	15
Yellow Bread	113	1	22

Beverages

	Cal	Fat	Cbs
Caffé Latte (Medium)	202	3	34
Caffé Mocha (Medium)	281	3	52
Cappuccino (Medium)	170	5	24
Caramel Latte Milkshake	559	30	68
Caramel, Vanilla or Hazelnut Latte (Medium)	226	6	33
• Coffee - 100% Colombian Decaf	0	0	0
Coffee - Gourmet House Blend Regular	2	0	0

• MOST HEALTHY   • LEAST HEALTHY

► EAT N' PARK (cont.)

	Cal	Fat	Cbs
Coffee Creamer (1 serving)	15	1	0
Cranberry Juice (Large)	198	0	51
Espresso Shot (Decaf)	0	0	0
Espresso Shot (Regular)	1	0	0
Fresh-Brewed Lipton Iced Tea	2	0	1
Hot Chocolate (Medium)	472	7	90
Iced Caffé Latte (no flavoring)	84	2	10
Iced Caramel, Vanilla or Hazelnut Latte	150	2	27
Iced Mocha Latte	163	2	28
Iced Oregon Chai Tea	93	3	12
Kids' Milkshake (Choco, Vanilla or Strawberry)	602	26	82
Lipton Brisk Raspberry Iced Tea	94	0	25
Lipton Hot Tea (Decaf)	2	0	1
Lipton Hot Tea (Regular)	2	0	0
• Mocha Java Milkshake	649	33	82
Old-Fash Milkshake (Choco, Vanilla, or Strwbry)	602	26	82
Oregon Chai Tea (Medium)	132	2	20
Oregon Chai Tea Milkshake	581	33	67
Skinny Shake	440	24	53
Sobe Lean Diet Cranberry Grapefruit	0	0	0
Vanilla Latte Milkshake	559	30	68

Breakfast

	Cal	Fat	Cbs
1 egg (poached)	77	5	1
1 egg (scrambled)	102	8	1
All-American Scrambler with bacon	619	29	55
All-American Scrambler with sausage	703	39	54
• Bacon (1 slice)	34	3	0
Baked Ham	110	4	1
Banana	90	0	23
Bananas Foster French Toast (2 slices)	495	15	82
Belgian Waffle	278	12	35
Blueberry Buttermilk Pancake (1 pancake)	84	1	16
Buttermilk Pancake (1 pancake)	76	1	15
Canadian-Style Bacon	86	4	1
Cheese Omelette	390	30	2
Chicken Fiesta Omelette	566	37	10
Eat'n Smart Smile	230	3	32
Egg Substitute, FF, No Cholesterol (1 serving)	67	4	1
Eggs Benedict	590	34	37
French Toast (1 slice)	141	5	17
Fruit Cup	59	0	15
Grilled Stickies and Eggs	790	47	65
Ham and Cheese Omelette	536	35	4
Hash Browns	201	8	28
Home Fries	208	12	24
Meat Lover's Omelette	726	55	3

● MOST HEALTHY   ● LEAST HEALTHY

EAT N' PARK (cont.)

	Cal	Fat	Cbs
Oatmeal	154	3	27
Oatmeal with Milk	202	4	33
Potato Pancakes	246	12	28
Raisin Bran Cereal with Milk	364	4	81
Sausage (1 piece)	107	10	0
Sourdough Toast	449	16	64
Strawberry Waffle	374	18	48
• T-Bone Steak and Eggs Smile	913	57	27
Veggie Omelette	415	30	8
Western Omelette	343	21	7

Burgers

	Cal	Fat	Cbs
Black Angus American Grill Burger	612	37	31
Black Angus BBQ Bacon & Cheddar Burger	865	53	53
Black Angus Mshr and Onion Burger	712	41	45
• Black Angus Superburger	1086	73	28
Classic Black Angus Bacon Chzburger	533	31	22
Classic Black Angus Burger	418	21	22
Classic Black Angus Cheeseburger	464	25	22
• Classic Gardenburger	220	4	33
Original Superburger	563	38	27

Children's

	Cal	Fat	Cbs
Breaded Cod	124	4	0
Breakfast Giggle w/ french toast & bacon	325	11	42
Breakfast Giggle w/ french toast & ssge	452	24	42
Breakfast Giggle w/ pancakes & bacon	234	9	28
Breakfast Giggle w/ pancakes & sausage	362	22	28
Breakfast Giggle w/ waffle & bacon	367	19	36
Breakfast Giggle w/ waffle & sausage	495	32	36
Breakfast Grin with bacon	393	27	21
Breakfast Grin with sausage	521	40	21
• Cereal with Milk	618	16	114
Cheeseburger	339	18	22
Chicken Fingers (2 fillets)	211	10	11
Grilled Cheese	523	39	22
Grilled Chicken	174	5	0
Hamburger	260	12	21
Hot Dog	359	24	24
• Jell-O	105	3	18
Mac'n Cheese	186	3	33
Oatmeal	358	15	47
Pizza	383	17	34
Spaghetti	322	3	60

Condiments

	Cal	Fat	Cbs
Alfredo Sauce	175	12	9
Beef Gravy	23	1	4
Blueberries	7	0	2

• MOST HEALTHY   • LEAST HEALTHY

▶ EAT N' PARK (cont.)

	Cal	Fat	Cbs
Butter (Whipped Blend)	96	11	0
Butter Swirl (was Butter, Cup, 5 grams)	36	4	0
Cheese sauce	150	12	4
Cocktail Sauce	66	0	17
Cream Cheese	99	10	1
Dill pickle slices	3	0	1
Grilled onions	22	1	3
Jelly	39	0	10
• Lettuce (Leaf)	1	0	0
Lettuce (Shredded)	4	0	1
Lite Soy Sauce	8	0	1
• Maple Syrup	222	0	60
Promise Spread	27	3	0
Red onions	12	0	3
Reduced-calorie Maple Syrup	30	0	13
Salsa	17	0	4
Sauce Supreme	125	13	2
Sugar-Free Pancake Syrup	38	0	16
Sweet'n Sour Sauce	81	2	16
Teriyaki Sauce	15	0	3
Tomatoes (2 slices)	5	0	1
Turkey Gravy	45	3	3

Desserts

	Cal	Fat	Cbs
Apple Pie (slice)	523	27	67
Banana Crème Pie (slice)	445	23	55
Blackberry Pie (slice)	566	28	75
Caramel Fudge Sundae	401	19	56
Cherry Pie (slice)	519	28	63
Chocolate Sundae	584	23	91
Coconut Crème Pie (slice)	487	27	55
Dutch Apple Pie (slice)	373	14	61
Grilled Stickies	585	31	64
Hot Fudge Sundae	490	21	71
Ice Cream (1 scoop)	114	6	13
Kids' Chocolate Sundae	315	13	47
Kids' Hot Fudge Sundae	286	13	39
Lemon Meringue Pie (slice)	260	13	31
Mini Dessert Bananas Foster	564	16	101
Mini Dessert Brownie	315	12	49
Mini Dessert Chocolate & Vanilla	190	6	30
Mini Dessert Smiley Cookie	251	4	55
Mini Dessert Strawberry Pie	313	6	64
Molten Lava Cake	233	8	38
New York-Style Cheesecake	460	33	36
No Sugar-Added Apple Pie (slice)	336	10	61
NSA Lactose-Free Vanilla Ice Cream (1 scoop)	130	8	15

● MOST HEALTHY   • LEAST HEALTHY

EAT N' PARK (cont.)

	Cal	Fat	Cbs
Orchard Fresh Pie (slice)	350	17	47
Oreo Crème Pie (slice)	501	29	60
Oreo Sundae	503	21	73
Peachberry Pie (slice)	388	19	51
Pumpkin Pie (slice)	400	19	50
• Sherbet	102	1	22
Strawberry Pie (slice)	296	12	45
Strawberry Sundae	584	19	106
• Turtle Sundae	935	49	111
Dinners			
Baked Cod (2 fillets)	432	25	6
Baked Lemon Sole (2 fillets)	387	20	11
Beef Liver and Onions	299	11	13
Breaded Fish Dinner (2 pieces)	926	45	56
Chargrilled Chicken (2 pieces)	348	9	0
Chargrilled Sockeye Salmon	287	15	0
Chesapeake Crab Stuffed Cod	278	8	20
Chicken and Broccoli Alfredo	630	19	66
Chicken Fillets (5 fillets)	529	26	28
Chicken Parmigiana (with Marinara Sauce)	959	37	100
• Chicken Parmigiana (with Meat Sauce)	985	40	95
Chicken Stir-Fry	392	8	47
• Cod Floridian (2 fillets)	241	3	8
Ground Sirloin	426	26	5
Mile-High Meatloaf	897	56	58
Nantucket Cod	419	28	13
Rosemary Chicken (2 pieces)	512	21	12
Seafood Pasta Bake	855	53	38
Sesame Pork Chops (2 chops)	400	23	3
Spaghetti (with Marinara Sauce)	694	9	129
Spaghetti (with Meat Sauce)	832	16	145
T-Bone Steak	576	39	1
Salads/Dressings			
Buffalo Chicken Salad	609	35	42
• Chicken Fajita Salad	732	43	41
Dressing Cajun Ranch (2 oz)	116	11	4
Dressing Fruit Salad Dip	143	14	6
• Dress Lite Burgundy Viniagrette (2 oz.)	36	2	5
Dress Poppy and Sesame Seed (2 oz.)	390	32	26
Fresh Fruit Salad	311	2	74
Garden Salad	93	3	15
Grilled Chicken and Strawberry Salad	216	6	13
Grilled Chicken Portobella Salad	320	11	23
Grilled Chicken Salad	444	19	30
Sandwiches			
BLT	491	15	66

• MOST HEALTHY   • LEAST HEALTHY

EAT N' PARK (cont.)

	Cal	Fat	Cbs
Buffalo Chicken Sandwich	740	41	59
• Chargrilled Chicken Sandwich	318	6	32
Chicken and Portobella Hoagie	847	56	47
Gourmet Grilled Cheese	793	58	27
Grilled Cheese Sandwich	727	39	65
Hot Turkey Sandwich	501	9	71
Philly Steak and Cheese	839	48	50
Reuben on Rye	729	50	31
Santa Fe Turkey and Bacon	878	60	45
Shredded Pot Roast Sandwich	530	31	28
Turkey Club	837	50	52
• Whale of a Cod Fish Sandwich	882	41	76

Sides

Applesauce	108	0	28
Baked Potato	190	0	44
Coleslaw	124	9	11
Cottage Cheese	115	2	5
• French Fries	352	19	43
Fresh Broccoli	39	0	8
Fruit Cup	59	0	15
Garden Rice	137	4	23
Macaroni and Cheese	254	12	26
Mashed Potatoes	286	24	17
• Mixed Vegetables	28	0	6
Onion Rings	244	16	23
Strawberries	54	1	13
White Rice	258	5	48

Soups (Bowl)

Chicken Noodle Soup	264	9	33
• Chili	208	6	26
Clam Chowder	231	14	19
• Cream of Broccoli Soup	380	21	44
Cream of Potato Soup	214	7	30
Stuffed Pepper Soup	240	5	38
Wedding Soup	211	5	26

EDO JAPAN

Bento Boxes

Beef Yakisoba Bento, 575 g	830	30	102
Chicken and Beef Bento, 566 g	880	26	120
Chicken Yakisoba Bento, 582 g	800	25	102
Seafood Grill Bento, 652 g	860	16	129
• Sizzling Shrimp Bento, 625 g	800	16	122
Sukiyaki Beef Bento, 571 g	900	28	120
Teriyaki Chicken Bento, 578 g	870	24	120

• MOST HEALTHY   • LEAST HEALTHY

EDO JAPAN (cont.)

	Cal	Fat	Cbs
Edo Extra's			
6 Extra Shrimp, 65 g	80	3	2
California Roll, 216 g	430	17	61
Extra Beef, 132 g	260	15	3
Extra Chicken, 139 g	220	11	3
• Rice Side Dish, 297 g	480	1	106
• Teriyaki Sauce, 60 ml	45	0	11
Tofu, 106 g	90	5	5
Vegetable Spring Roll, 45 g	120	6	14
Yakisoba Side Dish, 340 g	430	4	89
Teriyaki Dishes			
• Beef and Shrimp, 486 g	690	19	82
Beef Yakisoba, 425 g	540	18	62
Chicken and Beef, 416 g	590	14	80
Chicken and Shrimp, 493 g	660	15	82
Chicken Yakisoba, 432 g	510	14	62
Curry Chicken Bowl, 375 g	500	21	27
• Fresh Grilled Vegetables, 342 g	380	1	81
Ginger Pork, 414 g	650	23	82
Hawaiian Chicken, 440 g	590	12	85
Seafood Grill, 502 g	570	4	89
Sizzling Shrimp, 475 g	510	5	82
Sukiyaki Beef, 421 g	610	16	80
Teriyaki Chicken, 428 g	580	12	80
Tropical Teriyaki, 505 g	670	15	87
Udon Soup			
• Beef Udon, 947 g	580	17	72
Chicken Udon, 953 g	550	13	72
Shrimp Udon, 964 g	480	5	74
• Vegetable Udon, 909 g	370	2	77

EINSTEIN BROS. BAGELS

	Cal	Fat	Cbs
Bagel Dogs			
Original Asiago, 194 g	490	21	56
• Original Asiago Add Cheddar Chz, 212 g	560	27	56
• Original, 190 g	470	20	56
Original Add Cheddar Cheese, 209 g	550	26	56
Bagel Pretzels			
Asiago Cheese Bagel Pretzel, 108 g	300	7	52
• Cinnamon Sugar Bagel Pretzel, 116 g	320	5	66
Plain Bagel Pretzel, 101 g	270	5	52
• Salt Bagel Pretzel, 104 g	270	5	52
Bagels			
Asiago Cheese Bagel, 115 g	310	5	56
Blueberry Bagel, 108 g	300	1	65
Chocolate Chip Bagel, 106 g	280	3	56

• MOST HEALTHY   • LEAST HEALTHY

► EINSTEIN BROS. BAGELS (cont.)	Cal	Fat	Cbs
Cinnamon Raisin Swirl Bagel, 108 g	290	1	63
Cinnamon Sugar Bagel Chicago Style, 110 g	310	3	66
Cranberry Bagel, 108 g	270	1	60
Egg Bagel, 101 g	300	5	54
Everything Bagel, 105 g	270	2	56
Garlic Dip'd Bagel, 105 g	270	3	56
Good Grains Bagel, 106 g	280	3	58
Honey Whole Wheat Bagel, 103 g	260	1	57
Onion Bagel, 105 g	270	1	59
Onion Dip'd Bagel, 105 g	270	3	56
Plain Bagel, 101 g	260	1	56
Poppy Dip'd Bagel, 105 g	280	3	56
Potato Bagel, 100 g	270	4	52
• Power Bagel, Fruit & Nut, 113 g	310	5	61
• Pumpernickel Bagel, 101 g	240	2	53
Sesame Dip'd Bagel, 105 g	280	3	56
Sundried Tomato Bagel, 101 g	260	2	54
Bread Specialty			
Braided Challah Roll, 78 g	220	4	41
• Ciabatta Bread, 113 g	290	3	60
• Multi Grain Bread, 49 g	130	3	23
Breakfast Sandwiches			
• Bacon & Spinach Panini, 348 g	860	51	66
Egg Way with Bacon, 254 g	580	24	59
Egg Way with Black Forest Ham, 285 g	570	21	62
Egg Way with Sausage, 287 g	600	24	63
• Egg Way, Original, 247 g	530	20	62
Egg Way, Spinach Mshr & Swiss Omelette, 290 g	540	20	65
Sausage Ranchero Panini, 346 g	680	29	64
Vegetable Breakfast Panini, 415 g	730	36	68
Breakfast Wraps			
Santa Fe, 361 g	720	37	60
• Spicy Elmo, 318 g	720	41	56
Butter Blend Creamy Mustard Spread, 43	270	29	1
Deli Mustard, 5	5	0	0
Feta Pinenut Spread, 28	70	5	2
Honey Butter, 28	170	18	0
Hummus, 28	70	3	6
Peanut Butter, Creamy, 57	330	28	12
Roasted Garlic Horseradish Spread, 28	15	0	4
Spicy Roasted Tomato Spread, 30	140	14	3
Whole Kosher Pickle, 50	5	0	1
• Yellow Mustard, 5	0	0	0
Coffee Extras			
Half & Half, 1 fl.oz.	40	3	1
Light Whipped Cream, 2 Tbsp.	35	3	2

● MOST HEALTHY   ● LEAST HEALTHY

EINSTEIN BROS. BAGELS (cont.)	Cal	Fat	Cbs
On Top Reduced Fat Topping, 2 Tbsp.	20	2	2
Skim Milk, 8 fl.oz.	80	0	15
Syrup, Blackberry, 2 Tbsp.	100	0	25
Syrup, Caramel, 1 fl.oz.	100	0	25
Syrup, Cherry, 2 Tbsp.	100	0	25
Syrup, Chocolate, 2 Tbsp.	0	0	4
Syrup, Hazelnut, 1 fl.oz.	100	0	25
Syrup, Vanilla, 1 fl.oz.	100	0	25
• Syrup, Vanilla, Sugar Free, 1 fl.oz.	0	0	4
• Whole Milk, 8 fl.oz.	150	8	11
Coffee, Specialty (Medium)			
• Americano, 8 fl.oz.	1	0	0
Café Latte, 16 fl.oz.	200	8	20
Cafe Latte Nonfat, 16 fl.oz.	140	1	20
Café Latte Whole milk, 16 fl.oz.	250	12	21
Cappuccino, 16 fl.oz.	190	7	19
Cappuccino (Nonfat Milk), 15 fl.oz.	130	1	19
Cappuccino Whole Milk, 16 fl.oz.	190	9	17
Low Fat Mocha, 15 fl.oz.	350	15	42
Mocha, 15 fl.oz.	390	20	42
• Mocha Whole Milk, 16 fl.oz.	400	10	67
Condiments & Spreads			
Ancho Lime Salsa, 28 g	15	1	2
Ancho Mayo, 43 g	310	34	1
Cream Cheese			
Whipped Blueberry Reduced Fat, 20 g	70	5	6
Whipped Garden Veg Reduced Fat, 20 g	60	5	3
Whipped Garlic Herb Reduced Fat, 20 g	60	5	3
Whipped Honey Almond Red Fat, 20 g	70	5	6
Whipped Jalapeño Salsa Red Fat, 20 g	60	5	3
Whipped Onion and Chive, 20 g	70	6	3
• Whipped Plain, 20 g	70	7	1
• Whipped Plain Reduced Fat, 20 g	60	5	2
Whipped Smoked Salmon, 20 g	60	6	2
Whipped Strawberry Reduced Fat, 20 g	70	5	5
Whipped Sun Dried Tomato Basil Red. Fat, 20 g	60	5	2
Deli Melts			
Ham Deli Melt, 273 g	510	16	62
Pastrami Deli Melt, 273 g	540	17	64
Tuna Salad Deli Melt, 301 g	590	23	64
• Turkey Deli Melt, 273 g	510	15	62
• Veggie Deli Melt, 365 g	640	29	76
Deli Sandwiches			
• Deli Bacon, 261 g	830	52	52
Deli Chicken Salad, 274 g	460	18	47
Deli Ham, 261 g	520	26	48

EINSTEIN BROS. BAGELS (cont.)	Cal	Fat	Cbs
Deli Pastrami, 308 g	630	33	53
• Deli Tuna Salad, 268 g	440	15	50
Deli Turkey & Swiss, 316 g	690	41	49
Frozen Blended Drinks			
Café Caramel, 18 fl.oz.	620	9	100
Café Latte, 18 fl.oz.	400	10	65
Café Mocha, 18 fl.oz.	510	8	102
• Cookies &Cream, 18 fl.oz.	680	36	101
Strawberry, 18 fl.oz.	450	19	75
Vanilla, 18 fl.oz.	600	31	92
• Wild Berry, 18 fl.oz.	290	0	66
Gourmet Bagels			
Dutch Apple Bagel, 134 g	350	7	66
• Green Chile Bagel, 155 g	350	8	58
• Six-Cheese Bagel, 122 g	330	6	56
Spinach Florentine Bagel, 134 g	340	8	57
Iced Specialty Coffee			
Iced Americano, 0 fl.oz.	1	0	0
• Iced Coffee, 12 fl.oz.	0	0	0
Iced Latte, 16 fl.oz.	120	5	12
Iced Mocha, 16 fl.oz.	210	6	33
Iced Non Fat Latte, 16 fl.oz.	90	0	12
Low Fat Iced Mocha, 16 fl.oz.	180	3	32
Low Fat Mocha, Regular, 12 fl.oz.	190	3	34
Whole Milk Iced Latte, 16 fl.oz.	190	9	17
• Whole Milk Iced Mocha, 16 fl.oz.	390	9	66
Other Hot Beverages (Medium)			
Chai Tea w/ 2% milk, 16 fl.oz.	290	3	63
• Chai Tea w/ skim milk, 16 fl.oz.	270	0	63
Chai Tea w/ whole milk, 16 fl.oz.	310	4	63
Hot Chocolate, 12 fl.oz.	290	11	39
• Hot Chocolate w/ whole Milk, 12 fl.oz.	320	14	39
Pizza Bagels			
• Cheese, 179 g	420	12	63
Cheesy Garlic & Herb, 179 g	500	19	65
Pepperoni, 188 g	470	16	63
• Spinach and Mushroom, 271 g	580	25	70
Poured Beverages			
• Harney & Sons Tropical Berry Green Tea, 8 fl.oz.	0	0	0
Harney & Sons Tropical Green Tea, 8 fl.oz.	0	0	0
• Lemonade Blackberry, 16 fl.oz.	310	0	74
Spontaneitea Large, 24 fl.oz.	100	0	25
Salad Dressings			
Chile Lime Dressing, 32 g	60	4	5
Salads			
Bros Bistro Salad, 298 g	820	68	38

EINSTEIN BROS. BAGELS (cont.)	Cal	Fat	Cbs
• Bros Bistro Salad with Chicken, 397 g	940	71	39
Caesar Salad, 283 g	690	63	18
Caesar Salad with Chicken, 397 g	820	66	20
Chicken Chipotle Salad, 430 g	710	41	54
• Chipotle Salad, 331 g	590	38	53
Sandwich Fillings			
Cheese Provolone, 19 g	70	5	0
Cheese, American, 19 g	70	6	1
Cheese, Gorgonzola, 28 g	100	9	0
Cheese, Medium Cheddar, 19 g	80	6	0
Chz, Monterey Jack w/ Jalapeño Peppers, 19 g	70	5	0
Cheese, Swiss, 19 g	70	6	0
Chicken Breast, 113 g	140	5	1
• Chicken Salad, 113 g	210	14	2
Cold Smoked Salmon, 57 g	80	5	0
Ham, 85 g	90	3	0
Pastrami, 85 g	110	4	2
• Thick Cut Bacon, 14 g	60	5	1
Tuna Salad, 113 g	170	10	2
Turkey - Oven Roasted, 85 g	80	2	0
Turkey Sausage, 40 g	70	4	1
Sandwiches, Panini			
Italian Chicken Panini, 356 g	800	40	66
Turkey Club Panini, 376 g	790	41	66
Side Salads/Extras			
Bagel Croutons, 28 g	100	4	15
• Candied Walnuts, 43 g	260	22	9
Cole Slaw, 142 g	230	21	12
• Fruit Salad, 142 g	60	0	16
Sides			
Bagel Croutons, 34	150	12	9
Fruit and Yogurt Parfait, 340	230	2	42
• Fruit Salad, 312	140	0	36
Kettle Classic Natural Potato Chips, 28	150	9	15
• Traditional Potato Salad, 140	355	29	20
Soups (Cup)			
• Chicken Noodle, 248 g	120	4	14
Corn Crab Chowder, 248 g	280	18	18
Italian Wedding, 247 g	160	6	15
Seafood Minestrone, 248 g	130	5	16
Turkey Chili, 248 g	220	7	24
• Vegetarian Broccoli Cheese, 248 g	290	20	16
Specialty Sandwiches			
Club Mex on Challah, 302 g	750	49	46
Grilled Chicken, Bacon and Swiss, 309 g	750	46	45
Lox & Bagels, 281 g	520	21	66

• MOST HEALTHY   • LEAST HEALTHY

EINSTEIN BROS. BAGELS (cont.)	Cal	Fat	Cbs
• Rachel (Regular Size), 287 g	910	64	51
Reuben (Regular Size), 280 g	650	38	47
Roasted Turkey and Swiss, 308 g	690	41	49
Tasty Turkey on Asiago Bagel, 349 g	580	20	69
Turkey Rachel (Regular Size), 287 g	870	62	49
Turkey Reuben (Regular Size), 280 g	610	36	45
• Veg Out on Sesame Seed Bagel, 268 g	440	14	66
Sweets			
Blueberry Muffin, 142 g	480	22	65
• Chocolate Chip Coffee Cake, 174 g	760	34	110
Chocolate Mudslide Cookie, 78 g	320	17	46
Cinnamon Stix, 108 g	370	21	41
Cinnamon Walnut Strudel, 153 g	630	42	56
Fudge Brownie, 124 g	510	25	74
Heavenly Chocolate Chunk Cookie, 78 g	360	18	48
Iced Sugar Cookie, 106 g	480	15	76
Lemon Pound Cake, 141 g	440	16	69
Marshmallow Crispy Treat, 59 g	330	4	49
Mini Chocolate Mudslide Cookie, 39 g	160	8	23
Mini Heavenly Choco Chunk Cookie, 39 g	180	9	24
Mini Iced Sugar Cookie, 53 g	230	7	39
• Mini Oatmeal Raisin Cookie, 39 g	160	5	27
Mixed Berry Coffee Cake, 195 g	710	29	110
Oatmeal Raisin Cookie, 78 g	320	11	54
Strawberry White Choco Muffin, 156 g	550	25	78
Wraps			
California Chicken Wrap, 371 g	630	28	63
Chipotle Turkey Wrap, 369 g	730	37	70

EL POLLO LOCO

	Cal	Fat	Cbs
Beverages			
Horchata - 32 oz.	90	4	15
Bowls & Salads			
Chicken Caesar Bowl, 11 oz.	490	22	44
Chkn Caesar Salad (no dressing), 10 oz.	230	7	18
Chkn Tostada Salad (no dressing), 16 oz.	840	42	74
Chkn Tostada Salad (no drss, no shell), 10 oz.	410	13	39
Loco Salad w/ Creamy Cilantro Drss, 3 oz.	170	14	7
Small Garden Salad (no dressing), 4 oz.	70	4	8
• Small Garden Salad (no drss, no tortilla strips), 4 oz.	35	2	4
The Original Pollo Bowl®, 18 oz.	690	10	106
• Ultimate Pollo Bowl®, 24 oz.	1050	34	110
Burritos			
• BRC Burrito, 8 oz.	440	12	68
Classic Chicken Burrito®, 10 oz.	550	17	69
• Twice Grilled Burrito®, 15 oz.	840	39	56

• MOST HEALTHY   • LEAST HEALTHY

▶ EL POLLO LOCO (cont.)

	Cal	Fat	Cbs
Ultimate Grilled Burrito, 14 oz.	710	23	86
Desserts			
• Caramel Flan, 5 oz.	260	12	34
Two Churros, 2 each	300	18	32
• Vanilla Regular Cone, each	320	8	53
Vanilla Soft Serve - cup, 5 oz.	300	8	48
Dressings			
Regular Creamy Cilantro Dressing, 1 oz.	190	20	1
Flame-Grilled Chicken			
Chicken Breast, 4 oz.	220	9	0
Chicken Breast, Skinless, 4 oz.	180	4	0
Chopped Breast Meat, 3 oz.	100	2	0
• Leg, 2 oz.	90	4	0
• Thigh, 3 oz.	220	15	0
Wing, 1 oz.	90	5	0
Kid's Meal			
• BBQ Sauce (packet), 1 oz.	35	0	7
• Cheese Quesadilla, 5 oz.	420	23	35
Drumstick, 2 oz.	90	4	0
Popcorn Chicken, 3 oz.	200	12	10
Loco Value Menu			
• BRC Burrito, 8 oz.	440	12	68
Cheese Quesadilla, 5 oz.	420	23	35
Chkn Taquito w/ Avocado Salsa, 1 each	230	12	20
Chips & Guacamole, 3 oz.	250	14	26
• Leg, 2 oz.	90	4	0
Loco Salad w/ Creamy Cilantro Drss, 3 oz.	170	14	7
Taco al Carbon, 3 oz.	150	5	17
Two Churros, 2 each	300	18	32
Flame-Grilled Chicken			
Chicken Breast, 4 oz.	220	9	0
Chicken Breast, Skinless, 4 oz.	180	4	0
Chopped Breast Meat, 3 oz.	100	2	0
• Leg, 2 oz.	90	4	0
• Thigh, 3 oz.	220	15	0
Wing, 1 oz.	90	5	0
Kid's Meal			
• BBQ Sauce (packet), 1 oz.	35	0	7
• Cheese Quesadilla, 5 oz.	420	23	35
Drumstick, 2 oz.	90	4	0
Popcorn Chicken, 3 oz.	200	12	10
Loco Value Menu			
• BRC Burrito, 8 oz.	440	12	68
Cheese Quesadilla, 5 oz.	420	23	35
Chkn Taquito with Avocado Salsa, 1 each	230	12	20
Chips & Guacamole, 3 oz.	250	14	26

● MOST HEALTHY   • LEAST HEALTHY

► EL POLLO LOCO (cont.)

	Cal	Fat	Cbs
• Leg, 2 oz.	90	4	0
Loco Salad w/ Creamy Cilantro Drss, 3 oz.	170	14	7
Taco al Carbon, 3 oz.	150	5	17
Two Churros, 2 each	300	18	32
Mexican Favorites			
Chicken Soft Taco, 5 oz.	260	12	18
• Crunchy Chicken Taco, 3 oz.	190	8	16
• Grilled Chicken Nachos, 13 oz.	810	40	70
Grilled Chkn Tortilla Roll (no sauce), 6 oz.	390	16	37
Reg. Chkn Tortilla Soup (w/ tortilla strips), 11 oz.	210	9	18
Salsas & More			
Avocado Salsa, 2 oz.	40	4	2
Guacamole, 1 oz.	70	6	3
House Salsa, 2 oz.	10	0	2
› Jalapeño Hot Sauce (packet)	5	0	1
Pico de Gallo, 2 oz.	15	1	2
• Queso Sauce, 1 oz.	80	6	3
Salsa de Árbol, 2 oz.	10	0	2
Sides (Small Sides)			
BBQ Black Beans, 6 oz.	200	3	36
Cole Slaw, 4 oz.	130	10	9
Corn Cobbette, 5 oz.	90	1	19
• French Fries, 4 oz.	330	17	42
Fresh Vegetables (with margarine), 4 oz.	60	3	8
Fresh Vegetables (w/o margarine), 4 oz.	35	0	8
• Gravy, 1 oz.	10	0	2
Macaroni & Cheese, 6 oz.	280	17	28
Mashed Potatoes, 5 oz.	110	2	18
Pinto Beans, 6 oz.	200	4	29
Refried Beans (with Cheese), 6 oz.	270	7	36
Small Chicken Tortilla Soup, 7 oz.	160	8	14
Small Garden Salad (no dressing), 4 oz.	70	4	8
Sm Garden Salad (no drss, no tortilla strips), 4 oz.	35	2	4
Spanish Rice, 5 oz.	220	2	45
Tortillas & Chips			
(2) 6.5" Flour Tortillas, 2 each	210	7	30
• (2) 6" Corn Tortillas, 2 each	120	2	24
Tortilla Chips, 1 oz.	170	8	23

► FAMOUS DAVE'S

Other			
• BBQ Chkn w/ Jack Chz Snd (Lunch Portion)	480	14	57
Char-Grilled Chicken Sandwich	410	7	43
• Dave's Sassy BBQ Chkn Salad (Lunch Portion)	380	20	35
Dave's Sassy BBQ Pork Salad (Lunch Portion)	410	21	39
Georgia Chopped Pork Snd (Lunch Portion)	440	12	51

› MOST HEALTHY   • LEAST HEALTHY

FAMOUS DAVE'S (cont.)

	Cal	Fat	Cbs
Sweet & Sassy Grilled Salmon Fillet	450	26	11
Side			
Drunkin' Apples, 4 oz.	140	5	26
• Firecracker Green Beans, 6 oz.	60	3	7
Garlic Red Skin Mashed Potatoes, 4 oz.	90	4	13
• Wilbur Beans, 4 oz.	150	4	26

FATBURGER

	Cal	Fat	Cbs
Add-Ons			
American Cheese Add-on	70	5	1
Bacon Add-on	80	7	0
Cheddar Cheese Add-on	110	9	1
Chili Add-on	50	3	2
Chili Cheese Fat Fries	590	33	53
Chili Cheese Hot Dog	480	27	35
• Chili Cheese Skinny Fries	600	30	64
Chili Cup	200	11	10
Chili Cup with Cheese and Onions	320	20	12
Chili Fat Fries	480	24	52
Chili Skinny Fries	490	21	63
Egg Add-on	90	7	0
Fat Fries	380	18	47
Grilled Onions	120	14	1
• Lettuce	5	0	1
Onion Rings	540	29	64
Onions	5	0	1
Pickles	5	0	1
Skinny Fries	390	15	58
Shakes			
• Big Fat Float	390	12	73
Chocolate Shake	910	45	115
• Cookies & Ice Cream Shake	1180	59	163
Maui-Banana Shake	940	44	126
Peanut Butter Shake	950	53	114
Strawberry Shake	880	44	111
Vanilla Shake	890	44	113
Signature Items			
Baby Fat	400	21	37
Bacon and Egg Sandwich	350	16	37
Crispy Chicken Sandwich	560	27	53
• Fat Salad Wedge (no dressing)	60	4	5
Fat Salad Wedge w/ Chkn (no dressing)	210	6	8
Fatburger	590	31	46
Fatburger (no bun)	410	29	10
Fish Sandwich	560	31	55
Grilled Chicken Sandwich	430	14	42

FATBURGER (cont.)

	Cal	Fat	Cbs
Hot Dog	320	15	32
• Kingburger	850	41	44
Sausage and Egg Sandwich	780	53	47
Spicy Chicken Sandwich	520	21	58
Turkeyburger	480	21	50
Veggieburger	510	20	60

FAZOLI'S

Breadsticks

	Cal	Fat	Cbs
Breadstick, Dry (1 each), 1 oz.	100	2	20
Garlic Breadstick (1 each), 2 oz.	150	7	20

Classic Pasta

	Cal	Fat	Cbs
Classic Sampler Platter, 23 oz.	880	30	110
• Fettuccine w/ Alfredo - Reg, 20 oz.	900	27	126
Fettuccine w/ Marinara - Reg, 21 oz.	660	3	129
Fettuccine w/ Meat Sauce - Reg, 21 oz.	780	12	131
Penne w/ Alfredo - Reg, 20 oz.	900	27	126
Penne w/ Marinara - Reg, 21 oz.	660	3	129
Penne w/ Meat Sauce - Reg, 21 oz.	780	12	131
• Ravioli w/ Marinara Sauce, 12 oz.	490	15	69
Ravioli w/ Meat Sauce, 13 oz.	570	21	70
Spaghetti w/ Alfredo - Reg, 20 oz.	900	27	126
Spaghetti w/ Marinara - Reg, 21 oz.	660	3	129
Spaghetti w/ Meat Sauce - Reg, 21 oz.	780	12	131

Desserts

	Cal	Fat	Cbs
• Chocolate Chip Cannolis, 1 oz.	190	11	20
Chocolate Chunk Cookie, 4 oz.	510	26	68
• Chocolate Layer Cake, 7 oz.	700	38	87
Choco-Lato Mousse, 6 oz.	610	50	39
NY Style Chzcake w/ Strwbry Topping, 6 oz.	630	45	49
Turtle Cheesecake, 6 oz.	590	37	56

Drinks (Regular)

	Cal	Fat	Cbs
Italian Lemon Ice, 14 oz.	170	0	46

Kids Meals

	Cal	Fat	Cbs
Cheese Pizza, 4 oz.	270	11	32
Fettuccine Alfredo, 7 oz.	290	8	42
Meat Lasagna, 8 oz.	260	13	21
• Pepperoni Pizza, 4 oz.	310	14	32
Ravioli with Marinara Sauce, 6 oz.	250	7	35
Ravioli with Meat Sauce, 7 oz.	290	10	35
• Spaghetti with Marinara Sauce, 8 oz.	220	1	43
Spaghetti with Meat Sauce, 7 oz.	260	4	44
Spaghetti with Meatballs, 8 oz.	300	7	45

Oven-Baked Pasta

	Cal	Fat	Cbs
• Baked Spaghetti, 15.5 oz.	640	22	80
Baked Spaghetti with Meatballs, 19 oz.	890	39	86

● MOST HEALTHY   ● LEAST HEALTHY

FAZOLI'S (cont.)

	Cal	Fat	Cbs
Chicken Broccoli Penne Bake, 21 oz.	920	42	77
Chicken Parmigiano, 22 oz.	1000	39	108
Penne with Creamy Basil Chicken, 19 oz.	970	51	73
Rigatoni Romano, 17 oz.	880	44	76
• Tortellini Robusto, 18 oz.	1020	50	80
Twice Baked Lasagna, 18 oz.	700	39	47

Pasta Toppings

	Cal	Fat	Cbs
• Broccoli, 4 oz.	25	0	5
Broccoli and Fire-Rstd Tomatoes, 4 oz.	35	0	5
• Meatballs, 3 oz.	250	18	6
Sliced Grilled Chicken, 3 oz.	110	4	2
Sliced Italian Sausage, 2 oz.	200	16	3

Pizza

	Cal	Fat	Cbs
Cheese Slice, 4 oz.	270	11	32
Pepperoni Slice, 4 oz.	310	14	32

Salad Dressings

	Cal	Fat	Cbs
• Creamy Parm Peppercorn Ranch, 2 oz.	230	24	2
• Croutons (Pack), 1 oz.	70	3	8
Lemon Basil, 2 oz.	110	11	5
Red Wine Vinaigrette, 2 oz.	110	10	3

Salads

	Cal	Fat	Cbs
Chicken & Pasta Caesar, 13 oz.	470	15	38
Cranberry & Walnut Chicken, 12 oz.	390	14	27
• Crispy Chicken BLT, 13 oz.	480	26	31
Grilled Chicken Artichoke, 12 oz.	240	5	11
Side Caesar Salad, 4 oz.	40	2	4
• Side Garden Salad, 5 oz.	30	0	6
Side Italian Salad, 4 oz.	80	5	4
Side Pasta Salad, 6 oz.	300	12	38

Specialty Pasta

	Cal	Fat	Cbs
• Chicken Carbonara, 18 oz.	800	27	88
• Chicken Piccata, 18 oz.	870	43	86
Tortellini & Sun-Dried Tomato Rustico, 14 oz.	850	46	81

Submarinos®

	Cal	Fat	Cbs
Club Italiano, 13 oz.	780	36	68
• Fazoli's® Original, 13 oz.	880	50	68
• Ham and Swiss Supremo, 12 oz.	690	31	68
Italian Four Cheese & Tomato, 12 oz.	710	37	59
Roasted Red Pepper Chicken, 12 oz.	780	36	59
Smoked Turkey Basil, 13 oz.	750	37	68

FIREHOUSE SUBS

Beverages (Medium)

	Cal	Fat	Cbs
Sweet Tea	170	0	42
Unsweet Tea	0	0	0

• MOST HEALTHY   • LEAST HEALTHY

FIREHOUSE SUBS (cont.)

	Cal	Fat	Cbs
Breads			
• Sandwich bread (Kid's Menu)	220	3	44
Wheat 8"	230	3	46
• White 8"	240	3	46
Cheese			
• Cheddar, 2 slices	110	9	0
Monterey Jack, 2 slices	105	9	1
• Provolone, 2 slices	100	8	1
Swiss, 2 slices	110	8	1
Chili & Salads			
• Chief's Salad w/ Chicken Salad	740	58	16
Chief's Salad w/ Ham	360	18	16
Chief's Salad w/ Sliced Deli Chicken	320	14	12
Chiefs Salad w/ Tuna Salad	610	40	16
Chief's Salad w/ Turkey	300	15	12
Chili	370	28	17
• Pickle spear (1)	5	0	1
Desserts			
• Brownies (1)	420	18	63
• Chocolate Chip Cookie (1)	290	14	37
Macadamia Nut Cookie (1)	330	17	41
Oatmeal Raisin Cookie (1)	310	16	35
Peanut Butter Cookie (1)	360	26	25
Kid's Meals			
• Grilled cheese	380	25	23
Ham and cheese	240	8	28
Meatball and cheese	450	30	28
• Oreo cookies (2)	110	5	15
• Peanut butter and jelly	600	31	79
Roast beef and cheese	385	15	42
Turkey and cheese	230	6	25
Medium Subs			
• Chicken Salad, 4 oz.	760	46	63
Club On A Sub, 4 oz.	510	16	53
Corned Beef, 4 oz.	400	13	55
Engine Company, 4 oz.	390	6	52
Engineer, 4 oz.	380	5	55
Ham, 4 oz.	410	7	58
Hero, 4 oz.	430	7	54
Hook & Ladder, 4 oz.	410	7	68
Italian, 4 oz.	560	25	55
Meatball, 4 oz.	740	42	61
NY Steamer, 4 oz.	410	12	48
Pastrami, 4 oz.	420	8	58
Roast Beef, 4 oz.	410	6	48
Sliced Deli Chicken, 4 oz.	380	4	47

• MOST HEALTHY   • LEAST HEALTHY

FIREHOUSE SUBS (cont.)	Cal	Fat	Cbs
Smokehouse Beef & Cheddar, 4 oz.	740	36	63
Steak, 4 oz.	500	14	62
Tuna Salad, 4 oz.	610	28	62
Turkey, 4 oz.	370	4	54
• Veggie, 4 oz.	300	5	56

FIVE GUYS FAMOUS BURGERS & FRIES

Burgers

	Cal	Fat	Cbs
Bacon Burger, 279 g	780	50	39
• Bacon Cheeseburger, 317 g	920	62	40
Cheeseburger, 303 g	840	55	40
• Hamburger, 265 g	700	43	39

Dogs

	Cal	Fat	Cbs
• Bacon Cheese Dog, 200 g	695	48	41
Bacon Dog, 181 g	625	42	40
Cheese Dog, 186 g	615	41	41
• Hot Dog, 167 g	545	35	40

Fries

	Cal	Fat	Cbs
Regular Fries, 244 g	620	30	78

Other Sandwiches

	Cal	Fat	Cbs
Grilled Cheese, 110 g	430	26	41
Veggie Sandwich, 209 g	440	15	60

Toppings

	Cal	Fat	Cbs
• Bacon, 14 g / 2 slices	80	7	0
Cheese, 19 g/1 slice	70	6	1
Green Peppers, 25 g	5	0	2
• Jalapeños, 11 g	3	0	1
Lettuce, 30 g	4	0	1
Mushrooms, 25 g	10	0	1
Onions, 26 g	10	0	3
Tomatoes, 52 g	9	0	2

FOX'S PIZZA DEN

Cheese Pizza

	Cal	Fat	Cbs
9" Cheese Pizza, 1 slice	201	6	26
• 12" Cheese Pizza, 1 slice	171	5	22
14" Cheese Pizza, 1 slice	193	6	25
• 16" Cheese Pizza, 1 slice	210	7	27
12"x 24" Cheese Pizza, 1 slice	173	5	22

Pepperoni Pizzas

	Cal	Fat	Cbs
12" Pepperoni Pizza, 1 pizza	1420	53	170
• 16" Pepperoni Pizza, 1 pizza	2484	90	302
• 12" Pepperoni Slice, 1/8 pizza	178	7	21
16" Pepperoni Slice, 1/10 pizza	248	9	30

• MOST HEALTHY   • LEAST HEALTHY

▶ FRESHENS

	Cal	Fat	Cbs
MET-Rx Nutrition Boosters			
Cheddar Cheese Sauce, 2 oz.	34	2	5
Icing, 2 oz.	182	6	30
Immune Booster, 1 Tablet	N/A	N/A	1
• Marinara Sauce, 2 oz.	14	0	3
Memory Booster, 1 Tablet	N/A	N/A	2
Multivitamin, 1 Tablet	N/A	N/A	1
Nacho Cheese Sauce, 2 oz.	38	2	5
Pretzel Bites, 16 Bites	450	6	98
Protein Booster, 1 Scoop (10 g)	35	0	1
• Soft Pretzel, 1 Pretzel	450	6	98
Smoothies			
All That Razz, 21 oz.	360	0	79
Berry Breeze, 21 oz.	306	0	77
Blueberry Bay, 21 oz.	376	0	81
Carribbean Craze, 21 oz.	288	0	73
Jamaican Jammer, 21 oz.	355	1	78
Maui Beach, 21 oz.	90	0	48
Maui Mango, 21 oz.	292	0	74
Mystic Mango, 21 oz.	357	3	82
Orange Shooter, 21 oz.	334	3	77
Orange Sunrise, 21 oz.	353	3	81
Peach Passion, 21 oz.	152	0	32
Peach Sunset, 21 oz.	268	0	67
Peachy Pineapple, 21 oz.	327	0	69
• Pina Collider, 21 oz.	429	4	88
Pineapple Paradise, 21 oz.	331	4	77
Raspberry Royale, 21 oz.	270	0	67
• Strawberry Oasis, 21 oz.	89	0	49
Strawberry Shooter, 21 oz.	246	0	64
Strawberry Squeeze, 21 oz.	313	0	68
Strawberry Sunrise, 21 oz.	153	0	35

▶ FUDDRUCKERS

	Cal	Fat	Cbs
Build Your Own Specialty Burger			
Bacon Cheddar Burger w/ Bun, 1/2 lb	966	22	53
• Bacon Chdr Burger w/ Wheat Bun, 1/2 lb	886	20	45
The Works Burger w/ Bun, 1/2 lb	1022	22	60
The Works Burger w/ Wheat Bun, 1/2 lb	942	20	57
• Three Cheese Burger w/ Bun, 1/2 lb	1121	31	54
Three Chz Burger w/ Wheat Bun, 1/2 lb	1041	29	46
Burgers w/ Benefits			
Buffalo Burger w/ Wheat Bun	612	11	47
Elk Burger w/ Wheat Bun	469	6	47
Ostrich Burger w/ Wheat Bun	514	3	47
Salmon filet w/ Wheat Bun	523	3	59

● MOST HEALTHY   ● LEAST HEALTHY

FUDDRUCKERS (cont.)

	Cal	Fat	Cbs
• Turkey Burger w/ Wheat Bun	663	11	46
• Veggie Burger w/ Wheat Bun	395	2	67
Cold & Creamy Shakes			
Chocolate Shake	638	18	84
• Cookies n Cream Shake	677	18	89
• Strawberry Shake	630	18	86
Vanilla Shake	630	18	86
Fresh From the Oven			
• Brownie	488	7	40
Chocolate Chip Cookie	150	5	24
Crispy Squares	250	9	28
M & M Cookie	180	3	25
Oatmeal Raisin Cookie	170	4	22
Peanut Butter Cookie	200	5	19
Signature Buns	370	3	53
Snickerdoodle Cookie	180	5	24
Sugar Cookie	180	4	24
• The Daily Loaf, 1 Slice	80	1	13
Triple Chocolate Cookie	190	5	23
White Macadamia Nut Cookie	190	5	23
Fun & Tasty Kid's Meals			
Kid's Burger	463	7	40
• Kid's Cheeseburger	533	10	42
Kid's Chicken Bites	249	3	15
Kid's Grilled Cheese	341	8	31
Kid's Hotdog	445	9	41
Kid's Macaroni & Cheese	340	3	48
• Kid's Sliced Apples	33	0	8
Garden Fresh Salad			
Chicken Caesar Salad w/ Crispy Chicken	823	11	39
Chicken Caesar Salad w/ Grilled Chicken	735	9	17
Market Toss Salad w/ Crispy Chicken	598	10	36
Market Toss Salad w/ Grilled Chicken	511	9	15
Napa Valley Salad w/ Crispy Chicken	540	6	46
• Napa Valley Salad w/ Grilled Chicken	453	5	24
• Taco Salad w/ Crispy Chicken	959	15	86
Taco Salad w/ Grilled Chicken	786	13	64
Taco Salad w/ Nacho Beef	832	17	68
Hot & Delicious Sides			
BBQ Baked Beans	215	2	31
Chili Cheese Fries	551	12	50
Coleslaw	433	6	17
• Fruit Cup	60	0	16
• Onion Rings	566	6	58
Side Salad	96	5	8
Sweet Potato Fries	485	2	61

• MOST HEALTHY   ● LEAST HEALTHY

FUDDRUCKERS (cont.)

	Cal	Fat	Cbs
Wedge Cut Fries	296	3	36
Ice Cream Treats			
Hot Fudge & Caramel Sundae w/ Choco Ice Cream	544	11	85
w/ Strawberry Ice Cream	518	10	83
w/ Vanilla Ice Cream	637	14	94
• Ice Cream Brownie Blast	1365	27	171
Ice Crm Cookie Snd w/Choco Chip Cookies	540	18	80
w/ Chocolate Chunk Cookies	620	18	80
w/ Gourmet M & M Cookies	620	17	83
w/ Oatmeal Raisin Cookies	593	14	75
w/ Peanut Butter Cookie	673	17	67
w/ Snickerdoodle Cookies	620	17	80
w/ Sugar Cookies	620	15	80
w/ Triple Chocolate Cookies	647	18	77
w/ White Choco Macadamia Nut Cookies	647	18	77
• w/ Vanilla Ice Cream	70	2	8
The Original World's Greatest Hamburger			
The Original Burger w/ Bun, 1/2 lb	790	13	53
The Original Burger w/ Wheat Bun, 1/2 lb	710	12	45
Toppings			
• American Cheese, 2 Slices	140	6	4
Bacon	69	2	0
Bleu Cheese, Crumbles	76	4	0
Cheddar, 1 Slice	108	6	0
Grilled Mushrooms	35	0	2
Grilled Onions	44	0	6
Guacamole	38	0	2
Monterey Jack, 1 Slice	111	6	0
Pepper Jack, 1 Slice	111	6	0
Swiss, 1 Slice	111	5	1
Why Not Try Something Else			
3 Sliders w/ Bun	855	16	66
Chicken Tenders w/ Fries, 4 piece	708	6	68
• Crispy Fish Snd w/ Coleslaw, Tartar Sauce & Fries	1810	23	138
Dogzilla w/ Wedge Cut Fries	990	19	91
• Firehouse Boneless Wings, 9 wings	473	5	32
Fish n Chips	943	12	72
Grilled Chopped Steak w/ Side Salad	585	13	17
Mozz Sticks w/ Marinara Sauce, 6 Sticks	894	20	81
Original Chkn Snd, Crispy Chkn w/ Bun	719	6	77
Original Chkn Snd, Grilled Chkn w/ Bun	632	5	55
Ribeye Steak Sandwich	820	14	53
Tricked Out Nachos w/ Beef	1486	34	128
Tricked Out Nachos w/ Chicken	1439	31	124
Tricked Out Nachos w/ Chili	1399	32	135

• MOST HEALTHY   • LEAST HEALTHY

GIORDANO'S

	Cal	Fat	Cbs
• Small Cheese Stuffed Pizza, 7 oz.	550	25	57
Small Spinach Stuffed Pizza, 7 oz.	500	21	54
• Small Vegetarian Stuffed Pizza, 7 oz.	470	19	55

GLORIA JEAN'S

Blended Tea Lattes (Regular)

	Cal	Fat	Cbs
Mango Tea Latte, 24 oz.	316	12	55
• Chai Tea Latte, 24 oz.	174	3	31
• Green Tea Latte, 24 oz.	359	14	54

Chillers (Regular)

	Cal	Fat	Cbs
Chai Chiller, 24 oz.	416	14	66
• Crème Brulee Espresso Chiller, 24 oz.	319	9	52
Mocharetto Espresso Chiller, 24 oz.	405	13	66
Swiss Orange Mocha Espresso Chiller, 24 oz.	365	13	57
White Chocolate Oreo Chiller, 24 oz.	666	26	95
White Caramel Oreo Chiller, 24 oz.	821	26	133
Vanilla Caramel Chiller, 24 oz.	634	21	100
• Very Vanilla Chiller, 24 oz.	839	38	114

Cold Coffee Drinks (Regular)

	Cal	Fat	Cbs
Iced Café au Lait, 24 oz.	65	2	6
• Butter Rum Chiller, 24 oz.	656	19	112
Iced Coffee, 24 oz.	5	0	0
Iced Café Mocha, 24 oz.	397	17	51
Iced White Chocolate Mocha, 24 oz.	410	19	50
Iced Cappuccino Chiller, 24 oz.	484	16	66
Iced Latte, 24 oz.	200	8	19
• Iced Toddy, 24 oz.	2	0	0
Iced Toddy Supreme, 24 oz.	537	47	19

Cold Drinks (Regular)

	Cal	Fat	Cbs
Bulk Iced Tea, 24 oz.	5	0	1
• Italian Cream Soda, 24 oz.	397	13	70
Italian Cream Soda w/ Sugar-Free Syrup, 24 oz.	145	13	6
Italian Soda, 24 oz.	257	0	64
• Italian Soda with Sugar-Free Syrup, 24 oz.	0	0	0

Fruit Chillers (Regular)

	Cal	Fat	Cbs
• Bananaberry Split Chiller, 24 oz.	709	26	123
• Banana Chiller, 24 oz.	371	0	91
Banana Cream Chiller, 24 oz.	394	1	87
Raspberry Fruit Chiller, 24 oz.	371	0	91
Raspberries 'N Cream Chiller, 24 oz.	394	1	87
Strawberry Fruit Chiller, 24 oz.	371	0	91
Strawberries 'N Cream Chiller, 24 oz.	394	1	87
Wildberry Fruit Chiller, 24 oz.	371	0	91
Wildberries 'N Cream Fruit Chiller, 24 oz.	394	1	87

Hot Coffee Drinks (Regular)

	Cal	Fat	Cbs
Cafe Americano, 16 oz.	2	0	0

▷ GLORIA JEAN'S (cont.)

	Cal	Fat	Cbs
Cafe au Lait, 16 oz.	109	4	10
Cafe Breve, 16 oz.	314	28	10
Cafe Latte, 16 oz.	154	6	14
Vanilla Caramelatte, 16 oz.	376	10	64
Cafe Mocha, 16 oz.	388	16	51
White Chocolate Mocha, 16 oz.	401	18	49
Cappuccino, 16 oz.	124	5	11
Creme Brulee Latte, 16 oz.	352	11	54
• Espresso, 16 oz.	1	0	0
Espresso Con Pana, 16 oz.	20	2	1
Espresso Macchiato, 16 oz.	9	0	1
• Mocharetto, 16 oz.	506	16	81
Mocha Truffle, 16 oz.	320	13	43
Swiss Orange Mocha, 16 oz.	447	16	66

Holiday Drinks (Regular)

	Cal	Fat	Cbs
Butter Rum Latte, 16 oz.	580	17	100
White Chocolate Sleigh Ride, 16 oz.	582	19	91
Sleigh Ride Mocha, 16 oz.	538	17	87
• Sleigh Ride Chiller, 16 oz.	586	19	92
• Noel Nog, 16 oz.	516	29	52

Hot Drinks (Regular)

	Cal	Fat	Cbs
Hot Chai, 16 oz.	213	3	40
Hot Chocolate, 16 oz.	431	18	55
White Hot Chocolate, 16 oz.	445	20	54
• Hot Tea, 16 oz.	0	0	0
Irish Nut Crème, 16 oz.	403	13	60
Mocha Caramelatte, 16 oz.	416	12	65
• Mon Cheri Mocha, 16 oz.	450	14	70
Steamers, 16 oz.	336	11	49
Steamers With Sugar-Free Syrup, 16 oz.	210	11	17

Kids Drinks

	Cal	Fat	Cbs
• BananaBerry Chiller	330	13	47
• Grapple Fruit Chiller	330	13	45
Strawbical Fruit Chiller	330	13	47
WaterBerry Chiller	330	13	47

Mocha Chillers (Regular)

	Cal	Fat	Cbs
Banana Ana Mocha Chiller, 24 oz.	619	13	118
Banana Split Mocha Chiller, 24 oz.	701	13	138
• Coco Loco Mocha Chiller, 24 oz.	536	13	97
Cookies 'N Cream Mocha Chiller, 24 oz.	588	19	94
Cookies 'N Mint Mocha Chiller, 24 oz.	756	20	135
• English Toffee Twist Mocha Chiller, 24 oz.	776	17	124
Malted Mocha Chiller, 24 oz.	722	17	131
Mint Choco Bomb Mocha Chiller, 24 oz.	596	13	112
Nutty Mocha Frost Chiller, 24 oz.	750	22	130
Raspberry Dazzle Mocha Chiller, 24 oz.	619	13	118

● MOST HEALTHY • LEAST HEALTHY

GLORIA JEAN'S (cont.)

	Cal	Fat	Cbs
Strawberry Supreme Mocha Chiller, 24 oz.	619	13	118

Promotional Drinks (Regular)

	Cal	Fat	Cbs
• Iced Chai with Skim Milk, 24 oz.	193	0	41
Madagascar Vanilla Chiller, 24 oz.	662	35	91
• Chocolate Fudge Chiller, 24 oz.	664	28	108
Strawberry Vanilla Chiller, 24 oz.	550	13	101
Java Chiller, 24 oz.	459	18	70
Java Light Chiller, 24 oz.	255	6	41
Lite Mocha Chiller, 24 oz.	195	3	42

GODFATHER'S PIZZA

Desserts

	Cal	Fat	Cbs
• Apple Dessert (Medium), 93 g	200	1	38
Cherry Dessert (Medium), 93 g	210	1	39
Cinnamon Streusel (Medium), 74 g	230	1	40
• Monkey Bread - Cinn (Alum Pan), 286 g	830	5	139
Monkey Bread - Italian (Alum Pan), 248 g	690	5	105

Gluten-Free

	Cal	Fat	Cbs
Beef, 73 g	170	3	18
• Cheese, 61 g	140	2	18
Classic Combo, 83 g	180	3	19
• Meat Combo, 81 g	190	4	18
Pepperoni, 68 g	170	3	18
Sausage, 73 g	170	3	18

Golden (Medium)

	Cal	Fat	Cbs
All Meat Combo, 113 g	300	5	26
Bacon Cheeseburger, 111 g	270	5	26
• Cheese, 83 g	220	3	25
Combo, 117 g	290	5	27
Hawaiian, 99 g	230	4	27
Hot Stuff, 112 g	290	6	27
Humble Pie, 112 g	300	6	26
Pepperoni, 90 g	250	5	26
• Super Taco, 150 g	330	10	28
Super Combo, 135 g	320	8	28
Super Hawaiian, 107 g	250	4	27
Taco, 137 g	300	8	27
Veggie, 92 g	230	3	27

Mozza Loaded (Medium)

	Cal	Fat	Cbs
All Meat Combo, 128 g	350	7	27
Bacon Cheeseburger, 126 g	320	7	27
Cheese, 98 g	270	5	26
Combo, 131 g	340	7	28
• Hawaiian, 99 g	230	3	27
Hot Stuff, 126 g	340	7	27
Humble Pie, 127 g	350	8	27

● MOST HEALTHY   • LEAST HEALTHY

GODFATHER'S PIZZA (cont.)

	Cal	Fat	Cbs
Pepperoni, 105 g	300	6	26
Super Combo, 150 g	370	9	28
Super Hawaiian, 121 g	300	6	28
• Super Taco, 165 g	380	10	28
Taco, 151 g	350	9	28
Veggie, 106 g	280	5	27
Original (Medium)			
All Meat Combo, 142 g	370	6	35
Bacon Cheeseburger, 141 g	330	6	35
• Cheese, 103 g	260	3	34
Combo, 152 g	350	6	36
Hawaiian, 124 g	270	3	36
Hot Stuff, 144 g	360	6	35
Humble Pie, 145 g	360	6	35
Pepperoni, 110 g	290	5	34
Super Combo, 153 g	350	8	36
Super Hawaiian, 134 g	290	4	36
• Super Taco, 186 g	390	9	36
Taco, 171 g	360	8	36
Veggie, 139 g	270	4	36
Sides			
Breadsticks, 44 g	110	0	20
Breadsticks w/Cheese, 51 g	140	2	20
• Calzone - Cheese (Medium), 624 g	1660	24	200
Calzone - Combo (Medium), 624 g	1450	16	199
Calzone - Pepperoni (Medium), 553 g	1410	16	195
Cheesesticks (Medium), 67 g	200	3	24
Garlic Toast, 40 g	150	2	15
Garlic Toast w/Cheese, 54 g	210	4	16
• Hot Wings - breaded, 17 g	45	1	1
Potato Wedges, 454 g	690	8	96
Thin (Medium)			
All Meat Combo, 92 g	270	5	18
Bacon Cheeseburger, 95 g	260	6	18
• Cheese, 58 g	170	3	15
Combo, 92 g	240	3	17
Hawaiian, 78 g	190	3	16
Hot Stuff, 92 g	260	5	18
Humble Pie, 88 g	260	5	16
Pepperoni, 66 g	210	4	15
Super Combo, 116 g	290	6	19
Super Hawaiian, 90 g	220	4	19
• Super Taco, 131 g	300	8	19
Taco, 112 g	260	7	16
Veggie, 82 g	180	3	16

• MOST HEALTHY   • LEAST HEALTHY

GOLD STAR CHILI

	Cal	Fat	Cbs
Burritos			
• Chili Beef Burrito, 292 g	570	31	75
Chili Beef Burrito with Topper, 383 g	710	49	78
• Crispy Chicken Burrito, 277 g	840	34	62
Crispy Chicken Burrito with Topper, 334 g	790	56	84
Grilled Chicken Burrito, 268 g	580	29	59
Grilled Chicken Burrito w/ Topper, 325 g	730	51	72
Chilli by the bowl			
Chili (8 oz.), 227 g	213	50	8
Veggie Chili Bowl, 255 g	160	3	29
Gold Star Chili			
• Regular 2-Way, 340 g	420	24	58
Regular 2-Way bean, 425 g	489	21	71
Regular 2-Way onion, 383 g	436	23	62
• Regular 2-Way onion bean, 468 g	505	21	75
Gold Star Coney			
Cheese Coney, 160 g	343	47	31
Chili Cheese Sandwich, 132 g	288	39	30
• Chili Sandwich, 132 g	211	23	32
Coney, 146 g	286	42	30
• Low Carb Coney Bowl, 298 g	570	73	7
Sensational Entrée Sized Salads			
• Caesar Salad, 168 g	130	9	12
Cafe Salad, 224 g	160	15	15
Crispy Chicken Caesar Salad, 238 g	280	17	22
Crispy Chicken Cafe Salad, 295 g	310	23	24
Crispy Chkn Spring Harvest Salad, 315 g	360	26	32
Grilled Chicken Caesar Salad, 238 g	210	12	12
Grilled Chicken Cafe Salad, 295 g	250	18	15
Grilled Chkn Spring Harvest Salad, 315 g	300	20	33
Low Carb Chili Salad, 369 g	320	33	12
• South of the Border Chili Salad, 472 g	639	54	55
Spring Harvest Salad, 230 g	160	11	23
Sides			
Cheese Fries, 184 g	520	56	42
Chili Cheese Dip, 177 g	580	61	39
• Chili Cheese Fries, 269 g	596	55	46
Chili Cheese Nachos, 240 g	411	54	30
Fries, 149 g	366	46	44
Garlic Bread, 54 g	213	55	19
Garlic Bread w/ Cheese, 68 g	271	59	19
• Tex Mex (8 oz.), 227 g	210	38	17

• MOST HEALTHY   • LEAST HEALTHY

GOLDEN CORRAL

	Cal	Fat	Cbs
Brass Bell Bakery			
Apple Cobbler, 95 g	150	5	26
Apple Pie, 156 g	330	13	49
Banana Nut Bread, Garnished w/ Icing, 75 g	190	4	40
Banana Nut Bread, Garnished w/ Powdered Sugar, 68 g	170	4	35
Banana Pudding, 106 g	240	11	31
Bread Pudding, 100 g	240	12	30
Brownie, Fudgy, 41 g	140	6	20
Carrot Cake, 123 g	430	22	58
Cheesecake, New York Style Baked, 73 g	250	15	28
Cherry Cobbler, 95 g	180	5	31
Cherry Pie, 156 g	320	13	46
Choco Cake w/ Choco Frosting (Decorated w/ Cherries), 102 g	340	15	53
Chocolate Chess Mini Tarts, 90 g	340	18	40
Chocolate Soft Serve, 87 g	90	2	20
Coconut Cream Mini Tarts, 82 g	240	13	29
Fruit Mini Tarts, 118 g	220	9	31
German Chocolate Bars, 71 g	010	17	42
German Chocolate Cake, 107 g	370	18	52
• Gourmet Choco Cake w/ Choco Frosting, 147 g	590	31	83
Lemon Cream Mini Tarts, 91 g	240	11	34
No Sugar Added Blueberry Pie, 156 g	280	8	49
NSA Cheesecake, Strawberry, 66 g	220	15	21
NSA Chocolate Pudding, 108 g	110	5	13
NSA Peach Pie, 150 g	330	21	36
NSA Vanilla Nonfat Frozen Yogurt, 80 g	70	0	14
Orange Sherbet, 89 g	110	1	27
Peanut Butter Cream Mini Tarts, 99 g	340	21	32
Pecan Mini Tarts, 83 g	300	13	43
Pumpkin Mini Tarts, 91 g	220	10	30
Red Velvet Cake, 117 g	470	26	58
Shadow Cake, 112 g	430	20	62
Strawberry Shortcake, 83 g	200	7	33
Sugar Free Chocolate Chip Cookie, 22 g	90	5	15
• Sugar Free Strawberry/Cherry/Raspberry Gelatin, 85 g	10	0	1
Sugar Free Vanilla Cake, 77 g	200	12	28
Vanilla Soft Serve, 87 g	110	2	22
Breads			
Garlic Cheese Biscuits, 74 g	170	12	10
• Garlic Cheese Breadsticks, 45 g	120	5	13
• Homestyle Yeast Rolls, 63 g	180	4	31
Multigrain Rolls, 61 g	160	4	29
Skillet Cornbread, 56 g	120	3	22
Sourdough Rolls, 69 g	120	2	30
Cold Buffet			
Broccoli Salad, 54 g	110	8	9

• MOST HEALTHY   • LEAST HEALTHY

GOLDEN CORRAL (cont.)	Cal	Fat	Cbs
Cajun Potato Salad, 120 g	230	17	15
Coleslaw, 61 g	110	9	6
• Deviled Eggs, 31 g	70	5	1
Hot Bacon Dressing, 30 g	150	14	5
• Potato Salad, 120 g	250	19	16
Seafood Salad, 85 g	140	10	9
Shrimp and Seafood Salad, 85 g	140	8	6
Spinach Applewood Bacon Salad, 144 g	150	11	7
Tuna Salad, 103 g	200	14	5
Hot Buffet			
Apples, Escalloped, 113 g	130	2	29
Au Jus, 57 g	30	3	2
Awesome Pot Roast, 85 g	100	5	5
Baked Fish w/ Shrimp & Lemon Herb Sauce, 85 g	160	10	2
Baked Florentine Fish, 86 g	180	12	2
• BBQ Chicken (Leg Quarter), 221 g	490	22	21
BBQ Pork, 85 g	170	8	5
Bone-In Breaded Catfish, 85 g	210	14	7
Bourbon Street Chicken, 85 g	170	9	4
Breaded Catfish, 91 g	200	11	10
Breaded Scallops, 73 g	140	6	13
Broccoli & Rice, 115 g	120	5	16
Broccoli, Steamed, 78 g	25	0	6
Brown Gravy, 57 g	25	1	4
Brown Gravy with mushrooms, 57 g	25	1	4
• Cauliflower, Steamed, 78 g	20	0	3
Cheese Pizza, 79 g	170	7	21
Cheese Sauce, 57 g	80	5	4
Chicken Tenders, 81 g	170	8	6
Coconut Shrimp, 57 g	200	12	16
Collard Greens, 98 g	35	1	4
Corn on the Cob, 104 g	80	2	18
Crab Cakes, 55 g	180	15	8
Fried Chicken, 85 g	240	15	6
Golden Delicious Shrimp, 84 g	210	9	23
Green Beans, 121 g	35	2	4
Grilled Lemon Pepper Fish, 81 g	180	11	5
Ham (Pitt Style, Smoked), 85 g	110	6	1
Italian Red Sauce, 115 g	90	6	7
Linguine w/ Lemon Butter Herb Sauce, 164 g	270	17	23
Macaroni and Beef, 120 g	110	4	15
Macaroni and Cheese, 125 g	190	9	19
Mashed Potatoes, 100 g	140	7	18
Meatloaf (with Meatloaf Topping), 115 g	220	11	12
Mini Steakburgers, 102 g	280	15	16
Onions and Peppers, 57 g	30	2	4

• MOST HEALTHY • LEAST HEALTHY

GOLDEN CORRAL (cont.)

	Cal	Fat	Cbs
Pepperoni Pizza, 86 g	210	10	21
Popcorn Shrimp, 45 g	130	6	14
Poultry Gravy, 57 g	25	1	3
Rice Pilaf, 114 g	150	5	24
Rotisserie Chkn (Breast and Wing), 170 g	310	15	1
Salmon Lemonata, 85 g	130	10	3
Sautéed Mushrooms, 78 g	70	5	3
Shrimp Flatbread, 59 g	120	5	10
Shrimp Scampi, 76 g	170	13	3
Sirloin Steak, 128 g	230	9	1
Spicy Glazed Habanero Popcorn Shrimp, 85 g	210	7	30
Sweet and Sour Shrimp, 85 g	140	6	18
Sweet Homestyle Cornbread Stuffing, 93 g	130	6	17
Sweet Potato Casserole, 100 g	160	3	32
Tempura Battered Tilapia, 120 g	220	11	11
Tortellini & Shrimp in Lobster Sauce, 111 g	160	6	19
White Gravy, 57 g	45	3	4
White Rice, 114 n	100	0	23
Whole Carved Salmon, 85 g	120	6	1

Soup & Potato Bar

	Cal	Fat	Cbs
Chkn Noodle Soup – Soup and Potato Bar, 232 g	80	2	12
Clam Chowder – Soup and Potato Bar, 235 g	160	5	17
• Loaded Potato & Bacon Soup – Soup and Potato Bar, 240 g	250	14	21
Shrimp Jambalaya, 120 g	140	7	4
Timberline Chili, 248 g	230	9	26
• Vegetable Beef Soup, 227 g	80	1	14

Sunrise Breakfast Buffet

	Cal	Fat	Cbs
• Bacon and Chz Quiche (Whole, Sliced Quiche), 113 g	280	19	15
• Mini Cin-a-Gold Rolls, 65 g	230	9	35
Spinach Quiche, Whole, Sliced Quiche – Hot Bar, Breakfast, 102 g	230	16	14

GREAT STEAK & POTATO

Baked Potatoes

	Cal	Fat	Cbs
Broccoli & Cheese, 253 g	400	24	35
Cheese & Bacon, 223 g	530	35	29
• Plain, 170 g	160	0	36
Sour Cream & Chive, 209 g	350	23	32
The Great Potato - Chicken, 372 g	600	33	37
The Great Potato - Ham, 365 g	520	28	43
• The Great Potato - Steak, 386 g	620	38	37
The Great Potato - Turkey, 365 g	490	25	39
The King, 252 g	590	41	31

Breads/Tortillas

	Cal	Fat	Cbs
Bread, 7" Wheat, 113 g	310	4	56
Bread, 7" White, 113 g	290	3	55
• Pita, 79 g	220	5	38

• MOST HEALTHY   • LEAST HEALTHY

GREAT STEAK & POTATO (cont.)

	Cal	Fat	Cbs
• Tortilla, 117 g	370	9	60
Breakfast			
Potatoes, Deluxe Home, 344 g	390	23	44
• Potatoes, Fresh Cut Home, 301 g	380	23	42
Sandwich, Bacon, Egg & Cheese, 217 g	600	36	39
Sandwich, Egg & Cheese, 199 g	500	29	39
Sandwich, Ham & Cheese, 156 g	430	22	41
Sandwich, Ham, Egg & Cheese, 256 g	570	32	42
• Sandwich, Sausage, Egg & Chz, 256 g	700	47	39
Sandwich, Steak, Egg & Cheese, 284 g	600	34	40
Cheese			
• American, 1 oz.	100	9	1
• Philly Wiz, Cheese Sauce, 1 oz.	80	6	2
Provolone, 1 oz.	100	8	1
Swiss, 1 oz.	100	8	1
Fries and Sides (Regular)			
Coney Island Fry, 363 g	570	30	61
Great Fry, 292 g	440	20	60
• King Fry, 324 g	630	39	52
Nacho Fry, 335 g	510	27	53
• Potato Skins, 183 g	390	26	24
Wacker Fry, 278 g	490	27	51
Kids Meals			
Chicken Slider with Fry, 329 g	570	25	60
Grilled Cheese with Fry, 252 g	530	28	57
• Nuggets, Kids, 78 g	165	9	10
• Steak Slider with Fry, 336 g	580	28	60
Meats			
Chicken, serving, 113 g	140	3	0
Corned Beef, serving, 85 g	137	8	0
• Gyro Meat, serving, 113 g	210	12	5
Ham, serving, 113 g	120	4	6
Steak, serving, 128 g	160	7	0
• Turkey, serving, 113 g	90	1	2
Salads without dressing			
Great Salad, Grilled Chicken, 537 g	380	18	18
Great Salad, Grilled Ham, 537 g	360	20	24
• Great Salad, Grilled Steak, 551 g	400	23	18
Great Salad, Grilled Turkey, 537 g	330	17	20
Salad, Chef, 459 g	260	11	15
Salad, Garden, 345 g	60	1	13
• Salad, Side, 173 g	30	0	6
Wedge, Grilled Chicken, 421 g	270	12	11
Wedge, Grilled Steak, 435 g	290	16	11
Sandwiches			
Buffalo Chicken Upstate Philly, 7", 394 g	660	24	65

• MOST HEALTHY   • LEAST HEALTHY

GREAT STEAK & POTATO (cont.)

	Cal	Fat	Cbs
Cheeseburger, 291 g	640	35	41
Chicagoland Cheesesteak, 7", 378 g	680	29	63
• Chicken Philly Slider, 153 g	300	13	24
Great Steak Cheesesteak, 7", 387 g	740	37	62
Great Steak Cheesesteak, Wrap, 391 g	820	43	67
Gyro, 339 g	580	30	52
Ham Delight, 7", 373 g	710	33	71
Ham Explosion, 7", 415 g	710	34	70
Hamburger, 276 g	590	30	40
Kansas City (BBQ) Chzsteak, 7", 347 g	680	26	71
Original Chicken Philly, 7", 319 g	620	22	62
Original Chicken Philly, Wrap, 323 g	700	28	67
Original Philly Cheesesteak, 7", 336 g	650	26	62
Pastrami, 7", 380 g	790	41	65
Philly Burger, 404 g	820	50	47
Reuben, 7", 338 g	690	33	61
Steak Philly Slider, 160 g	310	15	24
Super Steak Cheesesteak, 7", 429 g	750	37	64
• Super Steak Cheesesteak, Wrap, 448 g	930	54	69
Teriyaki Chicken Philly, 7", 401 g	740	32	65
Turkey Philly, 7", 373 g	670	30	64
Ultimate Chicken Philly, 7", 415 g	730	33	64
Ultimate Chicken Philly, Wrap, 419 g	810	39	69
Veggie Delight, 7", 347 g	610	31	66
Wisconsin Inside-Out, 7", 177 g	560	27	57
Sauces/Dressings			
• Buffalo Sauce, 1 oz.	10	0	2
Marinara Dipping Sauce, 2 oz.	15	0	3
• Oil, serving, 0.3 oz.	60	7	0
Teriyaki Sauce, 1 oz.	25	0	3
Tzatziki Sauce, 1 oz.	50	4	2
Toppings - Baked Potato			
Bacon, 1 oz.	80	5	0
Broccoli, 4 ea	10	0	2
• Cheddar Cheese, 2 oz.	220	18	0
• Chives, 1 t.	0	0	0
Toppings - Sandwich			
Cucumber, 1 oz.	5	0	1
Green Pepper, 1 oz.	5	0	1
• Lettuce, 2 oz.	5	0	1
Mushrooms, 1 oz.	5	0	1
• Olives, 1 oz.	35	3	2
Onions, 2 oz.	20	0	4
Pineapple, 2 oz.	25	0	7
Sauerkraut, 2 oz.	10	0	2
Tomato Slices, 1 oz.	5	0	1

• MOST HEALTHY   • LEAST HEALTHY

▶ GREAT WRAPS

	Cal	Fat	Cbs
Breads			
• 12" Flour Tortilla	320	10	47
12" Honey Wheat Tortilla	300	8	50
12" Spinach Tortilla	290	9	43
12" Tomato Basil Tortilla	320	9	49
7" Pita	220	3	43
• Croutons, 1 oz.	75	10	9
Cheese			
• Cheddar Mix, 2 oz.	220	18	2
Crumbled Feta, 1 oz.	120	5	2
• Parmesan, 1 oz.	20	2	0
Pepper Jack, 2 oz.	220	18	2
Provolone, 2 oz.	200	16	2
Swiss, 2 oz.	160	12	0
Dressings			
• Cuban Sauce, 1 oz.	170	16	2
Feta, 2 oz.	160	16	4
• Zeke, 2 oz.	90	10	4
Fresh Veggies			
• Black Olives, 1 oz.	60	3	1
Chopped Cucumber, 1 oz.	3	0	1
Chopped Onion, 1 oz.	10	0	2
Chopped Pepperoncini, 1 oz.	5	0	0
Chopped Tomatoes, 2 oz.	10	0	0
Jalapeños, 1 oz.	17	1	1
Red Pepper, 1 oz.	20	1	2
Romaine, 2 oz.	10	N/A	1
• Shredded Lettuce, 2 oz.	0	0	0
Spinach, 1 oz.	5	0	1
Sprouts, 1 oz.	2	0	0
Meats			
• Bacon, 2 Slices	80	7	0
Chicken, 4 oz.	79	1	N/A
Chicken Tenderloin large, 4 oz.	90	3	N/A
• Gyro, 4 oz.	350	32	4
Ham, 2 oz.	80	2	2
Pork, 2 oz.	73	3	0
Steak, 4 oz.	110	4	1
Tuna, 4 oz.	105	2	0
Turkey, 4 oz.	80	0	4
Roasted Veggies			
Garlic Mushrooms, 1 oz.	5	2	1
• Green Pepper, 1 oz.	4	0	1
• Portabella Mushrooms, 3 oz.	81	14	5
Sauteed Onion, 1 oz.	27	1	3

• MOST HEALTHY   • LEAST HEALTHY

GREAT WRAPS (cont.)

	Cal	Fat	Cbs
Vegetarian Options			
Falafel, 2 oz.	340	7	56
Hummus, 2 oz.	140	8	14

GREEN BURRITO

	Cal	Fat	Cbs
Burritos			
Bean & Cheese Burrito, 407 g	820	37	100
Bean & Cheese Burrito - Chicken, 364 g	720	29	80
Bean & Chz Burrito - Ground Beef, 378 g	860	42	83
Bean & Cheese Burrito - Steak, 364 g	750	31	83
• Carne Asada Burrito, 312 g	680	30	65
Grilled Chicken Burrito, 485 g	1070	53	91
The Green Burrito®- Chicken, 612 g	900	32	120
The Green Burrito®- Steak, 612 g	930	34	122
Sides			
Chips, 57 g	300	17	35
• Chips & Cheese, 142 g	700	42	62
• Guacamole, 40 g	60	5	3
Pinto Beans & Cheese, 241 g	320	16	43
Rice, 198 g	340	10	58
Specialties			
Crisp Burritos (3 Pieces), 198 g	540	25	57
Enchiladas (2) - Cheese, 206 g	480	33	29
• Quesadilla - Cheese, 114 g	370	19	36
Quesadilla - Chicken, 199 g	460	21	38
Quesadilla - Steak, 199 g	490	24	40
Super Nachos - Chicken, 458 g	940	50	94
• Super Nachos - Ground Beef, 472 g	1080	63	97
Super Nachos - Steak, 458 g	970	53	97
Taco Salad - Chicken, 580 g	830	45	74
Taco Salad - Ground Beef, 594 g	970	58	76
Taco Salad - Steak, 580 g	860	48	76
Tacos			
• Fish Taco, 178 g	320	15	36
• Hard Taco - Chicken, 95 g	190	8	14
Hard Taco - Ground Beef, 95 g	240	14	15
Hard Taco - Steak, 95 g	200	10	16
Soft Taco - Chicken, 109 g	200	7	17
Soft Taco - Ground Beef, 109 g	250	13	18
Soft Taco - Steak, 109 g	220	9	18
Southwest Chicken Soft Taco, 116 g	300	19	17

HARDEE'S

	Cal	Fat	Cbs
Breakfast			
Bacon, Egg and Cheese Biscuit, 175 g	530	36	36
• Big Country® Brkfst Platter - Bacon, 369 g	910	48	91

• MOST HEALTHY   • LEAST HEALTHY

HARDEE'S (cont.)

	Cal	Fat	Cbs
Biscuit 'N' Gravy™, 251 g	530	33	48
Breaded Pork Chop Biscuit, 205 g	640	39	46
Chicken Fillet Biscuit, 226 g	600	34	50
Cinnamon 'N' Raisin™ Biscuit, 81 g	300	15	40
Country Ham Biscuit, 144 g	440	26	36
Country Steak Biscuit, 180 g	630	43	45
Frisco Breakfast Sandwich®, 185 g	400	18	27
Ham, Egg and Cheese Biscuit, 220 g	540	33	36
Jelly Biscuit, 137 g	520	34	44
Loaded Biscuit 'N' Gravy Brkfst Bowl™, 326 g	740	52	49
Loaded Breakfast Burrito, 265 g	760	49	39
Loaded Omelet Biscuit, 195 g	610	42	36
Low Carb Breakfast Bowl®, 208 g	620	50	6
Made from Scratch™ Biscuit, 109 g	370	23	35
Monster Biscuit™, 254 g	770	55	37
• Pancakes (3), 135 g	300	5	55
Pork Chop 'N' Gravy Biscuit, 234 g	680	42	48
Sausage and Egg Biscuit, 185 g	590	42	36
Sausage Biscuit, 142 g	530	38	36
Smoked Sausage Biscuit, 187 g	620	46	37
Sunrise Croissant™ with Ham, 163 g	400	23	27
Breakfast Sides			
Country Potatoes - Medium, 142 g	290	12	39
Grits, 142 g	110	5	16
Desserts			
Apple Turnover, 85 g	290	15	36
Chocolate Cake, 85 g	300	12	56
Chocolate Chip Cookie, 68 g	290	11	44
• Choco Chip Cookie - Fresh Baked, 52 g	250	14	30
• Hand-Scooped Malt, 414 g	780	35	98
Hand-Scooped Shake, 397 g	705	33	86
Peach Cobbler, small, 180 g	285	7	56
Single Scoop Ice Cream Cone, 126 g	285	13	37
Fried Chicken & Sides			
Cole Slaw, small, 113 g	170	10	20
• Fried Chicken Breast, 148 g	370	15	29
Fried Chicken Leg, 69 g	170	7	15
Fried Chicken Thigh, 121 g	330	15	30
Fried Chicken Wing, 66 g	200	8	23
• Mashed Potatoes, small, 142 g	90	2	17
Sides			
Crispy Curls™ - Medium, 132 g	410	20	52
• Natural-Cut French Fries - Med, 162 g	430	19	60
• Side Salad (no dressing), 191 g	120	7	7

► HARDEE'S (cont.)

	Cal	Fat	Cbs
Thickburgers® & Sandwiches			
1/3 LB Bacon Chz Thickburger®, 320 g	850	57	49
1/3 LB Cheeseburger, 240 g	620	33	51
1/3 LB Low Carb Thickburger®, 245 g	420	32	5
1/3 LB Mshr & Swiss Thickburger®, 259 g	650	36	47
1/3 LB Original Thickburger®, 343 g	770	48	53
2/3 LB Double Bacon Chz Thickburger®, 436 g	1200	84	50
2/3 LB Double Thickburger®, 445 g	1150	78	53
• 2/3 LB Monster Thickburger®, 386 g	1320	95	46
3 Piece Chicken Strips, 108 g	370	26	19
BBQ Chicken Sandwich, 271 g	400	6	62
Big Chicken Fillet Sandwich, 319 g	710	38	62
Big Hot Ham 'N' Cheese™, 232 g	460	20	40
Big Roast Beef™, 171 g	400	21	28
Charbroiled Chkn Club Snd, 306 g	630	32	54
Double Cheeseburger, 208 g	530	32	34
Fish Supreme Sandwich, 225 g	630	38	51
• Hot Ham 'N' Cheese™, 131 g	280	12	29
Jumbo Chili Dog, 145 g	400	26	25
Kids Meal - Cheeseburger, 215 g	560	29	59
Kids Meal - Chicken Strips, 149 g	450	27	40
Kids Meal - Hamburger, 203 g	520	25	59
Little Thick Cheeseburger, 167 g	450	23	38
Little Thickburger®, 220 g	570	39	35
Low Carb Charbroiled Chkn Club Snd, 250 g	360	23	14
Regular Roast Beef, 128 g	310	15	28
Six Dollar Thickburger®, 383 g	930	59	57
Small Cheeseburger, 139 g	350	19	32
Small Hamburger, 126 g	310	15	32
Spicy Chicken Sandwich, 153 g	440	21	41

► HARVEY'S

	Cal	Fat	Cbs
Beverages			
Chocolate Milkshake (14 oz.), 397 ml	730	33	91
Gatorade G2, 250 ml	30	0	7
Breakfast			
• Bacon (3 Strips), 9 g	40	4	0
• Breakfast Club Deluxe, 202 g	530	28	39
Breakfast Club, 157 g	400	19	36
Extra Egg, 50 g	90	6	0
Homefries, 116 g	300	19	29
Toast (2 Slices White), 71 g	180	2	35
Toast (2 Slices Whole Wheat), 71 g	170	2	32
Dipping Sauces			
Plum Sauce, 43 g	80	0	21
Sweet N' Sour Sauce, 43 g	80	1	17

• MOST HEALTHY   • LEAST HEALTHY

▶ HARVEY'S (cont.)

	Cal	Fat	Cbs
Garnishes			
Bacon, 3 g	15	1	0
Frank's Redhot Sauce, 8 ml	2	0	0
• Hot Peppers, 14 g	0	0	1
Lettuce, 28 g	4	0	1
Onions, 50 g	10	0	5
• Real Canadian Cheddar Chz Slice, 21 g	80	6	1
Tomato (Approx. 2 Slices), 50 g	10	0	2
Kids Combos			
• Cheeseburger Meal, 90 g	890	32	125
Chicken Strip Meal - 3 Pieces, 90 g	760	24	113
Hamburger Meal, 90 g	810	26	124
• Hot Dog Meal, 90 g	730	22	118
Main Menu Items			
Angus Burger, 213 g	560	26	47
Angus Burger with Cheese, 234 g	640	32	49
• Angus Burger w/ Chz & Bacon, 243 g	690	35	49
Angus Patty, 126 g	320	23	4
Chicken Strips - 3 Pieces, 114 g	320	15	27
Grilled Chicken, 165 g	290	5	28
Grilled Chicken Blt, 233 g	340	8	30
Grilled Chicken By Itself, 100 g	140	3	1
Hot Dog by Itself, 48 g	140	11	3
Hot Dog with Bun, 102 g	300	13	32
Original Bacon Cheeseburger, 168 g	500	26	39
Original Cheeseburger, 160 g	460	23	39
Original Hamburger, 139 g	380	16	37
Original Patty by Itself, 78 g	200	14	4
Veggie Burger, 138 g	290	10	33
• Veggie Burger By Itself, 73 g	130	7	6
Warm Grilled Chicken Blt Salad, 301 g	230	7	9
Warm Grilled Chicken Salad, 289 g	170	3	9
Salad Dressings			
Asian Sesame Dressing, 28 ml	60	3	9
Creamy Garlic Pprcrn Ranch Drss, 28 ml	108	11	2
Side Orders			
Fries - Regular, 120 g	320	13	49
Frings, 162 g	520	24	69
• Gravy, 92 g	30	1	6
Onion Rings - Regular, 72 g	270	15	33
• Poutine, 284 g	840	43	87
Side Garden Salad, 198 g	40	0	8

▶ HEAVENLY HAM

BBQ Heaven			
Heavenly BBQ	260	14	16

● MOST HEALTHY • LEAST HEALTHY

HEAVENLY HAM (cont.)

	Cal	Fat	Cbs
Onion Roll	230	5	39
Bone-In Hams			
Glaze and Visible Signs of Fat Rmvd, 3 oz.	159	3	4
Glazed, 3 oz.	190	11	4
Boneless Hams			
Glaze and Visible Signs of Fat Rmvd, 3 oz.	89	1	4
Glazed, 3 oz.	120	4	4
Breads			
Croissant	230	12	27
Focaccia Bread	220	4	40
• French Batard	210	1	46
Multigrain Batard	250	4	46
Onion Roll	230	5	39
• Sliced Wheat Bread	300	5	54
Cheeses			
Cheddar Cheese Slices	110	9	0
• Havarti Cheese	120	10	0
• Swiss Cheese Slices	110	8	2
Chicken Salad			
• Chicken Salad	230	17	8
Salad Mix	25	0	4
• Tomatoes	5	0	2
Classic Roast Beef			
Cheddar Cheese Slices	110	9	0
• French Batard	210	1	46
• Green Leaf Lettuce	0	0	0
Heavenly Roast Beef	80	3	2
Tomato Slices	5	0	2
Desserts			
Chocolate Chip, 1 cookie	270	12	40
• Fudge Brownie, 1 brownie	430	23	50
Heath Bar Crunch, 1 cookie	280	14	37
• Oatmeal Raisin Nut, 1 cookie	260	12	35
Peanut Butter, 1 cookie	290	18	29
White Choco Macadamia Nut, 1 cookie	290	15	35
Extras			
• Heavenly Seven Bean Soup, 1 cup	150	2	24
Spinach Dip, 2 Tbsp.	130	14	2
• Tomato & Cucumber Salad, 1/2 Cup	60	5	5
Paradise Club			
• Croissant	230	12	27
• Green Leaf Lettuce	0	0	0
Havarti Cheese	120	10	0
Heavenly Ham	45	1	2
Heavenly Peppered Bacon	70	6	2
Heavenly Smoked Turkey	30	0	2

• MOST HEALTHY   • LEAST HEALTHY

HEAVENLY HAM (cont.)

	Cal	Fat	Cbs
That Mustard	150	0	30
Tomato Slices	5	0	2

Sauces

	Cal	Fat	Cbs
Bistro Sauce, 1 oz.	120	13	1
• Dill Sauce, 2 oz.	170	19	1
• Horseradish Sauce, 1 oz.	60	6	1
Sweet Café Spread, 1 oz.	100	10	4
That Mustard, 1 oz.	150	0	30

Turkeys

	Cal	Fat	Cbs
Boneless Roasted Turkey Breast, 2 oz.	60	0	3
• Glazed Bnlss Smoked Tkey Breast, 3 oz.	60	0	3
• Whole Roasted Turkey, 3 oz.	160	10	0
Whole Smoked Turkey, 3 oz.	146	8	1

HIGH TECH BURRITO

	Cal	Fat	Cbs
Black Beans - 4.0 oz.	96	5	17
Brown Rice - 2.5 oz.	52	6	10
Chips - 3.0 oz.	140	55	17
Chips & Guac - 3.0 oz./3.5 oz.	204	108	21
Chips & Salsa - 3.0 oz./3.5 oz.	155	56	21
Flour Tortilla - 12"	274	70	45
Jack Cheese Shredded - 1 oz.	106	77	0
Lime Sour Cream - 2 oz.	58	40	3
• Mild Salsa - 2 oz.	12	1	3
• Saute Chicken Fajita	332	162	2
Spanish Rice - 2.5 oz.	83	3	18

HOMETOWN BUFFET

For nutritional information please see Country Buffet

HOOTERS

Entrees

	Cal	Fat	Cbs
Dozen Raw Oysters	115	4	7
• Garden Salad	115	2	22
• Grilled Big Fish Sandwich	435	5	46
Grilled Chicken Garden Salad	265	4	23
Grilled Chicken Sandwich	420	4	51
Snow Crab Legs	300	4	1
Steamed Shrimp	230	3	1

Side Dish

	Cal	Fat	Cbs
Baked Beans	115	1	24
• Dish Coleslaw	120	9	9
• Side Garden Salad	60	1	12

• MOST HEALTHY   • LEAST HEALTHY

HOT DOG ON A STICK

	Cal	Fat	Cbs
Cheese on a Stick			
American Cheese on a Stick, 82 g	270	14	26
Pepperjack Cheese on a Stick, 79 g	260	13	25
Hot Dogs			
• Beef Hot Dog on a Bun, 134 g	460	29	37
• Turkey Hot Dog on a Stick, 92 g	240	11	28
Veggie Dog on a Stick, 112 g	250	5	35
French Fries			
Fish & Zucchini Platter, 199 g	560	37	42
Fish & Zucchini Platter (Hawaii), 284 g	710	55	42
Fish Platter, 113 g	320	21	24
French Fries, 127 g	390	15	60
• Funnel Cake Sticks, 51 g	220	9	31
• Zucchini Platter, 279 g	780	68	35

HUNGRY HOWIE'S PIZZA

	Cal	Fat	Cbs
Boneless Wings			
Boneless Wings, 3 pieces	145	5	12
Howie Breads			
• Cajun Bread, 1/4 of brd	300	9	46
Cinnamon Bread, 1/4 of brd	313	9	59
Howie Bread, 1/4 of brd	300	9	46
• Three Cheeser Bread, 1/4 of brd	370	14	47
Howie Wings			
Howie Wings, 5 wings	180	13	0
Medium Pizza (8 Slices)			
Anchovies Topping Only, 1 Slice	44	3	0
Bacon Topping Only, 1 Slice	32	1	0
Banana Peppers Topping Only, 1 Slice	6	0	1
Beef Topping Only, 1 Slice	30	2	0
Black Olives Topping Only, 1 Slice	7	0	0
• Cheese Only Pizza, 1 Slice	191	6	23
Green Olives Topping Only, 1 Slice	7	0	0
Green Peppers Topping Only, 1 Slice	2	1	0
Ham Topping Only, 1 Slice	7	0	0
• Mushroom Topping Only, 1 Slice	2	0	0
Onions Topping Only, 1 Slice	2	1	0
Pepperoni Topping Only, 1 Slice	22	2	0
Pineapple Topping Only, 1 Slice	5	1	2
Sausage Topping Only, 1 Slice	27	2	0
Medium Thin Crust Low Carb (8 Slices)			
Anchovies Topping Only, 1 Slice	44	3	0
Bacon Topping Only, 1 Slice	32	1	0
Banana Peppers Topping Only, 1 Slice	6	0	1
Beef Topping Only, 1 Slice	30	2	0

• MOST HEALTHY   • LEAST HEALTHY

HUNGRY HOWIE'S PIZZA (cont.)	Cal	Fat	Cbs
Black Olives Topping Only, 1 Slice	7	0	0
• Cheese Only Pizza, 1 Slice	111	5	10
Green Olives Topping Only, 1 Slice	7	0	0
Green Peppers Topping Only, 1 Slice	2	1	0
Ham Topping Only, 1 Slice	7	0	0
• Mushroom Topping Only, 1 Slice	2	0	0
Onions Topping Only, 1 Slice	2	1	0
Pepperoni Topping Only, 1 Slice	22	2	0
Pineapple Topping Only, 1 Slice	5	1	2
Sausage Topping Only, 1 Slice	27	2	0
Oven Baked Subs			
Deluxe Italian Sub, 1/2 sub	506	18	61
Ham & Cheese Sub, 1/2 sub	475	15	61
Pizza Special Sub, 1/2 sub	606	24	68
• Pizza Sub, 1/2 sub	689	34	67
Steak & Cheese Sub, 1/2 sub	491	15	64
Turkey Club Sub, 1/2 sub	556	15	63
• Turkey Sub, 1/2 sub	466	13	63
Vegetarian Sub, 1/2 sub	530	21	64
Salads (Small)			
Antipasto, 2 per sld.	115	7	3
Chef, 2 per sld.	114	7	4
• Garden, 2 per sld.	20	0	3
• Greek, 2 per sld.	126	7	8
Sauces			
Dipping Sauce, 3 oz.	45	9	0

IN-N-OUT BURGER			
Burgers			
Cheeseburger Protein® Style, 300 g	330	25	11
Chzburger w/ mustard & ketchup, 268 g	400	18	41
Chzburger w/Onion, 268 g	480	27	39
Double-Double Protein® Style, 362 g	520	39	11
Double-Double w/ mustard & ketchup, 330 g	590	32	41
• Double-Double w/Onion, 330 g	670	41	39
• Hamburger Protein® Style, 275 g	240	17	11
Hamburger w/ mustard & ketchup, 243 g	310	10	41
Hamburger w/Onion, 243 g	390	19	39
Shakes			
• Chocolate Shake, 15 oz.	690	36	83
Strawberry Shake, 15 oz.	690	33	91
• Vanilla Shake, 15 oz.	680	37	78
Sides			
French Fries, 125 g	400	18	54

• MOST HEALTHY   • LEAST HEALTHY

ISLANDS RESTAURANTS

	Cal	Fat	Cbs
Appetizers			
• Beachside Sliders, 20 oz.	1490	62	170
Beachside Sliders Turkey, 20 oz.	1320	57	161
Buffalo Wings - BBQ, 9 oz.	570	44	3
Buffalo Wings - Teriyaki, 9 oz.	600	44	10
Buffalo Wings - Traditional Spicy, 9 oz.	620	48	8
Cheddar Fries, 6 oz.	550	42	33
Chips & Salsa, 6 oz.	380	18	53
Chips & Salsa w/ Guacamole, 5 oz.	320	17	39
Island Fries, 5 oz.	420	31	32
Nachos, 6 oz.	430	32	22
Onion Rings, 4 oz.	380	15	55
Quesadilla, 4 oz.	290	20	18
• Spinach-Artichoke Dip w/Chips, 4 oz.	290	19	25
Tiki Tenders, 7 oz.	480	26	46
Burgers			
Big Wave, 15 oz.	1020	67	66
Big Wave W/Cheese, 17 oz.	1230	92	66
Bleuhami, 17 oz.	1430	102	72
Hawaiian, 18 oz.	1450	102	79
Hula, 21 oz.	1520	110	72
Kilauea, 18 oz.	1560	115	79
Malibu, 18 oz.	1360	93	75
Maui, 18 oz.	1350	93	72
• Mavericks, 22 oz.	1570	91	128
Pipeline, 20 oz.	1410	99	75
Rincon, 19 oz.	1430	115	72
Sunset, 18 oz.	1250	83	75
Turkey, 15 oz.	815	42	67
• Veggie, 12 oz.	690	30	85
Dessert			
Chocolate Lava Dessert, 5 oz.	480	29	50
• Fudge Brownie, 7 oz.	750	39	94
Ice Cream Sundae, 5 oz.	340	20	35
Kona Pie, 4 oz.	350	23	34
Gremmie			
Gremmie Fries, 4 oz.	350	26	29
Jr. Quesadilla w/aplsc & carrots, 10 oz.	560	26	72
• Jr. Sundae, 3 oz.	220	15	17
Jr. Tiki Tenders w/aplsc & carrots, 12 oz.	630	24	69
Jr. Wave w/chz, aplsc & carrots, 14 oz.	760	40	65
Lil Chili Chz Dogger w/aplsc & carrots, 16 oz.	1050	71	66
Lil Dogger w/aplsc & carrots, 11 oz.	630	36	62
Macaroni & Cheese, 13 oz.	460	11	81
Sandcastle w/aplsc & carrots, 10 oz.	520	21	66

• MOST HEALTHY   • LEAST HEALTHY

ISLANDS RESTAURANTS (cont.)

	Cal	Fat	Cbs
Paradise's Bikini Beach			
No-Blame Grilled Veggie Tacos, 17 oz.	477	17	68
Northshore Tacos, Limited, 17 oz.	589	25	55
• Sleek Greek Salad™, 13 oz.	341	17	27
• Turkey Burger Lite, 22 oz.	670	20	84

Salads

	Cal	Fat	Cbs
China Coast, 27 oz.	1310	81	87
Garden Salad, 16 oz.	1330	99	83
• Greek Salad, 28 oz.	990	62	53
Jungle Caesar, 20 oz.	995	68	33
• Kaanapali Kobb, 30 oz.	1700	131	38
Wiqui Waqui, 31 oz.	1085	58	75

Sandwiches & Other Items

	Cal	Fat	Cbs
CA Flyer, 17 oz.	1230	55	115
Chicken Club Wrap, 23 oz.	960	77	72
Macaw, 17 oz.	1130	64	72
Moa Kai (Tuna), 14 oz.	1190	88	66
• Rotisseric Chicken, 29 oz.	1260	67	79
Sandpiper, 18 oz.	1000	51	72
• Shorebird, 18 oz.	950	49	65
Toucan, 16 oz.	1030	51	79
Tuna Wrap, 18 oz.	1090	80	60
Wedge, 13 oz.	1220	92	63

Soups

	Cal	Fat	Cbs
Tortilla Soup - Large, 22 oz.	610	38	40

Tacos

	Cal	Fat	Cbs
Baja - 2 Taco, 18 oz.	810	41	81
Cabo Loco - 2 Taco, 19 oz.	920	55	63
• Grilled Veggie - 2 Taco, 18 oz.	600	26	81
• Islands Fish - 2 Taco, 18 oz.	1020	67	85
Northshore - 2 Taco, 17 oz.	680	33	61
Yaki - 2 Taco, 19 oz.	790	34	90

JACK IN THE BOX

Breakfast

	Cal	Fat	Cbs
Bacon Breakfast Jack ®, 112 g	300	13	30
Bacon, Egg & Cheese Biscuit, 138 g	420	24	36
Breakfast Bowl, Denver, 311 g	790	57	44
• Breakfast Bowl, Hearty, 288 g	850	65	41
• Breakfast Jack ®, 124 g	280	11	30
Chorizo Sausage Burrito (no Salsa), 297 g	720	41	59
Chorizo Sausage Burrito (w/ Salsa), 321 g	730	41	61
Extreme Sausage® Sandwich, 210 g	660	47	32
French Toast Sticks (4 pc.), 141 g	600	33	68
Hash Brown Sticks (5 pc.), 83 g	280	19	26
Meaty Breakfast Burrito (no Salsa), 233 g	600	37	38

JACK IN THE BOX (cont.)

	Cal	Fat	Cbs
Meaty Breakfast Burrito (w/ Salsa), 257 g	610	37	40
Sausage Biscuit, 128 g	460	30	36
Sausage Breakfast Jack ®, 152 g	440	27	31
Sausage Croissant, 166 g	570	40	32
Sausage, Egg & Cheese Biscuit, 178 g	570	39	37
Sourdough Breakfast Sandwich, 151 g	410	21	34
Spicy Chicken Biscuit, 183 g	570	29	54
Steak & Egg Burrito (no Salsa), 296 g	810	50	55
Steak & Egg Burrito (w/ Salsa), 319 g	820	50	57
Supreme Croissant, 143 g	440	26	32
Ultimate Breakfast Sandwich, 225 g	510	24	41

Burgers & More

	Cal	Fat	Cbs
Bacon Ultimate Cheeseburger, 301 g	940	66	45
Big Cheeseburger, 200 g	610	38	44
Hamburger Deluxe w/ Cheese, 184 g	440	26	34
Hamburger Deluxe, 161 g	360	19	33
Hamburger w/ Cheese, 122 g	330	15	32
• Hamburger, 110 g	290	12	32
Jumbo Jack ® w/ Cheese, 260 g	620	39	45
Jumbo Jack®, 237 g	540	32	45
Junior Bacon Cheeseburger, 127 g	420	24	32
Mini Sirloin Burgers, 278 g	750	30	77
• Sirloin Cheeseburger w/ Bacon, 374 g	960	64	52
Sirloin Cheeseburger, 363 g	900	60	52
Sirloin Swiss & Grl Onion Burger w/ Bacon, 376 g	950	63	52
Sirloin Swiss & Grl Onion Burger, 364 g	880	59	52
Sourdough Jack®, 228 g	680	46	40
Sourdough Steak Melt, 228 g	650	38	38
Sourdough Ultimate Chzburger, 280 g	900	67	38
Ultimate Cheeseburger, 290 g	870	61	44

Cheeses

	Cal	Fat	Cbs
American Cheese, 11 g	40	4	0
• Real Swiss Cheese, 11 g	40	3	1
• Swiss Style Cheese, 18 g	70	6	0

Chicken & Fish

	Cal	Fat	Cbs
Chkn Fajita Pita made w/ Whole Grain, 192 g	320	11	33
Chkn Fajita Pita w/ Whole Grain (w/ Salsa), 215 g	330	11	35
Chicken Sandwich w/ Bacon, 158 g	480	26	42
Chicken Sandwich, 151 g	440	23	42
Crispy Chicken Strips (4 pc.), 195 g	560	24	53
• Fish and Chips w/ French Fries, 267 g	790	41	85
Fish Sandwich, 201 g	470	18	59
• Grilled Chicken Strips (4 pc.), 198 g	240	6	5
Homestyle Ranch Chicken Club, 265 g	700	33	65
Jack's Spicy Chicken ® w/ Cheese, 277 g	650	31	62
Jack's Spicy Chicken®, 254 g	570	25	60

• MOST HEALTHY   • LEAST HEALTHY

JACK IN THE BOX (cont.)

	Cal	Fat	Cbs
Mini Buffalo Ranch Chkn Snd, 291 g	740	28	90
Sourdough Grilled Chicken Club, 263 g	550	29	38
Dipping Sauces			
Buttermilk House Dipping Sauce, 25 g	130	13	3
• Fire Roasted Salsa, 21 g	5	0	1
Frank's ® Red Hot ® Sauce, 28 g	10	0	2
• Log Cabin ® Syrup, 62 g	190	0	49
Sweet & Sour Dipping Sauce, 28 g	45	0	11
Teriyaki Dipping Sauce, 28 g	60	1	11
Zesty Marinara Sauce, 25 g	15	0	4
Drinks			
• Iced Coffee, Caramel - 24 oz., 675 g	150	3	25
Iced Coffee, Original - 24 oz., 675 g	160	3	26
Iced Coffee, Vanilla - 24 oz., 675 g	160	3	27
Smoothie, Mango - 16 oz., 411 g	290	0	72
Smoothie, Strawberry - 16 oz., 394 g	270	0	67
Smoothie, Strwby Banana - 16 oz., 420 g	290	0	73
• Smoothie, Tropical - 16 oz., 481 g	330	0	81
Healthy Choices			
Chicken Teriyaki Bowl, 499 g	690	6	133
• Fruit Cup, 116 g	50	0	14
Grilled Chicken Salad, 400 g	240	8	15
Grl Chkn Strips w/ Teriyaki Dipping Sc, 226 g	300	6	18
Hamburger Deluxe, 161 g	360	19	33
Mango Smoothie - 16 oz., 411 g	290	0	72
• Steak Teriyaki Bowl, 499 g	750	11	133
Strwbry Banana Smoothie - 16 oz., 420 g	290	0	73
Kid's Meals			
Breakfast Jack ®, 124 g	280	11	30
Chicken Strips, Crispy (2 pc.), 98 g	280	12	26
• Chicken Strips, Grilled (2 pc.), 99 g	120	3	2
French Fries - Kids, 56 g	180	8	24
French Toast Sticks (2 pc.), 73 g	300	16	34
• Grilled Cheese, 94 g	330	16	34
Hamburger, 110 g	290	12	32
Hamburger w/ Cheese, 122 g	330	15	32
Other			
• Grape Jelly, 14 g	35	0	9
Grilled Onions, 20 g	10	0	2
• Malt Vinegar, 9 g	0	0	0
Pride Margarine Spread, 5 g	20	3	0
Red Onion (2 pc.), 9 g	5	0	1
Soy Sauce, 9 g	5	N/A	1
Strawberry Jelly, 14 g	35	0	9
Taco Sauce, 9 g	0	0	0

• MOST HEALTHY   • LEAST HEALTHY

JACK IN THE BOX (cont.)

	Cal	Fat	Cbs
Salads			
Bacon Ranch Dressing, 57 g	260	26	3
• Chkn Club Salad w/ Crispy Chkn Strips, 404 g	510	27	37
Chkn Club Salad w/ Grl Chkn Strips, 405 g	350	18	13
Creamy Southwest Dressing, 57 g	220	22	3
Gourmet Seasoned Croutons, 28 g	100	6	17
Grilled Chicken Salad, 400 g	240	8	15
Lite Ranch Dressing, 57 g	150	15	3
Low Fat Balsamic Vinaigrette, 57 g	35	2	5
• Side Salad, 115 g	20	0	4
SW Chkn Salad w/ Crispy Chkn Strips, 460 g	500	23	53
SW Chkn Salad w/ Grl Chkn Strips, 461 g	340	14	29
Spicy Corn Sticks, 28 g	140	7	18
Shakes & Desserts			
Cheesecake, 92 g	310	17	32
• Chocolate Overload Cake™, 93 g	300	7	57
Choco Shake w/ Whipped Topping, 376 g	800	38	101
Mini Churros (5 pç.), 86 g	350	19	43
• Oreo® Cookie Shake w/ Whipped Top, 362 g	810	43	92
Strwbry Shake w/ Whipped Top, 374 g	780	38	95
Vanilla Shake w/ Whipped Topping, 339 g	700	38	76
Snacks & Sides			
Bacon Cheddar Potato Wedges, 260 g	710	45	58
Beef Taco, 74 g	180	10	11
Egg Roll (1 pc.), 58 g	150	7	15
French Fries - Medium, 131 g	410	19	56
• Fruit Cup, 116 g	50	0	14
Mozzarella Cheese Sticks (3 pc.), 74 g	280	16	22
Onion Rings, 97 g	450	28	45
Pita Snack, Crispy Chicken, 158 g	410	19	43
Pita Snack, Fish, 155 g	390	20	40
Pita Snack, Grilled Chicken, 159 g	330	14	31
Pita Snack, Steak, 152 g	350	16	31
• Sampler Trio, 261 g	790	43	73
Seasoned Curly Fries - Medium, 130 g	430	25	46
Stuffed Jalapeños (3 pc.), 71 g	220	12	21
Something Different			
Chicken Teriyaki Bowl, 499 g	690	6	133
• Deli Trio Grilled Sandwich, 271 g	630	29	53
• Steak Teriyaki Bowl, 499 g	750	11	133
Tkey, Bacon and Cheddar Grilled Snd, 247 g	650	30	54
Substitute Sauces			
Chipotle Sauce (0.70 oz.), 20 g	110	12	1
Peppercorn Mayo (1.00 oz.), 28 g	190	20	1
Value Menu			
Big Cheeseburger, 200 g	610	38	44

• MOST HEALTHY   • LEAST HEALTHY

JACK IN THE BOX (cont.)	Cal	Fat	Cbs
Chicken Sandwich, 151 g	440	23	42
Grilled Cheese, 94 g	330	16	34
Hamburger Deluxe, 161 g	360	19	33
Hamburger Deluxe w/ Cheese, 184 g	440	26	34
Jumbo Jack®, 237 g	540	32	45
• Jumbo Jack® w/ Cheese, 260 g	620	39	45
Junior Bacon Cheeseburger, 127 g	420	24	32
• Side Salad, 123 g	50	3	5
Two Tacos, 147 g	360	21	33

JACK'S			
Breakfast			
Bacon Biscuit, 310 g	150	17	31
Bacon, Egg & Cheese Biscuit, 420 g	230	26	31
Biscuit, 250 g	110	12	31
Biscuit w/butter, 350 g	210	23	31
Bologna Biscuit, 370 g	200	23	33
Egg and Cheese Biscuit, 360 g	190	21	31
• Flapjacks, 330 g	70	8	57
Ham Biscuit, 310 g	130	14	31
Hash Browns, 440 g	250	27	45
Sausage Biscuit, 410 g	240	26	31
Sausage Gravy, 230 g	150	17	13
• Sausage, Egg & Cheese Biscuit, 520 g	320	35	32
Scrambled Eggs, 140 g	90	10	0
Single Gravy Biscuit, 420 g	220	24	40
Steak Biscuit, 480 g	250	28	43
Chicken & Sides			
Chicken Biscuit, 480 g	210	23	44
Healthy Choices			
Grits w/butter, 230 g	100	12	27

JAMBA JUICE			
• Acai Cup, 16 oz.	620	15	114
Berry Fulfilling, 403 g	177	1	38
Berry Topper Brkfst Meal, 12 oz.	360	8	67
Blueberry & Blackberry Oatmeal, 1 fl.oz.	290	4	59
Chunky Strwbry Smoothie w/ Organic Granola, 12 fl.oz.	450	14	68
Energy Boost, 1/2 tsp.	0	N/A	N/A
Jamba Light - Berry Fulfilling, 16 oz.	160	1	34
Jamba Oatmeal (fresh Banana), 1/2 cup	280	4	57
Mango Mantra, 16 oz.	170	1	36
Original Strawberry Nirvana, 16 oz.	170	0	36
Peach Perfection, 16 oz.	200	0	50
Peach Pleasure, 24 oz.	460	2	108
Peanut Butter Moo'd Smoothie, 16 fl.oz.	530	11	84

JAMBA JUICE (cont.)

	Cal	Fat	Cbs
Pomegranate Paradise, 16 oz.	260	1	64
Protein Boost, 8 g	28	0	0
Razzmatazz, 24 oz.	440	2	102
Strawberry Nirvana, 16 oz.	150	0	34
Strawberry Nirvana Smoothie, 16 oz.	170	0	36
Strawberry Wild, 24 oz.	410	1	98
• Wheatgrass Shot, 32 g	5	0	1
Baked Goods			
Apple Cinn Pretzel (1 Pretzel), 148 g	380	4	76
Cheddar Tomato Twist (1 bread), 91 g	240	5	38
• Omega-3 Choco Brownie Cookie (1 Cookie), 43 g	150	4	30
Omega-3 Oatmeal Cookie (1 Cookie), 43 g	150	6	26
Orange Dark Choco Chip Scone (1 Scone), 91 g	380	15	57
RedFat Blbry Lemon Loaf(1 bread), 85 g	290	8	53
Sourdough Parm Pretzel (1 Pretzel), 142 g	410	10	67
Tart Cherry Scone (1 Scone), 91 g	360	12	58
Zucchini Walnut Loaf (1 bread), 85 g	270	9	43
California Flatbreads			
• Four Cheesy (1flatbreads), 119 g	330	13	35
• MediterraneYUM (1flatbreads), 123 g	250	8	37
Smokehouse Chkn (1flatbreads), 131 g	300	8	41
Grab_N_Go Food			
Asian Style Chkn Wraps, 299 g	430	7	72
• Caesar The Day, 213 g	290	18	15
Chimichurri Chicken Wraps, 295 g	560	25	67
Gobble'licious, 263 g	570	28	49
Greeks Goodness Wraps, 318 g	500	20	70
• Greens and Grain Wraps, 308 g	620	12	108
Zesty Southwest Gr. Chicken Salad, 318 g	400	22	26

JIMBOY'S TACOS

	Cal	Fat	Cbs
Burgers			
• Cheese Burger	550	29	35
Hamburger	470	22	35
• Tacoburger	370	9	17
Burrito Bowls			
Carnitas	610	36	44
• Chicken	540	28	44
Fish	620	36	55
• Ground Beef	650	39	44
Shredded Beef	540	29	45
Steak	621	32	44
Burritos			
• Bean	530	28	55
Chicken	590	29	45
Ground Beef	610	32	50

• MOST HEALTHY   • LEAST HEALTHY

► JIMBOY'S TACOS (cont.)	Cal	Fat	Cbs
Shredded Beef	540	24	45
• Steak	750	40	46
Combo Burritos			
• Chicken	580	28	52
Ground Beef	620	33	57
Shredded Beef	585	28	53
• Steak	710	37	52
Dessert			
ChocoTaco	390	21	11
• Cinnamon Churros (3)	330	18	5
• Creme-Filled Churros (3)	405	20	5
Dinner Plates			
Bean Burrito	530	28	8
Bean Taco	190	12	4
Cheese Enchilada	350	20	11
Chicken Combo Burrito	580	28	8
Chicken Enchilada	460	21	11
Chicken Taco	200	11	4
Chile Relleno	300	24	8
Combination Dinner Plate Base	470	15	3
Ground Beef Combo Burrito	620	33	11
Ground Beef Enchilada	470	23	12
Ground Beef Taco	220	14	5
Shredded Beef Combo Burrito	585	28	9
Shredded Beef Enchilada	300	17	10
• Shredded Beef Taco	190	11	4
• Steak Combo Burrito	710	37	14
Steak Taco	190	10	3
El Gordos			
Chicken	400	20	29
• Ground Beef	460	25	35
Shredded Beef	400	19	30
• Steak	400	18	33
Enchiladas with Rice			
Cheese	350	20	28
Chicken	460	21	42
• Ground Beef	470	23	45
• Shredded Beef (Includes Rice)	300	17	16
Kid's Meals			
• Cheese Quesadilla & Chips	780	35	97
Ground Beef Taco & Chips	610	23	83
Jr. Bean Burrito & Chips	710	27	105
• Jr. Burger & Chips	320	15	25
Quesadillas			
• Cheese	400	25	27

JIMBOY'S TACOS (cont.)

	Cal	Fat	Cbs
Chicken	450	26	28
Ground Beef	480	29	31
Shredded Beef	460	26	28
• Steak	520	27	30
Salads			
Feta-Avocado Chicken Salad	710	43	40
Side Orders			
Corn Chips	280	15	36
Corn Tortilla 6"	60	1	12
Flour Tortilla 8"	170	4	28
• French Fries	700	34	89
Side Guacamole (2 oz.)	90	8	4
Side Nacho Cheese (2 oz.)	70	4	7
• Side Salsa Cruda (2 oz.)	10	0	2
Super Burritos			
• Carnitas	730	40	54
Chicken	630	31	58
Ground Beef	670	35	63
Shredded Beef	610	29	58
• Steak	600	28	59
Super Nachos			
Bean	850	48	96
• Chicken	780	45	81
Ground Beef	810	40	82
Shredded Beef	790	44	82
• Steak	1030	60	95
Taco Salads			
• Bean	530	29	50
Chicken	610	31	50
Ground Beef	660	37	56
Shredded Beef	615	31	51
• Steak	710	41	48
Tacos			
Bean	190	12	16
Carnitas Taco	200	5	15
Chicken	200	11	12
• Fish Taco	240	15	13
Ground Beef	220	14	15
Shredded Beef	190	11	13
• Steak	190	10	15
Taquitos			
Chicken	150	8	16
Ground Beef	230	17	16
The Works			
Guacamole & Sour Cream	90	8	3
Guacamole	35	3	0

• MOST HEALTHY　　• LEAST HEALTHY

JIMBOY'S TACOS (cont.)

	Cal	Fat	Cbs
Tostadas			
• Bean	290	20	23
Chicken	330	21	23
• Ground Beef	360	24	26
Shredded Beef	340	21	23
Value Menu			
Cheesy Bean Flautas	460	17	60
Cinnamon Crispies	130	6	28
• Fruit Cup	80	0	19
Ground Beef Jalapeño Poppers	220	9	25
Jr. Bean Burrito	390	21	41
Jr. Hamburger	470	22	35
• Parmesan Mini-Dillas	480	35	29
Side Guacamole	90	8	4
Vegetarian			
Bean Burrito	530	28	55
Bean Taco	190	12	16
Bean Tostada	290	20	23
Cheese Enchilada & Rice	350	20	28
Cheese Quesadilla	400	25	27
• Chile Relleno & Rice	530	32	40
Regular Nachos (Chips & Cheese)	360	19	43
• Side Pinto Beans	180	11	16
Side Spanish Rice	260	5	48
Veggie Burrito	500	17	72

JIMMY JOHN'S

	Cal	Fat	Cbs
8" Sub Sandwiches			
Big John®, 260 g	533	24	49
J.J.B.L.T, 233 g	634	35	49
Pepe®, 284 g	617	31	50
• Totally Tuna®, 368 g	648	31	54
• Turkey Tom®, 276 g	515	22	50
Vegetarian, 292 g	578	30	53
Vito, 286 g	600	28	52
Cookies			
Chocolate Chunk Cookie, 99 g	421	18	62
Raisin Oatmeal Cookie, 105 g	421	16	65
Giant Club Sandwiches			
Beach Club, 393 g	729	31	71
Billy Club, 390 g	800	34	68
• Bootlegger Club, 361 g	684	25	67
Club Lulu, 328 g	755	33	67
Club Tuna, 434 g	843	39	72
Country Club, 385 g	768	31	69
Gourmet Smoked Ham Club, 381 g	775	32	69

• MOST HEALTHY   • LEAST HEALTHY

JIMMY JOHN'S (cont.)

	Cal	Fat	Cbs
Gourmet Veggie Club, 358 g	773	38	71
Hunter's Club, 389 g	807	35	67
• Italian Night Club, 410 g	951	51	70
Ultimate Porker, 324 g	763	39	67
Low Fat/Low Carb Options			
Hunter's Club® Unwich, 311 g	470	35	4
The J.J. Gargantuan® Unwich, 440 g	742	54	7
Low-Fat Options			
4 Turkey Tom, 276 g	515	22	50
Slim 4 Turkey breast, 201 g	401	1	65
Pickles			
Pickle, Spear, 48 g	6	0	1
Plain Slims			
Slim 1 Ham & cheese, 225 g	508	10	66
Slim 2 Roast Beef, 201 g	424	3	64
Slim 3 Tuna salad, 278 g	722	31	68
• Slim 4 Turkey breast, 201 g	401	1	65
Slim 5 Salami, capicola cheese, 224 g	599	20	66
Slim 6 Double provolone, 194 g	545	16	65
• The J.J. Gargantuan, 498 g	991	54	54
Real Potato Chips			
• BBQ Jimmy Chips, 30 g	160	9	17
Jalapeño Chips, 30 g	150	7	18
Regular Chips, 30 g	160	8	18
Sea Salt & Vinegar Chips, 28 g	140	8	16
• Skinny Chips, 28 g	130	5	19

JOHNNY ROCKETS

Breakfast Menu			
Bacon, 34 g	180	14	1
Breakfast Sausage, 39 g	180	16	1
• Country Potatoes, 168 g	380	17	50
• Diced Ham, 28 g	50	3	1
Eggs - Over Easy, 56 g	90	7	0
Eggs - Over Hard, 56 g	90	6	2
Eggs - Scrambled, 56 g	90	6	1
Eggs Sunny Side Up, 56 g	90	7	1
French Toast, 67 g	150	4	23
Pancakes, 73 g	130	2	26
Plain Omlette, 116 g	220	17	1
Chicken			
• Chicken Club Sandwich, 369 g	930	51	58
Chicken Tenders, 227 g	610	33	39
• Grilled Chicken Breast, 283 g	560	25	47

JOHNNY ROCKETS (cont.)

	Cal	Fat	Cbs
Desserts			
• A la mode, 113 g	250	16	25
Apple Pie, 283 g	800	33	119
Single Scoop, 198 g	410	26	40
Super Sundae, 369 g	1110	74	120
The Perfect Brownie, 170 g	750	42	94
• The Perfect Brownie Sundae, 425 g	1464	91	176
Extra Extras			
American Cheese, 21 g	70	6	0
Ancho Chipotle, 21 g	80	6	5
Bacon, 17 g	90	7	1
Boca Patty, 99 g	100	2	8
Cheddar Cheese, 21 g	90	7	0
Chili, 85 g	155	12	5
Dijonnaise, 28 g	150	16	1
Egg, 57 g	70	5	1
Gourmet Blue Cheese, 21 g	150	16	1
Grilled Mushrooms, 28 g	33	3	1
Grilled Onions, 37 g	48	6	3
• Grilled Peppers & Onions, 28 g	20	1	3
Pepper Jack Cheese, 21 g	80	6	1
Pepper Relish Mayo, 42 g	187	18	7
Swiss Cheese, 21 g	62	5	0
Turkey Patty, 80 g	170	10	0
• Wheat Bun, 84 g	250	4	48
Flavor Shots			
Cherry, 21 g	22	0	2
• Chocolate, 21 g	60	0	13
• Lemon, 14 g	0	0	1
Vanilla, 21 g	21	0	5
Fountain			
Big Apple (Deluxe Shake), 454 g	890	54	89
• Butterfinger® (Deluxe Shake), 454 g	1020	65	85
Chocolate (Original Shake), 454 g	890	44	102
Choco PntBtr (Deluxe Shake), 454 g	890	50	96
Mocha Fudge (Deluxe Shake), 454 g	810	47	82
Oreo® Cookies & Crm (Delx Shake), 454 g	820	50	79
• Strawberry (Original Shake), 454 g	750	44	77
Strwbry-Banana (Delx Shake), 454 g	970	54	106
Vanilla (Original Shake), 454 g	840	44	100
Hamburgers			
#12, 340 g	900	59	55
• Bacon Cheddar Double, 510 g	1400	92	57
Bacon Cheddar Single, 311 g	860	53	42
Chili Cheese Hamburger, 311 g	850	50	53
Patty Melt, 255 g	690	37	49

JOHNNY ROCKETS (cont.)

	Cal	Fat	Cbs
Rocket Double®, 397 g	1020	63	52
Rocket Single®, 283 g	710	44	45
Route 66, 311 g	920	60	55
Smoke House Double, 397 g	1359	80	99
Smoke House Single, 283 g	950	55	68
St. Louis, 311 g	991	56	53
• Streamliner®, 311 g	410	8	57
The Original, 311 g	820	53	52

Other Favorites

	Cal	Fat	Cbs
Bacon, Lettuce & Tomato, 198 g	510	31	40
Chili Dog, 283 g	810	55	48
Egg Salad Sandwich, 311 g	870	64	46
Grilled Cheese, 142 g	540	29	48
• Hot Dog, 142 g	370	20	34
Philly Cheese Steak, 369 g	715	46	58
• Tuna Melt, 311 g	900	62	40
Tuna Salad Sandwich, 311 g	800	50	41

Rocket Kids Menu

	Cal	Fat	Cbs
• Chicken Tenders, 142 g	350	17	24
Grilled Cheese, 113 g	440	20	48
Hamburger, 113 g	370	19	32
Hot Dog, 142 g	450	26	39
Mini Hamburgers (2), 113 g	400	17	40
Mini Hot Dogs (2), 142 g	460	24	44
• Peanut Butter & Jelly, 142 g	490	19	66

Salads

	Cal	Fat	Cbs
Caesar Salad, 397 g	481	35	15
• Chkn Club Salad (w/chkn tenders), 425 g	620	37	27
Chkn Club Salad (w/grl breast), 425 g	480	26	8
• Garden Salad, 312 g	240	14	12
Grilled Chicken Caesar Salad, 255 g	343	31	13
Scoop Egg Salad, 170 g	470	42	2
Scoop Tuna Salad, 170 g	420	31	0

Starters

	Cal	Fat	Cbs
American Fries, 227 g	550	22	78
Cheese Fries, 283 g	780	44	72
Chili Bowl, 369 g	872	73	24
Chilli Fries, 425 g	1010	62	85
Half Rings & Half Fries, 227 g	680	31	88
• Mini Chili Dogs (3), 482 g	1470	105	78
Mini Hot Dogs (3), 227 g	690	36	66
Onion Rings, 227 g	790	36	80
Rocket Wings®, 255 g	640	36	26
Side Caesar Salad, 113 g	189	16	9
• Side Salad, 113 g	100	5	7
Sliders (traditional) (3), 227 g	750	42	63

• MOST HEALTHY   • LEAST HEALTHY

KENTUCKY FRIED CHICKEN

	Cal	Fat	Cbs
Beverages			
Manzanita Sol®, 20 fl.oz.	280	0	73
Miranda® Strawberry, 20 fl.oz.	280	0	73
Chicken			
• EC Chicken- Breast, 176 g	510	33	16
EC Chicken- Drumstick, 59 g	150	10	5
EC Chicken- Thigh, 110 g	340	24	10
EC Chicken- Whole Wing, 56 g	190	13	6
Grilled Chicken- Breast, 123 g	190	6	0
• Grilled Chicken- Drumstick, 42 g	70	4	0
Grilled Chicken- Thigh, 71 g	150	9	0
Grilled Chicken- Whole Wing, 37 g	80	5	0
OR Chicken- Breast, 164 g	320	15	4
OR Chicken- Drumstick, 53 g	120	7	3
OR Chicken- Thigh, 94 g	220	15	5
OR Chicken- Whole Wing, 48 g	140	8	4
OR Chkn-Breast w/o skin or breading, 116 g	150	3	0
Spicy Crispy- Breast, 178 g	420	25	12
Spicy Crispy- Drumstick, 55 g	160	10	5
Spicy Crispy- Thigh, 111 g	360	27	13
Spicy Crispy- Whole Wing, 51 g	170	12	6
Desserts			
Apple Turnover (1), 86 g	260	13	35
Brownie Minis (1 pack), 57 g	280	16	31
Café Valley Bakery® Choco Chip Cake, 76 g	280	9	47
Cookie Dough Pie Slice, 68 g	240	12	31
Dutch Apple Pie Slice, 108 g	320	14	47
Lemon Meringue Pie Slice, 81 g	250	7	42
Lil' Bucket™ Choco Crème Parfait Cup, 113 g	280	14	37
Lil' Bucket™ Lemon Crème Parfait Cup, 127 g	390	14	60
Lil' Bucket™ Strwbry Shortcake Parfait Cup, 99 g	230	8	39
• Pecan Pie Slice, 95 g	410	21	52
Sara Lee® Sweet Potato Pie Slice, 113 g	340	16	46
Strawberry Cream Chz Pie Slice, 78 g	270	15	31
Sweet Life® Choco Chip Cookie, 35 g	170	8	23
• Sweet Life® Oatmeal Raisin Cookie, 35 g	150	6	23
Sweet Life® Sugar Cookie, 35 g	160	7	22
Other			
• Cntry Fried Steak w/ Pprd White Gravy, 155 g	390	26	23
Cntry Fried Steak w/o Pprd White Gravy, 111 g	360	24	19
Colonel's Buttery Spread, 6 g	30	4	0
Fiery Buffalo Dipping Sauce Cup, 25 g	25	0	6
Honey Sauce Packet, 9 g	30	0	8
• Jalapeño Peppers, 32 g	20	2	1
KFC® Gizzards, 55 g	200	11	15
KFC® Livers, 55 g	180	11	11

● MOST HEALTHY • LEAST HEALTHY

KENTUCKY FRIED CHICKEN (cont.)

	Cal	Fat	Cbs
Sargento® Light String Cheese, 21 g	50	3	1
Sweet and Sour Dipping Sauce Cup, 25 g	45	0	12

Popcorn Chicken

	Cal	Fat	Cbs
Popcorn Chicken-Individual, 116 g	400	26	22

Pot Pie, Bowls, & Value Boxes

	Cal	Fat	Cbs
Chicken Pot Pie, 369 g	690	40	57
EC Drumstick Value Box, 172 g	440	24	41
EC Thigh Value Box, 223 g	630	38	47
Fiery Buffalo Hot Wings® Value Box, 190 g	500	27	46
Grilled Drumstick Value Box, 156 g	360	18	36
Grilled Thigh Value Box, 185 g	440	23	36
HBBQ Hot Wings® Value Box, 195 g	520	27	53
Hot Wings® Value Box, 169 g	470	27	41
• KFC Famous Bowls®-Mshd Potato w/Gravy, 525 g	700	32	77
OR Drumstick Value Box, 166 g	410	21	40
OR Thigh Value Box, 207 g	510	29	41
Popcorn Chicken Value Box, 218 g	660	38	55
Snack-Size Bowl, 232 g	320	15	34

Salads & More

	Cal	Fat	Cbs
Caesar Side Salad w/o Drss & Croutons, 76 g	35	2	2
• Crispy Chkn BLT Salad w/o Drss, 315 g	340	19	14
Crispy Chkn Caesar Salad w/o Drs & Croutons, 262 g	320	19	12
Grilled Chkn BLT Salad w/o Drss, 316 g	220	7	6
Grld Chkn Caesar Salad w/o Drs & Croutons, 263 g	200	6	4
• House Side Salad w/out Dressing, 87 g	15	0	2
Parmesan Garlic Croutons Pouch (1), 14 g	70	3	8

Sandwiches & Wraps

	Cal	Fat	Cbs
• Crispy Twister® w/ Crispy Strip, 238 g	590	31	49
Crispy Twister® w/ Crispy Strip w/o Sc, 216 g	480	20	48
Dbl Crunch Snd w/ Crispy Strip w/o Sc, 191 g	410	16	34
Double Crunch Snd w/ Crispy Strip, 214 g	520	28	35
Double Down, 241 g	540	32	11
Grilled Double Down, 253 g	460	23	3
Grilled Filet Sandwich, 197 g	390	15	27
Grilled Filet Snd w/o Sauce, 173 g	280	4	26
Grilled Twister®, 239 g	460	18	41
Grilled Twister® w/out Sauce, 217 g	360	8	40
Honey BBQ Sandwich, 162 g	310	4	42
KFC Snacker® w/ Crispy Strip, 115 g	300	14	28
KFC Snacker® w/ Crispy Strip w/o Sc, 105 g	250	9	27
KFC Snacker® w/ Crispy Strip, Buffalo, 115 g	260	9	30
KFC Snacker® w/ Crispy Strip, Ult Chz, 114 g	280	11	29
KFC Snacker®, Fish, 116 g	320	14	31
KFC Snacker®, Fish w/out Sauce, 105 g	290	12	29
KFC Snacker®, Honey BBQ, 98 g	210	3	32

• MOST HEALTHY   • LEAST HEALTHY

KENTUCKY FRIED CHICKEN (cont.)

	Cal	Fat	Cbs
Mini Melt, 108 g	250	7	31
OR Filet Sandwich, 197 g	480	24	37
OR Filet Sandwich w/out Sauce, 173 g	370	12	36
Tender Roast® Sandwich, 228 g	410	15	29
Tender Roast® Snd w/o Sauce, 204 g	300	4	28
Toasted Wrap w/ Crispy Strip, 133 g	360	20	27
Toasted Wrap w/ Grilled Filet, 134 g	300	14	24
Tst Wrap w/ Grilled Filet w/o Sauce, 120 g	240	8	23
Tst Wrap w/Tender Roast® Filet, 140 g	310	15	24
Tst Wrap w/ Crispy Strip w/o Sc, 119 g	300	14	27
Tst Wrap w/Tender Rst® Filet w/o Sc, 126 g	240	8	23

Sides (Individual)

BBQ Baked Beans, 130 g	200	2	39
Biscuit, 54 g	180	8	23
Cole Slaw, 130 g	180	11	19
Corn on the Cob (3"), 71 g	70	1	16
• Green Beans, 86 g	20	0	3
KFC® Cornbread Muffin, 52 g	210	9	28
KFC® Red Beans w/ Ssge and Rice, 144 g	160	3	26
Macaroni and Cheese, 137 g	180	9	21
Macaroni Salad, 180 g	180	9	20
Mashed Potatoes w/ Gravy, 145 g	120	4	19
Mashed Potatoes w/out Gravy, 102 g	90	3	15
Potato Salad, 128 g	200	10	24
• Potato Wedges, 102 g	260	13	33
Sweet Kernel Corn, 102 g	110	1	23
Three Bean Salad, 87 g	70	0	14

Strips & Filets

• Crispy Strips (3), 152 g	380	22	12
• KFC® Grilled Filet, 102 g	130	2	0
KFC® OR Filet, 96 g	170	7	4

Wings

Boneless Fiery Buffalo Wings (1), 34 g	80	4	6
Boneless HBBQ Wings (1), 33 g	80	4	7
Fiery Buffalo Hot Wings® (1), 29 g	80	5	5
Fiery Buffalo Wings (1), 28 g	80	5	4
Fiery Grilled Wings (1), 31 g	70	4	0
HBBQ Hot Wings® (1), 31 g	90	5	7
HBBQ Wings (1), 26 g	80	5	5
Hot Wings® (1), 22 g	70	5	3

KILWIN'S

Almond Bark - Milk Chocolate, 1 oz.	221	14	22
Almond Bark - White Chocolate, 1 oz.	221	13	24
Almond Butter Brickle, 1 oz.	218	14	23
Almond Cluster - Dark Choc, 1 oz.	221	16	18

• MOST HEALTHY   • LEAST HEALTHY

KILWIN'S (cont.)	Cal	Fat	Cbs
Almond Cluster - Milk Choc, 1 oz.	226	16	18
Almond Toffee Crunch, 1 oz.	220	15	20
Almond Toffee Crunch Bar, 1 oz.	192	13	18
Almonds - Dark Chocolate, 1 oz.	225	16	19
Almonds - Milk Chocolate, 1 oz.	219	15	20
Almonds roasted & salted, 1 oz.	210	12	23
Amaretto Truffle, 1 oz.	237	17	21
Apricots - Dark Chocolate, 1 oz.	140	5	24
Apricots - Milk Chocolate, 1 oz.	142	5	24
Bavarian Cream, 1 oz.	167	6	28
Black Licorice Twist, 1 oz.	143	0	39
Bombe' Truffle, 1 oz.	230	17	21
Brugg Truffle, 1 oz.	230	17	21
Butter Pecan Fudge, 1 oz.	242	17	22
Caramel Assortment, 1 oz.	184	9	26
Caramel Assortment, 1 oz.	233	16	22
Caramel Corn, 1 oz.	207	13	22
Caramel Sucker, 1 oz.	163	9	20
Caramel Topping, 1 oz.	107	5	15
Caramellows - Dark Chocolate, 1 oz.	173	9	23
Caramellows - Milk Chocolate, 1 oz.	178	8	24
Caramels - Dark Chocolate, 1 oz.	182	9	26
Caramels - Milk Chocolate, 1 oz.	185	8	27
Cashew Brittle, 1 oz.	195	10	28
Cashew Cluster - Dark Choc, 1 oz.	225	17	16
Cashew Cluster - Milk Choc, 1 oz.	228	17	16
Cashew Tuttles - Dark Chocolate, 1 oz.	205	13	21
Cashew Tuttles - Milk Chocolate, 1 oz.	207	13	21
Cashews - Dark Chocolate, 1 oz.	252	21	15
Cashews - Milk Chocolate, 1 oz.	222	16	18
Cashews - roasted & salted, 1 oz.	246	23	9
Chausse' Truffle, 1 oz.	240	17	20
Cherri Suisse Truffle, 1 oz.	232	16	21
Cherry Coins, 1 oz.	205	9	16
Cherry Cordial - Dark Chocolate, 1 oz.	173	7	28
Cherry Cordial Assortment, 1 oz.	175	7	28
Cherry Cordials - Milk Chocolate, 1 oz.	177	7	28
Choc Espresso Beans, 1 oz.	200	12	23
Choc Toffee Almonds, 1 oz.	220	15	18
Chocolate Berryblues, 1 oz.	170	9	21
Chocolate Blackberries, 1 oz.	220	16	18
Chocolate Bon Bon, 1 oz.	167	6	29
Chocolate Card "Thank You", 1 oz.	153	9	17
Chocolate Coffee Beans, 1 oz.	178	7	29
Chocolate Cream - Dark Chocolate, 1 oz.	166	6	28

KILWIN'S (cont.)

	Cal	Fat	Cbs
Chocolate Cream - Milk Chocolate, 1 oz.	168	6	28
Chocolate Fudge, 1 oz.	174	5	31
Chocolate Ice Cream Suckers, 1 oz.	135	4	26
Chocolate Jordan Almonds, 1 oz.	220	15	18
Chocolate Peanut Butter Fudge, 1 oz.	176	6	29
Chocolate Pecan Fudge, 1 oz.	169	5	31
Chocolate Star Pop, 1 oz.	231	14	23
Chocolate Walnut Fudge, 1 oz.	175	6	31
Cinn Rsted Almond, 1 oz.	137	0	34
Coconut Cluster - Dark Choc, 1 oz.	204	12	24
Coconut Cluster - Milk Choc, 1 oz.	209	12	24
Coconut Macaroon - Dark Choco, 1 oz.	233	13	28
Coffee Truffle, 1 oz.	233	16	21
Custom Coin Dark Mint Choc, 1 oz.	350	21	37
Custom Gold Coins Milk Choc, 1 oz.	229	14	25
Custom Silver Coins Milk Choc, 1 oz.	221	14	25
Dark Choc Sea Foam, 1 oz.	130	0	32
Dark Chocolate Almonds, 1 oz.	210	13	21
Dark Chocolate Bar, 1 oz.	310	21	28
Dark Chocolate Break-up, 1 oz.	210	13	23
Dark Chocolate Heart, 1 oz.	221	14	25
Family Assortment, 1 oz.	209	13	23
• Flavored Swizzle Stick, 1 oz.	50	0	14
Fontineau Truffle, 1 oz.	229	16	21
French Chocolate, 1 oz.	198	11	24
French Mint Truffle, 1 oz.	226	15	23
Gourmet Chocolate Nut Mix, 1 oz.	220	16	18
Gourmet Nut Mix, 1 oz.	220	15	18
Gummi Bears, 1 oz.	140	0	34
Gummi Pet Crocodile, 1 oz.	130	0	32
Gummy Bears, 1 oz.	158	0	40
Hazelnut Truffle, 1 oz.	233	17	21
Heavenly Hash, 1 oz.	183	8	26
Holland Mints, 1 oz.	160	5	32
Irish Cream Truffle, 1 oz.	233	16	21
Jamaican Truffle, 1 oz.	232	16	21
Jaw Breaker 2.25", 1 oz.	160	0	40
Katy Cream Assort, 1 oz.	174	7	28
Katy Kiss Cluster, 1 oz.	218	14	21
Kilwin's Dome Mk Choc, 1 oz.	231	14	24
Kilwin's Fudge Topping, 1 oz.	232	14	26
Kilwin's Square Mint, 1 oz.	231	14	24
Le Gran Truffle, 1 oz.	233	17	21
Licorice Bridge Mix, 1 oz.	130	1	31
Macadamia Nuts rstd & salt, 1 oz.	286	30	5
Macadamia Tuttles - Milk Choc, 1 oz.	222	16	20

• MOST HEALTHY   • LEAST HEALTHY

▶ KILWIN'S (cont.)

	Cal	Fat	Cbs
Macadamia Tuttles - White Choc, 1 oz.	216	15	21
Maple Cream - Dark Chocolate, 1 oz.	163	6	29
Maple Walnut Fudge, 1 oz.	168	4	32
Marshmallow - Dark Chocolate, 1 oz.	181	9	25
Marshmallow - Milk Chocolate, 1 oz.	186	9	25
Marzipan Bar, 1 oz.	150	3	30
Marzipan Fruits, 1 oz.	196	0	48
Milk Choc Alligator, 1 oz.	223	13	25
Milk Choc Almond Bar, 1 oz.	336	21	37
Milk Choc Crayons, 1 oz.	76	5	8
• Milk Choc Crisp Rice Bar, 1 oz.	350	22	34
Milk Choc Doctor Kit, 1 oz.	229	14	25
Milk Choc Hairdresser, 1 oz.	218	13	24
Milk Choc Malt Balls, 1 oz.	190	9	28
Milk Choc Mini Car, 1 oz.	229	14	25
Milk Choc Pansie, 1 oz.	229	14	25
Milk Choc Sea Foam, 1 oz.	180	10	26
Milk Chocolate Almonds, 1 oz.	200	15	19
Milk Chocolate Bar, 1 oz.	153	9	17
Milk Chocolate Break-up, 1 oz.	218	13	24
Milk Chocolate Cigar, 1 oz.	179	7	29
Milk Chocolate Coins, 1 oz.	153	9	17
Milk Chocolate Fish, 1 oz.	229	14	25
Milk Chocolate Golf Set, 1 oz.	218	13	24
Milk Chocolate Heart, 1 oz.	229	14	25
Milk Chocolate Maltballs, 1 oz.	190	9	26
Milk Chocolate Peanuts, 1 oz.	220	15	18
Milk Chocolate Raisins, 1 oz.	180	8	26
Milk Chocolate Tool Kit, 1 oz.	218	13	24
Milk Moose Sucker, 1 oz.	150	8	18
Mint Cookie Malt Balls, 1 oz.	140	1	31
Mint Smoothie Assortment, 1 oz.	180	8	26
Mint Smoothies - Dark Chocolate, 1 oz.	226	16	22
Mint Smoothies - Milk Chocolate, 1 oz.	229	16	22
Mixed Nuts - roasted & salted, 1 oz.	271	20	13
Mk Choc Caramel Apple, 1 oz.	220	12	25
Mk Choc Peanut Dino, 1 oz.	240	16	22
Molasses Chips - Dark Chocolate, 1 oz.	191	9	29
Molasses Chips - Milk Chocolate, 1 oz.	191	8	30
Natural Pistachios, 1 oz.	286	30	5
Nutcracker Sweets, 1 oz.	181	8	26
Orange Cream - Dark Chocolate, 1 oz.	161	5	30
Orange Cream - Milk Chocolate, 1 oz.	161	5	30
Orange Jellies - Dark Chocolate, 1 oz.	182	7	29
Orange Jellies - Milk Chocolate, 1 oz.	187	7	30
Orange Peel - Dark Chocolate, 1 oz.	167	8	26

• MOST HEALTHY   • LEAST HEALTHY

KILWIN'S (cont.)

	Cal	Fat	Cbs
Orange Peel - Milk Chocolate, 1 oz.	171	7	26
Oreo Cookie - White Chocolate, 1 oz.	209	11	27
Oreo Cookies - Milk Chocolate, 1 oz.	210	11	25
Pastel Choc Cherries, 1 oz.	200	10	26
Peanut Brittle, 1 oz.	186	14	21
Peanut Butter Cruncher Dark Choc, 1 oz.	214	13	23
Peanut Butter Cruncher Milk Choc, 1 oz.	218	13	23
Peanut Butter Cup, 1 oz.	180	5	33
Peanut Butter Fudge, 1 oz.	168	4	32
Peanut Butter Smoothie Dark Choc, 1 oz.	218	14	22
Peanut Butter Smoothie Milk Choc, 1 oz.	222	14	22
Peanut Cluster - Dark Chocolate, 1 oz.	217	15	18
Peanut Cluster - Milk Chocolate, 1 oz.	223	15	18
Peanut Corn, 1 oz.	166	4	32
Peanuts roasted & salted, 1 oz.	243	22	7
Pecan Bark - Dark Chocolate, 1 oz.	219	15	21
Pecan Bark - Milk Chocolate, 1 oz.	226	15	22
Pecan Brittle, 1 oz.	152	8	19
Pecan Cluster - Dark Chocolate, 1 oz.	235	18	17
Pecan Cluster - Milk Chocolate, 1 oz.	240	18	18
Pecan Streakers, 1 oz.	212	13	24
Pecan Tuttle Assortment, 1 oz.	175	7	28
Pecan Tuttles - Dark Chocolate, 1 oz.	223	16	19
Pecan Tuttles - Milk Chocolate, 1 oz.	226	16	19
Pecans - Dark Chocolate, 1 oz.	232	19	12
Pecans - Milk Chocolate, 1 oz.	247	21	15
Pecans roasted & salted, 1 oz.	232	20	7
Peppermint Patties Dark Choc, 1 oz.	177	8	28
Peppermint Patty, 1 oz.	200	9	33
Pretzels - Milk Chocolate, 1 oz.	199	9	27
Pretzels - White Chocolate, 1 oz.	199	9	28
Raisin Cluster - Dark Chocolate, 1 oz.	180	9	26
Raisin Cluster - Milk Chocolate, 1 oz.	186	9	27
Rasp & Blackberries, 1 oz.	190	10	25
Raspberry & Blackberry 10# case, 1 oz.	152	2	35
Raspberry Cream - Dark Chocolate, 1 oz.	159	5	29
Raspberry Cream - Milk Chocolate, 1 oz.	162	5	30
Raspberry Jellies - Dark Chocolate, 1 oz.	184	8	29
Raspberry Jellies - Milk Chocolate, 1 oz.	187	7	30
Raspberry Truffle, 1 oz.	230	17	21
Red Licorice Ropes, 1 oz.	160	0	39
Red Licorice Twist, 1 oz.	140	0	36
Royal Nut Assortment, 1 oz.	231	17	18
Salt Water Taffy, 1 oz.	130	8	15
Sanded Lemon Drops, 1 oz.	166	0	42
Sour Gummi Bears, 1 oz.	136	0	32

● MOST HEALTHY   ● LEAST HEALTHY

KILWIN'S (cont.)

	Cal	Fat	Cbs
Star of David, 1 oz.	180	11	20
Strawberry Bon Bon, 1 oz.	161	4	31
Sugar Free Caramel Corn, 1 oz.	224	15	20
Sugar Free Chocolate Fudge, 1 oz.	160	10	27
Sugar Free Chocolates, 1 oz.	147	9	17
Sugar Free Dark Pnut Cluster, 1 oz.	199	17	16
Sugar Free Festival Mints, 1 oz.	180	15	22
Sugar Free Hard Candy, 1 oz.	138	3	35
Sugar Free Milk Cashew Tuttle, 1 oz.	190	14	22
Sugar Free Milk Pecan Tuttles, 1 oz.	190	14	21
Sugar Free Milk Pnut Cluster, 1 oz.	187	16	16
Sugar Free Milk Squares, 1 oz.	159	14	21
Sugar Free Peanut Brittle, 1 oz.	154	4	36
Sugar Free Pnut Butter Fudge, 1 oz.	150	9	26
Sugar Free Pnut Cluster Asst, 1 oz.	190	16	18
Sugar Free Taffy, 1 oz.	160	0	40
Sugar Free Toffee Crunch, 1 oz.	164	8	27
Sugar Free Vanilla Fudge, 1 oz.	150	9	28
Sugar Free White Pnut Cluster, 1 oz.	197	15	18
Sugar Free White Squares, 1 oz.	175	13	26
Swedish Fish, 1 oz.	160	3	37
Tart Cherry Cluster - Milk Chocolate, 1 oz.	194	9	27
Truffle Assortment, 1 oz.	226	16	19
Tuxedo Espresso Beans, 1 oz.	190	9	26
Vanilla Butter Cream - Dark Choc, 1 oz.	166	6	28
Vanilla Butter Cream - Milk Choc, 1 oz.	168	6	28
White Chocolate Break-up, 1 oz.	218	12	26
White Chocolate Popcorn, 1 oz.	220	16	18
White Golf Ball, 1 oz.	223	12	27
White Moose Sucker, 1 oz.	164	10	18

KOHR BROS

The Original Light Frozen Custard

	Cal	Fat	Cbs
• Chocolate, 80 g	140	6	18
• Orange Sherbet, 87 g	104	2	21
Vanilla, 80 g	130	6	16

KOLACHE FACTORY

Croissants

	Cal	Fat	Cbs
• Ham & Cheese, 191 g	620	39	45
Ham & Egg, 194 g	610	38	46
• Italian Chicken, 213 g	550	32	46

Kolaches

	Cal	Fat	Cbs
Bacon & Cheese, 66 g	270	14	25
Bacon, Egg & Cheese, 142 g	400	19	38
BBQ Beef, 85 g	230	9	28

► KOLACHE FACTORY (cont.)

	Cal	Fat	Cbs
Cream Cheese, 85 g	220	9	30
Egg & Cheese, 142 g	410	20	39
Fruit (Average), 113 g	210	5	37
Ham & Cheese, 78 g	260	13	27
Italian Chicken, 85 g	230	9	25
Jalapeño & Cheese, 75 g	210	8	27
Philly Cheese Steak, 89 g	230	9	25
Pizza, 77 g	210	8	27
• Polish Sausage, 175 g	500	25	50
Potato Egg & Cheese, 142 g	350	14	42
Ranchero, 160 g	340	14	39
• Sausage, 52 g	160	7	21
Sausage & Cheese, 94 g	270	12	32
Sausage, Egg & Cheese, 146 g	400	19	38
Spinach, 94 g	290	6	27
Texas Hot Polish, 175 g	470	21	51
Specialties			
• Cinnamon Roll, 99 g	300	6	59
Cinnamon Twist, 119 g	570	20	92
• Sticky Bun, 147 g	600	32	74

► KOO KOO ROO

	Cal	Fat	Cbs
Chicken Bowls (w/o Sauce)			
Chargrilled Chicken Bowl, 1	569	19	57
Tostada Bowl (w/o shell), 1	528	22	45
Cold Side Dishes			
Tossed Salad (w/o dressing), 3 oz.	16	0	3
Dessert			
Kellogg's® Rice Krispies Treats®, 3 oz.	340	7	68
Fresh Roasted Turkey			
Hand Carved Turkey Sandwich, 1	599	32	31
• Sliced Turkey Breast, 1	182	8	0
• Traditional Turkey Dinner, 1	692	29	67
Hot Side Dishes			
Black Beans, 6 oz.	125	3	23
• Macaroni & Cheese, 6 oz.	340	17	32
Mashed Potatoes, 7 oz.	186	5	32
• Steamed Vegetables, 4 oz.	38	0	8
Stuffing, 5 oz.	111	7	11
Original Chicken			
1 Original Breast, 4 oz.	187	6	0
3 Piece Original Dark, 5 oz.	320	16	5
Rotisserie Chicken			
• Leg & Thigh, 9 oz.	300	18	1
Breast & Wing, 7 oz.	355	16	1
• Half Rotisserie Chicken, 11 oz.	655	34	2

● MOST HEALTHY   ● LEAST HEALTHY

▶ KOO KOO ROO (cont.)

	Cal	Fat	Cbs
Salads (w/o Dressing)			
BBQ Chicken Salad, 1	365	14	22
Chicken Caesar Salad, 1	286	11	13
Sandwiches			
• BBQ Chicken Sandwich, 1	562	12	71
• Chicken Caesar Sandwich, 1	781	36	63
Original Chicken Sandwich, 1	661	29	63
Wraps			
Caesar Chicken Wrap, 1	757	39	59

▶ KRISPY KREME DOUGHNUT

	Cal	Fat	Cbs
Doughnut Holes			
• Glazed Blueberry Doughnut Holes, 56 g	220	12	27
Glazed Cake Doughnut Holes, 56 g	210	10	29
Glazed Choco Cake Doughnut Holes, 56 g	210	10	29
Glazed Pumpkin Spice Doughnut Holes, 56 g	210	10	29
• Original Glazed Doughnut Holes, 54 g	200	11	25
Doughnuts			
• Apple Fritter, 101 g	380	20	47
Caramel Kreme Crunch, 98 g	380	19	49
Chocolate Glazed Cruller, 69 g	290	15	37
Chocolate Iced Cake, 71 g	280	14	36
Chocolate Iced Custard Filled, 86 g	300	17	35
Chocolate Iced Glazed, 66 g	250	12	33
Chocolate Iced Kreme Filled, 86 g	350	20	39
Chocolate Iced w/Sprinkles, 71 g	270	12	38
Cinnamon Apple Filled, 81 g	290	16	32
Cinnamon Bun, 67 g	260	16	28
Cinnamon Twist, 59 g	240	15	23
Dulce De Leche, 75 g	300	18	31
Glazed Chocolate Cake, 80 g	300	15	42
Glazed Cinnamon, 54 g	210	12	24
Glazed Cruller, 54 g	240	14	26
Glazed Kreme Filled, 86 g	340	20	39
Glazed Lemon Filled, 85 g	290	16	35
Glazed Pumpkin Spice, 80 g	300	14	42
Glazed Raspberry Filled, 85 g	300	16	36
Glazed Sour Cream, 80 g	300	13	43
Maple Iced Glazed, 66 g	240	12	32
New York Cheesecake, 90 g	340	20	34
Original Glazed, 52 g	200	12	22
Powdered Cake, 71 g	290	14	37
Powdered Strawberry Filled, 81 g	290	16	33
• Sugar, 49 g	200	12	21
Traditional Cake, 57 g	230	13	25

● MOST HEALTHY   ● LEAST HEALTHY

KRISPY KREME DOUGHNUT (cont.)

	Cal	Fat	Cbs
Fruity Chillers			
Orange You Glad Chiller, 12 oz.	180	0	43
Very Berry Chiller, 12 oz.	170	0	43
Kremey Chillers			
Berries & Kreme Chiller, 12 oz.	670	28	105
Chocolate, Chocolate Chiller, 12 oz.	630	28	95
• Lemon Sherbert Chiller, 12 oz.	670	29	104
Lotta Latte Chiller, 12 oz.	630	28	92
• Mocha Dream Chiller, 12 oz.	620	28	92
Oranges & Kreme Chiller, 12 oz.	670	28	49

KRYSTAL

	Cal	Fat	Cbs
Anytime Treats			
Apple Turnover, 81 g	220	8	34
Banana Freeze, 20 g	230	0	58
Blitz Energy Freeze, 20 g	320	0	78
Blitz Energy Drink (On The Rocks), 20 g	300	0	76
Blueberry Freeze, 20 g	230	0	58
Cherry Freeze, 20 g	230	0	58
Chocolate Milkquake, 466 g	880	50	92
Coca-Cola® Freeze, 20 g	170	0	44
Grape Freeze, 20 g	230	0	57
Lemon Icebox Pie, 106 g	320	9	56
• Oreo® Chocolate Sandwich Cookie, 22 g	100	5	16
Pomegranate Freeze, 20 g	230	0	57
Sour Green Apple Freeze, 20 g	230	0	57
Strawberry Freeze, 20 g	240	0	58
• Strawberry Milkquake, 456 g	900	48	105
Sweet Bites - 3 Piece, 45 g	210	14	22
Vanilla Milkquake, 546 g	850	49	87
Beverages			
Hot Chocolate (2 Singles), 16 g	160	2	35
Land O' Lakes Grip'n Go® 2% Milk, 12 g	190	7	19
Breakfast			
4 Pancakes, 117 g	280	8	44
4-Carb Scrambler W/Bacon, 209 g	450	31	2
4-Carb Scrambler W/Sausage, 260 g	620	52	3
Bacon Biscuit, 81 g	330	17	32
Bacon Egg Cheese on Toast, 130 g	330	16	24
Bacon on Toast, 65 g	220	10	24
Bacon, Egg, Cheese Biscuit, 146 g	440	24	34
• Big Stack Breakfast, 287 g	780	51	45
Biscuit, 71 g	260	13	32
Chik Biscuit, 129 g	400	18	43
Custom Breakfast, 265 g	600	43	59
Egg Biscuit, 127 g	340	18	34

KRYSTAL (cont.)

	Cal	Fat	Cbs
Egg on Toast, 110 g	230	9	26
Express Breakfast, 374 g	550	29	51
Gravy Biscuit, 184 g	350	18	41
Grits, 257 g	160	2	33
Grits W/Margarine, 257 g	160	2	33
Kryspers, 57 g	150	7	19
Krystal Sunriser, 84 g	200	11	16
One Egg Custom Brkfst (Senior), 172 g	420	28	29
Original Scrambler W/Bacon, 283 g	330	16	27
Original Scrambler W/Sausage, 309 g	420	26	27
Pancake Scrambler, 152 g	380	25	23
Sausage Biscuit, 107 g	420	28	32
Sausage Egg Cheese on Toast, 172 g	520	35	34
Sausage Gravy Scrambler, 334 g	630	41	46
Sausage on Toast, 90 g	300	20	24
Sausage, Egg, Cheese Biscuit, 172 g	520	35	34
Southwestern Scrambler, 363 g	440	26	32
• Toast, 53 g	150	5	24

Lunch & Dinner

B.A. Burger, 210 g	550	35	46
B.A. Chili Cheese, 167 g	390	20	38
• B.A. Double Bacon Cheese, 303 g	850	59	48
Bacon Cheese Krystal, 79 g	200	11	20
BBQ Bacon & Cheese B.A., 241 g	640	36	58
Cheese Krystal, 73 g	160	8	20
Chik Club, 128 g	320	16	29
Chik'n Bites - Small, 88 g	200	7	20
Chili Cheese Fries, 232 g	570	29	62
Chili Cheese Krystal, 115 g	290	19	22
Chili Cheese Pup, 83 g	230	14	16
Chili Pup, 69 g	170	10	16
Corn Pup, 68 g	240	14	22
Crispy Chicken Salad, 313 g	370	21	20
Double Cheese Krystal, 138 g	350	17	34
Double Krystal, 123 g	290	13	33
Krystal, 65 g	130	6	20
Krystal Chik, 104 g	300	16	27
Large Chili, 340 g	300	11	33
Medium Fries, 119 g	310	13	46
Plain Pup, 54 g	150	8	15
Ranch Chili Cheese Fries, 275 g	760	49	64
• Side Salad, 114 g	70	5	4

L&L HAWAIIAN BARBECUE

BBQ Chicken, 1 piece, 89 g	180	N/A	4
BBQ Chicken (regular)	1180	N/A	101

• MOST HEALTHY   • LEAST HEALTHY

L&L HAWAIIAN BARBECUE (cont.)	Cal	Fat	Cbs
BBQ Hamburger	405	N/A	31
BBQ Short Ribs (regular)	1130	N/A	100
BBQ Mix	1280	N/A	107
Brown Rice, 1 scoop	160	N/A	33
Cheeseburger	475	N/A	30
Chicken Katsu, 1 piece	350	N/A	20
• Chicken Katsu (regular)	1690	N/A	148
Chicken Musubi	263	N/A	39
French Fries	450	N/A	62
Fried Shrimp	1230	N/A	148
Garlic Ahi, 1 piece, 68 g	130	N/A	0
Garlic Ahi (regular)	920	N/A	89
Garlic Shrimp	740	N/A	92
Hamburger	425	N/A	29
Hamburger Steak (regular)	1445	N/A	104
Healthy BBQ Chicken	363	N/A	42
Healthy Garlic Ahi	313	N/A	38
Healthy Garlic Shrimp	213	N/A	41
Healthy Salmon Patty	363	N/A	40
Kalua Pork & Cabbage (regular)	1090	N/A	93
Katsu Musubi	335	N/A	45
• Katsu Sauce 97 g	100	N/A	25
Loco Moco (regular)	1385	N/A	103
Macaroni Salad, 1 scoop	350	N/A	23
Mahi, 1 piece, 70 g	145	N/A	5
Mahi Mahi (regular)	1020	N/A	103
Mahi Mahi Sandwich	315	N/A	31
Saimin	383	N/A	79
Seafood Combo	1404	N/A	127
Short Rib, 1 piece, 49 g	160	N/A	4
Spam Musubi	293	N/A	37
Tartar Sauce 41 g	190	N/A	3
Teri Beef Sandwich	280	N/A	32
Teri Beef, 1 piece, 61 g	110	N/A	6
Teriyaki Beef (regular)	980	N/A	107
White Rice, 1 scoop	150	N/A	33

LA ROSA'S PIZZERIA

Appetizers

Barbecue Wings (1 piece), 46 g	105	6	4
Blue Cheese Dipping Cup, 42 g	230	24	2
Boneless Wings-BBQ (1 piece), 40 g	75	3	8
Boneless Wings-Hot (1 piece), 40 g	78	5	6
Boneless Wings-Med (1 piece), 41 g	80	5	5
Cheesy Flatbread (1/4 total), 104 g	354	22	26
Chicken Tenders, 243 g	541	31	30

• MOST HEALTHY   • LEAST HEALTHY

LA ROSA'S PIZZERIA (cont.)

	Cal	Fat	Cbs
Diablo Sauce (2 oz cup), 64 g	206	15	17
• Four Taste Sampler, 669 g	1569	99	82
French Fry Basket, 295 g	533	32	70
French Fry Basket w/ Prov, 385 g	862	56	73
Garlic Sauce Dipping Sauce, 51 g	360	40	0
Hot Wings (1 piece), 45 g	104	7	2
Medium Wings (1 piece), 46 g	105	7	2
Mozzarella Cheese Sticks, 181 g	636	43	36
Onion Twists (Regular), 207 g	462	27	48
• Pizza Sauce Dipping Cup, 57 g	50	2	7
Seasoned Kitchen Chips (Reg), 170 g	433	26	47

Calzones

	Cal	Fat	Cbs
• 3 Meat & 3 Cheese, 441 g	1080	55	102
3 Veggie & 3 Cheese, 438 g	860	34	105
Cheese, 364 g	840	34	101
Cheese & Pepperoni, 375 g	960	45	101
Philly Cheesesteak Calzone, 348 g	872	39	90
Philly Chicken Calzone, 341 g	745	24	90
• Pizza Sauce Dipping Cup, 57 g	50	2	7
Ranch Dipping Cup, 42 g	230	24	2
Sausage Pelucci Calzone, 425 g	1042	52	92

Desserts

	Cal	Fat	Cbs
Blonde Brownie Dessert Mini, 36 g	159	9	19
• Fudge Brownie Dessert Mini, 40 g	150	7	22
Graeter's Big Scoop cup, 210 g	600	42	56
Hot Fudge Brownie (1/2 portion), 223 g	758	40	99
• Italian Crème Cake, 257 g	998	57	112
Pizza Frite (1/2 portion), 122 g	342	6	64
Raspberry Swirl Dessert Mini, 62 g	185	13	15

Focaccia Style Pizza (Medium)

	Cal	Fat	Cbs
Florentine (1/10), 94 g	240	13	24
Roma (1/10), 94 g	300	18	23

Fresh Baked Breads

	Cal	Fat	Cbs
Breadsticks (5), 309 g	998	13	190
• Breadsticks w/Provolone (5), 389 g	1293	35	193
Garlic Bread (2), 66 g	240	9	35
Garlic Bread w/Provolone (2), 104 g	390	21	35
Garlic Sauce Dipping Sauce, 51 g	360	40	0
• Pizza Sauce Dipping Cup, 57 g	50	2	7

Fresh Salads and Soup

	Cal	Fat	Cbs
Antipasto for One, 271 g	317	21	12
Baked Onion Soup, 272 g	304	16	28
Grilled Chicken Salad, 318 g	296	12	11
• JoJo's BLT Salad (w/dressing), 257 g	505	35	9
• Minestrone Soup, 336 g	130	2	22
Tossed Salad, 205 g	163	9	10

● MOST HEALTHY   • LEAST HEALTHY

▶ LA ROSA'S PIZZERIA (cont.)

	Cal	Fat	Cbs
Tuna Salad Plate, 336 g	433	28	16
Hand Tossed Pizzas (Medium)			
• Cheese, 96 g	230	8	29
• Big 4 Meat, 124 g	326	15	29
Big 4 Pick 4, 119 g	278	11	30
Big 4 Veggie, 126 g	238	7	30
Double Pepperoni, 111 g	298	14	29
Hoagys			
Baked Buddy Hoagy, 248 g	665	28	62
Baked Royal Hoagy, 254 g	601	22	62
• Chicken Italiano Hoagy, 427 g	778	28	65
Fillet of Haddock Hoagy, 302 g	630	15	81
Link Sausage Hoagy, 273 g	621	24	64
Meatball Hoagy, 334 g	689	26	77
Original Steak Hoagy, 321 g	727	35	65
Philly Chicken Hoagy, 264 g	451	4	64
Philly Steak Hoagy, 263 g	621	25	64
Tuna Hoagy, 273 g	588	20	66
• Turkey Hoagy, 306 g	418	2	66
Ingredients and Dressings for Hoagys			
Kitchen Chips, 28 g	150	9	15
Mushroom Sauce, 60 g	20	0	4
• Pesto Mayonnaise, 74 g	290	26	15
• Pickle Chips, 39 g	5	0	1
Pizza Sauce, 57 g	50	2	7
Provolone, 28 g	103	7	1
Red Onion Slices, 14 g	6	0	1
Sharp White Cheddar, 26 g	92	8	1
Tomato Slices, 51 g	11	0	2
Just Right Combo Meals			
1/2 Baked Buddy, 124 g	333	14	31
1/2 Lasagna, 300 g	368	19	31
1/2 Original Steak Hoagy, 161 g	364	18	33
• 1/2 Ziti Chicken Alfredo, 298 g	491	21	51
Sm Spag + 1 meatball, 227 g	437	12	67
• Small Salad-no dressing, 163 g	155	9	10
Kid's Meals			
Cheese Sticks & Potatoes, 286 g	536	28	55
Chicken Tenders & Potatoes, 299 g	492	26	49
• Mac 'n Cheese, 310 g	378	12	58
Smiley Pizza Cheese, 382 g	726	30	79
• Smiley Pizza Pepperoni, 396 g	796	36	79
Spaghetti and Meatball, 311 g	515	10	86
Pan Crust Pizzas (Medium)			
Big 4 Meat, 126 g	323	15	29
Big 4 Pick 4, 121 g	275	11	30

• MOST HEALTHY   • LEAST HEALTHY

LA ROSA'S PIZZERIA (cont.)

	Cal	Fat	Cbs
• Big 4 Veggie, 128 g	235	7	30
Cheese, 105 g	300	16	30
• Double Pepperoni, 121 g	370	22	30
Pasta Dinners			
Add Chkn Strips w/Traditional Sc, 283 g	284	10	21
Add Link Ssge w/Traditional Sc, 283 g	416	26	21
Add Meatballs (3) w/Traditional Sc, 264 g	381	23	25
Cheese Ravioli, 496 g	661	26	80
Lasagna w/ Meat Sauce, 599 g	735	38	61
Meat Ravioli, 496 g	621	22	102
• Minestrone Soup, 336 g	130	2	22
Spaghetti & Meatballs, 640 g	870	28	119
Spaghetti or Ziti w/Alfredo Sauce, 546 g	976	50	104
Spaghetti or Ziti w/Meat Sauce, 546 g	698	18	104
Spaghetti or Ziti w/Traditional Sc, 546 g	640	12	113
Tossed Salad – no dressing, 205 g	163	9	10
• Ziti Chicken Alfredo, 596 g	982	42	102
Ziti Sausage Pelucci, 624 g	766	20	115
Salad Dressing			
LaRosa's Creamy Garlic, 43 g	250	26	3
LaRosa's Italian, 43 g	230	26	2
Traditional Crust Pizzas (Medium)			
• Big 4 Meat, 104 g	286	16	20
Big 4 Pick 4, 100 g	238	12	20
• Big 4 Veggie, 106 g	198	8	21
Cheese, 76 g	200	10	19
Double Pepperoni, 94 g	280	16	20

LAMAR'S

Bizmarks			
• Bavarian Cream	620	22	101
• Blueberry Filled	520	20	81
Cherry Filled	550	19	88
Lemon Filled	530	21	80
Cake Donuts			
Apple Spiced	340	17	44
Blueberry	350	17	47
Chocolate Iced	330	18	37
• Old Fashioned Sour Cream	420	18	60
• White Iced	320	17	38
Lamar's Bars			
• Caramel Iced (Unfilled)	430	18	59
Chocolate Iced (Bavarian Cream Filled)	600	22	96
Chocolate Iced (Chocolate Fluff Filled)	800	35	118
Chocolate Iced (Unfilled)	540	22	81
• Chocolate Iced (White Fluff Filled)	810	35	120

LAMAR'S (cont.)

	Cal	Fat	Cbs
Specialty Donuts			
Cinnamon Roll	690	25	106
• Cinnamon Roll (Raisin Nut)	850	27	137
Cinnamon Twist	770	26	120
• German Chocolate Knot	480	27	54
Yeast Raised Donuts			
Ray's Chocolate Glazed	290	11	44
Ray's Original Glazed	220	10	31

LITTLE CAESARS

	Cal	Fat	Cbs
14" Round HOT-N-READY® Pizza			
Just Cheese, 113 g	240	9	30
Pepperoni, 120 g	280	11	30
3 Meat Treat® (1/8 pizza)			
3 Meat Treat® (8 slices), 138 g	350	18	30
Baby Pan!Pan!®			
Cheese and Pepperoni, 140 g	360	18	33
Just Cheese, 133 g	320	15	33
Caesar Dips®			
• Buffalo, 43 g	140	2	4
Buffalo Ranch, 43 g	230	4	3
• Buttery Garlic, 43 g	380	9	0
Cheezy, 43 g	210	4	3
Chipotle, 43 g	220	4	2
Caesar Wings®			
• Barbecue, 33 g	70	4	3
Hot, 33 g	60	5	1
Mild, 30 g	60	4	1
• Oven Roasted, 26 g	50	4	0
Crazy Bread®			
Crazy Bread®, 38 g	100	3	15
Crazy Sauce®			
Crazy Sauce®, 113 g	45	0	10
Deep Dish Pizza (1/8 pizza)			
Just Cheese, 138 g	320	13	38
Pepperoni, 145 g	360	16	38
Hula Hawaiian™ (1/8 pizza)			
Pineapple and Canadian Bacon, 150 g	280	9	34
Pineapple and Ham, 150 g	270	9	33
Little Caesars Pepperoni Chz Bread®			
Little Caesars Pepp Chz Bread® (10 pieces), 49 g	150	8	13
Ultimate Supreme (1/8 pizza)			
Ultimate Supreme (8 slices), 151 g	310	14	31
Vegetarian (1/8 pizza)			
Vegetarian (8 slices), 154 g	270	10	32

• MOST HEALTHY   • LEAST HEALTHY

LONG JOHN SILVER'S

	Cal	Fat	Cbs
Chicken			
Chicken Plank®, 52 g	140	8	9
Desserts			
• Chocolate Cream Pie, 74 g	280	17	28
• Pineapple Cream Pie, 89 g	300	17	35
Turtle Pie, 77 g	290	16	34
Dollar Stretcher Menu			
Baja Fish Taco, 112 g	350	22	28
Chicken & Fries, 137 g	370	18	42
Double Jr. Fish Sandwich, 168 g	440	22	46
• Four Battered Shrimp, 56 g	170	12	10
Jr. Fish Sandwich, 117 g	310	14	37
Popcorn Shrimp, 83 g	270	16	23
Six Hushpuppies, 83 g	360	19	56
Small Golden Fries, 85 g	230	10	33
Three Shrimp & Fries, 127 g	360	19	41
• Two Jr. Fish & Fries, 187 g	490	26	51
Zesty Chicken Sandwich, 118 g	350	18	35
Fish And Seafood			
Battered Fish, 92 g	260	16	17
Battered Shrimp, 42 g	130	9	8
• Breaded Clam Strips, 85 g	320	19	29
Buttered Langostino Lobster Bites, 91 g	230	9	24
Crispy Breaded Fish, 75 g	190	10	17
Grilled Pacific Salmon, 128 g	150	5	2
• Grilled Tilapia, 116 g	110	3	1
Langostino Lobster Stuffed Crab Cake, 62 g	170	9	16
Popcorn Shrimp, 83 g	270	16	23
Shrimp Scampi, 130 g	200	13	3
Sandwiches, Bowls, & More			
Chicken Sandwich, 137 g	360	15	40
Fish Sandwich, 176 g	470	23	49
Freshside Grille® Smart Choice Salmon, 304 g	280	7	27
Freshside Grille® Smart Choice Shrimp Scampi, 306 g	330	15	29
• Freshside Grille® Smart Choice Tilapia, 292 g	250	5	27
Salmon Bowl with Sauce, 426 g	460	8	65
Salmon Bowl without Sauce, 383 g	380	8	47
Shrimp Bowl with Sauce, 389 g	390	5	65
Shrimp Bowl without Sauce, 346 g	310	5	47
• Ultimate Fish Sandwich®, 206 g	530	27	50
Sauces/Condiments			
Cocktail Sauce, 28 g	25	0	6
• Ginger Teriyaki Sauce, 43 g	80	0	18
Louisiana Hot Sauce, 5 g	0	0	0
• Malt Vinegar, 14 g	0	0	0
Marinara, 28 g	15	0	4

• MOST HEALTHY　• LEAST HEALTHY

LONG JOHN SILVER'S (cont.)

Sides

	Cal	Fat	Cbs
Breaded Mozzarella Sticks, 50 g	150	9	13
Breadstick, 58 g	170	4	29
Broccoli Cheese Bites, 93 g	230	12	25
Broccoli Cheese Soup, 210 g	220	18	8
Cole Slaw, 113 g	200	15	15
Corn Cobbette with Butter Oil, 102 g	150	10	14
Corn Cobbette without Butter Oil, 95 g	90	3	14
Crumblies®, 28 g	170	12	14
Fries- Platter Portion, 85 g	230	10	34
Hushpuppy, 23 g	60	3	9
• Jalapeño Cheddar Bites, 82 g	240	14	23
• Jalapeño Peppers, 37 g	15	0	2
Rice, 142 g	180	1	37
Vegetable Medley, 113 g	50	2	8

MACARONI GRILL

Classico Italian

	Cal	Fat	Cbs
Chicken Marsala, Lunch	620	34	46
Chicken Parmigiana	850	37	76
Chicken Scaloppine, Lunch	740	45	46
Eggplant Parmigiana	800	47	65
Fettuccine Alfredo	780	46	71
Fettuccine Alfredo w/ Chicken	910	48	71
Fettuccine Alfredo w/ Shrimp	825	46	71
• Lasagna Al Forno	560	30	43
• Mama's Trio	1280	67	74
Parmesan-Crusted Sole, Lunch	1190	71	101
Spaghetti & Meatballs (Bolognese sauce)	880	37	87
Spaghetti & Meatballs (Tomato sauce)	720	27	85
Spaghetti Bolognese	570	19	72

Create Your Own Handcrafted Pasta

	Cal	Fat	Cbs
Alfredo	180	13	14
Arrabbiata Sauce (Spicy Red Sauce)	320	21	12
• Bolognese (Meat Sauce)	160	11	11
Pasta	390	4	79
Pomodoro (Tomato Basil)	360	29	18
• Sauces	610	59	9

Desserts

	Cal	Fat	Cbs
Amaretto Apple Crispetti	1210	41	200
• Italian Sorbetto w/ Biscotti	220	2	48
Lemon Passion	940	53	104
N.Y. Cheesecake Plain	1090	73	93
• N.Y. Chzcake w/ Caramel Fudge Sauce	1650	95	179
Simple Lemon Pound Cake	250	11	35
Smothered Chocolate Cake	1580	102	147

• MOST HEALTHY   • LEAST HEALTHY

MACARONI GRILL (cont.)

	Cal	Fat	Cbs
Tiramisu	1120	80	88
Dressings & Sauces			
• Mediterranean Vinaigrette, 1 fl.oz.	130	14	3
Parmesan Peppercorn Dressing, 1 fl.oz.	120	12	2
• Pizzaiola Sauce, 1 fl.oz.	40	4	3
Fresh Antipasti			
Calamari Fritti	650	43	42
Crab-Stuffed Mushrooms	310	24	4
Fresh Mozzarella Fritta	680	44	39
• Mediterranean Olives	140	13	4
Mozzarella Alla Caprese	330	16	33
Prosciutto e Parmigiano	470	25	21
Roasted Vegetables	330	19	32
Romano's Sampler	800	52	50
• Spinach Artichoke Dip	810	35	94
Tomato Bruschetta	560	17	77
Fresh Italian Sandwiches			
Grilled Chicken Sandwich	670	20	66
Imported Prosciutto Sandwich	630	23	68
Grilled Specialties (Includes Sides)			
Calabrese Strip	1130	65	47
Center-Cut Filet	760	39	36
Grilled Halibut	770	34	58
• Grilled Pork Chops	1380	77	96
Grilled Salmon	750	35	55
Honey Balsamic Chicken, Lunch	540	13	54
• Simple Salmon	420	22	6
Handcrafted Pasta			
• Capellini Pomodoro	390	14	55
• Carmela's Chicken Rigatoni	1080	58	100
Chicken Cannelloni	600	29	42
Lobster Ravioli	520	30	32
Mushroom Ravioli	790	44	70
Pasta Milano	750	24	93
Penne Rustica	980	38	94
Pollo Caprese	550	20	45
Pollo Limone Rustica	990	50	79
Sausage Salentino	900	50	67
Seafood Linguine	650	22	75
Shrimp Portofino - Lunch	560	34	37
Kid's			
Beef Kabob w/ Fresh Broccoli	150	6	4
Chicken Strips w/ Fresh Broccoli	390	22	23
Crispy Fish Filet w/ Salad	340	24	16
Grilled Cheese Sandwich w/ Salad	440	30	27
Grilled Chicken & Broccoli	310	7	28

• MOST HEALTHY   • LEAST HEALTHY

MACARONI GRILL (cont.)

	Cal	Fat	Cbs
Kid's Cheese Pizza	470	14	60
• Vanilla Gelato w/ Strawberries	110	4	17
• Kid's Pepperoni Pizza	530	20	60
Macaroni & Cheese	400	9	64
Pasta Pomodoro	340	12	48
Side Fries	250	9	40
Spaghetti & Meatball w/ Tomato Sauce	430	17	51
Spaghetti w/ Meat Sauce	390	13	46

Mediterranean Lunch

	Cal	Fat	Cbs
• 1/2 Grilled Chicken Sandwich Only	330	10	33
• 1/2 Imported Prosciutto Sandwich Only	320	11	34
Fresh Greens	320	26	20

Neapolitan Pizza

	Cal	Fat	Cbs
• Italian Sausage	970	39	95
• Margherita	720	20	95
Pepperoni	920	37	102
Prosciutto e Arugula	900	34	94
Quattro Formaggio	950	34	111
Roasted Vegetali	800	27	102

Rosemary Spiedini (Includes Sides)

	Cal	Fat	Cbs
Aged Beef Tenderloin Spiedini	410	12	27
Center-Cut Lamb Spiedini	500	24	29
Grilled Chicken Spiedini	360	10	17
• Italian Sausage Spiedini	720	40	43
• Jumbo Shrimp Spiedini	230	5	15

Toppings

	Cal	Fat	Cbs
Fresh Broccoli	10	0	1
Fresh Mushrooms	10	0	0
Fresh Spinach	20	0	3
• Grape Tomatoes	5	0	0
Handmade Meatballs	310	18	15
• Italian Sausage	330	22	3
Roasted Chicken	130	2	0
Roasted Garlic Cloves	60	1	11
Sauteed Shrimp	45	0	0
Sun-Dried Tomatoes	60	0	11

Zuppa Della Casa & Insalata

	Cal	Fat	Cbs
Amalfi Chicken Soup	420	12	45
• Caesar Salad	260	20	14
Chicken Caesar	650	42	29
Fresh Greens	320	26	20
• Parmesan-Crusted Chicken	960	63	49
Pasta e Fagioli Soup	330	14	39
Scallops & Spinach Salad	360	18	16
Warm Spinach Salad	330	20	21

• MOST HEALTHY   • LEAST HEALTHY

MAGGIE MOO'S ICECREAM

	Cal	Fat	Cbs
Basic Flavors			
• Low Fat/Lactose Free, 72 g	90	3	15
NSA, 64 g	110	4	28
Sorbet/Fat Free, 85 g	120	0	30
Udderly Cream, 80 g	180	11	18
Zoomers (Medium)			
Caramel Coffee, 24 oz.	680	21	123
Creamy Mango, 24 oz.	652	4	142
Iced Cream Coffee, 24 oz.	530	19	92
Mocha Coffee, 24 oz.	780	22	149
• Peach Orange - Blossom, 24 oz.	500	14	94
• Pineapple Coconut-Colada, 24 oz.	800	41	109
Raspberry Pomegranate, 24 oz.	765	1	151
Strawberry Banana, 24 oz.	620	19	116
Triple Berry Pomegranate, 24 oz.	765	2	154

MANCHU WOK

	Cal	Fat	Cbs
Appetizers			
Chicken Egg Roll, 70 g	150	7	17
• Seafood Rangoon, 85 g	300	21	20
• Vegetable Egg Roll, 70 g	150	6	20
Beef Dishes			
Beef & Broccoli, 142 g	180	13	12
Black Pepper Beef, 142 g	180	14	8
• Pepper Steak, 142 g	170	12	10
• Spicy Beef, 142 g	180	14	10
Chicken Dishes			
Black Pepper Chicken, 142 g	170	11	9
Chicken & Mushrooms, 142 g	160	11	8
• Chicken with Snow Peas, 142 g	140	9	11
General Tso's Chicken, 142 g	360	21	31
Green Bean Chicken, 142 g	160	10	10
• Honey Garlic Chicken, 142 g	430	21	50
Kung Pao Chicken, 142 g	180	12	12
Orange Chicken, 142 g	400	21	42
Oriental Grilled Chicken, 142 g	240	9	20
Pineapple Chicken, 142 g	170	9	19
Sesame Chicken, 142 g	370	14	46
Spicy Chicken, 142 g	150	9	10
Sweet & Sour Chicken Tenders, 142 g	340	18	17
Pork			
BBQ Pork, 142 g	240	11	16
Sweet & Sour Pork, 142 g	360	19	37
Rice & Noodles			
Fried Rice, 227 g	410	13	65
• Noodles (Lo Mein), 227 g	300	17	33

● MOST HEALTHY • LEAST HEALTHY

MANCHU WOK (cont.)	Cal	Fat	Cbs
• Shanghai Noodles, 227 g	410	14	56
Steamed Rice, 227 g	370	0	84
Vegetables			
Mixed Vegetables, 142 g	130	10	11

MAX & ERMA'S

	Cal	Fat	Cbs
Appetizers			
Black Bean Roll-Ups	577	10	95
Low-Fat Tex Mex Dressing, 2 tbsp.	23	0	2
Beverages			
Fruit Smoothie	124	0	29
Entrees			
Black Bean Veggie Burger	649	28	79
Caribbean Chicken: Lunch Portion	536	20	59
Salads			
• Baby Greens Salad	119	11	6
Half Hula Bowl	319	5	46
• Hula Bowl	583	10	78
Sides			
Fruit Salad, 5 oz.	54	0	17
Garlic Breadstick, 1 Breadstick	150	6	20

MAZZIO'S PIZZA

	Cal	Fat	Cbs
Calzone Rings & Quesapizza			
4 Meat/Four Chz Calzone w/o Sc, 96 g	274	11	33
Chicken Quesapizza w/o Sauce, 113 g	317	13	33
• Ham Bacon & Chdr Calzone w/o Sc, 90 g	244	8	32
Pepperoni Calzone w/o Sauce, 87 g	260	10	33
• Pepperoni Quesapizza w/o Sauce, 99 g	332	16	32
Deep Pan 1 Topping Pizzas (Medium - 8 Slices)			
• Canadian Bacon, 137 g	330	14	38
Cheese, 130 g	332	15	38
Chicken, 144 g	338	14	38
Hamburger (Beef), 144 g	359	17	38
Pepperoni, 131 g	352	17	37
• Sausage, 144 g	374	19	38
Deep Pan Pricebuster Pizzas (Medium - 8 Slices)			
• Cheesebuster, 130 g	348	16	38
• Meatbuster, 146 g	385	20	38
Supremebuster, 144 g	356	17	38
Deep Pan Specialty Pizzas (Medium - 8 Slices)			
4 Meat, 151 g	403	21	38
California Alfredo, 144 g	383	19	38
Chicken Club, 150 g	355	16	38
Combo, 160 g	381	19	39
• Greek, 142 g	414	24	38

• MOST HEALTHY • LEAST HEALTHY

▶ MAZZIO'S PIZZA (cont.)

	Cal	Fat	Cbs
Lucky 7 Pizza, 162 g	353	17	39
Mazzio's "Works", 171 g	406	21	39
Mexican, 183 g	413	21	42
• Veggie, 152 g	331	15	39
Dippin' Sauces			
• Marinara, 60 g	29	1	5
Buffalo, 57 g	19	N/A	4
Chocolate, 57 g	177	1	43
Picante, 60 g	20	N/A	4
• Vanilla, 57 g	181	N/A	45
Dippin' Zone: Chicken			
• Boneless Dippin' Chicken (10 ct), 51 g	122	6	7
• Rst & BBQ Tossed Wings (10 ct), 82 g	191	12	7
Wings of Fire (10 ct) w/o Sauce, 71 g	161	11	1
Dippin' Zone: Fries			
Cheese Fries, 179 g	432	26	35
Full Order, 133 g	279	14	34
Dippin' Zone: Italian			
Artichoke Spin Dip with Bread, 87 g	245	16	18
Breadsticks w/o Sauce, 52 g	150	3	26
• Cheese Dippers w/o Sauce, 128 g	405	18	47
Garlic Cheese Toast w/o Sauce, 54 g	205	13	16
Garlic Toast w/o Sauce, 40 g	160	10	15
• Mozzarella Sticks w/o Sauce, 57 g	181	12	10
Toasted Ravioli w/o Sauce, 43 g	118	5	13
Dippin' Zone: Ribs			
Rib Dippers 3/4 lb Tossed w/ BBQ, 138 g	458	32	13
Dippin' Zone: Southwestern			
• Cheese Nachos w/ jalapeños, 113 g	423	30	19
Meat Nachos (Beef w/ jalapeños), 142 g	484	34	20
Meat Nachos (Chkn w/ jalapeños), 135 g	448	30	20
• Meat Nachos (Ssge w/ jalapeños), 142 g	504	37	20
Dippin' Zone: Sweet			
Cinnamon Sticks w/o Sauce, 145 g	626	36	70
French Bread Pizzas			
Deli (1 Bread), 201 g	480	20	60
• Greek (1 Bread), 257 g	623	31	61
• Hawaiian (1 Bread), 208 g	449	13	62
Pepperoni (1 Bread), 179 g	495	21	58
Southwestern Chicken (1 Bread), 230 g	532	20	61
Hot Toasted Sandwiches			
Chkn, Bacon & Swiss (Focaccia), 392 g	1021	70	48
• Chkn, Bacon & Swiss (Hoagie), 510 g	1362	72	120
Ham & Cheddar (Focaccia), 351 g	747	47	47
Ham & Cheddar (Hoagie), 470 g	1088	50	119
• Kosher Pickle Spear, 28 g	5	N/A	1

• MOST HEALTHY   • LEAST HEALTHY

MAZZIO'S PIZZA (cont.)	Cal	Fat	Cbs
Mazzio's Sub (Focaccia), 344 g	768	49	45
Mazzio's Sub (Hoagie), 462 g	1109	52	117
Potato Chips (Lays), 28 g	152	10	15
Turkey & Swiss (Focaccia), 376 g	718	38	46
Turkey & Swiss (Hoagie), 494 g	1059	40	118
Tuscan Smash (Focaccia), 354 g	645	34	45
Tuscan Smash (Hoagie), 473 g	986	36	117
Original Crust: 1 Topping Pizzas (Medium - 8 Slices)			
• Canadian Bacon, 113 g	231	9	30
Cheese, 105 g	234	9	30
Chicken, 120 g	239	7	31
Hamburger (Beef), 120 g	260	10	31
Pepperoni, 106 g	254	10	30
• Sausage, 120 g	276	12	31
Original Crust: Pricebuster Pizzas (Medium - 8 Slices)			
• Cheesebuster, 105 g	249	9	30
• Meatbuster, 121 g	286	13	31
Supremebuster, 119 g	257	10	31
Original Crust: Specialty Pizzas (Medium - 8 Slices)			
4 Meat, 126 g	305	15	31
California Alfredo, 119 g	285	13	30
Chicken Club, 125 g	257	9	31
Combo, 135 g	282	12	31
• Greek, 117 g	315	17	30
Lucky 7 Pizza, 137 g	255	10	32
Mazzio's "Works", 146 g	307	14	31
Mexican, 158 g	314	14	35
• Veggie, 127 g	232	8	31
Signature Pastas			
Chicken Parmesan, 614 g	947	27	135
Chicken Spinach Artichoke Pasta, 463 g	1005	38	113
Chicken-Fried Chicken Alfredo, 479 g	1290	69	120
Fettuccine Alfredo, 343 g	1061	56	107
• Garlic Toast (1 Piece), 40 g	160	10	15
• Greek Pasta, 458 g	1456	94	107
Lasagna Red & White, 669 g	984	62	64
Lasagna with Alfredo, 598 g	1264	94	55
Lasagna with Marinara, 740 g	704	30	73
Lasagna with Meat Sauce, 712 g	949	52	64
Spaghetti with Marinara, 449 g	641	8	120
Spaghetti with Meat Sauce, 428 g	825	25	113
Spag w/ Meatballs (4) & Marinara, 562 g	972	34	126
Spag w/ Meatballs (4) & Meat Sauce, 541 g	1156	50	119
Thin Crust: 1 Topping Pizzas (Medium - 8 Slices)			
• Canadian Bacon, 91 g	179	8	18
Cheese, 84 g	182	9	18

• MOST HEALTHY　　• LEAST HEALTHY

MAZZIO'S PIZZA (cont.)

	Cal	Fat	Cbs
Chicken, 98 g	187	8	19
Hamburger (Beef), 98 g	208	11	19
Pepperoni, 85 g	202	11	18
• Sausage, 98 g	224	12	19

Thin Crust: Pricebuster Pizzas (Medium - 8 Slices)

	Cal	Fat	Cbs
• Cheesebuster, 84 g	197	9	19
• Meatbuster, 100 g	234	13	19
Supremebuster, 98 g	205	11	19

Thin Crust: Specialty Pizzas (Medium - 8 Slices)

	Cal	Fat	Cbs
4 Meat, 105 g	253	15	19
California Alfredo, 98 g	233	13	18
Chicken Club, 104 g	205	9	19
Combo, 114 g	231	13	19
• Greek, 96 g	263	17	19
Lucky 7 Pizza, 116 g	203	10	20
Mazzio's "Works", 125 g	255	15	20
Mexican, 136 g	262	14	23
• Veggie, 105 g	180	8	19

MCDONALD'S

Breakfast

	Cal	Fat	Cbs
Bacon, Egg & Cheese Biscuit, 140 g	420	23	37
Bacon, Egg & Chz McGriddles®, 164 g	420	18	48
• Big Breakfast w/ Hotcakes, 420 g	1090	56	111
Big Breakfast®, 269 g	740	48	51
Biscuit, 76 g	260	12	33
Egg McMuffin®, 137 g	300	12	30
English Muffin, 56 g	160	3	27
• Grape Jam, 14 g	35	0	9
Hash Brown, 56 g	150	9	15
Hotcake Syrup, (1 pkg) 60 g	180	0	45
Hotcakes & Ssge w/o Syrup & Mrgrn, 192 g	520	24	61
Hotcakes w/o Syrup & Margarine, 151 g	350	9	60
McSkillet™ Burrito w/ Sausage, 238 g	610	36	44
McSkillet™ Burrito w/ Steak, 250 g	570	30	44
Sausage Biscuit, 117 g	430	27	34
Sausage Biscuit w/ Egg, 163 g	510	33	36
Sausage Burrito, 109 g	300	16	26
Sausage McGriddles®, 141 g	420	22	44
Sausage McMuffin®, 111 g	370	22	29
Sausage McMuffin® w/ Egg, 162 g	450	27	30
Sausage Patty, 41 g	170	15	1
Ssge, Egg & Chz McGriddles®, 201 g	560	32	48
Scrambled Eggs (2), 96 g	170	11	1
Southern Style Chicken Biscuit, 143 g	410	20	41
Strawberry Preserves, 14 g	35	0	9

▶ MCDONALD'S (cont.)

	Cal	Fat	Cbs
Whipped Margarine (1 pat), 6 g	40	5	0
Chicken and Sauces			
Chicken McNuggets® (4 piece), 64 g	190	12	11
• Chkn Selects® Prem Breast Strips (3 pc), 131 g	400	24	23
SW Chipotle Barbeque Sauce, 5 g	60	0	15
Spicy Buffalo Sauce, 35 g	60	6	1
• Sweet 'N Sour Sauce, 28 g	50	0	12
Desserts/Shakes			
• Apple Dippers, 68 g	35	0	8
Baked Hot Apple Pie, 77 g	250	13	32
Chocolate Chip Cookie, 33 g	160	8	21
Choco Triple Thick® Shake, 444 ml	580	14	102
Cinnamon Melts, 114 g	460	19	66
Fruit 'n Yogurt Parfait (7 oz), 149 g	160	2	31
Fruit 'n Yogurt Parfait (w/o granola), 142 g	130	2	25
Hot Caramel Sundae, 182 g	340	8	60
Hot Fudge Sundae, 179 g	330	10	54
Kiddie Cone, 29 g	45	1	8
Low Fat Caramel Dip, 21 g	70	1	15
McDonaldland® Cookies, 57 g	260	8	43
• McFlurry® w/ M&M'S® Candies, 348 g	620	20	96
McFlurry® w/ OREO® Cookies, 337 g	550	17	88
Oatmeal Raisin Cookie, 33 g	150	6	22
Peanuts (for Sundaes), 7 g	45	4	2
Strawberry Sundae, 178 g	280	6	49
Strawberry Triple Thick® Shake, 444 ml	560	13	97
Sugar Cookie, 33 g	160	7	21
Vanilla Red Fat Ice Cream Cone, 90 g	150	4	24
Vanilla Triple Thick® Shake, 444 ml	550	13	96
French Fries			
Medium French Fries, 4.1 oz.	380	19	48
McCafe Frappes (Medium)			
Frappe Caramel, 16 fl.oz. cup	550	24	76
Frappe Mocha, 16 fl.oz. cup	560	24	78
Salad Dressings			
Newman's Own® Creamy SW Drss, 2 fl.oz.	100	6	11
Salads			
Butter Garlic Croutons, 14 g	60	2	10
Prem Bacon Ranch Salad (w/o chkn), 223 g	140	7	10
Prem Bacon Ranch Salad w/ Crispy Chkn, 324 g	370	20	20
Prem Bacon Ranch Salad w/Grld Chkn, 321 g	260	9	12
Premium Caesar Salad (w/o chkn), 213 g	90	4	9
Premium Caesar Salad w/ Crispy, 314 g	330	17	20
Prem Caesar Salad w/Grilled Chkn, 311 g	220	6	12
Premium SW Salad (w/o chkn), 231 g	140	5	20
• Premium SW Salad w/ Crispy Chkn, 353 g	430	20	38

MCDONALD'S (cont.)

	Cal	Fat	Cbs
Premium SW Salad w/ Grilled Chkn, 350 g	320	9	30
• Side Salad, 87 g	20	0	4
Snack Size Fruit & Walnut Salad, 163 g	210	8	31

Sandwiches

	Cal	Fat	Cbs
• Angus Bacon & Cheese, 291 g	790	39	63
Angus Deluxe, 314 g	750	39	61
Angus Mushroom & Swiss, 283 g	770	40	59
Big Mac®, 214 g	540	29	45
Big N' Tasty®, 206 g	460	24	37
Big N' Tasty® w/ Cheese, 220 g	510	28	38
Cheeseburger, 114 g	300	12	33
Chipotle BBQ Snack Wrap® (Crispy), 120 g	330	15	35
Chipotle BBQ Snack Wrap® (Grilled), 125 g	260	9	28
Double Cheeseburger, 165 g	440	23	34
Double Quarter Pounder w/ Chz, 279 g	740	42	40
Filet-O-Fish®, 142 g	380	18	38
• Hamburger, 100 g	250	9	31
Honey Mustard Snack Wrap® (Crispy), 118 g	330	16	34
Honey Mustard Snack Wrap® (Grilled), 124 g	260	9	27
Mac Snack Wrap†, 126 g	330	19	26
McChicken®, 143 g	360	16	40
McDouble, 151 g	390	19	33
McRib ®†, 209 g	500	26	44
Premium Crispy Chkn Classic Snd, 230 g	530	20	59
Premium Crispy Chkn Club Snd, 254 g	630	28	60
Prem Crispy Chkn Ranch BLT Snd, 240 g	580	23	62
Premium Grilled Chkn Classic Snd, 226 g	420	10	51
Premium Grilled Chkn Club Snd, 250 g	530	17	52
Prem Grilled Chkn Ranch BLT Snd, 236 g	470	12	54
Quarter Pounder® w/ Cheese+, 198 g	510	26	40
Quarter Pounder®+, 169 g	410	19	37
Ranch Snack Wrap® (Crispy), 117 g	340	17	33
Ranch Snack Wrap® (Grilled), 122 g	270	10	26
Southern Style Crispy Chkn Snd, 161 g	400	17	39

MR. GOODCENTS

Bread

	Cal	Fat	Cbs
Mr. Goodcents White Half Bread, 128 g	270	2	57
• Mr. Goodcents Wheat Half Bread, 128 g	270	3	55
• Mr. Goodcents Satisfier Bread, 51 g	110	2	18

Cold Subs (Half Sub)

	Cal	Fat	Cbs
Centsable Sub Wheat Bread, 227 g	480	20	58
Centsable Sub White Bread, 227 g	490	19	60
Cheese Mix Wheat Bread, 213 g	560	26	58
Cheese Mix White Bread, 213 g	560	25	60
Ham & Cheese Wheat Bread, 227 g	400	10	59

• MOST HEALTHY   • LEAST HEALTHY

MR. GOODCENTS (cont.)

	Cal	Fat	Cbs
Ham & Cheese White Bread, 227 g	400	9	61
Italian Sub Wheat Bread, 213 g	640	37	55
Italian Sub White Bread, 213 g	640	36	57
Mr. Goodcents Org Wheat Bread, 213 g	510	25	56
Mr. Goodcents Org White Bread, 213 g	520	24	58
Oven Rst Chkn Breast White Bread, 213 g	350	5	57
Oven Rst Chkn Breast Wheat Bread, 213 g	350	6	55
Penny Club Wheat Bread, 213 g	350	6	57
Penny Club White Bread, 213 g	350	5	59
• Pepperoni & Cheese Wheat Bread, 227 g	740	46	55
Pepperoni & Cheese White Bread, 227 g	740	45	57
Roast Beef Wheat Bread, 213 g	350	6	55
Roast Beef White Bread, 213 g	350	5	57
Tuna Salad Wheat Bread, 213 g	490	21	63
Tuna Salad White Bread, 213 g	490	20	64
Turkey Wheat Bread, 213 g	350	6	58
Turkey White Bread, 213 g	350	5	60
Veggie Sub Wheat Bread, 212 g	290	4	58
• Veggie Sub White Bread, 212 g	290	3	60
Desserts			
• Baked Brownie, 65 g	260	10	41
• Giant Chocolate Chip Cookie, 71 g	420	22	52
Giant Peanut Butter Cookie, 71 g	340	20	36
Dress Options (Amount on 8" Sub)			
American Cheese, 14 g	40	3	1
Bacon (3 slices), 14 g	60	5	0
Black Olives, 7 g	30	2	2
Cheddar Cheese, 14 g	60	5	0
• Jalapeños, 7 g	0	0	0
Mozzarella Cheese, 14 g	40	3	0
Pepper Jack Cheese, 14 g	50	4	1
Provolone Cheese, 14 g	50	4	0
Regional Peppers (Banana), 7 g	0	0	0
• Spicy Ranch, 14 g	70	7	1
Standard Dress, 21 g	30	2	2
Standard Dress, no oil, 19 g	10	0	2
Swiss Cheese, 14 g	50	4	0
Flatbread Pizza			
• Chz w/ Red Sauce Flatbread Pizza, 248 g	530	22	63
Chz w/ White Sc Flatbread Pizza, 234 g	720	41	65
• Chkn Alfredo Flatbread Pizza, 291 g	770	42	65
Pepperoni Flatbread Pizza, 276 g	670	35	63
Hot Subs (Half Sub)			
Chkn Bacon Ranch Wheat Bread w/ Chdr, 255 g	630	29	57
Chkn Bacon Ranch White Bread w/ Chdr, 255 g	630	28	59
Chkn Parm Sub Wheat Bread w/ Mozz, 255 g	490	13	62

• MOST HEALTHY   • LEAST HEALTHY

▶ MR. GOODCENTS (cont.)

	Cal	Fat	Cbs
• Chkn Parm Sub White Bread w/ Mozz, 255 g	490	12	63
• Meatball Wheat Bread w/ Mozz., 298 g	670	33	65
Meatball White Bread w/ Mozz., 398 g	670	32	67
Philly Jack 'n Cheese on Wheat, 269 g	490	16	60
Philly Jack 'n Cheese on White, 269 g	490	15	62

Pasta

	Cal	Fat	Cbs
Alfredo Sauce on Mostaccioli, 397 g	1290	80	106
Chz Tortellini with Alfredo Sauce, 420 g	1110	81	64
Chz Tortellini with Red Sauce, 420 g	330	6	51
• Chkn Alfredo on Mostaccioli, 510 g	1370	79	112
Chkn Parmesan on Mostaccioli, 525 g	660	10	100
• Garlic Bite (1), 51 g	160	6	24
Red Sauce on Mostaccioli, 397 g	520	4	100
Red Sauce on Mostaccioli w/Meatball, 369 g	610	20	79

Satisfier

	Cal	Fat	Cbs
Centsable Sub Satisfier, 136	280	16	20
Cheese Mix Satisfier, 136	400	25	21
Ham & Cheese Satisfier, 143	240	9	22
Italian Sub Satisfier, 136	480	36	18
Mr. Goodcents Original Satisfier, 136	350	24	19
Oven Roasted Chkn Breast Satisfier, 136	180	5	18
Penny Club Satisfier, 136	190	5	20
• Pepperoni & Cheese Satisfier, 143	570	45	18
Roast Beef Satisfier, 136	180	5	18
Tuna Salad Satisfier, 136	330	20	25
Turkey Satisfier, 136	180	5	21
• Veggie Sub satisfier, 115	120	3	21

Sides

	Cal	Fat	Cbs
Baked Lays KC Masterpiece, 31 g	140	4	25
• Baked Lays Original, 28 g	130	2	26
Baked Lays Sour Cream & Onion, 31 g	140	4	24
Cheetos Snacks, 56 g	320	20	31
Doritos Black Pepper Jack, 49 g	260	14	32
Doritos Cool Ranch, 49 g	260	13	31
Doritos Nacho Cheese, 49 g	250	14	30
• Fritos Corn Chips, 28 g	320	20	32
Lay's Classic Potato Chips, 42 g	230	15	23
Lay's Sour Cream & Onion, 28 g	240	15	23
Meatballs (3), 85 g	230	17	5
Miss Vickie's Jalapeño, 0 g	190	11	22
Sun Chips Harvest Cheddar, 28 g	210	9	29
Sun Chips Original, 28 g	210	10	27

Soups (8 oz.)

	Cal	Fat	Cbs
Broccoli Cheese Soup, 227 g	360	22	32
Chicken Noodle Soup, 227 g	120	1	22

• MOST HEALTHY   • LEAST HEALTHY

MR. PITA

	Cal	Fat	Cbs
9" Regular Size			
• Cranberry Turkey	424	1	77
Grilled Chicken & Broccoli	373	4	57
Grilled Chicken Caesar	353	4	50
Grilled Hawaiian Chicken	375	4	57
• Grilled Raspberry Chicken	342	3	56
Ultra Combo (Chicken/Turkey)	354	3	56
Ultra Grilled Chicken	367	4	56
Ultra Supreme	350	3	56
Ultra Turkey	343	1	56

MR. SUB

	Cal	Fat	Cbs
Breakfast Sandwiches			
Bacon & Egg, 177 g	365	16	36
Egg & Cheese, 195 g	435	21	36
• Ham & Cheese, 195 g	350	13	39
• Sausage & Egg, 224 g	505	30	36
Steak & Egg, 195 g	355	13	37
Cheese			
• Chedr Chz for sm Ult Chdr Club sub, 28 g	120	9	0
Cheddar/Mozz. Chz Shred for wraps, 15 g	50	4	1
Feta Cheese for Greek salad, 30 g	85	7	1
Parmesan for Caesar salads, 15 g	60	4	1
• Process Slice for most small subs, 12 g	40	3	2
Classic Subs			
• Assorted Cold Cuts, 180 g	290	9	38
Italian Salami, 158 g	280	10	35
• Maple Baked Ham, 174 g	250	4	40
Cookies			
Carnival, 38 g	160	7	23
• Double Chocolate Chip, 38 g	180	9	23
Milk Chocolate Chunk, 38 g	170	8	22
• Oatmeal Raisin, 38 g	160	6	23
Triple Chocolate Chip, 38 g	170	8	23
More Subs You Love			
BBQ Rib, 141 g	360	17	34
BLT, 133 g	260	8	34
• Breaded Chicken, 203 g	370	13	46
Great Canadian Club, 184 g	300	8	38
Grilled Chicken, 181 g	260	5	38
Louisiana Chicken, 161 g	290	8	35
Meatball, 146 g	360	15	38
Montreal Style Corned Beef, 154 g	280	7	34
Philly Style Steak no Cheese, 133 g	260	5	34
Philly Style Steak with Cheese, 145 g	300	8	36
Pizza Supremo, 110 g	270	10	34

● MOST HEALTHY   • LEAST HEALTHY

MR. SUB (cont.)

	Cal	Fat	Cbs
Roast Beef, 154 g	280	8	35
Santa Fe Spicy Chicken, 203 g	370	13	46
Seafood with Crab, 174 g	300	10	43
Smoked Turkey Breast, 160 g	230	4	36
• Veggie, 118 g	180	2	34
White Albacore Tuna, 174 g	280	8	37
Panini Grilled Subs			
Classic Reuben, 182 g	290	7	35
• Grilled Buffalo Chicken, 181 g	260	5	38
Tuna Melt, 156 g	340	10	34
• Ultimate Cheddar Club/Cheese, 226 g	440	18	38
Ultimate Club no Cheddar, 198 g	320	9	38
Plain Buns and Tortillas			
Cheese Tortilla, 65 g	190	5	31
• Regular Tortilla, 65 g	200	5	32
Sm Greek Ssn Red Salt Sub Bun, 75 g	200	4	35
Sm Mozza-Chdr Red Salt Sub Bun, 77 g	200	4	33
• Small Multigrain Red Salt Sub Bun, 70 g	170	2	32
Small White Red Salt Sub Bun, 70 g	170	2	32
Sm Whole Wheat Red Salt Sub Bun, 70 g	170	2	32
Sun Dried Tortilla, 65 g	190	5	32
Whole Wheat Tortilla, 65 g	180	5	30
Salads			
Albacore Tuna, 240 g	140	6	8
Classic Caesar, 122 g	70	5	2
• Garden, 184 g	35	1	6
• Grilled Chicken Caesar, 185 g	160	7	6
Maple Baked Ham, 225 g	85	2	10
Mediterranean Greek, 227 g	70	3	8
Seafood with Crab, 240 g	150	8	15
Smoked Turkey Breast, 226 g	80	2	8
Sauces			
• Louisiana Sauce, 10 g	5	0	1
Meatball Sauce, 30 g	15	0	4
• Mr Sub Secret Sauce, 10 g	40	5	0
Pizza Sauce, 10 g	5	0	1
Soup			
Chicken Noodle, 250 g	110	3	17
Chicken with Rice, 250 g	90	2	15
Chilli With Beef, 250 g	198	1	34
Cream of Broccoli, 250 g	170	10	16
Cream of Mushroom, 250 g	170	10	16
Cream of Potato & Leek, 250 g	190	9	23
Cream of Tomato, 250 g	150	6	20
Creamy Tomato & Rst Red Pepper, 250 g	110	3	19
• Garden Vegetable, 250 g	60	0	13

• MOST HEALTHY   • LEAST HEALTHY

▶ MR. SUB (cont.)	Cal	Fat	Cbs
• Hearty Chilli with Beef, 250 g	231	2	36
Italian Wedding, 250 g	140	4	24
Mediterranean Chicken, 250 g	110	4	15
Minestrone, 250 g	80	0	17
Paste Fagioli, 250 g	150	2	28
Vegetable Beef & Barley, 250 g	90	1	18
Toppings (in grams)			
Bacon (2 strips), 10 g	50	4	0
Banana Peppers, 10 g	2	0	0
• Croutons (14 g), 14 g	60	2	10
Cucumbers (3 slices), 10 g	2	0	0
• Dill Pickles (3 slices), 10 g	1	0	0
Green Olives, 10 g	10	1	1
Green Pepper, 10 g	2	0	1
Iceberg Lettuce, 28 g	4	0	3
Jalapeño Peppers, 10 g	2	0	0
Red Onions, 10 g	4	0	1
Sliced Mushrooms, 10 g	3	0	1
Tomatoes (3 wheels), 30 g	5	0	4
Wraps			
Albacore Tuna, 248 g	460	16	52
Louisiana Chicken, 190 g	430	15	48
Roast Beef, 218 g	440	14	49
• Seafood with Crab, 218 g	470	19	61
Smoked Turkey Breast, 220 g	360	9	51
• Veggie, 164 g	310	8	49

▶ MRS. FIELDS			
Bite-Size Nibbler® Cookies			
Cinnamon Sugar, 37 g	170	8	22
• Debra's Special Nibbler, 38 g	170	7	23
• Peanut Butter, 38 g	180	10	20
Semi-Sweet Chocolate, 38 g	170	8	24
Triple Chocolate, 38 g	170	9	23
White Chunk Macadamia, 38 g	180	9	23
Brownies			
Butterscotch Blondie, 76 g	350	14	52
Double Fudge, 76 g	360	20	45
Pecan Fudge, 76 g	360	20	46
• Special Walnut Fudge & Blondie, 76 g	330	16	43
Toffee Fudge, 76 g	360	19	47
• Walnut Fudge, 76 g	360	20	45
Mrs. Fields® Cakes			
Chocolate Chip, 83 g	350	17	45
Mrs. Fields® Cookies			
• Butter, 44 g	200	8	29

• MOST HEALTHY   • LEAST HEALTHY

MRS. FIELDS (cont.)

	Cal	Fat	Cbs
• Cut Out, 90 g	400	19	56
Debra's Special, 44 g	200	9	28
Peanut Butter, 44 g	210	12	24
Semi-Sweet Choco w/ Walnuts, 44 g	220	11	29
Semi-Sweet Chocolate, 44 g	210	10	29
Triple Chocolate, 44 g	210	11	28
White Chunk Macadamia, 44 g	230	12	27

Mrs. Fields® Muffins

	Cal	Fat	Cbs
• Blueberry, 21 g	70	3	10
• Chocolate Chip, 21 g	80	4	11
Mandarin Orange, 21 g	80	3	9
Raspberry, 21 g	70	3	10

NOAH'S BAGELS

Bagel Dogs

	Cal	Fat	Cbs
• Asiago Bagel Dog, 201 g	510	21	59
Everything Bagel Dog, 201 g	510	20	59
• Original Bagel Dog, 197 g	490	20	59

Bagels

	Cal	Fat	Cbs
Asiago Cheese Topped Bagel, 120 g	330	6	57
Blueberry Bagel, 106 g	270	1	59
Cheddar Bagel Shtick - Kosher, 120 g	330	6	57
Chocolate Chip Bagel, 106 g	290	4	60
Chopped Garlic Bagel, 110 g	290	3	58
Cinnamon Raisin Bagel, 106 g	270	1	58
Cinnamon Sugar Bagel, 115 g	310	3	64
Cracked Pepper Bagel, 106 g	280	4	55
• Cranberry Orange Bagel, 99 g	250	1	54
Egg Bagel, 106 g	290	3	57
Everything Bagel, 110 g	280	2	57
Good Grains, 110 g	280	2	58
Onion Bagel, 106 g	270	2	57
Plain Bagel, 106 g	270	1	57
• w/ Peanut Butter & Jelly, 177 g	550	15	90
Poppyseed Bagel, 110 g	290	3	57
Power Bagel, 113 g	310	5	61
Pumpernickel Bagel, 106 g	260	2	57
Sesame Seed Bagel, 110 g	290	3	57
Sourdough Bagel, 106 g	280	4	55
Sun-Dried Tomato Bagel, 106 g	270	2	57
Whole Wheat Bagel, 106 g	260	1	57
w/Sesame Seeds & Sunflower Seeds, 125 g	370	11	61

Breads

	Cal	Fat	Cbs
• Bialy, Traditional - Kosher, 149 g	380	4	77
Braided Challah, 57 g	160	3	29
Challah Roll, 84 g	230	4	44

• MOST HEALTHY   • LEAST HEALTHY

NOAH'S BAGELS (cont.)	Cal	Fat	Cbs
Ciabatta Bread, 113 g	290	3	60
Corn Meal Rye Bread, 57 g	150	2	31
Harvest Grain Bread, 65 g	180	2	36
Marble Rye Bread, 49 g	160	1	30
• Potato Bread, 49 g	140	2	28
Breakfast Sandwiches / Wraps			
Egg Mit Cheese & Tomato, 284 g	530	21	61
Egg Mit Lox & Chives, 251 g	490	17	59
Egg Mit Plain, 223 g	450	14	59
Egg Mit Spinach Mshr & Swiss, 277 g	530	20	61
Egg Mit Turkey Sausage, 282 g	590	24	61
Egg Mit w/Cheese, 242 g	520	20	60
Egg Mit, Artichoke & Tomato, 341 g	620	28	67
Egg Mit, Bacon & Cheddar, 262 g	620	28	61
Egg Spinach, Bacon Panini, 334 g	790	43	65
Egg White Florentine Wedge w/Tkey Ssge, 279 g	390	17	34
Egg White on Plain Bagel - no Chz, 207 g	310	1	57
• Egg Whites - no Cheese, 106 g	50	0	1
• Egg Whites - w/ Cheese, 120 g	90	3	2
Egg Whites Snd w/Tkey Ssge, 265 g	390	5	59
Egg, Vegetarian Omelette Panini, 391 g	670	31	66
Lox & Bagel, 319 g	520	21	65
Santa Fe Breakfast Wrap, 411 g	750	34	77
• Veggie Breakfast Wrap, 442 g	810	41	77
Cream Cheese			
Whipped Blueberry Reduced Fat, 20 g	70	5	6
Whipped Garden Veg Reduced Fat, 20 g	60	5	3
Whipped Garlic Herb Reduced Fat, 20 g	60	5	3
Whipped Honey Almond Red Fat, 20 g	70	5	6
Whipped Jalapeño Salsa Red Fat, 20 g	60	5	3
Whipped Onion and Chive, 20 g	70	6	3
• Whipped Plain, 20 g	70	7	1
Whipped Plain Reduced Fat, 20 g	60	5	2
Whipped Smoked Salmon, 20 g	60	6	2
Whipped Strawberry Reduced Fat, 20 g	70	5	5
• Whpd Sundried Tomato & Basil RedFat, 20 g	60	5	2
Deli Melts			
Hummus Melt, 290 g	570	19	76
Pastrami Melt, 271 g	530	17	61
Roast Beef Melt, 271 g	530	17	60
• Tuna Melt, 328 g	630	31	62
• Turkey Melt, 271 g	490	15	59
Veggie Melt, 349 g	590	25	70
Deli Sandwich			
Ancho Chkn Bacon Signature Snd, 365 g	680	29	67

• MOST HEALTHY   • LEAST HEALTHY

NOAH'S BAGELS (cont.)

	Cal	Fat	Cbs
Blackened Chicken Club, 294 g	630	33	53
California Chicken Sandwich, 282 g	460	16	53
Deli Chicken Salad, 289 g	490	20	49
Deli Cornbeef, 396 g	740	34	61
Deli Roast Beef, 396 g	730	34	60
Deli Tuna Salad, 368 g	510	20	63
Deli Turkey, 412 g	710	30	66
Deli Turkey Pesto Club, 309 g	670	40	46
Deli Whitefish, 346 g	850	55	68
Deli, Egg Salad - Kosher, 327 g	650	6	68
Deli, Pastrami, 396 g	750	34	62
• Mediterranean Tkey Snd on Whole Wheat, 303 g	380	12	43
• Rachel Sandwich, 394 g	1030	68	53
• Reuben Sandwich, 394 g	770	41	47
Veg Out Sandwich, 287 g	490	14	75
Gourmet Bagels			
Cinnamon Knot Bagel - Kosher, 134 g	380	2	84
• Dutch Apple Bagel, 141 g	340	3	72
Jalapeño Cheddar Bagel - Kosher, 139 g	340	7	58
Red Pepper Pesto Bagel - Kosher, 205 g	410	14	62
Six-cheese Bagel, 127 g	340	6	57
Spinach Florentine Bagel, 139 g	350	8	58
• Three Cheese Bagel - Kosher, 170 g	490	18	58
Tuscan Pesto Bagel, 170 g	430	16	59
Other Hot Beverages (Regular)			
Hot Choco, Low Fat, 12 fl.oz.	270	8	37
• Hot Choco, Nonfat, 12 fl.oz.	220	2	37
• Hot Choco, Whole, 12 fl.oz.	290	11	35
Panini Sandwiches			
Albacore Tuna Panini, 386 g	690	36	62
Italian Chicken Panini, 354 g	810	40	67
• Kosher Vegetarian on Plain Bagel, 394 g	860	41	79
Mediterranean Panini, 301 g	550	18	77
• Tomato Mozzarella Panini, 223 g	440	16	59
Turkey Club Panini, 376 g	790	41	66
Pizza Bagels			
• Artichoke & Spinach, 340 g	670	32	70
Artichoke, Tom & Red Onion - Kosher, 316 g	550	20	67
• Cheese - Kosher, 177 g	420	11	60
Cheesy Garlic & Herb, 177 g	500	19	62
Mushroom - Kosher, 241 g	540	21	62
Pepperoni, 194 g	500	19	60
Spinach & Mushroom - Kosher, 269 g	580	25	63
Tomato & Rosemary - Kosher, 247 g	540	20	63
Salad Dressings			
Harvest Chicken Salad Dressing, 30 g	90	8	3

NOAH'S BAGELS (cont.)

	Cal	Fat	Cbs
Raspberry Vinaigrette Dressing, 32 g	160	14	8

Salads

	Cal	Fat	Cbs
Caesar Salad, 298 g	600	53	23
• Caesar Side Salad, 128 g	280	27	7
Chicken Caesar Salad, 397 g	720	54	23
City Salad, 326 g	830	68	39
• City Salad with Chicken, 425 g	950	71	40
Mediterranean Salad w/ Grilled Chkn, 376 g	390	27	22
Southwestern Chicken Salad, 430 g	710	41	54

Sandwich Fillings

	Cal	Fat	Cbs
American Cheese, 19 g	70	6	1
Cheddar Cheese, 19 g	80	6	0
Chicken Breast, 113 g	140	5	1
• Chicken Salad, 142 g	260	17	3
Cold Smoked Salmon, 57 g	80	5	0
Corned Beef, 85 g	110	4	1
Gorgonzola Cheese, 28 g	100	9	0
Ham, 85 g	90	3	0
Pastrami, 85 g	110	4	2
Pepper Jack Cheese, 19 g	70	5	0
Provolone Cheese, 19 g	70	5	0
Roast Beef, 85 g	100	4	1
Swiss Cheese, 19 g	70	6	0
• Thick Cut Bacon, 14 g	60	5	1
Tuna Salad, 142 g	220	18	3
Turkey Breast, 85 g	80	2	0
Turkey Sausage, 40 g	70	4	1

Sides & Salad Extras

	Cal	Fat	Cbs
Ancho Salsa, 71 g	40	2	6
Bagel Croutons, 28 g	100	4	15
Candied Walnuts, 43 g	260	22	9
• Egg Salad, 142 g	330	29	3
Fresh Fruit Cup, 312 g	140	0	36
Fruit and Yogurt Parfait, 340 g	230	2	42
Homestyle Cole Slaw, 85 g	190	17	8
Kettle Classic Natural Potato Chips, 49 g	260	16	26
• Pickle - Kosher, 50 g	5	0	1
Redskin Potato Salad, 85 g	160	12	13
Tim's Chips - Kosher, 28 g	140	9	15
Tuna Salad, 142 g	280	20	3

Soups (Cup)

	Cal	Fat	Cbs
Broccoli Cheese, 248 g	290	20	16
• Chicken Noodle, 248 g	110	4	13
Italian Wedding, 247 g	160	6	15
• Tortilla Soup, 248 g	300	19	19
Turkey Chili, 248 g	220	7	24

● MOST HEALTHY   • LEAST HEALTHY

NOAH'S BAGELS (cont.)

	Cal	Fat	Cbs
Specialty Coffee (Regular)			
• Americano, 8 fl.oz.	0	0	0
Cafe Latte Nonfat, 12 fl.oz.	110	0	17
Café Latte, Low Fat, 12 fl.oz.	160	7	17
Cafe Latte, Whole, 12 fl.oz.	200	10	16
Cappuccino Low Fat, 12 fl.oz.	120	5	13
Cappuccino Nonfat, 12 fl.oz.	90	0	13
Cappuccino, Whole, 12 fl.oz.	150	8	13
Espresso, 2 fl.oz.	0	0	0
Macchiato, Low Fat, 12 fl.oz.	270	5	49
Macchiato, Nonfat, 12 fl.oz.	230	0	49
• Macchiato, Whole, 12 fl.oz.	290	8	47
Mocha, Low Fat, 12 fl.oz.	230	5	39
Mocha, Nonfat, 12 fl.oz.	190	0	39
Mocha, Whole, 12 fl.oz.	270	9	38
Spreads			
Butter, 14 g	110	11	0
Butter Spread, 28 g	170	18	0
• Garlic Mayo, 43 g	270	27	8
Grape Jam, 43 g	110	0	28
• Honey, 28 g	90	0	23
Hummus, 57 g	90	4	11
Peanut Butter, Crunchy, 32 g	210	16	6
Red Pepper Pesto Spread, 43 g	220	24	1
Strawberry Jam, 43 g	110	0	28
Sweets			
Apple Cinnamon Coffee Cake, 188 g	700	28	108
• Babka - Chocolate - Kosher, 56 g	100	4	16
Babka - Cinnamon - Kosher, 56 g	100	4	16
Blueberry Coffee Cake, 195 g	710	29	109
Blueberry Muffin, 142 g	480	22	65
• Chocolate Chip Coffee Cake, 174 g	760	34	110
Chocolate Chip Cookie, 78 g	360	18	48
Chocolate Mudslide Cookie, 78 g	320	17	46
Cinnamon Twists, 108 g	370	21	41
Cinnamon Walnut Strudel, 153 g	630	42	56
Cranberry Orange Muffin, 129 g	460	22	63
Marshmallow Crispy Treat, 111 g	410	7	86
Mini Chocolate Chip Cookie, 39 g	180	9	24
Mini Chocolate Mudslide Cookie, 39 g	160	8	23
Mini Iced Sugar Cookie, 53 g	230	7	39
Mini Oatmeal Raisin Cookie, 39 g	160	5	27
Oatmeal Raisin Cookie, 78 g	320	11	54
Peanut Butter Power Cookie, 61 g	260	12	35
Rugelach - Chocolate - Kosher, 28 g	110	5	18
Rugelach - Cinnamon - Kosher, 28 g	110	5	16

• MOST HEALTHY   • LEAST HEALTHY

NOAH'S BAGELS (cont.)	Cal	Fat	Cbs
Snickerdoodle Cookie, 78 g	400	18	56
Strawberry White Choco Muffin, 156 g	550	25	78
Sugar Cookie w/ Icing, 106 g	480	15	76

Wraps

	Cal	Fat	Cbs
Albacore Tuna Wrap, 350 g	540	26	57
Ancho Chicken Caesar Wrap, 357 g	770	42	61
• Ancho Chkn Wedge w/rst onion & chili rajas, 260 g	350	14	40
Balsamic Chicken Wrap, 385 g	570	21	61
• Chicken Caesar Wrap, 357 g	790	46	62
Southwestern Turkey Wrap, 383 g	750	37	73
Veggie Wrap, 279 g	460	17	64

NOODLES & COMPANY

American

	Cal	Fat	Cbs
Buttered Noodles	620	16	84
Caesar Salad	320	28	11
• Chicken Noodle Soup	300	4	44
Mushroom Stroganoff	780	31	100
Spaghetti	670	18	101
• Spaghetti & Meatballs	900	35	104
Wisconsin Mac & Cheese	900	31	119

Asian

	Cal	Fat	Cbs
Bangkok Curry	490	13	85
• Chinese Chop Salad	310	15	40
• Indonesian Peanut Saute	950	23	165
Japanese Pan Noodles	690	9	133
Pad Thai	700	20	117
Thai Curry Soup	480	19	70

Extras & Desserts

	Cal	Fat	Cbs
Chocolate Chunk Cookie	360	8	65
Ciabatta Roll	160	2	31
Cucumber Tomato Salad	80	0	18
Flat Bread	210	4	37
Potstickers	340	9	49
• Rice Krispy Treat	530	19	90
Snoodledoodle Cookie	350	7	65
Tossed Green Salad	60	6	3
• Tossed Green Salad w/Fat Free Asian	30	0	7

Mediterranean

	Cal	Fat	Cbs
Pasta Fresca	780	22	111
Penne Rosa	810	26	119
• Pesto Cavatappi	910	30	124
• The Med Salad	310	13	39
Tomato Bisque	420	23	45
Whole Grain Tuscan Linguine	770	26	108

● MOST HEALTHY   • LEAST HEALTHY

NOODLES & COMPANY (cont.)

	Cal	Fat	Cbs
Proteins			
Braised Beef	190	10	0
Chicken Breast	130	3	0
• Meatballs	230	17	3
Organic Tofu	180	11	4
Parmesan-Crusted Chicken Breast	190	8	1
Sautéed Beef	210	12	1
• Sautéed Shrimp	35	0	0

NOTHING BUT NOODLES

	Cal	Fat	Cbs
Add-Ons			
• Beef, 2 bowl	110	4	0
Chicken, 2 bowl	100	3	0
• Shrimp, 2 bowl	53	1	1
Tofu, 2 bowl	60	4	1
Baked Dish			
• Eggplant Parmesan, 2 bowl	725	37	79
• Lobster Ravioli, 2 bowl	637	81	21
Stuffed Shells, 2 bowl	701	57	28
Desserts			
Almonds drzl w/ non- alc Amaretto Liqueur, 1 bowl	113	3	20
Cannoli, 1 bowl	374	17	44
Chocolate Syrup, 1 bowl	100	0	23
Cotton Candy, 1 bowl	65	0	17
Key Lime Pie, 1 bowl	590	33	67
• New York Cheesecake, 1 bowl	770	53	59
• Strawberry Puree, 1 bowl	65	0	8
Triple Chocolate Cake, 1 bowl	710	33	106
Dressings			
• Oriental Salad Dressing, 2 bowl	135	10	12
Poppy Seed, 2 bowl	70	6	5
• Rst Garlic Balsamic Vinaigrette, 2 bowl	30	3	2
Kids			
Alfredo, 1 bowl	719	55	39
• Buttery Noodles, 1 bowl	723	49	51
Macaroni & Cheese, 1 bowl	454	26	38
• Spaghetti, 1 bowl	290	6	47
Noodle Bowls - American			
• Beef Stroganoff, 2 bowl	508	31	33
Buttery Noodles, 2 bowl	651	44	46
Santa Fe Pasta, 2 bowl	705	54	40
• Southwest Chipotle, 2 bowl	713	58	41
Spicy Cajun Pasta, 2 bowl	660	50	44
Noodle Bowls - Asian			
• Pad Thai Noodles, 2 bowl	602	10	118
• Sesame Lo Mein, 2 bowl	411	11	64

• MOST HEALTHY • LEAST HEALTHY

NOTHING BUT NOODLES (cont.)	Cal	Fat	Cbs
Spicy Japanese Noodles, 2 bowl	419	8	74
Thai Peanut, 2 bowl	568	20	89
Noodle Bowls - Italian			
Basil Pesto, 2 bowl	574	42	36
Cappelini Primavera, 2 bowl	500	28	56
• Fettuccini Alfredo, 2 bowl	723	56	36
Margherita Pasta, 2 bowl	474	31	36
Marinara Pasta, 2 bowl	487	11	77
• Three-Cheese Macaroni, 2 bowl	446	21	45
Pasta-Less Bowls			
Cheesy Chicken & Vegetables, 2 bowl	318	21	6
• Chicken Pomodoro, 2 bowl	452	34	7
Primavera Chkn & Veg Wrap, 2 bowl	318	15	26
• Shrimp Pesto Florentine, 2 bowl	308	25	5
Thai Curry Beef & Vegetables, 2 bowl	443	30	16
Rice Dishes			
General Tso's Chicken, 2 bowl	760	44	69
• Kung Pao Chicken, 2 bowl	935	51	89
• Thai Peanut Stir Fry, 2 bowl	595	27	59
Salads			
BBQ Chicken Salad, 2 bowl	205	15	11
Caesar Salad, 2 bowl	247	19	14
Chopped Salad, 2 bowl	229	15	10
Cranberry Spinach Salad, 2 bowl	154	10	18
Garden Fresh Salad, 2 bowl	110	5	12
• Greek Salad, 2 bowl	409	31	26
Hunk of Lettuce, 2 bowl	229	21	7
Mandarin Orange Salad, 2 bowl	205	14	13
Oriental Salad, 2 bowl	187	11	20
Pear & Balsamic Spinach Salad, 2 bowl	395	28	38
Spicy Cucumber & Chicken Salad, 2 bowl	284	15	10
Steak Salad, 2 bowl	135	19	7
Sun-Dried Tomato, 2 bowl	271	12	32
Soups			
Tomato Bisque, 2 bowl	253	23	9
Starters			
Cucumber Side Salad, 1 bowl	193	16	13
• Fresh Mozzarella, 1 bowl	767	27	134
• Garlic Breadsticks, 1 bowl	106	4	0
Mozzarella Cheese Bread, 1 bowl	633	17	86
Potstickers, 2 bowl	479	33	39
Thai Lettuce Wraps, 2 bowl	361	23	15

O'CHARLEY'S			
À La Carte			
Asparagus, 1 serv	80	6	4

• MOST HEALTHY • LEAST HEALTHY

O'CHARLEY'S (cont.)

	Cal	Fat	Cbs
Bacon 1 slice, 1 serv	45	4	0
• Bacon Chips for Baked Potato, 1 tsp.	10	0	0
Beer Battered Onion Rings, 1 serv	380	26	32
Broccoli, 1 serv	140	10	11
Broccoli Cheese Casserole, 1 serv	270	16	20
French Fries, 1 serv	390	24	40
Pice Pilaf, 1 serv	190	5	30
• Sweet Potato Fries 5 oz., 1 serv	470	31	46

Appetizers

	Cal	Fat	Cbs
Authentic Spinach & Artichoke Dip, 1 serv	780	44	86
Barbacoa Quesadilla, 1 serv	1170	73	64
Barbacoa Shredded Beef Tacos, 1 serv	850	39	76
Chicken Tenders, 1 serv	800	57	29
Chkn Tenders and Naked Twisted Chips w/o Sauces, 1 serv	1150	60	110
Chkn Tenders w/ Buffalo Sauce, 1 serv	810	53	31
Chkn Tenders w/ Chipotle BBQ Sauce Appetizer, 1 serv	1040	37	119
Chkn Tenders w/ Honey Mustard w/o Side, 5 Tenders	1090	61	82
Chips and Salsa, 1 serv	520	18	82
Loaded Baked Potato, 1 serv	480	29	54
Onion Rings, 1 serv	380	26	32
Over-Loaded Potato Skins, 1 serv	1260	98	43
• Plain Potato, 1 serv	240	5	50
Southern Fried Chkn Tacos, 1 serv	1150	52	120
Southwestern Chz Dip & Chips, 1 serv	820	45	84
Southwestern Chz Dip & Chips, 1 serv	820	45	84
Southwestern Chkn Quesadilla, 1 serv	1060	60	64
Southwestern Twisted Chips, 1 serv	1280	89	111
Spicy Jack Cheese Wedges, Seven each	880	60	55
Sweet Potato Fries 4.5 oz., 1 serv	470	31	46
• Top Shelf Combo Appetizer, 1 serv	1880	130	105

Brunch

	Cal	Fat	Cbs
Brunch Grillers w/o fries, 1 serv	1160	69	85
Brunch Jelly, 1 serv	50	0	13
Brunch Quesadilla, 1 serv	1220	82	65
Brunch Quesadilla w/bacon, 1 serv	1370	95	65
Brunch Toast with Jelly, 1 serv	260	10	38
Build Your Own Waffle Base, 1 serv	460	20	57
Build Your Own Waffle, Side of Choco Chips Semi Sweet, 1 serv	210	12	27
Build Your Own Waffle, Side of Chopped Pecans, 1 serv	210	21	4
• Build Your Own Waffle, Side of Fresh Strawberries, 1 serv	10	0	3
Build Your Own Waffle, Side of Reeses Peanut Butter Cups, 1 serv	160	10	18
Cajun Chicken Omelette, 1 serv	870	63	13
Cajun Shrimp and Grits, 1 serv	920	55	62
Eggs (2) & Bacon (3), 1 serv	420	36	2
Eggs (2) & Sausage (2), 1 serv	500	42	2
Eggs two w/o sides, 1 serv	290	24	2

• MOST HEALTHY   • LEAST HEALTHY

▶ O'CHARLEY'S (cont.)

	Cal	Fat	Cbs
Ham & Cheese Omelette, 1 serv	1210	76	76
• O'Charley's Signature Overloaded Brunch Platter, 1 serv	1690	103	116
Pancakes (3) with Syrup, 1 serv	520	18	84
Prime Rib Omelet w/o sides, 1 serv	1420	91	78
Sausage, One Pattie	110	9	0
Seasoned Brunch Potatoes, 1 serv	430	27	40
Smashed Potatoes, 1 serv	370	12	47
Spinach Mshr Omelet w/o sides, 1 serv	1110	67	80
Steak & Eggs, 1 serv	1260	78	57
Toast, 1 serv	220	9	28
Ultimate Open-Faced Omelette, 1 serv	1230	75	85

Butcher's Cut Premium Steaks

	Cal	Fat	Cbs
Filet Mignon, 1 serv	450	28	0
Grilled Top Sirloin 7 oz., 1 serv	430	28	1
Louisiana Sirloin, 1 serv	680	40	3
• O'Charley's Butchers Cut Premium USDA Choice Steak 5 oz, 1 serv	260	14	0
Prime Time Prime Rib 10 oz., 1 serv	670	43	3
• Steak Tips Monterey, 1 serv	960	61	48
Your Favorite Ribeye Steak, 1 serv	810	55	0

Chicken & Ribs

	Cal	Fat	Cbs
Bistro Chicken Sandwich, 1 serv	770	44	51
Boneless Buffalo O'Tenders, 1 serv	880	66	27
• Chicken Harvest Pot Pie, 1 serv	1220	57	116
Chicken Minis, 1 serv	800	35	86
Chicken Tenders, 1 serv	850	57	34
• Chicken Tortilla Soup, Cup, One cup	150	9	12
Chipotle BBQ Ribs Half, One half rack	780	47	48
Chipotle Chicken O Tenders, 1 serv	720	31	64
Grilled Baja Chicken, 1 serv	1010	36	103
Grilled Chicken Breast, 1 serv	170	5	2
Grilled Chicken Dinner, 1 serv	500	17	31
Grilled Chicken Sandwich, 1 serv	610	27	52
Grilled Chicken Tacos, 1 serv	870	40	73
Key West Citrus Chicken, 1 serv	840	22	94
Lemon Artichoke Chicken, 1 serv	920	55	55
O'Charley's Baby Back Ribs Half Rack, One half rack	740	48	38
Outrageous Chkn & Spinach Lasagna, 1 serv	1210	73	72
Teriyaki Sesame Chicken, 1 serv	1030	25	151

Desserts

	Cal	Fat	Cbs
• Cinnamon Sugar Donuts, One serving	1130	54	139
• Key Lime Pie, One slice	610	23	91
Ooey Gooey Caramel Pie, One slice	730	28	106
Ultimate Chocolate Choco Cake, One slice	1080	59	151

Dressing

	Cal	Fat	Cbs
Cranberry Orange Vinaigrette 2 oz., 1 serv	130	10	15
Greek Feta Vinaigrette 2 oz., 1 serv	620	64	7

• MOST HEALTHY • LEAST HEALTHY

O'CHARLEY'S (cont.)

	Cal	Fat	Cbs
• Pico de Gallo, 1/4 Cup	10	0	2
• Three Cheese Shrimp Dip, One serving	870	49	86

Fresh Burgers

	Cal	Fat	Cbs
Better Cheddar Bacon Burger, 1 serv	990	57	55
Better with Bacon Patty Melt, 1 serv	1110	64	63
Classic Burger, 1 serv	740	37	54
Classic Burger with Cheddar, 1 serv	900	50	55
Firecracker Burger Wrap, 1 serv	1150	71	73
Grilled Turkey Burger, 1 serv	890	54	54
• Hamburger, 1 serv	710	36	50
Mushroom Swiss Bacon Burger, 1 serv	1130	77	53
• O'Charley's Grillers, 1 serv	1260	64	112
Philly Burger, 1 serv	1230	77	71
Three Cheese Bacon Burger, 1 serv	930	54	51
Wild West Burger, 1 serv	1210	79	67

Hearty Favorites

	Cal	Fat	Cbs
Club Sandwich, One serving	990	58	82
1/2 White Cheddar Grilled Chz w/ Bacon & Tomato	500	31	30

Kid's Menu

	Cal	Fat	Cbs
Jr. Brunch Eggs Only, One serving	200	19	1
Jr. Brunch Fries, One serving	330	21	31
Jr. Brunch Plate, One serving	800	50	70
Jr. Cheeseburger, One serving	650	33	57
Jr. Chicken Tenders, One serving	210	12	8
Jr. Corn Dogs, One serving	500	38	32
Jr. French Fries, One serving	310	19	31
Jr. French Toast, One serving	1040	50	117
Jr. Fruit Cup Peaches, One serving	70	0	18
Jr. Fruit Cup Pears, One serving	70	N/A	18
• Jr. Fruit Cup Pineapple, One serving	60	N/A	16
Jr. Grilled Chicken, One serving	240	11	0
Jr. Grilled Steak, One serving	260	14	0
Jr. Hamburger, One serving	540	24	57
Jr. Macaroni and Cheese, One serving	360	23	27
Jr. Pancakes, One serving	670	18	121
Jr. Pasta, One serving	260	5	46
Jr. Pizza, One serving	440	21	45
Jr. Shrimp, One serving	310	18	25
• Jr. Waffle, One serving	1070	48	146

Pasta

	Cal	Fat	Cbs
12-Spice Chicken Pasta, One serving	1390	77	103
• Baked Penne Italiano, One serving	1700	99	142
Baked Shrimp Scampi Pasta, One serving	1090	63	95
Bayou Shrimp Pasta, One serving	1640	87	155
• Cajun Chicken Pasta, One serving	1080	47	94

▶ O'CHARLEY'S (cont.)

	Cal	Fat	Cbs
Chicken Parmesan Pasta, One serving	1500	77	138
Jambalaya Pasta, One serving	1340	77	108
Meatballs and Spaghetti, One serving	1400	73	127
Prime Rib Pasta, One serving	1530	101	90
Sandwiches			
Bacon & Chz Trio Chkn Snd, One serv	860	46	51
• Buffalo Kickin Sandwich, One serv	1180	74	79
Cheeseburger w/Cheddar, One serv	860	48	51
Chzburger w/Monterey Jack, One serv	850	47	51
Cheeseburger w/Swiss, One serv	850	46	51
Classic Cuban Sandwich, One serv	910	58	51
• Half-Club Sandwich, One serv	510	30	42
Prime Rib Philly Sandwich, One serv	980	56	82
Roast Beef Ciabatta Snd, One serv	880	47	74
Savory Signatures			
• Baked Potato (loaded), One serv	590	40	52
Baked Potato (plain), One serv	240	5	50
Half White Cheddar Grilled Chz, One serv	410	23	29
• Over-Loaded Potato Soup, Cup, One serv	160	9	16
Seafood			
• Bayou Salmon, One serv	1570	97	84
Caribbean Combo, One serv	810	39	62
Catfish Lunch, One serv	1170	99	37
Catfish Platter, One serv	1430	121	46
Cedar Planked Salmon, One serv	530	32	2
• Cedar Planked Tilapia, One serv	280	11	2
Chipotle BBQ Salmon 6 oz., One serv	430	22	17
Fresh Atlantic Grilled Salmon, 6 oz.	370	22	2
w/Chipotle-BBQ Sauce, 9 oz.	610	33	17
Fried Shrimp Dinner, One serv	740	47	35
Grilled Shrimp Dinner, One serv	290	7	32
Hand Battered Fish n' Chips, One serv	1140	85	43
Teriyaki Sesame Tilapia, One serv	850	24	102
Side Items			
• Broccoli, One serving	140	10	10
Broccoli Cheese Casserole, One serving	230	14	17
• Smashed Potatoes, One serving	370	12	47
Signature Salads			
Apple Crunch Salad, One serv	920	56	79
• Black & Bleu Caesar Salad, One serv	1050	79	22
Cajun Chicken Salad, One serv	740	49	17
California Chkn Salad w/o Dressing, One serv	700	37	48
California Shrimp Salad w/o Dressing, One serv	700	42	53
Classic Caesar Salad, One serv	450	39	16
w/ Grilled Chicken, One serv	680	50	16
w/ Grilled Salmon, One serv	880	69	16

• MOST HEALTHY   • LEAST HEALTHY

O'CHARLEY'S (cont.)

	Cal	Fat	Cbs
House Salad, One serv	230	11	19
• House Salad w/o Dressing, One serv	120	6	12
Original Southern Fried Chkn Salad w/o Dressing, One serv	900	42	74
Pecan Chkn Tender Salad w/o Dressing, One serv	1020	60	81
Tortilla Chkn Salad w/o Dressing, One serv	610	27	41

Soup of the Day

	Cal	Fat	Cbs
• Broccoli & Three Cheese Soup, One cup	200	15	9
Chicken Harvest Soup, One Cup	160	8	12
Chicken Tortilla Soup, One cup	150	9	12
Chili, Cup, One Cup	150	5	19
Clam Chowder, One cup	200	12	14
Pepper Steak Soup, Cup	130	8	8
Roasted Tomato Basil Soup, One cup	130	9	10
• Southwestern Steak Soup, One cup	100	5	10
Wild Mushroom Cream Soup, One Cup	150	14	7

OLD SPAGHETTI FACTORY

Appetizers

	Cal	Fat	Cbs
Broccoli-small, 213 g	300	28	10
Olive Tapenade, 51 g	190	12	19
• Shrimp Spinach and Artichoke Dip, 67 g	150	10	10
• Sicilian Garlic Cheese Bread, 114 g	328	19	28
Toasted Beef Ravioli, 110 g	200	5	30
Toasted Cheese Ravioli, 109 g	210	6	30

Classics

	Cal	Fat	Cbs
Italian Sausage w/ Meat Sauce, 538 g	940	36	107
MF Clam/Meat, 425 g	640	12	105
MF Clam/Mizithra Chz & Brown Butter, 403 g	850	36	101
MF Marinara/Clam, 425 g	610	10	106
MF Marinara/Meat, 425 g	590	7	107
MF Marinara/Mizithra Chz & Brown Butter, 403 g	800	35	103
MF Marinara/Mushroom, 425 g	580	8	107
MF Meat/Mizithra Chz & Brown Butter, 403 g	820	34	102
MF Mushroom/Clam, 425 g	630	13	105
MF Mushroom/Meat, 425 g	610	10	105
MF Mshrm/Mizithra Chz & Brown Butter, 446 g	850	37	105
Pot Pourri, 460 g	780	26	106
Spaghetti and Sicilian Meatballs, 595 g	960	31	114
Spaghetti w/ Clam Sauce, 425 g	660	14	104
• Spaghetti w/ Marinara Sauce, 425 g	560	5	108
Spaghetti w/ Meat Sauce, 425 g	610	9	105
• Spag. w/ Mizithra Chz & Brown Butter, 382 g	1040	59	99
Spag. w/ Sauteed Mushroom Sc, 510 g	670	16	111

Desserts

	Cal	Fat	Cbs
• Chocolate Truffle Mousse Cake, 250 g	850	41	118
• Italian Cream Sodas, 213 g	140	4	25

● MOST HEALTHY   • LEAST HEALTHY

OLD SPAGHETTI FACTORY (cont.)

	Cal	Fat	Cbs
Masterpiece Shake, 241 g	700	39	81
Mud Pie, 169 g	490	20	70
Spumoni Ice Cream, 85 g	180	9	21
Vanilla Ice Cream, 85 g	170	9	21
Factory Favorites			
Baked Lasagna-Dinner, 500 g	800	43	61
Breast of Chicken Fettucine, 519 g	1040	58	96
Chicken Marsala, 497 g	970	53	75
Chicken Parmigiana, 546 g	830	32	80
• Fettuccine Alfredo, 406 g	1080	70	91
• Spinach and Cheese Ravioli, 314 g	480	16	63
Spinach Tortellini w/Alfredo Sc, 343 g	930	55	86
Factory Platters			
Lasagna & Eggplant Parm, 869 g	1060	47	112
Lasagna & Chicken Marsala, 785 g	1080	60	69
• Ravioli & Spaghetti w/ Meat Sauce, 598 g	880	22	133
Spaghetti w/ Meat Sauce, Ssg & Mtbls, 708 g	1360	64	114
Manicotti &spag. w/Mizithra Chz & Butter, 368 g	930	45	100
• Spinach Tortellini Half Lasagna & Chkn Marsala, 768 g	1450	80	113
Hearty Meal Entrees			
• Hearty Marinara Sauce, 709 g	940	8	180
Hearty Clam Sauce, 709 g	1110	23	173
Hearty Italian Ssg w/ Meat Sauce, 823 g	1350	42	177
Hearty Meat Sauce, 709 g	1020	15	176
• Hearty Mizithra Chz and Brown Butter, 638 g	1750	101	164
Hearty Pot Pourri, 745 g	1280	43	176
Hearty Sauteed Mshr Sauce, 851 g	1120	26	184
Hearty Sicilian Meatballs, 879 g	1350	36	186
Kid's Meals			
• Applesauce, 85 g	40	0	10
Grilled Cheese Sandwich, 130 g	480	30	40
Kid's Macaroni and Cheese, 226 g	390	10	59
Kid's Ravioli, 286 g	420	14	55
Kid's Spaghetti Marinara w/ Sicilian Meatball, 368 g	570	16	75
• Kid's Fettuccine Alfredo, 293 g	770	48	68
Kid's Juice Bar, 68 g	60	0	15
Kid's Marinara, 283 g	370	4	72
Kid's Spaghetti w/Brown Butter & Mizithra Chz, 248 g	660	37	65
Kid's Spaghetti w/Clam Sauce, 283 g	440	9	69
Kid's Spaghetti w/Meat Sauce, 283 g	410	6	70
Other Items			
Bay Shrimp Crostini Appetizer, 264 g	720	41	54
• Burger Sliders, 674 g	1770	107	65
• Chz Manicotti w/Marinara Sauce, 346 g	490	21	54
Chicken Caesar - half order, 284 g	590	46	16

• MOST HEALTHY • LEAST HEALTHY

OLD SPAGHETTI FACTORY (cont.)

	Cal	Fat	Cbs
Cobb Salad – half order, 448 g	740	61	19
Eggplant Parmigiana, 709 g	670	8	126
Factory Burger w/chips, 472 g	1370	84	71
Garlic Fries Appetizer, 524 g	1410	107	106
Meatball Sandwich, 402 g	1060	58	79
Portuguese Linguica Appetizer, 499 g	1080	75	52
Rock Shrimp Salad – half order, 308 g	510	4	16
Sausage Sandwich, 345 g	860	51	74
Pastabilities			
Angel Hair, 228 g	420	2	82
Fettuccine/Penne, 228 g	420	2	85
• Gluten Free, 256 g	470	1	104
Spaghetti, 256 g	460	3	93
• Whole Wheat, 228 g	390	2	85
Salads			
BLT Salad, 440 g	1000	85	23
Caesar Upgrade, 200 g	440	37	14
Caesar Salad (no chicken), 412 g	820	72	25
• Chicken Caesar Salad, 582 g	1110	90	28
House Salad-1000 Island, 142 g	230	17	16
House Salad-Balsamic, 128 g	260	21	15
House Salad-Blue Cheese, 142 g	280	24	13
House Salad-Caesar, 142 g	330	30	13
House Salad-Creamy Pesto, 142 g	280	24	13
• House Salad-FF Honey Mustard, 128 g	120	3	21
Sandwiches			
Chkn Smoked Mozzarella Panini, 411 g	1340	75	114
• Sicilian Style Snd - Meatball, 468 g	1280	68	104
• Sicilian Style Snd - Sausage, 468 g	1380	83	100
Seniors Meals			
Caesar Salad (no chicken), 291 g	560	48	17
Chicken Caesar Salad, 433 g	730	53	22
Italian Sausage w/ Meat Sauce, 397 g	740	33	72
Pot Pourri, 283 g	520	19	69
• Spaghetti Marinara, 283 g	370	4	72
• Spaghetti Marinara w/ Sicilian Meatballs, 453 g	770	29	78
Spaghetti Mizithra & Brown Butter, 248 g	660	37	65
Spaghetti w/Clam Sauce, 283 g	440	9	69
Spaghetti w/Meat Sauce, 283 g	410	6	70
Spaghetti w/Mushroom Sauce, 340 g	450	10	74
Sides			
• Alfredo Sauce, 6 oz.	640	67	7
Clam Sauce, 6 oz.	200	12	9
Creamy Pesto Dressing, 43 g	190	21	1
Marinara Sauce, 6 oz.	90	3	13

OLD SPAGHETTI FACTORY (cont.)

	Cal	Fat	Cbs
• Marsala Sauce, 6 oz.	70	4	6
Meat Sauce, 6 oz.	140	7	11
Sausage, 128 g	340	27	3
Sauteed Mushroom Sauce, 255 g	200	14	15
Sicilian Meatballs (2), 170 g	420	27	7
Signature Selections			
Baked Chicken, 522 g	1030	62	71
Chicken Penne, 548 g	910	32	105
Crab Ravioli, 312 g	810	46	73
• Garlic Mizithra, 425 g	1240	77	103
Jumbo Tortellini w/ Flat Iron Steak, 421 g	940	54	185
Lasagna Vegetariano, 588 g	830	48	68
Meatloaf Italian Style, 526 g	1180	68	83
• Spaghetti Vesuvius, 425 g	720	21	105
Soups			
Chicken Mulligatawny, 9 oz.	260	19	20
• Clam Chowder Soup, 9 oz.	370	25	19
Cream of Broccoli, 9 oz.	240	19	21
• Minestrone Soup, 9 oz.	60	2	10

OLIVE GARDEN

Antipasti (Appetizers)	Cal	Fat	Cbs
Alfredo Dipping Sauce	380	35	9
Breadstick (with garlic-butter spread)	150	2	28
Bruschetta	610	13	100
Calamari	890	54	64
Add Marinara Sauce	70	3	10
Add Parmesan-Peppercorn Sauce	300	30	6
Caprese Flatbread	600	36	46
Grilled Chicken Flatbread	760	44	47
Hot Artichoke-Spinach Dip	650	31	68
Italiano: Add Marinara Sauce	70	3	10
Italiano: Add Parm-Peppercorn Sauce	300	30	6
• Italiano: Add Tomato Sauce	45	2	6
Italiano: Calamari	440	27	32
Italiano: Chicken Fingers	330	16	22
Italiano: Fried Mozzarella	370	22	26
Italiano: Fried Zucchini	370	20	42
Italiano: Stuffed Mushrooms	410	28	19
Italiano: Toasted Beef & Pork Ravioli	360	16	39
• Lasagna Fritta	1030	63	82
Marinara Dipping Sauce	70	3	10
Mussels di Napoli	180	8	13
Sicilian Scampi	500	22	43
Smoked Mozzarella Fonduta	940	48	72
Stuffed Mushrooms	410	28	19

• MOST HEALTHY   • LEAST HEALTHY

▶ OLIVE GARDEN (cont.)

	Cal	Fat	Cbs
Carne (Beef & Pork)			
Chianti Braised Short Ribs	1060	58	71
• Mixed Grill	770	24	48
• Pork Milanese	1510	87	118
Steak Gorgonzola-Alfredo	1310	73	82
Steak Toscano	880	43	45
Children's Entrée			
Children's Grilled Chicken	210	6	12
Cucina Classica (Classic Recipes)			
Capellini Pomodoro	840	17	141
Chicken Parmigiana	1090	49	79
Eggplant Parmigiana	850	35	98
Fettuccine Alfredo	1220	75	99
Five Cheese Ziti al Forno	1050	48	112
Lasagna Classico	850	47	39
• Linguine alla Marinara	430	6	76
Spaghetti & Italian Sausage	1270	67	97
Spaghetti & Meatballs	1110	50	103
Spaghetti with Meat Sauce	710	22	94
• Tour of Italy	1450	74	97
Desserts			
Chocolate Milkshake	520	22	72
Strawberry Milkshake	500	24	62
• Sundae	180	9	21
• Vanilla Milkshake	530	23	73
Dolci (Desserts)			
Black Tie Mousse Cake	760	48	73
Chocolate Gelato	620	25	49
Lemon Cream Cake	610	35	69
• Tiramisu	510	32	48
Torta di Chocolate	800	51	75
White Chocolate Raspberry Cheesecake	890	62	70
• Zeppoli	920	35	131
add Chocolate Sauce	210	3	44
Entrées			
Cheese Pizza (cheese & sauce only)	470	14	66
Cheese Ravioli with Tomato Sauce	300	8	43
Chicken Fingers	330	16	22
• Add Broccoli	25	0	4
Add Fries	400	21	47
• Fettuccine Alfredo	800	48	60
Grilled Chicken with Pasta & Broccoli	310	5	33
Herb-Grilled Salmon	510	26	5
Macaroni & Cheese	340	6	58
Mixed Grill	745	24	25
Mixed Grill (all chicken)	630	20	27

• MOST HEALTHY   • LEAST HEALTHY

OLIVE GARDEN (cont.)

	Cal	Fat	Cbs
Pennine Rigate	561	19	90
Spaghetti with Tomato Sauce	250	3	45
Steak Toscano	760	46	9
Frozen Specialties			
• Chocolate Almond Amore	600	21	135
Frozen Tiramisu	410	14	95
Mango Daiquiri	240	0	10
Peach Bellini	170	0	0
Peach Daiquiri	270	0	10
Strawberry Bellini	220	0	0
Strawberry Daiquiri	250	0	15
Strawberry Frozen Margarita	340	0	25
Strawberry Siciliano	360	10	50
Strawberry-Mango Frozen Margarita	350	0	20
Tangerine Palermo	410	12	50
• Wild Berry Bellini	160	0	10
Wild Berry Daiquiri	270	0	5
Wild Berry Frozen Margarita	290	0	20
Insalate (Salads)			
Caesar Salad without croutons	800	61	8
Garden-Fresh Salad without croutons	300	24	16
Martinis			
Chocolate Martini	260	4	45
• Mango Martini	180	0	0
Pomegranate Margarita Martini	290	0	5
Sour Apple Martini	210	0	0
• Strawberry-Limoncello Martini	300	0	15
Pasta Ripiena (Filled Pastas)			
• Braised Beef & Tortellini	740	41	60
Cheese Ravioli With Marinara Sauce	530	18	64
Cheese Ravioli With Meat Sauce	600	22	65
• Ravioli di Portobello	450	19	53
Manicotti Formaggio	680	33	58
Pesce (Fish & Seafood)			
Grilled Shrimp Caprese	900	40	82
• Herb-Grilled Salmon	510	26	5
Parmesan Crusted Tilapia	590	25	42
• Seafood Alfredo	1020	52	88
Seafood Portofino	800	33	85
Shrimp & Asparagus Risotto	620	30	44
Shrimp Primavera	730	12	110
Pizze (Pizzas)			
• Chicken Alfredo Pizza	1180	40	144
Create Your Own Pizza w/ chz & sauce	910	28	129
Add Pepperoni	120	11	0
Add Italian Sausage	130	11	1

OLIVE GARDEN (cont.)

	Cal	Fat	Cbs
• Add Mushrooms	5	0	1
Add Onions	15	0	4
Add Bell Peppers	10	0	2
Add Black Olives	45	4	3
Add Roma Tomatoes	10	0	2

Pollo (Chicken)

	Cal	Fat	Cbs
Chicken & Gnocchi Veronese	1030	58	72
• Chicken & Shrimp Carbonara	1440	88	80
Chicken Alfredo	1440	82	103
Chicken Marsala	770	37	59
Chicken Scampi	1020	53	84
Garlic-Herb Chicken con Broccoli	960	41	90
Stuffed Chicken Marsala	800	36	40
• Venetian Apricot Chicken	380	4	32

Pollo e Pesce (Chicken & Seafood)

	Cal	Fat	Cbs
Grilled Chicken Spiedini	460	13	26
Shrimp Primavera	510	9	79

Signature Cocktails

	Cal	Fat	Cbs
Berry Sangria Glass	230	0	15
Italian Margarita	240	0	10
Lime-Mint Fresco	230	0	45
• Limoncello Lemonade	260	0	5
Peach Fresco	200	1	10
Peach Sangria Glass	250	0	50
Sicilian Citrus Fresco	210	0	10
Strawberry Fresco	230	0	5
Tropical Sangria Glass	220	0	10
Venetian Sunset	190	0	10

Zuppe e Insalate (Soups & Salads)

	Cal	Fat	Cbs
Chicken & Gnocchi (One serving)	250	8	29
Garden-Fresh Salad (One serving w/ drss)	350	26	22
Garden-Fresh Salad (One serving w/o drss)	120	4	17
• Grilled Chicken Caesar	850	64	14
• Minestrone (One serving)	100	1	18
Pasta e Fagioli (One serving)	130	3	17
Zuppa Toscana (One serving)	170	4	24

ON THE BORDER MEXICAN GRILL

Appetizers

	Cal	Fat	Cbs
• Border Sampler, 1 Serving	2000	134	105
Chkn Flautas w/ Original Queso, 4 Each	1070	66	69
Chips and Salsa, 1 Basket	430	22	52
Empanadas Chkn w/ Org Queso, 5 Each	1170	82	72
Empanadas Grnd Beef w/ Org Queso, 5 Each	1210	86	72
Fajita Quesadillas - Chicken, 1 Serving	1230	84	59

• MOST HEALTHY   • LEAST HEALTHY

ON THE BORDER MEXICAN (cont.)

	Cal	Fat	Cbs
Fajita Quesadillas - Steak, 1 Serving	1220	90	58
Firecracker Stfd Jalapeños w/ Queso, 1 Srv	1950	134	123
Grande Fajita Nachos - Chkn, 1 Serving	1540	84	88
Grande Fajita Nachos - Steak, 1 Serving	1520	94	87
Guacamole Live! w/o Chips, 1 Serving	570	50	34
• Guacamole w/o Chips, 1 Serving	200	16	15
Original Queso Carne Style w/o Chips, 1 Cup	330	24	10
Original Queso w/o Chips, 1 Cup	240	18	8
OTB Dip Trio w/o Chips, 1 Serving	450	33	22
Ult Loaded Queso w/o Chips, 1 Serving	770	52	36

Border Lunch - Favorites

	Cal	Fat	Cbs
• Border's Best Lunch Chkn Fajitas w/o Tort. & Cndmnt, 1 Srv	430	14	44
Border's Best Lunch Steak Fajitas w/o Cndmnt, 1 Srv	560	26	42
Brisket Tacos, 1 Serving	970	39	126
Chile con Carne for Chimi/Burrito, 1 Srv	100	5	7
• Dos XX Fish Tacos, 1 Serving	1660	110	131
Fresh Sour Crm Sc for Chimi/Burrito, 1 Srv	80	6	5
Little Bordurrito Chkn w/o drss, 1 Srv	1060	59	90
Little Bordurrito Steak w/o drss, 1 Srv	1050	64	90
Lunch Beef Burrito w/o Sauce, 1 Serving	750	26	89
Lunch Chkn Burrito w/o Sauce, 1 Serving	690	22	90
Lunch Chimichanga Chkn w/o Sauce, 1 Srv	920	48	90
Lunch Chimichanga Grnd Beef w/o Sc, 1 Srv	1050	62	90
Queso for Chimi/Burrito, 1 Serving	150	11	5
Ranchero Sauce for Chimi/Burrito, 1 Srv	60	3	8

Border Lunch Create Your Own Combo

	Cal	Fat	Cbs
• Black Beans w/ Cheese, 1 Serving	130	3	20
Chkn Flautas w/ Chile con Queso, 1 Serving	330	21	19
Chicken Tortilla Soup, 1 cup	330	18	26
• Chz Stfd Chile Relleno w/ Ranchero Sc, 1 Srv	680	57	28
Crispy Taco Chicken, 1 Serving	260	12	19
Crispy Taco Ground Beef, 1 Serving	320	19	19
Empanadas Beef w/ Chile con Queso, 1 Srv	540	39	30
Empanadas Chkn w/ Chile con Queso, 1 Srv	520	37	30
Enchilada Chkn w/ Sour Cream Sc, 1 Srv	210	11	18
Enchilada Chz & Onion w/ Chile con Carne, 1 Srv	360	24	20
Enchilada Grnd Beef w/ Chile con Carne, 1 Srv	260	15	20
House Salad -No Dressing, 1 Serving	200	12	20
Mexican Rice, 1 Serving	280	4	53
Pork Tamale w/ Chile con Carne, 1 Serving	290	20	14
Refried Beans w/ Cheese, 1 Serving	230	10	24
Soft Taco -Chicken, 1 Serving	240	11	24
Soft Taco -Ground Beef, 1 Serving	310	18	24

Border Lunch Soup, Salads & Starters

	Cal	Fat	Cbs
Chicken Tortilla Soup, 1 Cup	330	18	26
Chile con Carne Style w/o Chips, 1 Cup	330	24	10

• MOST HEALTHY   • LEAST HEALTHY

ON THE BORDER MEXICAN (cont.)

ON THE BORDER MEXICAN (cont.)	Cal	Fat	Cbs
Chile con Queso w/o Chips, 1 Cup	240	18	8
Chips and Salsa, 1 Basket	430	22	52
Guacamole w/o chips, 1 Serving	200	16	15
• House Salad -No dressing, 1 Serving	200	12	20
• Lunch Fajita Nachos -Chicken, 1 Serving	1060	59	60
Lunch Fajita Nachos -Steak, 1 Serving	1050	66	60
Lunch Taco Salad w/ Chkn-No drss, 1 Srv	880	60	57
Lunch Taco Salad w/ Grnd Beef-No drss, 1 Srv	940	67	57
Quesa. Combo -Chkn, 1 Serving	600	39	28
Quesadilla Combo -Steak, 1 Serving	590	42	28

Burritos & Chimis

	Cal	Fat	Cbs
• Big Chkn Bordurrito w/Side Salad-No Drss, 1 Srv	1780	85	170
Big Steak Bordurrito w/Side Salad-No Drss, 1 Srv	1760	96	170
Chile con Carne for Chimi/Burrito, 1 Srv	100	5	7
Classic Chicken Burrito w/o sc, 1 Srv	910	33	106
Classic Chimi. Chicken w/o Sauce, 1 Srv	1290	75	106
Classic Chimi. Grnd Beef w/o Sc, 1 Srv	1400	87	106
Classic Shrd Beef Burrito w/o Sc, 1 Srv	1010	38	103
Fresh Sour Crm Sc for Chimi/Burrito, 1 Srv	80	6	5
Queso for Chimi/Burrito, 1 Serving	150	11	5
• Ranchero Sc for Chimi/Burrito, 1 Srv	60	3	8
3 Sauce Fajita Chkn Burrito, 1 Serving	1240	48	119
3 Sauce Fajita Steak Burrito, 1 Srv	1220	59	119

Choose Your Condiments

	Cal	Fat	Cbs
Guacamole, 1 Serving	40	4	3
Homemade Flour Tortillas, 3 Each	270	11	56
• Mexican Rice, 1 Serving	280	4	53
Mixed Cheese, 1 Serving	110	9	1
• Pico de Gallo, 1 Serving	10	1	1
Sour Cream, 1 Serving	60	5	2

Choose Your Sauce

	Cal	Fat	Cbs
Chipotle Honey Sauce, 1 Serving	230	4	48
• Habanero Fire Sauce, 1 Serving	120	9	9
Tequila Lime Chile Sauce, 1 Serving	170	14	6

Choose Your Veggie

	Cal	Fat	Cbs
• Baja Blend Veggies, 1 Serving	210	15	17
Classic Veggies, 1 Serving	90	5	11
• El Diablo Veggies, 1 Serving	50	2	8

Create Your Own Combo

	Cal	Fat	Cbs
Chkn Flautas w/ Chile con Queso, 1 Srv	330	21	19
Chicken Tortilla Soup, 1 cup	330	18	26
• Chz Stfd Chile Relleno w/Ranchero Sc, 1 Srv	680	57	28
Crispy Taco - Chicken, 1 Serving	260	12	19
Crispy Taco - Ground Beef, 1 Serving	320	19	19
Empan. Chkn w/ Chile con Queso, 1 Srv	520	37	30

• MOST HEALTHY   • LEAST HEALTHY

ON THE BORDER MEXICAN (cont.)	Cal	Fat	Cbs
Empan. Grnd Beef w/ Chile con Queso, 1 Srv	540	39	30
Enchil. Chkn w/ Sour Cream Sauce, 1 Srv	210	11	18
Enchil. Chz & Onion w/ Chile con Carne, 1 Srv	360	24	20
Enchil. Grnd Beef w/ Chile con Carne, 1 Srv	260	15	19
• House Salad - No Dressing, 1 Serving	200	12	20
Pork Tamale w/ Chile con Carne, 1 Srv	290	20	14
Soft Taco - Chicken, 1 Serving	240	11	24
Soft Taco - Ground Beef, 1 Serving	310	18	24
Desserts			
Border Brownie Sundae w/ Vanilla Ice Crm, 1 Srv	1310	73	160
Chocolate Turtle Empanadas, 1 Serving	1200	72	136
Kahlua® Ice Cream Pie, 1 Serving	820	42	99
Sizzling Apple Crisp, 1 Serving	1120	45	177
• Sopapillas (5), 1 Serving	1350	44	236
• Sopapillas 2 w/ Choco syrup, 1 Serving	540	18	92
Sopapillas 2 w/ Honey, 1 Serving	630	17	118
Enchiladas			
Enchilada Suizas, 1 Serving	1000	44	110
Grilled Enchil. - Avocado w/ Red Chile Pesto, 1 Serving	1040	55	107
Grilled Enchilada - Pepper Jack Chkn, 1 Serving	1090	50	102
• Grilled Enchilada - Smoky Beef Brisket, 1 Serving	970	46	97
Ranchiladas, 1 Serving	1480	83	105
3 Enchil. Dinner Chkn w/ Sour Crm Sauce, 1 Srv	1080	47	118
• 3 Enchil. Dinner Chz & Onion w/Chile con Carne, 1 Srv	1590	95	123
3 Enchil. Dinner Grnd Beef w/ Chile con Carne, 1 Srv	1240	60	122
Fajita Grill			
• Grld Veg. w/ Portobello Mshr, 1 Serving	210	14	21
Mesquite-Grilled Chicken, 1 Serving	300	16	4
Mesquite-Grilled Steak, 1 Serving	370	27	2
• Pulled Pork (Carnitas), 1 Serving	760	69	2
Seasoned, Sauteed Shrimp, 1 Serving	420	33	3
Fresh Grill (Served As Listed)			
• Add Bacon Wrapped Shrimp Skewer, 1 Serving	460	40	3
Carne Asada, 1 Serving	940	35	105
Chicken Salsa Fresca, 1 Serving	520	9	60
Jalapeño-BBQ Salmon, 1 Serving	590	21	45
• Queso Chicken, 1 Serving	1130	50	115
Tomatillo Chicken, 1 Serving	850	24	108
Kid's Menu			
Cheeseburger, 1 Serving	550	41	24
Chicken Tenders, 1 Serving	540	36	44
Corn Dog, 1 Serving	280	17	25
Sundae w/ Choco Syrup, 1 Serving	360	18	51
Sundae w/ Strawberry Purée, 1 Serving	320	18	41
Grilled Chicken, 1 Serving	90	1	2
Grilled Chicken Sandwich, 1 Serving	340	17	25

• MOST HEALTHY   • LEAST HEALTHY

ON THE BORDER MEXICAN (cont.)

	Cal	Fat	Cbs
Hamburger, 1 Serving	450	32	23
Black Beans, 1 Serving	130	3	20
French Fries, 1 Serving	250	10	36
• House Salad - No dressing, 1 Serving	10	0	2
Mexican Rice, 1 Serving	280	4	53
Mixed Vegetables, 1 Serving	180	14	13
Refried Beans, 1 Serving	230	10	24
Mexican Plate Chz Enchiladas, 1 Srv	340	24	18
Mexican Plate Chicken Taco, 1 Serving	240	11	24
Mexican Plate Crispy Chkn Taco, 1 Srv	260	12	19
Mex Plate Crispy Grnd Beef Taco, 1 Srv	320	19	19
Mex Plate Soft Grnd Beef Taco, 1 Srv	310	18	24
Nachos - Bean & Cheese, 1 Serving	780	43	59
Nachos - Cheese, 1 Serving	550	36	31
• Quesadilla, 1 Serving	850	67	36

OTB Taco Stand

	Cal	Fat	Cbs
Brisket Tacos w/ Jalapeño BBQ Sauce, 1 Srv	1280	55	155
• Dos XX® Fish Tacos w/Crmy Red Chile Sauce, 1 Srv	2240	152	170
Grld Mahi Mahi Tacos w/Crmy Red Chile Sauce, 1 Srv	1200	61	116
Ld Carne Asada Tacos w/ Crmy Red Chile Sauce, 1 Srv	1510	93	114
Street-Style Mini Tacos - Chkn, 1 Srv	1020	50	96
Street-Style Mini Tacos - Steak, 1 Srv	1080	60	93
SW Chkn Tacos w/ Crmy Red Chile Sauce, 1 Srv	1460	85	132
Taco Melt - Beef (Crispy), 1 Serving	860	45	79
Taco Melt - Beef (Soft), 1 Serving	920	45	109
• Taco Melt - Chicken (Crispy), 1 Serving	770	34	79
Taco Melt - Chicken (Soft), 1 Serving	820	34	109

Side Items & Extras

	Cal	Fat	Cbs
Black Beans w/ Cheese, 1 Serving	130	3	20
Fat-Free Mango Citrus Vinaigrette, 1 Srv	45	0	11
Guacamole, 1 Serving	40	4	3
• Mexican Rice, 1 Serving	280	4	53
• Pico de Gallo, 1 Serving	10	1	1
Refried Beans w/ Cheese, 1 Serving	230	10	24
Smoked Jalapeño Vinaigrette, 1 Serving	230	23	8
Sour Cream, 1 Serving	60	5	2
Vegetables - Grilled, 1 Serving	70	0	16
Vegetables - House, 1 Serving	180	14	13

Signature Fajitas

	Cal	Fat	Cbs
• Al Carbon Fajitas -Chicken, 1 Serving	230	5	11
Al Carbon Fajitas -Steak, 1 Serving	300	15	9
Monterey Ranch Chicken, 1 Serving	660	42	13
• The Ultimate Fajita, 1 Serving	1100	91	26

Soup & Salads

	Cal	Fat	Cbs
Sizzling Fajita Salad w/Chkn - No Drss, 1 Srv	700	45	25
Chicken Tortilla Soup, 1 cup	330	18	26

• MOST HEALTHY   • LEAST HEALTHY

ON THE BORDER MEXICAN (cont.)	Cal	Fat	Cbs
Citrus Chipotle Chkn Salad w/Mango Citrus Vingrt, 1 Srv	290	4	42
Grande Taco Salad w/ Chkn - No Drss, 1 Srv	1280	84	83
• Grande Taco Salad w/ Grnd Beef - No Drss, 1 Srv	1370	95	83
• House Salad - No Dressing, 1 Serving	200	12	20
Sizzling Fajita Salad - Steak - No Dres, 1 Srv	820	57	24

ORANGE JULIUS

Add a Banana
1 Banana, 126 g	110	0	29

Fruit Drinks
Bananarilla®, 20 oz.	400	9	82
Blackberry, 20 oz.	350	8	68
Cranberry Banana Julius ®, 20 oz.	170	1	43
• Cranberry Orange Julius ®, 20 oz.	150	1	37
Cranberry Pineapple Julius ®, 20 oz.	170	1	43
Mango Julius®, 20 oz.	190	1	48
Orange Julius®, 20 oz.	160	1	41
Peach Julius®, 20 oz.	170	1	43
Piña Colada, 20 oz.	330	8	64
Pineapple Julius®, 20 oz.	150	1	38
Pomegranate Julius®, 20 oz.	200	1	50
Raspberry Julius®, 20 oz.	220	1	56
Strawberry Banana, 20 oz.	380	8	75
Strawberry Lemonade Julius®, 20 oz.	260	1	67
Tripleberry®, 20 oz.	380	8	78
• Tropical, 20 oz.	430	9	89

Hot Dogs
Bacon Cheese Dog, 160 g	490	33	24
Cheese Dog, 153 g	460	31	24
Chicago Dog, 268 g	430	27	29
Chili Melt Dog, 165 g	470	33	25
Chili Slaw Dog, 184 g	470	31	28
Pepperoni Cheese Dog, 163 g	460	31	26
Relish Dog, 156 g	420	27	28
Reuben Dog, 196 g	520	36	24
• Sauerkraut Dog, 167 g	410	27	24
Southwest Chili Dog, 190 g	500	34	27
• Triple Cheese Dog, 176 g	540	38	24

Light Premium Fruit Smoothies
• Strawberry Delight™, 20 oz.	250	0	60
Berry-Pom Twilight™, 20 oz.	230	0	55
• Tropical Sunlight™, 20 oz.	220	0	55

Nutrition Boosts
• Fiber Plus, 6 g	5	0	4
Heart Health, 4 g	15	0	3
Joint Care, 6 g	20	0	5

ORANGE JULIUS (cont.)

	Cal	Fat	Cbs
• Protein, 19 g	90	3	8
Other Beverages			
Cool Cappuccino, 20 oz.	370	13	56
• Cool Mocha, 20 oz.	490	16	78
• Eggnog, 20 oz.	330	12	53
Other Food			
Nachos - Large, 226 g	550	29	700
Salted Pretzel, 66 g	160	1	34
Pitas			
• Chicken Caesar Pita, 187 g	470	23	45
• Chicken Fajita Pita, 222 g	380	1	49
Garden Veggie Pita, 208 g	460	26	49
Santa Fe Grilled Chicken Pita, 208 g	470	22	47
Steak Fajita Pita, 229 g	400	14	51
Turkey Club Pita, 201 g	460	23	46
Premium Fruit Smoothies			
3-Berry Blast, 20 oz.	460	0	108
• Berry Banana Squeeze, 20 oz.	270	0	106
Berry Lemon Lively, 20 oz.	440	0	70
Blackberry Storm, 20 oz.	680	15	128
Blackberry Toner, 20 oz.	410	0	94
• Cocoa Latte Swirl, 20 oz.	960	0	75
Cran Orange Chill Tart 'N' Berry™, 20 oz.	410	0	92
Mango Passion, 20 oz.	370	1	97
Orange Swirl™, 20 oz.	540	23	156
Peach White Tea, 20 oz.	320	12	103
Peaches & Cream, 20 oz.	360	0	86
Pomegranate & Berries, 20 oz.	400	0	92
Raspberry Créme, 20 oz.	650	15	118
Raspberry Crush, 20 oz.	390	1	98
Raspberry White Tea, 20 oz.	410	0	100
Strawberry Sensation, 20 oz.	430	0	89
Strawberry Xtreme, 20 oz.	390	3	99
Tropical Tango, 20 oz.	380	10	99
Tropi-Colada, 20 oz.	530	0	83

OUTBACK STEAKHOUSE

Add On Mates	Cal	Fat	Cbs
Grilled Scallops	336	23	12
Lobster & Mushroom Topping	395	36	8
• Lobster Tail	530	47	5
• Sautéed Mushrooms	134	3	18
Shrimp scampi	313	20	17
Three grilled shrimp	162	9	7
Aussie-tizers® to Share (Per Serving)			
• Alice Springs Chkn Quesadilla® - Regular	535	33	32

• MOST HEALTHY   • LEAST HEALTHY

OUTBACK STEAKHOUSE (cont.)

	Cal	Fat	Cbs
Aussie Cheese Fries - Regular	356	25	23
Bloomin' Onion	261	14	31
Gold Coast Coconut Shrimp	142	5	17
Grilled Shrimp on the Barbie	320	21	6
Kookaburra Wings Medium	520	45	7
• Seared Ahi Tuna - Regular	111	6	4
Burgers & Sandwiches			
Bacon Cheese Burger & Aussie Fries	1483	99	88
• Grld Chkn & Swiss Snd & Aussie Fries	1050	52	93
Roasted Filet Sandwich & Aussie Fries	1117	39	131
• The Bloomin' Burger® & Aussie Fries	1527	91	119
The Outbacker Burger & Aussie Fries	1113	64	86
Freshly Made Sides			
Aussie Fries	354	19	43
Blue Cheese Pecan Chopped Salad	523	36	35
Caesar Salad	330	27	16
Classic Blue Cheese Wedge Salad	357	24	26
Dressed Baked Potato	520	26	65
Fresh Seasonal Veggies	143	11	11
Fresh Steamed Green Beans	134	10	9
Garlic Mashed Potatoes	374	25	33
House Salad - Blue Cheese	331	26	18
Potato Boats	165	2	32
Potato Wedges	278	15	33
• Side Bread & Butter	117	6	12
• Sweet Potato	593	21	99
Irresistible Desserts			
• Carrot Cake	112	3	22
Chocolate Thunder From Down Under®	478	38	34
Classic Cheesecake	184	9	26
• Classic Cheesecake Sample	991	34	171
Nutter Butter® Peanut Butter Pie Sample	880	56	89
Sweet Adventure Sampler Trio™	599	30	81
Joey Menu			
Boomerang Cheese Burger	436	15	37
Grilled Cheese-A-Roo	394	25	29
• Joey Grilled Chicken On The Barbie	209	8	0
Joey Sirloin	240	12	0
Junior Ribs	636	53	1
Kookaburra Chkn Fingers & Aussie Fries	1030	60	90
Mac A Roo 'N Cheese	402	31	16
• Spotted Dog Sundae -Chocolate Sauce	1216	94	89
Outback Favorites			
Alice Springs Chicken® & Aussie Fries	1657	113	74
• Baby Back Ribs & Aussie Fries	2367	179	67
Back Back Ribs & Aussie Fries	1403	99	66

● MOST HEALTHY   ● LEAST HEALTHY

OUTBACK STEAKHOUSE (cont.)

	Cal	Fat	Cbs
Filet w/Mshrm Sauce & Ssnl Veg & Garlic Msh Pot.	867	54	52
• Grld Chkn on the Barbie & Fresh Ssnl Veg	587	26	32
New Zealand Rack of Lamb & Ssnl Veg & Msh Pot.	1821	149	49
No Rules Parm Pasta - Chkn & Scallops	1379	77	96
Rstd Pork Tenderloin & Stmd Green Beans & Msh Pot.	855	43	73

Perfect Combinations

Filet & Shrimp Scampi & Garlic Msh Pot.	995	63	52
• OB Special® 6 oz & Grld Shrimp on the Barbie	554	35	8
• Ribs & Alice Springs Chkn® & Aussie Fries	1626	118	50
Teriyaki Filet Medallions & Fresh Stmd Green Beans	618	27	52

Signature Steaks

Chargrilled Ribeye, 10 oz.	787	63	2
New York Strip, 14 oz.	713	37	1
New York Strip, 8 oz.	567	37	92
Outback Special®, 9 oz.	445	23	1
Prime Rib, 8 oz.	537	45	2
Ribeye 10, oz.	882	74	1
• Teriyaki Marinated Sirloin, 9 oz.	418	12	17
• The Melbourne, 20 oz.	1010	58	1
Victoria's Filet®, 6 oz.	518	42	1

Soups & Salads

Chicken Caesar Salad	1045	74	27
Classic Roasted Filet Wedge Salad	563	30	27
• Queensland Salad - Bleu Cheese	1076	82	28
Shrimp Caesar Salad	713	53	27
• Walkabout Soup® of the Day Crm of Brcli, cup	282	21	16

Straight From the Sea

Atlantic Salmon & Fresh Seasonal Veggies	728	57	13
Fresh Tilapia w/Pure Lump Crab Meat & Fresh Ssnl Veg	653	40	20
• Lobster Tails	640	48	6
Shrimp En Fuego Fettuccine	1187	55	95

PANDA EXPRESS

Appetizers

Chicken Egg Roll, 3 oz. / 1 roll	200	12	16
• Chicken Potsticker, 3 oz. / 3 pcs	220	11	23
Cream Cheese Rangoon, 2 oz. / 3 pcs	190	8	24
• Veggie Spring Roll, 3 oz. / 2 rolls	160	7	22

Beef

• Beijing Beef, 6 oz.	850	50	67
• Broccoli Beef, 5 oz.	150	6	12
Mongolian Beef, 7 oz.	230	11	17

Chicken

Black Pepper Chicken, 6 oz.	250	14	12
• Broccoli Chicken, 6 oz.	180	9	11
Kung Pao Chicken, 6 oz.	300	19	13

• MOST HEALTHY   • LEAST HEALTHY

▶ PANDA EXPRESS (cont.)	Cal	Fat	Cbs
Mandarin Chicken, 6 oz.	310	16	8
Mushroom Chicken, 6 oz.	220	13	9
• Orange Chicken, 5 oz.	400	20	42
Pineapple Chicken, 6 oz.	240	12	19
Potato Chicken, 5 oz.	220	11	18
String Bean Chicken, 5 oz.	190	10	11
Sweet & Sour Chicken, 6 oz.	400	17	46
Chicken Breast			
Pineapple Chicken Breast, 6 oz.	220	8	20
• String Bean Chicken Breast, 6 oz.	170	7	13
• SweetFire Chicken Breast™, 6 oz.	440	18	53
Thai Cashew Chicken Breast, 6 oz.	280	19	21
Pork			
BBQ Pork, 5 oz.	360	19	13
Sweet & Sour Pork, 6 oz.	400	23	36
Rice & Noodles			
• Chow Mein, 8 oz.	400	12	61
• Fried Rice, 10 oz.	570	18	85
Steamed Rice, 9 oz.	420	0	93
Sauces & Cookies			
• Fortune Cookies, 8 g / 1 pc	32	0	7
• Mandarin Sauce, 2 oz.	160	0	40
Potsticker Sauce, 2 oz.	45	0	10
Sweet & Sour Sauce, 2 oz.	80	0	21
Shrimp			
Crispy Shrimp, 4 oz. / 6 pcs	260	13	26
• Honey Walnut Shrimp, 4 oz.	370	23	27
Kung Pao Shrimp, 6 oz.	250	15	14
• Tangy Shrimp, 6 oz.	190	7	19
Soup			
Egg Flower Soup, 10 oz.	90	2	15
Hot & Sour Soup, 11 oz.	90	4	12
Veggies			
Eggplant & Tofu, 6 oz.	310	24	19
Mixed Veggies (Entree), 4 oz.	35	0	7
▶ **PANERA BREAD**			
Artisan Breads			
• Ciabatta, 6 oz.	460	6	84
• Country Loaf, 2 oz.	140	1	27
Country Miche, 2 oz.	140	1	28
Focaccia, 2 oz.	180	5	28
Focaccia w/ Asiago Cheese, 2 oz.	160	5	23
French Baguette, 2 oz.	150	1	30
French Miche, 2 oz.	140	1	28
Sesame Semolina Loaf, 2 oz.	140	1	29

• MOST HEALTHY   • LEAST HEALTHY

PANERA BREAD (cont.)

	Cal	Fat	Cbs
Sesame Semolina Miche, 2 oz.	140	1	30
Stone-Milled Rye Loaf, 2 oz.	140	1	28
Stone-Milled Rye Miche, 2 oz.	140	1	27
Three Cheese Demi, 2 oz.	160	2	29
Three Cheese Loaf, 2 oz.	140	2	26
Three Cheese Miche, 2 oz.	150	2	27
Three Seed Demi, 2 oz.	160	4	27
Whole Grain Baguette, 2 oz.	150	2	30
Whole Grain Loaf, 2 oz.	140	1	27
Whole Grain Miche, 2 oz.	140	2	28

Artisan Pastries

	Cal	Fat	Cbs
Cheese, 4 oz.	400	23	41
• Cherry, 5 oz.	450	22	55
• Chocolate, 4 oz.	350	20	38
Fresh Apple, 5 oz.	380	19	51
Pecan Braid, 4 oz.	440	25	46

Bagels

	Cal	Fat	Cbs
Asiago Cheese, 4 oz.	330	6	55
Blueberry, 4 oz.	330	2	67
Chocolate Chip Bagel, 4 oz.	370	6	69
• Cinnamon Crunch, 5 oz.	430	8	81
Cinnamon Swirl & Raisin, 4 oz.	320	3	65
Everything, 4 oz.	300	3	59
French Toast, 4 oz.	350	5	67
Jalapeño & Cheddar Bagel, 4 oz.	310	3	56
• Plain, 4 oz.	290	2	59
Sesame, 4 oz.	310	3	59
Whole Grain, 5 oz.	370	4	70

Baked Egg Soufflés

	Cal	Fat	Cbs
Four Cheese, 6 oz.	480	31	34
Spinach & Artichoke, 6 oz.	540	35	36
Spinach & Bacon, 7 oz.	580	39	34
• Turkey Sausage & Potato, 6 oz.	450	29	35

Brownies & Blondies

	Cal	Fat	Cbs
Chocolate Fudge Brownie, 4 oz.	410	14	64
Macadamia Nut Blondie, 4 oz.	460	21	62

Cafe Sandwiches

	Cal	Fat	Cbs
Full Mediterranean Veg on Tom Basil, 14 oz.	610	13	100
Full Napa Almond Chkn Salad on Sesame Semolina, 12 oz.	680	26	87
Full Salmon Club Croissant, 10 oz.	770	52	37
• Full Sierra Tkey on Focaccia w/ Asiago Chz, 14 oz.	970	54	80
Full Smkd Ham & Swiss on Stone-Milled Rye, 14 oz.	700	28	65
• Full Smkd Tkey Breast on Country, 12 oz.	560	17	68
Full Tuna Salad on Honey Wheat, 12 oz.	750	47	64

Cakes

	Cal	Fat	Cbs
Cinnamon Coffee Crumb Cake, 4 oz.	470	25	54

• MOST HEALTHY   • LEAST HEALTHY

PANERA BREAD (cont.)

	Cal	Fat	Cbs
• Lemon Poppyseed, 5 oz.	450	20	62
• Pineapple Upside-Down, 6 oz.	510	22	75
Cookies			
Bunny shaped Shortbread Cookie, 3 oz.	370	19	45
Chocolate Chipper, 3 oz.	440	23	59
Chocolate Duet w/ Walnuts, 3 oz.	450	24	55
Oatmeal Raisin, 3 oz.	370	14	57
• Shortbread, 3 oz.	350	21	36
• Toffee Nut, 3 oz.	460	19	59
Flavorful Cream Cheese Spreads			
• Plain, 1 oz.	100	10	1
Reduced Fat Hazelnut, 1 oz.	80	6	3
Reduced Fat Honey Walnut, 1 oz.	80	6	4
Reduced Fat Plain, 1 oz.	70	6	1
Reduced Fat Raspberry, 1 oz.	70	5	4
Reduced Fat Sun-Dried Tomato, 1 oz.	70	6	2
• Reduced Fat Veggie, 1 oz.	60	5	1
Frozen Drinks			
• Caramel, 16 fl.oz.	600	22	97
Low Fat Black Cherry Smoothie, 16 fl.oz.	290	2	63
• Low Fat Mango Smoothie, 16 fl.oz.	230	2	51
Low Fat Strwbry Smoothie w/ Ginseng, 16 fl.oz.	260	2	59
Mango, 18 fl.oz.	330	10	61
Mocha, 16 fl.oz.	570	21	92
Granola Parfait			
Strawberry Granola Parfait, 8 oz.	280	12	41
Grilled Breakfast Sandwiches			
Asiago Chz Bagel Brkfst Snd w/Bacon, 8 oz.	610	27	56
Asiago Chz Bagel Brkfst Snd w/Egg & Chz, 7 oz.	480	18	55
• Asiago Chz Bagel Brkfst Snd w/ Sausage, 8 oz.	650	33	56
Bacon, Egg & Cheese on Ciabatta, 7 oz.	510	24	44
• Breakfast Power Sandwich, 6 oz.	360	14	36
Egg & Cheese on Ciabatta, 6 oz.	380	14	43
Jalapeño & Cheddar Bagel Snd w/ Bacon, 7 oz.	590	25	58
Jalapeño & Cheddar Bagel Snd w/ Egg & Chz, 6 oz.	460	15	57
Jalapeño & Cheddar Bagel Snd w/ Ssge, 8 oz.	630	30	58
Jalapeño & Cheddar Bagel Snd w/Smkd Ham, 7 oz.	490	15	58
Sausage, Egg & Chz on Ciabatta, 8 oz.	550	30	44
Hand-Tossed Salads			
Full Asian Sesame Chicken, 11 oz.	400	20	29
Full BBQ Chopped Chicken, 15 oz.	500	22	47
Full Caesar, 10 oz.	390	27	25
Full Chicken Caesar Salad, 13 oz.	510	29	26
Full Chopped Chicken Cobb, 16 oz.	500	36	8
Full Classic Cafe, 10 oz.	170	11	18
• Full Fresh Fruit Cup - Small, 5 oz.	60	0	16

● MOST HEALTHY   • LEAST HEALTHY

PANERA BREAD (cont.)

	Cal	Fat	Cbs
• Full Fuji Apple w/ Chicken, 14 oz.	520	31	33
Full Greek, 14 oz.	380	34	14
Full Mediterranean Salmon Salad, 14 oz.	480	30	27
Full Salmon Caesar Salad, 12 oz.	480	34	15
Hot Panini			
• Cuban Chicken Panini, 13 oz.	860	37	86
Full Frontega Chicken® on Focaccia, 13 oz.	860	39	80
• Full Smokehouse Turkey™ on Three Chz, 11 oz.	720	29	66
Full Tomato & Mozz. on Ciabatta, 12 oz.	770	29	96
Full Turkey Artichoke on Focaccia, 14 oz.	750	27	88
Iced Drinks			
Iced Chai Tea Latte, 16 fl.oz.	160	4	26
Iced Green Tea - Grande, 16 fl.oz.	90	0	23
Muffins & Muffies			
Apple Crunch Muffin, 5 oz.	470	12	83
Carrot Walnut Muffin, 5 oz.	440	19	62
Chocolate Chip Muffie, 3 oz.	280	12	40
Cranberry Orange Muffin, 5 oz.	480	19	71
• Pumpkin Muffie, 3 oz.	270	10	42
• Pumpkin Muffin, 6 oz.	530	20	81
Wild Blueberry Muffin, 5 oz.	390	15	58
Panera Kids™			
Panera Kids Deli Snd - Roast Beef, 5 oz.	320	10	35
Panera Kids Deli Snd - Smkd Ham, 5 oz.	300	9	34
Panera Kids Deli Snd - Smkd Tkey, 5 oz.	300	10	35
Panera Kids Grilled Chz Snd, 4 oz.	300	12	35
• Panera Kids Mac & Cheese, 8 oz.	490	30	37
• Panera Kids Organic Yogurt (blbry, strwbry), 2 oz.	70	1	12
Panera Kids PntBtr & Jelly Snd, 5 oz.	410	18	56
Salad Dressings			
• Full Red-Sugar Asian Sesame Vinaigrette, 2 oz.	90	8	6
• Full White Balsamic Apple Vinaigrette, 2 oz.	150	12	11
Tangerine Honey Vinaigrette, 2 oz.	100	7	10
Scones			
• Cinnamon Chip, 5 oz.	530	26	66
Orange, 5 oz.	470	11	87
Strawberries & Cream, 4 oz.	420	19	57
• Wild Blueberry, 4 oz.	390	16	56
Signature Sandwiches			
• Full Asiago Rst Beef on Asiago Chz, 13 oz.	690	27	64
Full Bacon Tkey Bravo® on Tom Basil, 14 oz.	840	32	87
Full Chkn Caesar on Three Chz, 13 oz.	710	32	66
Full Chipotle Chkn on Artisan French, 13 oz.	990	56	69
• Full Italian Combo on Ciabatta, 18 oz.	1040	45	94
Soups & More			
Baked Potato, 12 oz.	340	22	29

• MOST HEALTHY   • LEAST HEALTHY

PANERA BREAD (cont.)

	Cal	Fat	Cbs
Broccoli Cheddar, 12 oz.	290	16	24
Cream of Chicken & Wild Rice, 12 oz.	320	17	33
French Onion, 13 oz.	240	12	24
Low Fat Garden Veg w/ Pesto, 12 oz.	160	4	28
• Low-Fat Chicken Noodle, 12 oz.	110	4	10
Low-Fat Vegetarian Black Bean, 12 oz.	170	4	29
New England Clam Chowder, 12 oz.	450	34	29
• Signature Mac & Cheese - Small, 8 oz.	490	30	37
Vegetarian Creamy Tomato Soup, 13 oz.	370	23	39

Specialty Breads

	Cal	Fat	Cbs
Asiago Cheese Demi, 2 oz.	160	4	22
Asiago Cheese Loaf, 2 oz.	160	4	23
Cinnamon Raisin Loaf, 2 oz.	180	3	34
Honey Wheat Loaf, 2 oz.	170	3	30
Hot Cross Buns, 1 bun	220	5	37
Sourdough Roll, 3 oz.	200	1	39
• Sourdough Soup Bowl, 8 oz.	590	3	118
Sourdough XL Loaf, 2 oz.	140	1	28
• Tomato Basil Loaf, 2 oz.	140	1	27
White Whole Grain Loaf, 2 oz.	140	3	26

Specialty Pastries

	Cal	Fat	Cbs
• Bear Claw, 5 oz.	460	24	54
French Croissant, 3 oz.	310	18	30
• Pastry Ring - Apple Cherry Chz, 3 oz.	220	10	27

Sweet Rolls

	Cal	Fat	Cbs
• Cinnamon Roll, 6 oz.	620	24	89
Cobblestone, 7 oz.	650	13	123
• Pecan Roll, 6 oz.	720	38	88

PAPA GINO'S

Appetizers (Small)

	Cal	Fat	Cbs
BBQ Chick Tenders, 234 g	520	18	55
Buff. Chick.Tender, 234 g	450	19	36
• Cheese Breadsticks, 378 g	970	39	116
Chicken Tender, 188 g	430	18	36
Chicken Wings BBQ, 257 g	640	32	58
Chicken Wings Buffalo, 328 g	930	76	33
Chicken Wings Honey BBQ, 257 g	650	34	62
Chicken Wings Plain, 172 g	480	32	24
Chkn Wings Plain w/ Honey Mustard, 257 g	650	36	65
Chicken Wings Plain w/ Ranch, 257 g	720	51	30
Chicken Wings Spicy BBQ, 257 g	580	33	41
Chicken Wings Teriyaki, 257 g	660	32	64
Cinnamon Stick Icing, 71 g	240	1	57
Cinnamon Sticks, 204 g	620	19	100
French Fries, 347 g	540	23	80

• MOST HEALTHY   • LEAST HEALTHY

PAPA GINO'S (cont.)

	Cal	Fat	Cbs
• Marinara Dip Sauce, 31 g	20	1	3
Mozzarella Sticks, 313 g	950	59	69
Entree			
Papa Platter-Penne, 550 g	990	32	135
Papa Platter-Spaghetti, 550 g	990	32	135
Pasta Trio Plate, 570 g	990	34	138
Penne, 474 g	650	11	118
Penne Alfredo, 417 g	900	36	111
Penne Alfredo Chicken Broccoli, 573 g	1050	42	116
• Ravioli, 383 g	590	24	71
Spag & Meatballs, 556 g	890	29	123
Spaghetti, 474 g	650	11	118
Spaghetti Alfredo, 417 g	900	36	111
Spaghetti Alfredo Chkn Broccoli, 573 g	1050	42	116
• Spaghetti Chick Parm, 663 g	1070	39	129
Kids			
• Cheese Slice, 158 g	310	9	42
Chicken Tender Meal, 258 g	510	21	54
• Hot Dog Meal, 273 g	620	35	64
Penne, 252 g	330	6	61
Pepperoni Slice, 172 g	380	16	42
Spaghetti & Meatball, 295 g	460	15	63
Large Thin Crust Pizza (Per Slice)			
BBQ Chicken, 130 g	270	7	38
Buffalo Chicken, 127 g	240	7	31
• Cheese, 113 g	220	6	31
Chicken and Roasted Garlic, 159 g	290	10	34
Chicken Pepper, 162 g	270	9	32
Hawaiian, 140 g	240	6	35
Meat Combo, 142 g	320	15	32
• Papa Roni, 140 g	320	15	32
Pepperoni, 123 g	270	11	31
Super Veggie, 178 g	240	7	35
The Works, 159 g	300	12	33
Pasta			
Single Breadsticks, 75 g	190	8	23
Pizza Slices (Per Slice)			
Cheese, 158 g	310	9	42
Pepperoni, 172 g	380	16	42
Rustic			
BBQ Chicken, 99 g	240	9	28
Buffalo Chicken, 97 g	220	9	23
• Cheese, 88 g	200	9	23
Chicken and Roasted Garlic, 116 g	240	10	25
Chicken Pepper, 119 g	230	10	24
Hawaiian, 106 g	220	9	26

• MOST HEALTHY   • LEAST HEALTHY

PAPA GINO'S (cont.)

	Cal	Fat	Cbs
Meat Combo, 109 g	280	15	24
• Papa Roni, 108 g	280	15	24
Pepperoni, 97 g	240	12	24
Super Veggie, 131 g	230	9	26
The Works, 116 g	250	13	24
Salads			
Buffalo Chicken Tender, 325 g	330	15	29
Caesar, 234 g	190	10	19
• Chicken Bacon Cheddar, 415 g	530	33	22
Chicken Caesar, 365 g	320	11	14
Chicken Tender, 308 g	320	14	29
• Garden, 289 g	180	8	25
Single Breadsticks, 75 g	190	8	23
Side			
• Meatballs (2), 128 g	280	21	9
Penne, 252 g	330	6	61
• Penne Alfredo, 209 g	450	18	55
Spaghetti, 252 g	330	6	61
Spaghetti Alfredo, 209 g	450	18	55
Slice Pizza Large			
BBQ Chicken, 186 g	390	9	56
• Breakfast Bacon/Egg, 224 g	560	29	46
Breakfast Egg & Cheese, 222 g	460	20	46
Breakfast Saus Egg & Cheese, 217 g	480	22	47
Breakfast Veg Egg & Cheese, 271 g	450	18	50
Buffalo Chicken, 181 g	350	9	46
Chicken Pepper, 228 g	390	12	48
Hawaiian, 198 g	340	9	52
Meat Combo, 201 g	460	20	47
Papa Roni, 198 g	460	21	48
Pepperoni, 176 g	380	14	47
• Super Veggie, 245 g	340	9	51
The Works, 224 g	420	16	49
Slice Pizza Thick Crust			
BBQ Chicken, 207 g	470	9	70
• Breakfast Bac Egg & Cheese, 267 g	680	31	63
Breakfast Egg & Cheese, 246 g	560	20	63
Breakfast Saus Egg & Cheese, 260 g	600	25	63
Breakfast Veg Egg & Cheese, 313 g	570	21	67
Buffalo Chicken, 202 g	430	10	61
Cheese, 201 g	450	13	62
Chicken and Roasted Garlic, 243 g	480	12	65
Chicken Pepper, 249 g	470	13	63
• Hawaiian, 220 g	430	9	66
Meat Combo, 222 g	540	21	62
Papa Roni, 220 g	540	21	62

• MOST HEALTHY   • LEAST HEALTHY

PAPA GINO'S (cont.)

	Cal	Fat	Cbs
Pepperoni, 200 g	480	15	64
Super Veggie, 268 g	430	10	66
The Works, 245 g	500	17	64
Sub Panini			
Basil Chicken, 399 g	1080	60	85
• Eggplant, 378 g	860	40	95
Italian Deli, 309 g	1050	69	69
• Sausage & Pepper, 445 g	1150	69	75
Subs (Large)			
Chicken Cutlet, 345 g	930	38	105
• Chicken Parmesan, 476 g	1090	44	113
• Vegetarian, 447 g	710	15	112
Subs (Small)			
BLT, 298 g	720	35	71
• Hot Dog, 128 g	400	25	31
• Italian, 313 g	910	48	69
Lobster Roll, 234 g	550	34	31
Meatball, 298 g	740	32	76
Meatball Parmesan, 326 g	840	41	76
Steak, 252 g	630	25	65
Steak & Cheese, 280 g	720	32	68
Super Steak, 429 g	760	32	76
Tuna, 241 g	740	39	67
Turkey, 224 g	460	4	72
Turkey Club, 333 g	630	23	70
Toppings (Per Large Slice)			
• Bacon, 13 g	80	7	0
Black Olives, 11 g	15	1	1
Broccoli, 20 g	5	0	1
Capicola, 6 g	5	0	0
Extra Cheese, 12 g	35	3	0
Green Pepper, 12 g	0	0	1
Hamburger, 19 g	50	4	0
Mushrooms, 12 g	5	0	0
Onions, 12 g	5	0	1
Pepperoni, 7 g	35	3	0
Sausage, 21 g	70	6	0
• Sliced Tomato, 7 g	0	0	0

PAPA JOHN'S PIZZA

BBQ Chicken & Bacon Pizza

	Cal	Fat	Cbs
Original Crust Pizza, 150 g	350	12	44
Thin Crust Pizza, 114 g	29	13	29
Cheese Pizza			
Original Crust Pizza, 125 g	290	10	37
Thin Crust Pizza, 90 g	230	12	22

• MOST HEALTHY • LEAST HEALTHY

PAPA JOHN'S PIZZA (cont.)

	Cal	Fat	Cbs
Garden Fresh Pizza			
Original Crust Pizza, 161 g	280	9	39
Thin Crust Pizza, 125 g	220	11	24
Hawaiian BBQ Chicken Pizza			
Original Crust Pizza, 164 g	350	12	46
Thin Crust Pizza, 127 g	290	13	31
Pepperoni Pizza			
Original Crust Pizza, 130 g	330	14	37
Thin Crust Pizza, 94 g	270	16	22
Sausage Pizza			
Original Crust Pizza, 134 g	330	15	37
Thin Crust Pizza, 97 g	270	16	22
Side Items			
Apple Pie, 190 g	480	10	90
BBQ Wings, 79 g	190	12	6
Breadsticks, 115 g	290	5	54
Buffalo Wings, 79 g	170	13	3
Cheesesticks, 136 g	370	16	41
• Chicken strips, 74 g	130	5	10
Chocolate Pastry Delights, 35 g	200	11	25
• Cinnamon Sweetsticks, 192 g	580	16	98
Cinnapie, 167 g	560	19	90
Garlic Parmesan Breadsticks, 124 g	340	10	54
Honey Chipotle Wings, 79 g	190	12	8
Spicy Italian Pizza			
Original Crust Pizza, 147 g	380	18	38
Thin Crust Pizza, 111 g	320	20	22
Spinach Alfredo Pizza			
Original Crust Pizza, 116 g	290	11	36
Thin Crust Pizza, 79 g	230	13	20
The Meats Pizza			
Original Crust Pizza, 148 g	370	17	38
Thin Crust Pizza, 112 g	310	19	22
The Works Pizza			
Original Crust Pizza, 157 g	230	120	39
Thin Crust Pizza, 121 g	270	15	23
Tuscan Six Cheese Pizza			
Original Crust Pizza, 133 g	320	13	38
Thin Crust Pizza, 96 g	260	14	22

PAPA MURPHY'S

	Cal	Fat	Cbs
Calzones			
Chicken Florentine, 218 g	470	20	46
Combo, 184 g	450	21	46
• Italian, 209 g	470	21	47
• Marinara Sauce Cup, 14 g	10	0	2

• MOST HEALTHY   • LEAST HEALTHY

PAPA MURPHY'S (cont.)

	Cal	Fat	Cbs
Veggie, 197 g	410	17	46
Family Size Stuffed Pizza			
5-Meat, 1 slice, 143 g	370	16	39
Big Murphy, 1 slice, 157 g	370	16	40
• Chicago Style, 1 slice, 149 g	370	16	40
• Chicken & Bacon, 1 slice, 151 g	370	15	39
Medium Size Original Crust Pizzas			
50/50, 1 slice, 97-131 g	280	14	26
All Meat, 1 slice, 113 g	290	14	25
Barbeque Chicken, 1 slice, 117 g	280	10	30
Cheese, 1 slice, 90 g	230	9	25
Cowboy, 1 slice, 125 g	290	15	26
Forty-Niner, 1 slice, 109 g	290	15	25
Gourmet Chicken Garlic, 1 slice, 112 g	260	12	25
Gourmet Classic Italian, 1 slice, 125 g	280	13	26
Gourmet Supreme, 1 slice, 98 g	250	11	26
Gourmet Vegetarian, 1 slice, 113 g	250	11	25
Hawaiian, 1 slice, 114 g	240	10	28
Herb Chkn Mediterranean, 1 slice, 102 g	270	12	27
• Murphy's Combo, 1 slice, 131 g	300	15	27
Papa's Favorite, 1 slice, 138 g	300	15	27
Papa-Roni, 1 slice, 100 g	270	14	25
Pepperoni, 1 slice, 97 g	260	13	25
Perfect, 1 slice, 97-114 g	250	11	26
Rancher, 1 slice, 114 g	270	13	26
Specialty of the House, 1 slice, 121 g	270	13	26
• Taco Grande, 1 slice, 101 g	220	10	23
Vegetarian Combo, 1 slice, 136 g	250	11	27
Veggie Mediterranean, 1 slice, 92 g	260	11	27
Side Items			
Apple Dessert Pizza, 97 g	240	5	46
Caesar Salad, 120 g	50	2	4
Cheesy Bread (without Sauce), 75 g	220	7	31
Cherry Dessert Pizza, 97 g	240	5	44
Chicken Caesar Salad, 170 g	140	5	5
Cinnamon Wheel, 82 g	250	7	42
Club Salad, 189 g	140	8	6
Cookie Dough w/ Hershey's Choco Chips, 28 g	120	6	17
Cream Cheese Frosting, 11 g	50	3	4
Croutons, 18 g	90	4	11
Garden Salad, 206 g	100	6	8
Italian Salad, 186 g	140	10	7
• Lasagna, 184 g	330	18	26
• Marinara Sauce Cup for Chzy Bread, 14 g	10	0	2
Thin Crust Pizzas			
50/50, 1 slice, 64-91 g	185	11	14

• MOST HEALTHY   • LEAST HEALTHY

PAPA MURPHY'S (cont.)

	Cal	Fat	Cbs
All Meat, 1 slice, 76 g	190	11	13
Barbeque Chicken, 1 slice, 79 g	180	8	17
• Cheese, 1 slice, 58 g	140	7	13
Chicken Bacon Artichoke, 1 slice, 78 g	180	9	13
Cowboy, 1 slice, 86 g	190	11	14
• Forty-Niner, 1 slice, 91 g	240	14	17
Gourmet Chicken Garlic, 1 slice, 76 g	170	9	13
Gourmet Classic Italian, 1 slice, 85 g	190	10	14
Gourmet Supreme, 1 slice, 64 g	160	8	14
Gourmet Vegetarian, 1 slice, 76 g	160	9	12
Hawaiian, 1 slice, 77 g	160	7	15
Herb Chkn Mediterranean, 1 slice, 68 g	180	9	15
Meat, 1 slice, 76 g	190	11	13
Murphy's Combo, 1 slice, 91 g	200	12	14
Papa's Favorite, 1 slice, 96 g	200	12	15
Pepperoni, 1 slice, 64 g	170	9	13
Rancher, 1 slice, 77 g	180	10	14
Specialty of the House, 1 slice, 82 g	180	10	14
Taco Grande, 1 slice, 87 g	180	10	16
Vegetarian Combo, 1 slice, 72 g	160	8	15
Veggie Mediterranean, 1 slice, 59 g	170	9	15
Veggie, 1 slice, 72 g	160	9	13

PEI WEI ASIAN DINER

Caramel Chicken

	Cal	Fat	Cbs
Beef (stock velveted), 2 per dish	360	12	36
• Beef, 2 per dish	570	31	54
Chicken (stock velveted), 2 per dish	370	14	37
Chicken, 2 per dish	490	23	44
• Shrimp (stock velveted), 2 per dish	310	12	36
Shrimp, 2 per dish	360	17	40
Vegs & Tofu (stock velveted), 2 per dish	390	17	43
Vegetables & Tofu, 2 per dish	420	21	45

Dan Dan Noodles

	Cal	Fat	Cbs
Chicken, 2 per dish	390	10	53

First Tastes & Add Ons

	Cal	Fat	Cbs
Crab Wontons (2), 1 per dish	170	10	13
• Crispy Potstickers (2), 1 per dish	150	8	12
Edamame, 2 per dish	160	7	9
• Hot & Sour Soup (bowl), 2 per dish	310	13	20
Pei Wei Spring Rolls (2), 1 per dish	210	7	35
Thai Wonton Soup (bowl), 2 per dish	200	8	21

Ginger Broccoli

	Cal	Fat	Cbs
Beef (stock velveted), 2 per dish	270	10	16
• Beef, 2 per dish	320	17	21
Chicken, 2 per dish	290	12	17

● MOST HEALTHY • LEAST HEALTHY

PEI WEI ASIAN DINER (cont.)

	Cal	Fat	Cbs
• Shrimp, 2 per dish	220	10	16
Vegetables & Tofu, 2 per dish	310	16	25
Gluten Free			
• Asian Chopped Chkn Salad, 2 per dish	230	12	10
Served w/ - Sweet Chile Sauce, 2 oz.	140	0	17
• Vietnamese Chkn Salad Rolls, 3 per dish	130	7	9
Honey Seared			
Beef (stock velveted), 2 per dish	300	3	38
Beef, 2 per dish	340	10	42
Chicken (stock velveted), 2 per dish	280	4	39
Chicken, 2 per dish	420	12	51
• Shrimp (stock velveted), 2 per dish	230	3	38
• Shrimp, 2 per dish	430	15	51
Vegs & Tofu (stock velveted), 2 per dish	330	8	45
Vegetables & Tofu, 2 per dish	370	13	48
Japanese Teriyaki Bowl with White Rice			
Beef (stock velveted), 2 per dish	500	8	75
Beef, 2 per dish	550	13	81
Chicken (stock velveted), 2 per dish	530	9	78
Chicken, 2 per dish	560	13	80
• Shrimp (stock velveted), 2 per dish	490	8	78
Shrimp, 2 per dish	530	12	80
Vegs & Tofu (stock velveted), 2 per dish	560	13	84
• Vegetables & Tofu, 2 per dish	600	17	86
Kid's Wei Honey Seared			
• Beef, 2 per dish	140	4	16
• Chicken, 2 per dish	180	5	21
Shrimp, 2 per dish	150	5	19
Kid's Wei Lo Mein			
Beef, 2 per dish	170	11	7
• Chicken, 2 per dish	180	11	6
• Shrimp, 2 per dish	110	8	5
Kid's Wei Teriyaki			
Beef, 2 per dish	235	11	21
• Chicken, 2 per dish	245	11	20
• Shrimp, 2 per dish	180	8	19
Lemon Pepper			
Beef (stock velveted), 2 per dish	260	10	18
• Beef, 2 per dish	480	29	36
Chicken (stock velveted), 2 per dish	280	12	19
Chicken, 2 per dish	400	21	26
• Shrimp (stock velveted), 2 per dish	210	10	18
Shrimp, 2 per dish	260	16	21
Vegs & Tofu (stock velveted), 2 per dish	290	16	26
Vegetables & Tofu, 2 per dish	330	20	27

• MOST HEALTHY   • LEAST HEALTHY

◢ PEI WEI ASIAN DINER (cont.)

	Cal	Fat	Cbs
Lo Mein Noodles			
Beef (stock velveted), 2 per dish	510	15	64
Beef, 2 per dish	540	20	68
Chicken (stock velveted), 2 per dish	520	16	65
Chicken, 2 per dish	560	20	67
• Shrimp (stock velveted), 2 per dish	480	15	64
Shrimp, 2 per dish	520	18	67
Vegs & Tofu (stock velveted), 2 per dish	550	20	71
• Vegetables & Tofu, 2 per dish	590	24	73
Mandarin Kung Pao			
Beef (stock velveted), 2 per dish	350	17	18
• Beef, 2 per dish	570	36	24
Chicken (stock velveted), 2 per dish	350	19	17
Chicken, 2 per dish	480	28	27
• Shrimp (stock velveted), 2 per dish	300	17	18
Shrimp, 2 per dish	400	28	22
Vegs & Tofu (stock velveted), 2 per dish	380	22	26
Vegetables & Tofu, 2 per dish	410	26	28
Mongolian			
Beef (stock velveted), 2 per dish	280	10	19
• Beef, 2 per dish	320	17	23
Chicken, 2 per dish	290	12	20
• Shrimp, 2 per dish	230	10	19
Vegetables & Tofu, 2 per dish	310	16	26
Noodle & Rice Bowls			
Beef (stock velveted), 2 per dish	490	11	65
Beef, 2 per dish	520	16	68
Chicken, 2 per dish	500	12	66
• Shrimp, 2 per dish	460	11	65
• Vegetables & Tofu, 2 per dish	530	16	72
Orange Peel			
Beef (stock velveted), 2 per dish	350	10	42
• Beef, 2 per dish	560	30	59
Chicken (stock velveted), 2 per dish	330	12	35
Chicken, 2 per dish	450	21	42
• Shrimp (stock velveted), 2 per dish	270	10	34
Shrimp, 2 per dish	320	16	38
Vegs & Tofu (stock velveted), 2 per dish	340	15	41
Vegetables & Tofu, 2 per dish	380	20	43
Pad Thai			
Beef (stock velveted), 2 per dish	710	18	105
• Beef, 2 per dish	790	26	109
Chicken, 2 per dish	720	20	105
• Shrimp, 2 per dish	680	18	105
Vegetables & Tofu, 2 per dish	750	23	111

• MOST HEALTHY   • LEAST HEALTHY

▶ PEI WEI ASIAN DINER (cont.)

	Cal	Fat	Cbs
Pei Wei Spicy			
Beef (stock velveted), 2 per dish	400	11	47
• Beef, 2 per dish	660	30	74
Chicken (stock velveted), 2 per dish	410	12	48
Chicken, 2 per dish	530	22	56
• Shrimp (stock velveted), 2 per dish	320	8	47
Shrimp, 2 per dish	400	16	51
Vegs & Tofu (stock velveted), 2 per dish	430	16	55
Vegetables & Tofu, 2 per dish	460	20	57
Pei Wei Spicy Salad			
Chicken, 2 per dish	550	24	60
Shrimp, 2 per dish	430	19	56
Rice & Noodles			
Brown Rice, 2 per dish	170	2	37
Egg Noodles, 2 per dish	220	3	39
• Fried Rice, 2 per dish	410	17	52
• Rice Noodles, 2 per dish	130	0	31
White Rice, 2 per dish	200	0	44
Rice & Noodles for Kid's wei			
Brown Rice, 2 per dish	100	1	20
Egg Noodles, 2 per dish	100	2	18
• Fried Rice, 2 per dish	320	17	32
• Rice Noodles, 2 per dish	60	0	14
White Rice, 2 per dish	110	0	24
Sauces & Sides			
Fried Wonton Strips, 1 cup	130	5	16
Lettuce Wrap Sauce, 2 oz. vol	50	3	3
Lime Vinaigrette, 1 oz. vol	110	10	4
• Potsticker Sauce, 2 oz. vol	30	1	3
Rice Sticks, 1 cup	130	0	33
• Sesame Ginger Dressing, 2 oz. vol	220	21	6
Side of Vegetables, 6 oz.	35	0	7
Sweet Chile Sauce, 2 oz. vol	140	0	17
Thai Peanut Sauce, 2 oz. vol	160	10	16
Spicy Korean			
Beef (stock velveted), 2 per dish	310	13	18
• Beef, 2 per dish	360	20	22
Chicken, 2 per dish	330	15	19
• Shrimp, 2 per dish	260	13	18
Vegetables & Tofu, 2 per dish	340	18	26
Sweet & Sour			
Beef (stock velveted), 2 per dish	240	1	34
Beef, 2 per dish	290	8	39
Chicken (stock velveted), 2 per dish	250	3	35
Chicken, 2 per dish	360	10	48
• Shrimp (stock velveted), 2 per dish	170	1	34

• MOST HEALTHY • LEAST HEALTHY

PEI WEI ASIAN DINER (cont.)	Cal	Fat	Cbs
• Shrimp, 2 per dish	370	13	47
Vegs & Tofu (stock velveted), 2 per dish	250	6	41
Vegetables & Tofu, 2 per dish	310	10	44
Thai Blazing Noodles			
Beef (stock velveted), 2 per dish	510	8	84
• Beef, 2 per dish	590	15	89
Chicken, 2 per dish	520	9	85
• Shrimp, 2 per dish	490	8	84
Vegetables & Tofu, 2 per dish	550	13	91
Thai Coconut Curry			
Beef (stock velveted), 2 per dish	350	19	20
• Beef, 2 per dish	390	25	24
Chicken, 2 per dish	360	20	21
• Shrimp, 2 per dish	280	18	20
Vegetables & Tofu, 2 per dish	380	24	27
Thai Dynamite			
Beef (stock velveted), 2 per dish	210	8	11
Beef, 2 per dish	260	15	15
Chicken (stock velveted), 2 per dish	230	10	12
Chicken, 2 per dish	330	17	24
• Shrimp (stock velveted), 2 per dish	160	8	11
• Shrimp, 2 per dish	350	20	24
Vegs & Tofu (stock velveted), 2 per dish	240	13	18
Vegetables & Tofu, 2 per dish	280	17	20
Wraps, Salads & Rolls			
Asian Chp Chkn Salad (w/o drss), 2 per dish	170	4	12
Asian Chopped Chicken Salad, 2 per dish	390	25	17
Minced Chkn w/ Cool Lettuce Wraps, 2 per dish	310	11	36
Pe Wei Spicy Shrimp Salad, 2 per dish	430	19	56
Pei Wei Spicy Chkn Salad (w/o drss), 2 per dish	505	19	60
• Pei Wei Spicy Chicken Salad, 2 per dish	560	24	62
• Vietnamese Chkn Salad Rolls, 3 per dish	130	7	9

PENN STATION			
Cheeses			
• American	100	5	1
• Provolone	100	8	1
Swiss	100	8	1
Condiments/Toppings			
• Olive Oil & Vinegar	96	11	0
Oregano	16	2	0
Parmesan Cheese	25	2	0
Pizza Sauce	18	0	4
• Sauerkraut	16	0	4
Teriyaki	28	0	5

• MOST HEALTHY   • LEAST HEALTHY

PENN STATION

Ingredient	Cal	Fat	Cbs
Bread (Small 7")	273	2	54
Wrap (10")	207	6	34

Meats

	Cal	Fat	Cbs
• Artichokes	8	0	2
Bacon	55	4	0
Chicken	47	1	0
Chicken Salad	66	5	3
Corned Beef	73	2	1
Ham	33	1	0
• Pepperoni	140	13	0
Salami	120	11	0
Sausage	90	7	1
Steak	38	2	0
Tuna Salad	60	4	3
Turkey (white)	25	0	0

Veggies

	Cal	Fat	Cbs
• Banana Peppers (Grilled)	1	0	0
Green Peppers (Grilled)	4	0	1
Lettuce	5	0	1
Mushrooms (Grilled)	3	0	0
Red Onions	17	0	3
Tomato	5	0	1
• Yellow Onions (Grilled)	21	0	5

PEPE'S MEXICAN

Pepe's Beef Menu Items

	Cal	Fat	Cbs
Beef & Bean Burrito, 228 g	510	24	52
Beef & Bean Tostada, 186 g	380	23	26
Beef Flauta - Plain, 57 g	160	9	10
Beef Flauta w/ Cheese and Sauce, 80 g	190	12	11
Beef Taco Crisp, 138 g	210	11	16
Beef Taco Salad w/Salsa - no shell, 475 g	330	19	20
• Beef Taco Salad with 4 oz. Salsa, 536 g	550	26	52
Beef Taco Soft Corn, 161 g	250	10	28
Beef Taco Soft Flour, 146 g	250	11	24
Refried Beans w/ Mexican Chz, 126 g	300	20	22
• Spanish Rice w/ Ranchera Sauce, 112 g	140	6	21

Pepe's Burrito

	Cal	Fat	Cbs
• Beef & Bean Burrito, 228 g	510	24	52
Chicken & Bean Burrito, 228 g	480	21	51
• Pork & Bean Burrito, 228 g	470	19	51

Pepe's Chicken Menu Items

	Cal	Fat	Cbs
Chicken & Bean Burrito, 228 g	480	21	51
Chicken & Bean Tostada, 186 g	360	21	21
• Chicken Enchilada Suiza, 124 g	190	9	15

• MOST HEALTHY   • LEAST HEALTHY

PEPE'S MEXICAN (cont.)

	Cal	Fat	Cbs
Chicken Flauta - Plain, 57 g	190	10	16
Chicken Flauta w/ Chz and Sauce, 80 g	230	13	17
Chicken Taco Crisp, 138 g	190	9	15
Chkn Taco Salad w/Salsa - no shell, 475 g	300	16	19
• Chicken Taco Salad w/ 4 oz. Salsa, 536 g	520	23	51
Chicken Taco Soft Corn, 161 g	230	8	27
Chicken Taco Soft Flour, 146 g	230	9	23

Pepe's Flauta

	Cal	Fat	Cbs
• Beef Flauta - Plain, 57 g	160	9	10
Beef Flauta w/ Chz and Sauce, 80 g	190	12	11
Chicken Flauta - Plain, 57 g	160	10	16
• Chicken Flauta w/ Sauce & Chz, 80 g	230	13	17

Pepe's Pork Menu Items

	Cal	Fat	Cbs
Pork & Bean Burrito, 228 g	470	19	51
Pork & Bean Tostada, 186 g	350	20	26
Pork Enchilada Suiza, 124 g	190	8	15
• Pork Taco Crisp, 135 g	170	6	16
Pork Taco Salad w/Salsa - no shell, 475 g	290	13	19
• Pork Taco Salad with 4 oz. Salsa, 536 g	500	20	52
Pork Taco Soft Corn, 160 g	220	6	27
Pork Taco Soft Flour, 145 g	220	7	24

Pepe's Salads

	Cal	Fat	Cbs
Beef Taco Salad w/Salsa - no shell, 475 g	330	19	20
• Beef Taco Salad with 4 oz. Salsa, 536 g	550	26	52
Chkn Taco Salad w/Salsa - no shell, 475 g	300	16	19
Chicken Taco Salad w/ 4 oz. Salsa, 536 g	520	23	51
• Pork Taco Salad w/Salsa - no shell, 475 g	290	13	19
Pork Taco Salad w/Salsa - 4 oz. Salsa, 536 g	500	20	52

Pepe's Taco

	Cal	Fat	Cbs
Beef Taco Crisp, 138 g	210	8	16
Beef Taco Soft Corn, 161 g	250	10	28
• Beef Taco Soft Flour, 146 g	250	11	24
Chicken Taco Crisp, 138 g	190	9	15
Chicken Taco Soft Corn, 161 g	230	8	27
Chicken Taco Soft Flour, 146 g	230	9	23
• Pork Taco Crisp, 135 g	170	6	16
Pork Taco Soft Corn, 160 g	220	6	27
Pork Taco Soft Flour, 145 g	220	7	24

Pepe's Tostada

	Cal	Fat	Cbs
• Beef & Bean Tostada, 186 g	380	23	26
Chicken & Bean Tostada, 186 g	360	21	21
• Pork & Bean Tostada, 186 g	350	20	26

PETER PIPER PIZZA

14" Large Pizza (Original)

	Cal	Fat	Cbs
Cheese, 105 g	300	10	36

• MOST HEALTHY   • LEAST HEALTHY

PETER PIPER PIZZA (cont.)

	Cal	Fat	Cbs
• Ham & Pineapple, 116 g	280	7	38
• Pepperoni & Sausage, 112 g	310	11	37
Pepperoni, 116 g	310	10	38
Sausage, 111 g	300	9	37

14" Large Specialty Pizza (Original)

	Cal	Fat	Cbs
5 Meat Supreme, 127 g	350	13	38
• California Veggie, 91 g	200	6	23
Chicago Classic, 121 g	300	10	38
• New York 3 Chz w/ Pepperoni, 127 g	380	16	38
Smokehouse, 130 g	370	15	38
The Werx, 140 g	320	11	38

Appetizers & Dessert

	Cal	Fat	Cbs
Breadsticks, 69 g	250	10	36
Chicken Strips, 138 g	300	9	26
Cinnamon Crunch Dessert, 86 g	220	2	49
• Garlic Cheese Bread, 92 g	310	14	37
• Wings, 48 g	110	8	0

Salad

	Cal	Fat	Cbs
Chicken Caesar, 229 g	200	8	10
• Family, 371 g	290	16	14
Garden, 250 g	50	0	10
Italian Chef, 114 g	20	0	4
• Side, 145 g	20	0	4

PETRO'S

Baked Potatoes

	Cal	Fat	Cbs
Broccoli 3 Cheese	657	30	77
Butter Sour Cream	482	18	74
• Lite	363	0	74
Loaded	679	33	78
• Loaded w/chili	780	37	90

Chili (Medium)

	Cal	Fat	Cbs
• Chicken	275	4	43
Original	370	14	42
• Veggie	385	11	58

Garden Salads

	Cal	Fat	Cbs
Garden Salads	43	1	8

Hot Dogs

	Cal	Fat	Cbs
Chili	315	17	28
Chili/Cheese	347	19	29
• Loaded	352	19	30
• Plain	266	14	22
Slaw	352	16	23

Lite Pasta Petro® (Medium)

	Cal	Fat	Cbs
Lite Pasta Petro®	494	4	80

PETRO'S (cont.)	Cal	Fat	Cbs
Lite Petro® (Medium)			
Lite Petro®	532	16	66
Pasta Petro® (Medium)			
Pasta Petro®	627	27	68
Petro Salads			
Grilled Chicken	742	41	42
Original	570	36	42
Petro® (Medium)			
• Chicken	665	36	59
Original	734	43	58
• Veggie	745	41	70
Tostitos™ Chips			
• Loaded Tostitos™ / Ultimate Nachos	880	51	79
Queso	500	27	60
Ransalsa	560	35	61
• Salsa	413	18	62

PHILLY CONNECTION			
Original Cheesesteak Sandwich			
7 inch (Small)	455	11	55
10 inch (Regular)	623	15	73

PICCADILLY			
Low Carb Items			
Baby Lima Beans, 5 oz.	105	6	10
Baked Cajun Bnlss Chkn Breast, 1 orders	379	19	9
Black Beans and Rice, 5 oz.	80	0	17
Blackened Bnlss Chkn Breast, 1 orders	297	14	3
Broccoli Florets, 3 oz.	92	7	6
• Broiled Chicken Half, 1 halves	1545	105	14
Buttered Baby Carrots, 3 oz.	84	6	8
Buttered Cabbage, 3 oz.	66	5	6
Buttered Okra, 3 oz.	78	6	6
Caesar Salad, 3 oz.	165	13	8
Cajun Baked Tilapia, 1 orders	332	20	4
Cauliflower w/ Cheese Sauce, 1 orders	173	10	5
Chicken and Dumplings, 8 oz.	285	10	7
Chicken Tetrazzini, 1 orders	376	21	18
Corn Bread Dressing, 5 oz.	143	7	14
Corn Sticks, 1 each	157	9	16
Cream of Broccoli Soup, 1 orders	151	10	16
French Style Baked Yellow Squash, 1 orders	97	4	14
Fried Butterflied Shrimp, 12 piece	139	15	0
Green Bean Supreme, 5 oz.	113	7	16
Green Beans, 1 orders	37	2	5
Greens, Turnip w/Diced Turnips, 1 orders	62	2	11

PICCADILLY (cont.)

	Cal	Fat	Cbs
Ham Steak, 3 oz.	107	6	1
Italian Salad Bowl, 1 orders	101	6	6
Large Angus Chop Steak, 10 oz.	884	65	5
Meat Sauce and Spaghetti, 1 orders	457	33	11
Mediterranean Style Tilapia, 8 oz.	240	8	8
Piccadilly Fruit Salad, 6 oz.	72	0	18
Roast Beef, 6 oz.	640	53	0
Sliced Bacon, 10 order	249	20	1
Small Angus Chopped Steak, 5 oz.	434	31	0
Smothered Okra, 5 oz.	109	8	10
Southwestern Boneless Chkn Breast, 1 orders	604	33	17
Spinach Salad, 1 orders	93	5	7
• Spring Salad Bowl, 3 oz.	18	0	4
Sweet Yellow Corn, 5 oz.	122	6	17
Tilapia with Shrimp Cream Sauce, 9 oz.	278	6	10
Tomato, Cucumber and Onion Salad, 4 oz.	42	0	10
Vegetable Soup, 8 fl.oz.	45	0	9
Yellow Squash and Zucchini, 1 orders	86	5	11

Popular Items

	Cal	Fat	Cbs
Ambrosia Fruit Salad, 7 oz.	287	14	43
Baked Macaroni and Cheese, 5 oz.	310	17	26
Beef Liver with Onion Sauce, 1 orders	363	20	22
Biscuits, 2 oz.	241	15	23
Black Forest Cake, 1 slice	330	14	49
Blackberry Cobbler, 8 oz.	658	25	101
Blackened Pork Chop w/ Fettuccine Alfredo, 8 oz.	658	30	35
Blackened Shrimp w/ Fettuccine, 13 oz.	827	40	73
Black-Eyed Peas, 1 orders	193	2	32
Bread Pudding with Rum Sauce, 7.5 oz.	807	23	107
Breaded Okra, 3.25 oz.	242	13	26
Broccoli and Rice, Au Gratin, 5 oz.	387	17	42
Buttermilk Chess Pie, 1 slice	635	30	87
Candied Sweet Potatoes, 4.5 oz.	304	0	77
Caramel Custard, 1 each	445	7	84
Carrot Souffle, 5 oz.	392	17	58
Cheese Grits, 1 orders	1004	71	45
Cheesecake, 1 slice	649	41	55
Cherry Cobbler, 8 oz.	506	20	76
Chicken Cacciatore, 14 oz.	896	18	139
Chicken Florentine, 8 oz.	464	9	44
Chicken Parmigiana, 1 orders	1238	36	135
Chkn Teriyaki w/ Polynesian Rice, 1 orders	659	16	79
• Chicken-Rice Soup, 1 cup	100	0	20
Chocolate Cake, 1 slice	377	16	55
Chocolate Cream Pie, 1 slice	693	48	66
Coconut Cream Pie, 1 slice	549	33	59

• MOST HEALTHY   • LEAST HEALTHY

PICCADILLY (cont.)

	Cal	Fat	Cbs
Crawfish Etouffee, 1 orders	555	14	84
Cupcakes, 1 each	171	8	24
Custard Pie, 1 slice	348	13	49
French Fried Potatoes, 4.5 oz.	219	10	31
Fresh Strawberry and Banana, 10 oz.	380	1	52
Fried Chicken, 2 pieces	797	46	33
Garlic Bread, 1 slice	205	10	25
Grits, 1 orders	355	16	49
Italian Boneless Chkn Breast, 1 orders	819	62	25
Italian Cream Cake, 1 slice	715	38	85
Italian Delight Cake, 1 slice	563	35	62
Italian Rotini Salad, 4 oz.	283	19	26
Lemon Icebox Pie, 1 slice	589	31	71
• Lemon Pepper Chicken Half, 1 halves	1546	105	22
Mashed Potatoes, 5 oz.	117	4	19
Meatballs and Spaghetti, 12 oz.	814	40	80
Mexican Corn Bread, 1 each	213	13	20
Mexican Style Pinto Beans, 5 oz.	384	15	66
Mississippi Mud Pie, 1 slice	439	29	43
Neptune Salad, 5 oz.	244	14	25
New Orleans Style Sauteed Shrimp, 5 oz.	837	40	78
Old Fashion Brownie, 1 slice	1005	35	176
Parmesan Crusted Tilapia, 1 each	351	9	27
Pea Salad, 5 oz.	291	17	20
Peach Cobbler, 8 oz.	545	22	82
Peanut Butter Choco Satin Pie, 6 slice	758	54	62
Pecan Pie, 1 slice	675	28	99
Potato Salad, 4 oz.	168	7	24
Pumpkin Pie, 1 slice	310	11	48
Red Beans with Rice/Sausage, 5.5 oz.	806	42	76
Red Velvet Cake, 1 slice	833	54	83
Roasted New Potatoes, 5 oz.	198	7	31
Salmon Pattie, 1 orders	231	9	24
Seafood Gumbo, 1 orders	227	6	32
Sesame Glaze Boneless Chkn Breast, 9 oz.	717	34	57
Shrimp and Corn Soup, 1 cup	201	10	19
Shrimp Creole and Rice, 1 orders	1065	32	176
Shrimp Diablo, 10 oz.	443	10	54
Shrimp Scampi and Fettuccini, 1 orders	648	42	35
Smothered Pork Chop, 8 oz.	732	34	46
Soft Roll, 2 oz.	211	8	30
Southern Fried Fish, 2 pieces	451	26	20
Southwest Fiesta Chkn Salad, 1 orders	698	37	35
SW Style Pork Chop w/Mexican Rice, 8 oz.	954	31	113
Spiced Beets, 4 oz.	144	0	34
Strawberry Shortcake, 1 orders	351	14	55

• MOST HEALTHY   • LEAST HEALTHY

PICCADILLY (cont.)

	Cal	Fat	Cbs
Sweet Potato Pie, 1 slice	473	21	68
Tomato-Macaroni Soup, 1 cup	111	1	22
Turkey and Dressing, 1 orders	377	14	43
Waffles, 1 each	129	4	19
Watermelon, 11 order	170	1	43

PIZZA HUT

9" Personal PANormous™ Pizza

	Cal	Fat	Cbs
Cheese Only, 402 g	1100	45	124
Dan's Original, 477 g	1270	62	124
Ham & Pineapple, 421 g	1020	37	128
Hawaiian Luau, 446 g	1150	49	129
Italian Sausage & Red Onion, 464 g	1210	56	128
• Meat Lover's®, 491 g	1470	80	123
Pepperoni & Mushroom, 419 g	1050	42	123
Pepperoni, 387 g	1100	48	121
Spicy Sicilian, 463 g	1220	57	126
Supreme, 488 g	1270	62	125
Triple Meat Italiano, 447 g	1280	62	123
• Veggie Lover's®, 463 g	1010	38	127

12" Fit 'n Delicious® Pizza

	Cal	Fat	Cbs
Chicken, Mushrooms & Jalapeño, 93 g	170	5	22
• Chkn, Red Onion & Green Pepper, 95 g	180	5	23
• Diced Red Tomato, Mshr & Jalapeño, 87 g	150	4	23
Green Pepper, Red Onion & Diced Red Tomato, 89 g	150	4	24
Ham, Pineapple & Diced Red Tomato, 84 g	160	5	24
Ham, Red Onion & Mushroom, 84 g	160	5	23

12" Medium Hand-Tossed Style Pizza

	Cal	Fat	Cbs
Cheese Only, 84 g	220	8	26
Dan's Original, 103 g	260	12	26
Ham & Pineapple, 91 g	200	7	27
Hawaiian Luau, 98 g	240	10	27
Italian Sausage & Red Onion, 99 g	240	11	27
• Meat Lover's®, 105 g	300	16	25
Pepperoni & Mushroom, 91 g	210	8	26
Pepperoni, 83 g	230	10	25
Spicy Sicilian, 99 g	250	11	26
Supreme, 106 g	260	12	26
Triple Meat Italiano, 96 g	260	12	25
• Veggie Lover's®, 102 g	200	7	27

12" Medium Pan Pizza

	Cal	Fat	Cbs
Cheese Only, 91 g	240	11	27
Dan's Original, 110 g	280	14	27
Ham & Pineapple, 97 g	230	9	28
Hawaiian Luau, 104 g	260	12	28
Italian Sausage & Red Onion, 106 g	270	13	28

• MOST HEALTHY   • LEAST HEALTHY

▷ PIZZA HUT (cont.)

	Cal	Fat	Cbs
• Meat Lover's®, 113 g	330	18	27
Pepperoni & Mushroom, 97 g	240	10	27
Pepperoni, 90 g	250	12	26
Spicy Sicilian, 106 g	270	13	27
Supreme, 112 g	290	14	27
Triple Meat Italiano, 103 g	290	15	27
• Veggie Lover's®, 107 g	230	9	28

12" Medium Thin 'N Crispy® Pizza

	Cal	Fat	Cbs
Cheese Only, 65 g	190	8	22
Dan's Original, 85 g	240	12	22
Ham & Pineapple, 73 g	180	6	23
Hawaiian Luau, 81 g	220	10	24
Italian Sausage & Red Onion, 81 g	220	10	23
• Meat Lover's®, 85 g	280	16	22
Pepperoni & Mushroom, 73 g	190	8	22
Pepperoni, 63 g	200	9	21
Spicy Sicilian, 81 g	220	10	22
Supreme, 88 g	240	12	23
Triple Meat Italiano, 76 g	240	12	22
• Veggie Lover's®, 86 g	180	6	23

12" Pizza Mia™ Pizza

	Cal	Fat	Cbs
Cheese Only, 74 g	200	7	24
Pepperoni, 72 g	200	8	24

14" Large Stuffed Crust Pizza

	Cal	Fat	Cbs
Cheese Only, 132 g	350	14	39
Dan's Original, 159 g	420	21	39
Ham & Pineapple, 143 g	340	13	41
Hawaiian Luau, 151 g	380	16	41
Italian Sausage & Red Onion, 153 g	390	18	40
• Meat Lover's®, 165 g	480	26	39
Pepperoni & Mushroom, 142 g	350	15	39
Pepperoni, 134 g	380	17	38
Spicy Sicilian, 153 g	400	19	40
Supreme, 163 g	420	21	40
Triple Meat Italiano, 151 g	420	21	39
• Veggie Lover's®, 155 g	330	13	40

Appetizers

	Cal	Fat	Cbs
Baked Hot Wings (2 pieces), 44 g	100	6	1
Baked Mild Wings (2 pieces), 44 g	110	7	1
Breadsticks (each), 44 g	150	7	19
• Cheese Breadsticks (each), 56 g	180	7	20
• Marinara Dipping Sauce (3 oz), 85 g	60	0	12

Bone Out Wings

	Cal	Fat	Cbs
• All American, 54 g	150	8	11
Buffalo Burnin Hot, 73 g	190	8	18
Buffalo Medium, 73 g	190	9	18

• MOST HEALTHY   • LEAST HEALTHY

▶ PIZZA HUT (cont.)

	Cal	Fat	Cbs
Buffalo Mild, 73 g	190	9	18
Cajun, 77 g	200	8	21
• Garlic Parmesan, 71 g	260	19	11
Honey BBQ, 82 g	220	8	27
Spicy Asian, 80 g	210	8	24
Spicy BBQ, 81 g	200	8	21
Crispy Bone In Wings			
• All American, 55 g	200	14	8
Buffalo Burnin Hot, 75 g	230	15	16
Buffalo Medium, 75 g	230	15	16
Buffalo Mild, 75 g	230	15	16
Cajun, 79 g	240	14	19
• Garlic Parmesan, 72 g	300	25	9
Honey BBQ, 83 g	260	14	24
Spicy Asian, 82 g	250	14	21
Spicy BBQ, 82 g	240	14	19
Desserts			
White Icing Dipping Cup (2 oz), 57 g	170	0	44
• Hershey's® Choco Sauce (1.5 oz), 43 g	120	3	24
• Hershey's® Choco Dunkers® (2 pc), 60 g	200	9	26
Cinnamon Sticks (2 pieces), 55 g	170	6	26
P'Zone® Pizza			
Classic, 235 g	630	23	77
• Marinara Dipping Sauce (3 oz), 85 g	60	0	12
• Meaty, 246 g	710	31	76
Pepperoni, 219 g	630	24	76
Side items			
Apple Pie (2 pies), 87 g	330	17	40
• Fried Cheese Sticks (4 pcs), 119 g	380	24	29
• Wedge Fries (1/2 order), 123 g	320	18	35
Stuffed Pizza Rollers			
Marinara Dipping Sauce (3 oz), 85 g	60	0	12
Stuffed Pizza Rollers, 76 g	230	10	24
Traditional Wings			
• All American, 39 g	80	5	0
Buffalo Burnin Hot, 59 g	110	6	8
Buffalo Medium, 59 g	110	6	8
Buffalo Mild, 59 g	110	6	8
Cajun, 63 g	120	5	11
• Garlic Parmesan, 56 g	180	16	1
Honey BBQ, 67 g	140	5	16
Spicy Asian, 65 g	130	5	13
Spicy BBQ, 66 g	120	5	11
Tuscani Pastas			
• Bacon Mac N Cheese, 324 g	520	22	54
Chicken Alfredo, 323 g	630	33	56

• MOST HEALTHY   • LEAST HEALTHY

	Cal	Fat	Cbs
PIZZA HUT (cont.)			
Lasagna, 321 g	600	33	43
Meaty Marinara, 315 g	520	24	50
PIZZA PIZZA			
Bone-in Chicken			
9 cut breast, 1 pc 150 g	350	21	13
• 9 cut drumstick, 1 pc 80 g	160	9	6
9 cut keel, 1 pc 140 g	270	13	7
• 9 cut thigh, 1 pc 155 g	440	34	9
9 cut wing, 1 pc 80 g	190	12	10
Breads - sides			
Garlic Bread/Toast, 2 pieces	240	9	36
Garlic Stick, 2 sticks	360	12	54
Chicken Item			
Classic Wings, 200 g	380	26	6
• Crispy Breaded Wings, 276 g	740	50	28
• Boneless Chicken Bites, 100 g	200	8	19
Chicken Strips, 138 g	290	13	21
Shrimp, 40 g	220	12	18
Chips			
Doritos Collision, 45 g	230	12	28
Doritos Nachos Cheese, 45 g	230	12	29
• Lay's Classic, 43 g	240	15	22
Miss Vickie's Sea Salt & malt Vinegar, 43 g	230	13	25
• Rold Gold Pretzels, 50 g	190	1	41
Sunchips Country BBQ, 43 g	210	9	29
Classic Pizzas (Medium)			
Bacon Double Cheeseburger, 99 g	230	9	28
• Big Bacon Bonanza, 106 g	290	15	28
Canadian Eh!, 113 g	230	9	29
• Cheese, 89 g	190	5	29
Classic Super, 112 g	200	6	29
Garden Veggie, 111 g	190	5	29
New York Pepperoni, 95 g	210	9	28
Pepperoni, 96 g	190	6	29
Sausage Mushroom Melt, 114 g	280	8	27
Spicy BBQ Chicken, 117 g	220	5	34
Sweet Heat, 108 g	200	5	30
Tropical Hawaiian, 113 g	280	14	29
Classic Pizzas (Slice)			
Bacon Double Cheeseburger, 295 g	690	27	84
Big Bacon Bonanza, 312 g	820	41	83
Canadian Eh!, 324 g	680	27	86
• Cheese, 258 g	560	14	83
Classic Super, 324 g	600	18	87
Garden Veggie-Classic Dough, 358 g	600	16	89

• MOST HEALTHY   • LEAST HEALTHY

PIZZA PIZZA (cont.)

	Cal	Fat	Cbs
Garden Veggie, 358 g	600	17	86
New York Pepperoni, 281 g	610	24	84
Pepperoni, 286 g	590	18	85
• Sausage Mushroom Melt, 314 g	830	22	82
Spicy BBQ Chicken, 357 g	670	15	103
Sweet Heat, 324 g	610	15	89
Tropical Hawaiian, 331 g	820	39	86

Dipping Sauces

	Cal	Fat	Cbs
• Creamy garlic, 57 g	360	39	2
Honey garlic sauce, 70 g	110	0	26
Hot wing sauce, 63 g	70	0	16
Italian Marinara, 57 g	30	1	4
Jalapeño cheddar, 57 g	210	20	4
Mild wing sauce, 63 g	70	0	17
Peppercorn ranch, 57 g	300	32	2
Plum Sauce, 57 g	100	0	24
• Poutine sauce, 57 g	15	0	3
Seafood sauce, 57 g	70	0	16
Sweet Chili Thai, 57 g	110	0	25

Gluten Free Crust

	Cal	Fat	Cbs
Crust Only, 38 g	80	2	16

Pasta

	Cal	Fat	Cbs
• Cheese Tortollini Alfredo, 340 g	710	41	71
Mac and Cheese, 340 g	680	34	75
• Penne Bolognese, 340 g	440	9	71

Salads

	Cal	Fat	Cbs
Caesar Salad, 186 g	110	4	14
• Garden Salad, 326 g	50	0	11
• Mediterranean Greek Salad, 361 g	170	11	12

Sauces

	Cal	Fat	Cbs
Bruschetta, 50 g	55	6	3
• Classic tomato, 50 g	20	0	5
Homestyle Pizzaletto, 60 g	40	2	5
• Pesto, 50 g	183	17	0

Signature Pizzas (Medium)

	Cal	Fat	Cbs
Bacon Chicken Mushroom Melt, 114 g	280	8	28
Chicken Bruschetta Parm, 93 g	180	6	21
Grilled Veggie and Goat Cheese, 122 g	210	6	30
Loaded Classic, 120 g	230	10	29
• Meat Supreme, 131 g	280	12	29
Mediterranean Vegetarian, 112 g	200	5	31
• Pesto Amore, 85 g	170	7	19
Pesto Con Pollo, 102 g	230	8	28
Philly Cheese Steak, 119 g	230	7	30
Sweet Chili Chicken, 92 g	180	5	27

• MOST HEALTHY   • LEAST HEALTHY

PIZZA PIZZA (cont.)

	Cal	Fat	Cbs
Signature Pizzas (Slice)			
• Bacon Chicken Mushroom Melt, 332 g	850	24	85
Chicken Bruschetta Parm, 334 g	700	22	88
Grilled Veggie and Goat Cheese, 378 g	660	20	91
Loaded Classic, 347 g	670	28	88
Meat Supreme, 361 g	760	31	86
Mediterranean Vegetarian, 346 g	620	17	93
Pesto Amore, 301 g	650	23	82
Pesto Con Pollo, 324 g	750	28	85
Philly Cheese Steak, 346 g	690	21	90
• Quattro Formaggio, 298 g	610	18	87
Sweet Chili Chicken, 308 g	660	16	101
Snack Item			
Apple Pie/Turnover, 85 g	220	8	34
Onion Rings, 4 oz.	253	12	33
• Reg. Fries, 5 oz.	290	12	42
• Two-Bite Brownies, 18 g (one)	85	5	10
Stuffed Sandwich			
Bacon Cheeseburger, 156 g	350	13	43
• Basic Cheese and Sauce, 142 g	290	8	42
Classic Super, 177 g	310	10	44
Garden Veggie, 174 g	300	8	44
Mediterranean Vegetarian, 185 g	310	8	48
Pepperoni, 162 g	320	11	44
• Tropical Hawaiian, 220 g	600	37	44

PLANET SMOOTHIE

	Cal	Fat	Cbs
Cool Blended Smoothies			
• P B & J	700	32	98
Shag-a-delic	300	0	77
The Last Mango	340	1	85
• Twig & Berries	280	0	74
Vinnie del Rocco	370	0	92
Energy Smoothies			
Berry Bada-Bing	350	1	92
Chocolate Elvis	430	17	68
Frozen Goat	220	1	55
• Grape Ape	210	0	54
• Java the Nut	480	23	61
Road Runner	300	0	75
Spazz	270	0	69
Kids Smoothies			
Bonzai Berry (12 oz)	210	0	55
Captain Kid (12 oz)	180	0	46
• Peanut Butter Dream (12 oz)	270	17	27
Plain Jane (12 oz)	170	0	42

● MOST HEALTHY   • LEAST HEALTHY

PLANET SMOOTHIE (cont.)

	Cal	Fat	Cbs
• Purple Primate (12 oz)	160	0	40
Strawberry Shortcake (12 oz)	160	0	41
Twig Jr. (12 oz)	200	0	53
Protein Smoothies			
Big Bang -protein blast	370	0	80
Big Bang -workout blast	340	0	87
Chocolate Chimp -protein blast	220	2	38
• Chocolate Chimp -workout blast	190	2	45
Merlin's Mix -pineapple (32 oz)	330	2	29
Merlin's Mix -straw/banana (32 oz)	390	2	47
• Merlin's Mix -strawberry (32 oz)	460	2	65
Mr. Mongo -chocolate (protein blast)	300	2	59
Mr. Mongo -chocolate (workout blast)	270	2	66
Mr. Mongo -strawberry (protein blast)	370	0	82
Mr. Mongo -strawberry (workout blast)	350	0	89
Weight Loss Smoothies			
Billy Bob Banana	260	1	66
Leapin' Lizard	250	0	64
Lunar Lemonade -raspberry	250	0	63
Lunar Lemonade -strawberry	250	0	63
Mediterranean Monster	260	0	68
Rasmanian Devil	270	0	70
• Two Piece Bikini -chocolate	220	5	52
• Two Piece Bikini -strawberry	290	0	72
Wellness Smoothies			
Acai	370	7	76
Acai Bowl	370	10	66
• Earth Quaker	490	2	118
Hangover Over	310	0	83
Screamsicle	290	0	73
Thelma & Louise	260	0	65
Werewolf	270	0	69
Yo' Adriane	320	0	83
• Zeus Juice	250	0	64

POLLO TROPICAL

	Cal	Fat	Cbs
Condiments			
Chimichurri, 1 oz.	110	11	3
• Cilantro Garlic, 1 oz.	160	17	1
Curry Mustard Sauce, 1 oz.	150	17	0
• Fuego Salsa, 1 oz.	5	0	1
Guava BBQ Sauce, 1 oz.	50	0	12
Mojo Sauce, 1 oz.	80	9	1
Salsa, 1 oz.	5	0	1
Desserts/Frozen Beverages			
• Flan, 4 oz.	210	9	26

POLLO TROPICAL (cont.)	Cal	Fat	Cbs
Guava Cheesecake, 5 oz.	310	17	36
Key Lime Pie, 4 oz.	320	13	59
Mango Tropichiller® Crm Smoothie, 17 oz.	330	8	63
Mango Tropichiller®, 16 oz.	290	0	72
Piña Colada Tropichiller® Crm Smoothie, 17 oz.	330	9	65
Piña Colada Tropichiller®, 16 oz.	310	4	76
Strwbry Tropichiller® Crm Smoothie, 17 oz.	330	8	63
Strawberry Tropichiller®, 16 oz.	290	0	72
• Tres Leches, 5 oz.	380	9	76
Entrées Only			
1/4 Chicken dark meat w/o skin, 3 oz.	180	9	0
1/4 Chicken dark meat, 4 oz.	270	17	0
1/4 Chicken white meat w/o skin, 5 oz.	230	7	0
1/4 Chicken white meat, 6 oz.	350	17	0
1/4 rack Ribs, 2 oz.	200	15	1
Boneless Chicken Breasts (2), 6 oz.	230	4	0
• Churrasco Steak, 4 oz.	170	7	4
• Roast Pork, 6 oz.	400	22	1
Fajitas			
Chicken, 29 oz.	1150	35	151
Steak, 29 oz.	1140	40	154
Kids Meals			
1/4 Chicken dark meat w/skin, 13 oz.	650	23	75
• Cheese Quesadilla (each), 14 oz.	820	38	93
• Chicken Breast, 13 oz.	500	8	75
Salads, Soups, Wraps & Sandwiches			
• Caesar Salad, 3 oz.	140	12	4
• Caribbean Cobb Chicken Salad, 22 oz.	950	41	57
Chicken Caesar Salad, 15 oz.	750	46	13
Chicken Caesar Wrap, 5 oz.	360	18	29
Chicken Chipotle Sandwich, 7 oz.	480	19	44
Classic Chicken Sandwich, 7 oz.	480	18	46
Cuban Wrap, 5 oz.	400	21	30
Guava Pork BBQ Sandwich, 6 oz.	460	14	52
Large Caribbean Chicken Soup, 17 oz.	250	4	43
Side Dishes			
Balsamic Tomatoes (Regular Side), 5 oz.	110	8	9
Black Beans w/ Mojo (Regular Side), 5 oz.	120	4	23
Boiled Yuca w/ Mojo (Regular Side), 11 oz.	340	9	68
Caesar Salad (Regular Side), 4 oz.	210	19	6
• Chicken Gravy (Regular Side), 2 oz.	38	3	3
• Coleslaw (Regular Side), 8 oz.	570	51	29
Curly Fries (Regular Side), 0 oz.	0	0	0
Dinner Roll, 1 oz.	90	1	17
Flour Tortilla, 1 oz.	100	3	16
Garlic Mashed Potatoes (Reg.), 8 oz.	280	12	38

• MOST HEALTHY   • LEAST HEALTHY

POLLO TROPICAL (cont.)

	Cal	Fat	Cbs
Kernel Corn (Regular Side), 8 oz.	240	7	37
Macaroni & Cheese (Regular Side), 9 oz.	410	23	36
Red Beans w/ Mojo (Regular Side), 9 oz.	250	5	40
White Rice (Regular Side), 8 oz.	330	5	67
Yellow Rice w/ Vegs (Regular Side), 8 oz.	240	4	48

Tropical Favorites

	Cal	Fat	Cbs
• Cheezy Yuca Bites (6 pieces), 7 oz.	290	14	32
• Fried Yuca (5 pieces), 6 oz.	500	24	69
Sweet Plantains (5 pieces), 5 oz.	310	8	63

Tropichops® (Regular)

	Cal	Fat	Cbs
Chkn w/White Rice & Black Beans, 17 oz.	530	10	90
• Chkn w/Yellow Rice & Vegetables, 10 oz.	330	5	51
• Pork w/White Rice & Black Beans, 18 oz.	680	22	92
Pork w/Yellow Rice & Vegetables, 13 oz.	490	18	54
Ropa Vieja (shredded beef), 19 oz.	600	16	98
Vegetarian, 19 oz.	580	12	110

POPEYE'S CHICKEN & BISCUITS

Big Deals

	Cal	Fat	Cbs
Chicken Biscuit, 102 g	350	20	30
• Delta Mini, 101 g	300	13	30
• Loaded Chicken Wrap, 170 g	400	17	44

Big Easys

	Cal	Fat	Cbs
Chicken Bowl, 368 g	570	29	44
Crispy Chicken Sandwich, 227 g	560	23	56

Cajun Wings

	Cal	Fat	Cbs
Cajun Wing segments, 244 g	595	43	19

Louisiana Legends

	Cal	Fat	Cbs
• Chicken Etouffee, 151 g	160	10	6
• Chicken Sausage Jambalaya, 151 g	220	11	20
Crawfish Etouffee, 151 g	180	5	25
Smothered Chicken, 151 g	210	8	24

Louisiana Travelers

	Cal	Fat	Cbs
Mild Tenders, 174 g	375	17	24
• Nuggets, 71 g	220	12	13
• Spicy Tenders, 174 g	405	17	30

Mild Chicken

	Cal	Fat	Cbs
• Breast, 179 g	350	20	8
• Leg, 63 g	110	7	3
Thigh, 111 g	280	20	7
Wing, 59 g	150	10	5

Mild Chicken (Skinless & Breading Removed)

	Cal	Fat	Cbs
Breast, 123 g	120	2	0
Leg, 52 g	50	2	0
• Strips, 94 g	130	3	3
Thigh, 72 g	80	4	0

• MOST HEALTHY   • LEAST HEALTHY

POPEYE'S CHKN & BISCUITS (cont.)

	Cal	Fat	Cbs
• Wing, 42 g	40	2	0

Naked Chicken Strips
Naked, 118 g	220	10	2

Sandwiches
• Deluxe Mild w/mayo or Deluxe spicy, 265 g	630	31	53
Deluxe Mild wo/mayo, 237 g	480	15	54
• Po Boy Sandwich, 113 g	330	17	36

Seafood
Butterfly Shrimp, 102 g	310	19	22
Popcorn Shrimp, 85 g	280	16	22

Sides
Biscuits, 60 g	240	13	26
Cajun Rice, 117 g	170	6	22
Cinnamon Apple Turnover, 86 g	250	12	34
Coleslaw, 138 g	260	23	14
Corn on the Cobb, 284 g	190	2	37
French Fries, 88 g	310	17	35
• Green Beans, 100 g	70	1	14
Mashed Potatoes & Gravy, 142 g	120	4	18
Mashed Potatoes No Gravy, 113 g	100	3	17
Red Beans & Rice, 174 g	320	19	31

Spicy Chicken
• Breast, 179 g	360	22	8
• Leg, 63 g	100	5	3
Thigh, 111 g	300	24	7
Wing, 59 g	140	9	5

Spicy Chicken (Skinless & Breading Removed)
Breast, 123 g	120	2	1
Leg, 52 g	50	2	0
• Strips, 94 g	150	4	5
Thigh, 72 g	80	3	2
• Wing, 42 g	40	2	0

PORT OF SUBS

Chicken
• Buffalo Chicken Griller, 5" Griller	245	13	37
• Chipotle Chicken Griller, 5" Griller	261	12	38
Teriyaki Chicken Griller, 5" Griller	259	15	41

Cold Submarine Sandwiches
Bacon Lettuce & Tomato, 8 oz.	519	30	43
• Ham American, 10 oz.	382	20	45
Ham Salami Capicolla Pepp Provolone, 10 oz.	532	26	45
Ham Salami Provolone, 9 oz.	469	21	45
Ham Turkey Provolone, 10 oz.	434	15	46
Peppered Pastrami Swiss, 9 oz.	439	17	44
Peppered Pastrami Turkey Swiss, 8 oz.	511	26	44

• MOST HEALTHY   • LEAST HEALTHY

▶ PORT OF SUBS (cont.)

	Cal	Fat	Cbs
Roast Beef Provolone, 10 oz.	421	14	43
Roast Beef Turkey Provolone, 10 oz.	421	14	45
Roasted Chicken Breast Provolone, 10 oz.	410	13	45
Salami Pepperoni Provolone, 8 oz.	511	27	45
Salami Provolone, 8 oz.	479	25	45
Salami Turkey Provolone, 9 oz.	465	20	46
Smoked Ham Swiss, 10 oz.	447	17	45
Smkd Ham Tkey Smokey Cheddar, 10 oz.	431	15	47
Tuna (without cheese), 9 oz.	422	18	45
Turkey Provolone, 11 oz.	421	14	47
• Vegetarian, 11 oz.	599	33	49
Cookies			
• Brownies, 5 oz.	300	10	48
Chocolate Chunk Cookie, 5 oz.	560	19	72
Oatmeal Raisin Cookie, 5 oz.	500	23	68
• White Chunk Macadamia Nut Cookie, 5 oz.	580	31	70
Eating Light			
• Ham Turkey, 10 oz.	328	5	46
Peppered Pastrami, 8 oz.	293	4	44
Roast Beef, 9 oz.	315	4	43
Roast Beef Turkey, 9 oz.	315	4	45
Roasted Chicken Breast, 9 oz.	304	3	44
Smoked Ham, 8 oz.	301	4	44
Smoked Ham Turkey, 10 oz.	320	5	46
Turkey, 10 oz.	315	4	47
• Vegetarian (without cheese), 7 oz.	238	2	44
Fresh Salads			
Caesar Salad, 6 oz.	333	30	7
Chef Salad, 11 oz.	388	25	13
Garden Salad, 8 oz.	93	5	10
• Grilled Chicken Caesar Salad, 13 oz.	541	34	15
Grilled Chicken Salad, 13 oz.	300	10	16
Tuna Salad, 11 oz.	311	23	12
Kid's Meal Sandwich			
• Grilled Cheese, 3 oz.	112	10	5
Ham, 3 oz.	200	3	4
• Salami, 3 oz.	254	9	4
Turkey, 3 oz.	190	3	4
Sides			
Macaroni Salad, 145 g	330	22	28
Potato Salad, 145 g	230	12	28
Sliced Fresh GRILLERS™			
• BBQ Pork Griller, 299 g	782	18	104
Grilled Chicken Griller, 245 g	518	13	58
Hot Pastrami Griller, 245 g	538	15	58
Italian Griller, 218 g	553	21	58

• MOST HEALTHY   • LEAST HEALTHY

PORT OF SUBS (cont.)	Cal	Fat	Cbs
• Meatball, 245 g	440	31	51
N.Y. Steak & Cheese Griller, 245 g	615	18	57

PRET A MANGER

Bagels

	Cal	Fat	Cbs
Classic Bagel & Cream Cheese, 146 g	390	10	63
• Energy Bagel, 4 oz.	340	5	66
• Smoked Salmon & Cream Cheese, 176 g	440	15	63

Baguette

	Cal	Fat	Cbs
• American Tuna Baguette, 233 g	620	30	63
Bag. of the Week: Aged Chdr & Chutney, 295 g	610	25	67
w/ Chicken Caesar, 303 g	580	20	68
w/ Turkey & Bacon, 300 g	590	20	67
w/ Smkd Salmon & Cream Chz, 235 g	520	20	64
Brkfst Bag. - Classic Egg & Bacon, 138 g	370	20	37
• w/ - Cream Chz, Tomato & Basil, 141 g	270	10	39
w/ - Classic Egg & Rstd Tomato, 153 g	360	20	42
Brie & Basil, 261 g	500	20	58
Chicken Mozzarella, 323 g	500	16	68
Pret's Famous Ham & Cheese, 227 g	560	20	55
Roasted Beef, Arugula & Parmesan	460	0	0

Cookies, Cakes & Treats

	Cal	Fat	Cbs
Banana Cake	420	24	48
Carrot Cake	460	29	47
Chocolate Brownie	390	20	51
• Chocolate Cake	470	19	71
Chocolate Chunk Cookie	310	16	43
Fruit & Oat Slice	430	19	57
Harvest Cookie	350	8	24
Love Bar	460	25	54
Love Bite	250	13	30
Mini Brownie	200	11	25
• Nuts & Bolts	160	NA	NA
Raspberry Bar	390	18	55
Royale Cookie	330	NA	NA

Croissants & Pastries

	Cal	Fat	Cbs
• Almond Croissant, 95 g	410	23	41
Ham, Swiss & Rstd Tomato Croissant, 137 g	400	22	34
• Pain au Chocolat, 82 g	300	15	34
Plain Croissant, 85 g	300	16	32

Hot Wraps

	Cal	Fat	Cbs
• Jalapeño Chicken Hot Wrap, 312 g	400	21	46
Spicy Falafel Hot Wrap, 280 g	540	24	61
• Swedish Meatball Ragu Hot Wrap, 334 g	700	37	49

Muffins & Hot Oatmeal

	Cal	Fat	Cbs
Blueberry Muffin, 135 g	360	9	68

• MOST HEALTHY   • LEAST HEALTHY

► PRET A MANGER (cont.)

	Cal	Fat	Cbs
• Bran Muffin, 135 g	290	9	53
Cranberry & Orange Muffin, 125 g	370	12	62
Hot Oatmeal, 485 g	590	12	97

Pret Yogurt Pots

	Cal	Fat	Cbs
• LF Yogurt, Banana & Honey Pret Pot, 312 g	480	20	83
LF Yogurt, Blbry & Granola Pret Pot, 259 g	360	20	47
Low Fat Yogurt Yoga Bunny Pret Pot, 187 g	250	12	28

Salad & Sushi

	Cal	Fat	Cbs
Chicken & Avocado Salad, 350 g	430	28	41
Chicken Caesar Salad, 278 g	400	16	24
Pret's Cobb & Greens Salad, 313 g	430	24	30
Red, White and Greens Salad, 230 g	300	17	14
• Salmon & Brown Rice Salad, 240 g	560	25	59
• Salmon Snack Box, 171 g	290	8	39
Shrimp & Salmon Sushi, 298 g	480	7	78
Tofu & Veggie Sushi, 240 g	360	5	63
Tuna Nicoise Salad, 498 g	310	15	16

Sandwiches

	Cal	Fat	Cbs
Aged Cheddar & Chutney, 268 g	550	30	52
American Tuna, 204 g	560	30	46
• Avocado & Parmesan, 293 g	570	27	59
Balsamic Chicken & Avocado, 259 g	520	25	58
BLT, 219 g	510	25	50
Chicken & Bacon, 254 g	480	20	58
Chicken, Apple & Cranberry, 226 g	490	20	60
Classic Turkey Club, 336 g	520	21	59
Corned Beef & Pickle Deli, 202 g	460	20	48
Egg Salad, Spinach & Parmesan, 285 g	570	26	53
Pret's Egg Salad & Arugula, 183 g	460	20	47
Snd of the Week: w/ Chkn Caesar, 254 g	440	15	51
w/ Falafel, Tomato & Spinach, 327 g	460	10	81
w/ Hummus & Roasted Tomato, 296 g	490	20	71
w/ Red, White & Greens, 274 g	380	10	25
w/ Smoked Salmon & Egg, 213 g	490	25	49
w/Tuna Nicoise, 300 g	550	30	20
• Slim Snd of the Week: Bacon & Avocado	275	N/A	N/A
w/ Cream Cheese & Veggie	295	N/A	N/A
Slow Roasted Beef & Horseradish Sauce, 196 g	490	15	49
Smoked Ham & Egg, 196 g	450	16	48

Soups (Medium)

	Cal	Fat	Cbs
Angus Steak Chili with Beans, 12 oz.	345	11	35
Beef Barley & Vegetables, 12 oz.	165	5	18
Chicken Noodle, 12 oz.	165	3	20
Chunky Tomato Stew, 12 oz.	135	5	20
• Corn Chowder, 12 oz.	38	17	51
Cream of Pea & Bacon, 12 oz.	465	21	38

• MOST HEALTHY   • LEAST HEALTHY

PRET A MANGER (cont.)	Cal	Fat	Cbs
Hungarian Mushroom, 12 oz.	285	20	18
Malaysian Chicken, 12 oz.	390	20	36
Miso Soup	45	1	6
Moroccan Lentil, 12 oz.	435	20	54
• New England Clam Chowder, 12 oz.	525	36	32
Souper Reuben, 12 oz.	300	17	23
Sweet Butternut Squash, 12 oz.	270	15	32
Tomato Bisque, 12 oz.	315	18	29
Veggie Split, 12 oz.	330	5	29

PRETZEL TIME

Blended Drinks

	Cal	Fat	Cbs
Cool Cappuccino, 20 fl.oz.	640	21	107
Mango Madness, 729 g	520	16	89
Mocha Mania, 20 fl.oz.	620	20	106
• Power Pomegranate, 729 g	490	16	86
• Rockin' Raspberry, 20 fl.oz.	650	20	117
Strawberry Banananza, 20 fl.oz.	650	20	115

Lemonade

	Cal	Fat	Cbs
Original Lemonade, 44 oz.	380	0	91

Pretzel

	Cal	Fat	Cbs
Caramel Crunch Pretzel, 119 g	300	4	58
Cinnamon Sugar Pretzel, 110 g	330	4	65
• Everything Pretzel, 131 g	420	10	72
Garlic Pretzel, 119 g	310	4	60
Iced Cinnamon Swirl Pretzel, 110 g	330	4	65
Parmesan Pretzel, 113 g	310	4	60
Ranch Pretzel, 119 g	320	5	60
Salted Pretzel, 119 g	310	4	59
• Unsalted Pretzel, 119 g	280	1	59

Pretzel Bites

	Cal	Fat	Cbs
• Cinnamon Sugar Pretzel Bites, 110 g	330	4	65
• Salted Pretzel Bites, 100 g	250	1	52
Unsalted Pretzel Bites, 100 g	250	1	52

Pretzel Dogs

	Cal	Fat	Cbs
Pretzel Dogs, 158 g	480	29	38

PRETZELMAKER

Blended Drinks

	Cal	Fat	Cbs
Cool Cappuccino, 20 fl.oz.	640	21	107
Mango Madness, 729 g	520	16	89
Mocha Mania, 20 fl.oz.	620	20	106
• Power Pomegranate, 729 g	490	16	86
• Rockin' Raspberry, 20 fl.oz.	650	20	117
Strawberry Banananza, 20 fl.oz.	650	20	115

• MOST HEALTHY   • LEAST HEALTHY

PRETZELMAKER (cont.)	Cal	Fat	Cbs
Lemonade			
Original Lemonade, 44 oz.	380	0	91
Pretzel			
Caramel Crunch Pretzel, 119 g	300	4	58
Cinnamon Sugar Pretzel, 110 g	330	4	65
• Everything Pretzel, 131 g	420	10	72
Garlic Pretzel, 119 g	310	4	60
Iced Cinnamon Swirl Pretzel, 110 g	330	4	65
Parmesan Pretzel, 113 g	310	4	60
Ranch Pretzel, 119 g	320	5	60
Salted Pretzel, 119 g	310	4	59
Unsalted Pretzel, 119 g	280	1	59
Pretzel Bites			
• Cinnamon Sugar Pretzel Bites, 110 g	330	4	65
• Salted Pretzel Bites, 100 g	250	1	52
Unsalted Pretzel Bites, 100 g	250	1	52
Pretzel Dogs			
Pretzel Dogs, 158 g	480	29	38

QDOBA MEXICAN GRILL			
3 Cheese Nachos			
Grilled Chicken, 13 oz.	970	46	84
Grilled Steak, 13 oz.	970	44	88
• Grilled Vegetables, 13 oz.	710	33	92
• Ground Beef, 13 oz.	1070	60	84
Pulled Pork, 14 oz.	910	35	102
Shredded Beef, 14 oz.	970	42	92
Burritos			
• Flour Tortilla Burrito, 4 oz.	330	8	54
Grilled Chicken, 7 oz.	520	18	55
Grilled Steak, 7 oz.	520	17	57
Grilled Vegetables, 7 oz.	390	12	59
• Ground Beef, 7 oz.	570	25	55
Pulled Pork, 8 oz.	490	13	64
Shredded Beef, 8 oz.	520	16	59
Chips & Dips Section			
• 3-Cheese Queso, 6 oz.	470	29	43
Fiery Habanero, 4 oz.	295	13	40
Guacamole, 6 oz.	450	27	46
Mango Salsa, 4 oz.	310	13	44
• Pico de Gallo, 4 oz.	290	13	38
Roasted Chile Corn, 4 oz.	340	14	48
Salsa Roja, 4 oz.	295	13	41
Salsa Verde, 4 oz.	295	13	40
Grilles Quesadilla			
Cheese Only, 8 oz.	770	44	55

• MOST HEALTHY   • LEAST HEALTHY

QDOBA MEXICAN GRILL (cont.)

	Cal	Fat	Cbs
Grilled Chicken, 11 oz.	960	54	56
Grilled Steak, 11 oz.	960	53	58
Grilled Vegetables, 11 oz.	830	48	60
• Ground Beef, 11 oz.	1010	61	56
Pulled Pork, 12 oz.	930	49	65
Shredded Beef, 12 oz.	960	52	60

Signature Flavors

	Cal	Fat	Cbs
Ancho Chile BBQ Burrito, 6 oz.	280	12	19
• Fajita Ranchera Burrito, 6 oz.	205	9	5
Grilled Veggie Burrito, 7 oz.	250	13	8
Mexican Gumbo, 12 oz.	280	14	12
Poblano Pesto Burrito, 6 oz.	250	14	6
• Queso Burrito, 6 oz.	290	17	6

Taco Salad

	Cal	Fat	Cbs
Grilled Chicken, 7 oz.	205	10	4
Grilled Steak, 7 oz.	205	9	6
• Grilled Vegetables, 7 oz.	75	4	4
• Ground Beef, 7 oz.	255	17	4
Pulled Pork, 8 oz.	175	5	13
Shredded Beef, 8 oz.	205	8	8

Tacos

	Cal	Fat	Cbs
Grilled Chicken, 2 oz.	120	7	8
Grilled Steak, 2 oz.	120	6	9
• Grilled Vegetables, 2 oz.	80	4	10
• Ground Beef, 2 oz.	140	9	9
Pulled Pork, 2 oz.	110	5	11
Shredded Beef, 2 oz.	120	6	10

Tortilla Soup

	Cal	Fat	Cbs
Grilled Chicken, 9 oz.	150	8	9
Tortilla Soup, 8 oz.	90	5	9

QUIZNO'S SUB

Classic Subs (Regular)

	Cal	Fat	Cbs
Classic Club	510	13	62
• Classic Italian	640	31	60
Honey Bacon Club	510	13	63
Honey Bourbon Chicken	440	7	59
The Traditional	450	9	63
Turkey Bacon Guacamole	590	19	64
• Turkey Ranch & Swiss	430	8	63
Veggie	460	16	59

Everyday Value Deli Subs (Regular)

	Cal	Fat	Cbs
Honey-Cured Ham & Swiss	430	9	61
Oven Roasted Turkey and Cheddar	420	8	62
Roast Beef & Cheddar	430	7	63
• Tuna Melt	870	58	59

• MOST HEALTHY   • LEAST HEALTHY

QUIZNO'S SUB (cont.)

	Cal	Fat	Cbs
Flatbread Sammies			
Alpine Chicken Sammie	240	6	26
Bistro Steak Sammie	200	4	28
Cantina Chicken Sammie	220	5	27
• Italiano Sammie	290	14	26
Roadhouse Steak Sammie	210	4	29
Sonoma Turkey Sammie	200	5	28
• Veggie Sammie	190	6	27
Qkidz Subs and Sammies			
• Cheesy Sammie	230	10	25
• Cheesy Sub	220	10	21
• Ham & Cheese Sub	140	3	21
Ham and Cheese Sammie	170	4	25
Turkey & Cheese Sub	140	3	22
Turkey and Cheese Sammie	170	4	26
Regular chopped salads			
Chicken Caesar Regular Chopped Salad	230	9	8
Chicken Taco Regular Chopped Salad	230	7	8
Chili Taco Regular Chopped Salad	230	11	20
Classic Cobb Regular Chopped Salad	250	13	9
Honey Mustard Chkn Reg Chopped Salad	260	12	9
• Pan Asian Regular Chopped Salad	170	3	7
• Rspbry Chipotle Chkn Reg Chopped Salad	310	16	8
Savory Soups (Cup)			
Broccoli Cheese Soup	130	9	9
• Chicken Noodle Soup	60	1	8
• Chili	140	4	15
Tomato Basil Soup	80	4	6
Signature Subs (Regular)			
Baja Chicken	550	17	57
Bourbon Grille Steak	610	22	61
• Chicken Carbonara	550	17	56
Double Cheese Cheesesteak	610	22	62
Honey Mustard Chicken	560	17	59
Mesquite Chicken	560	17	59
Prime Rib and Peppercorn	610	22	62
• Steakhouse Beef Dip	620	24	60
Toasty Bullets			
Beef Bacon & Cheddar Bullet	280	7	38
Italian Bullet	340	15	35
Pesto Turkey Bullet	260	7	37
• Tuna Melt Bullet	350	19	35
Turkey Club Bullet	270	7	37
Toasty Torpedoes			
Beef Bacon & Cheddar Torpedo	620	16	85
Italian Torpedo	730	31	80

• MOST HEALTHY   • LEAST HEALTHY

QUIZNO'S SUB (cont.)

	Cal	Fat	Cbs
• Torpedo	570	14	84
• Tuna Melt Torpedo	750	38	79
Turkey Club Torpedo	600	16	83

RANCH 1

Dressings/Sauces

	Cal	Fat	Cbs
Dressing, Chipotle Ranch, 1 oz.	165	18	1
Dressing, Sesame Ginger, 1 oz.	59	3	8
Sauce, Ancho Chile Pepper, 1 oz.	134	14	1
Sauce, Pepper & Onion Saute, 1 oz.	143	16	1
• Sauce, Roasted Red Pepper, 1 oz.	232	26	0
Sauce, Spicy, 1 oz.	34	0	8
• Sauce, Teriyaki, 1 oz.	24	0	5

Fries

	Cal	Fat	Cbs
Fries, Cheese, Reg, 9 oz.	493	27	54
Fries, Medium, 6 oz.	381	21	43

Individual Items

	Cal	Fat	Cbs
• Chicken, Crispy, 5 oz.	326	15	22
Chicken, Grilled, 4 oz.	146	6	0
Chicken, Popcorn, 4 oz.	325	12	30
Green Mix for Sandwiches, 3 oz.	31	2	2
Peppers & Onions, 2 oz.	27	2	3
Rice, 4 oz.	97	0	21
Roll, 6", 3 oz.	175	1	35
Steamed Vegetables, 3 oz.	27	0	6
• Tomato, Onion & Carrot Fajita Mix, 3 oz.	20	0	5
Tortilla Strips, 1 oz.	93	4	12

Other Items

	Cal	Fat	Cbs
Bowl, Chicken Teriyaki, 19 oz.	504	7	78
Chicken on Mixed Greens, 21 oz.	340	19	17
Chicken Tenders, 6 oz.	387	14	32
Chicken, Popcorn - Small, 6 oz.	325	12	30
Fajitas, Chicken, 10 oz.	540	24	53
• Platter, Chicken - Rice, 11 oz.	273	6	28
• Wrap, Grilled Chicken Caesar, 13 oz.	746	41	55

Salads - Completed

	Cal	Fat	Cbs
Salad, Grilled Chicken Caesar, 13 oz.	429	30	14
• Salad, Mandarin Chicken, 19 oz.	817	43	78
• Salad, Mixed Greens w/ Chkn no dress, 16 oz.	317	19	14
Salad, Southwest Chicken, 18 oz.	744	50	44

Sandwiches

	Cal	Fat	Cbs
Chicken & Cheese, 11 oz.	389	12	39
Chicken Philly, 9 oz.	410	13	40
• Crispy Chicken, 11 oz.	711	39	60
Crispy Spicy Chicken, 11 oz.	543	17	68
Grilled Spicy Chicken, 10 oz.	363	7	46

• MOST HEALTHY   • LEAST HEALTHY

▶ RANCH 1 (cont.)

	Cal	Fat	Cbs
Ranch 1 Classic, 9 oz.	683	47	37
• Ranch 1 Classic w/o sauce, 8 oz.	335	9	37
Teriyaki Chicken, 10 oz.	404	7	56

▶ RED LOBSTER

Accompaniments

	Cal	Fat	Cbs
Baked Potato	190	1	40
Caesar Salad	270	21	13
Cheddar Bay Biscuit™ (each)	150	8	16
Coleslaw	200	15	13
• Creamy Langostino Lobster Baked Potato	370	12	48
Creamy Langostino Lobster Mashed Potatoes	360	22	23
Fresh Asparagus (seasonal)	60	3	5
• Fresh Broccoli	45	1	6
Freshly Cooked Potato Chips	300	19	28
Fries	330	17	40
Garden Salad	90	3	13
Home-Style Mashed Potatoes	180	9	22
Wild Rice Pilaf	180	3	34

Add to Any Meal

	Cal	Fat	Cbs
• Maine Lobster Tail	60	1	0
• North Pacific King Crab Legs, 1/2 lb	130	1	1
Snow Crab Legs, 1/2 lb	80	1	0

Chef's Creations

	Cal	Fat	Cbs
• Mediterranean Shrimp Fresh Fish Topping	200	10	11
Seaport Lobster and Shrimp	610	19	44
• Wood-Grilled Tilapia w/ Spicy Soy Broth	630	20	64

Create Your Own Feast

	Cal	Fat	Cbs
Fried Crawfish	750	47	49
Fried Oysters	590	32	58
Garlic Shrimp Scampi	190	13	1
Garlic-Grilled Jumbo Shrimp	110	3	3
• Parrot Isle Jumbo Coconut Shrimp	780	44	72
Seafood-Stuffed Flounder	160	5	6
Shrimp Linguini Alfredo	550	29	41
• Steamed Snow Crab Legs	80	1	0
Walt's Favorite Shrimp	470	26	34
Wood-Grilled Fresh Salmon	210	9	0
Wood-Grilled Peppercorn Sirloin	280	10	0

Create Your Own Festival of Shrimp

	Cal	Fat	Cbs
BBQ Bacon-Wrapped Shrimp	450	25	36
• Cajun Shrimp	290	8	35
Coconut Shrimp Bites	290	18	19
Crab-and-Seafood-Stuffed Shrimp	380	24	17
Garlic-Cream Shrimp	380	14	44
• Wood-Grilled Pecan-Crusted Shrimp	470	23	48

• MOST HEALTHY   • LEAST HEALTHY

▶ RED LOBSTER (cont.)

	Cal	Fat	Cbs
Create Your Own Lunch			
• Bay Scallops-Broiled	70	1	2
Bay Scallops-Fried	140	7	9
Chicken Breast Strips	410	24	28
Crunch-Fried Fish	410	24	27
• Fried Crawfish	420	26	28
Hand-Breaded Shrimp	130	8	7
Lightly Breaded Clam Strips	370	22	31
Desserts			
• Chocolate Wave	1490	81	172
Key Lime Pie	580	22	88
NY-Style Cheesecake w/ Strawberries	520	36	39
Surf's Up Sundae	770	31	117
Warm Apple Crumble à la Mode	1070	51	142
• Warm Chocolate Chip Lava Cookie	170	9	20
Dressings & Dipping Sauces			
Cocktail Sauce, 2 oz.	40	0	9
Marinara Sauce, 2 oz.	25	1	4
• Pico de Gallo, 2 oz.	10	0	2
Piña Colada Sauce, 2 oz.	80	4	12
• Remoulade, 2 oz.	230	22	6
Sweet and Spicy Glaze, 2 oz.	100	0	24
Drinks			
• Casco Bay Coolers Banana Bay Choco Smoothie	460	14	78
Casco Bay Coolers Bry Strwbry Banana Smoothie	340	9	63
Casco Bay Coolers Cherry Wave Slushy	290	0	73
Casco Bay Coolers Sunset Strawberry Smoothie	250	6	47
• Red Rockin' Shirley T	170	0	43
Kid's Entrees			
Broiled Fish	150	1	3
• Chicken Fingers	410	24	28
Grilled Chicken	210	4	14
Macaroni & Cheese	280	7	42
Popcorn Shrimp	140	7	13
• Snow Crab Legs	80	1	0
Light House Menu			
Chilled Jumbo Shrimp Cocktail	120	1	9
Fresh Asparagus (Seasonal)	60	3	5
Fresh Broccoli	45	1	6
Garden Salad (Before Dressing)	90	3	13
• Petite Shrimp Salad Topping	15	0	0
Rainbow Trout, Wood-Grilled Broiled	220	10	6
• Salmon, Wood-Grilled or Broiled	270	9	6
Steamed Live Maine Lobster, 1 1/4 lb	45	0	0
Tilapia, Wood-Grilled or Broiled	210	3	9

● MOST HEALTHY • LEAST HEALTHY

▶ RED LOBSTER (cont.)

	Cal	Fat	Cbs
Lobster, Crab & Shrimp			
Chef's Sig. Lobster and Shrimp Pasta, Half Portion	510	25	43
Crab Linguini Alfredo, Half Portion	560	25	47
• Live Maine Lobster, 1 1/4 lb	45	0	0
North Pacific King Crab Legs	390	4	2
• Parrot Isle Jumbo Coconut Shrimp	980	55	90
Rock Lobster Tail	90	1	0
Rockzilla	130	2	0
Shrimp Your Way Coconut Shrimp Bites	290	18	19
Shrimp Your Way Fried Shrimp	190	11	9
Shrimp Your Way Popcorn Shrimp	180	9	16
Shrimp Your Way Scampi	130	9	1
Snow Crab Legs-1 pound	160	1	0
Stuffed Maine Lobster	240	7	12
Walt's Favorite Shrimp	700	39	52
Lunch Classics			
• Cajun Chkn Linguini Alfredo, Lunch Portion	630	27	45
Crunchy Popcorn Shrimp	280	14	26
Farm-Raised Catfish, Blackened	190	9	0
Farm-Raised Catfish, Fried	220	12	3
Flounder, Broiled	150	1	0
Flounder, Fried	210	8	2
Garlic Shrimp Scampi	130	9	1
Hand-Breaded Shrimp	230	13	11
Maple-Glazed Chicken	410	7	55
Sailor's Platter	300	7	9
Seafood-Stuffed Flounder	160	5	6
Shrimp Linguini Alfredo-Lunch Portion	550	29	41
Walleye-Beer Battered	350	21	12
Walleye-Blackened	150	4	5
• Walleye-Broiled	130	2	0
Walleye-Fried	300	15	18
Monday and Tuesday Specials			
• Shrimp Lover's Mon & Tues Coconut Shrimp Bites	290	18	19
Shrimp Lover's Mon & Tues Fried Shrimp	190	11	9
Shrimp Lover's Mon & Tues Popcorn Shrimp	180	9	16
• Shrimp Lover's Mon & Tues Scampi	130	9	1
Nonalcoholic Drinks			
Bahama Mama	230	0	57
Berry Mango Daiquiri	210	0	52
Classic Margarita - Frozen	280	0	69
• Classic Margarita - On the Rocks	150	0	22
Piña Colada	280	7	52
Raspberry Margarita	330	0	81
• Sail Away Smoothie - Banana Bay Choco	460	14	78

RED LOBSTER (cont.)	Cal	Fat	Cbs
Sail Away Smoothie - Berry Strawberry Banana	340	9	63
Sail Away Smoothie - Sunset Strawberry	250	6	47
Strawberry Daiquiri	230	0	56
Strawberry Margarita	340	0	85
Sunset Passion Colada	330	8	62
Tropical Freeze - Orange	250	6	49
Tropical Freeze - Pineapple	250	5	50

Quick Catches for Lunch

	Cal	Fat	Cbs
Beer-Battered Shrimp and Chips	540	35	40
Coastal Soup & Salad w/ Bayou Seafood Gumbo	660	20	81
Coastal Soup & Salad w/ Crmy Potato Bacon Soup	700	29	84
Coastal Soup & Salad w/ New England Clam Chowder	710	30	79
Coastal Soup & Salad w/ Seafood Gumbo	680	22	87
Coastal Soup & Salad w/ Spicy Shrimp Soup	630	20	81
Crunch-Fried Fish Sandwich	730	37	67
Hand-Tss Caesar Salad w/ Wood-Grl Chkn	670	52	14
Hand-Tss Caesar Salad w/ Wood-Grl Shrimp	620	34	47
Shrimp & Wood-Grl Chkn w/ Hand-Breaded Shrimp	520	18	43
Shrimp & Wood-Grl Chkn w/ Wood-Grl Shrimp Skewer	380	8	34
Shrimp & Wood-Grl Chkn w/ Garlic Shrimp Scampi	380	8	36
Shrimp Jambalaya	590	51	14
Wood-Grl Chkn BLT, w/ Fresh Cooked Chips	1030	55	68
• Wood-Grl Salmon BLT, w/ Fresh Cooked Chips	1110	59	68
• Wood-Grilled Shrimp Skewers	360	7	47

Seaside Starters

	Cal	Fat	Cbs
Buffalo Chicken Wings	680	39	0
Chicken Breast Strips	410	24	28
Chilled Jumbo Shrimp Cocktail	120	1	9
Clam Strips	370	22	31
Crispy Calamari and Vegetables	760	49	58
Fried Crawfish	1190	69	104
Fried Oysters	590	31	66
• Hand-Shucked Oysters - 1 Dozen	100	3	7
Lobster Nachos	1090	64	94
Lobster Pizza	720	30	69
• Lobster, Artichoke and Seafood Dip	1200	74	101
Lobster, Crab & Seafood Stuffed Mshr	380	21	20
Mango-Jalapeño Shrimp Skewers	560	22	58
Mozzarella Cheesesticks	340	20	24
New England Seafood Sampler	760	43	45
Pan-Seared Crab Cakes	280	14	13
Parrot Isle Jumbo Coconut Shrimp	590	33	54
Peach-Bourbon BBQ Scallops	430	27	24
Steamed Clams	430	15	10
Stuffed Mushrooms	220	12	12
Wood-Grilled Shrimp Bruschetta	650	26	58

• MOST HEALTHY   • LEAST HEALTHY

RED LOBSTER (cont.)

	Cal	Fat	Cbs
Shrimp			
Crunchy Popcorn Shrimp	560	27	51
Shrimp Linguini Alfredo, Half Portion	550	29	41
Shrimp Your Way Coconut Shrimp Bites	290	18	19
Shrimp Your Way Fried Shrimp	190	11	9
Shrimp Your Way Popcorn Shrimp	180	9	16
• Shrimp Your Way Scampi	130	9	1
• Walt's Favorite Shrimp	700	39	52
Signature Combinations			
• Admiral's Feast	1500	87	110
• Broiled Seafood Platter	280	8	11
Seaside Shrimp Trio	1030	57	68
Ultimate Feast®	620	30	29
Soups and Salads			
Bayou Seafood Gumbo, Cup	190	6	15
Creamy Potato Bacon Soup, Cup	220	15	19
• Manhattan Clam Chowder, Cup	80	1	12
• New England Clam Chowder, Cup	230	17	13
Seafood Gumbo, Cup	230	8	25
Spicy Shrimp Soup, Cup	160	6	15
Specialty Drinks			
• Alotta Colada	700	16	95
Bahama Mama	350	0	62
Berry Mango Daiquiri	350	0	51
Big Berry Daiquiri	350	0	65
• Mango Mai Tai	190	0	34
Mudslide	520	21	52
Piña Colada	320	6	55
Red Passion Colada	310	5	55
Strawberry Daiquiri	250	0	46
Sunset Passion Colada	360	0	35
Triple Berry Sangria	200	8	63
Traditional Favorites			
Broiled Seafood Platter	280	8	11
Cajun Chkn Linguini Alfredo, Half Portion	630	27	45
Flounder-Broiled	320	2	10
Flounder-Fried	440	16	5
Seafood-Stuffed Flounder	320	11	13
• Walleye-Beer Battered	700	42	24
Walleye-Blackened	300	7	9
• Walleye-Broiled	260	4	0
Walleye-Fried	600	29	35
Wood-Fire Grilled Shellfish			
• Garlic-Grilled Jumbo Shrimp	370	9	40
Maui Luau Shrimp and Salmon	760	16	82
Peach-Bourbon BBQ Shrimp and Scallops	540	27	36

• MOST HEALTHY   • LEAST HEALTHY

▶ RED LOBSTER (cont.)	Cal	Fat	Cbs
Wood-Grl Lobster, Shrimp & Scallops	500	11	42
Wood-Grilled Scallops, Shrimp and Chkn	600	13	42
Wood-Fire Grilled Steak and Chicken			
Center-Cut NY Strip Steak, 14 oz.	590	33	0
Maple-Glazed Chicken	570	9	62
NY Strip and Rock Lobster Tail	690	35	0
• Steak Lobster-and-Shrimp Oscar	1170	77	20
• Wood-Grl Peppercorn Sirloin & Shrimp	560	21	25
Wood-Grilled, Broiled or Blackened			
Arctic Char, Half Portion	340	15	13
Barramundi, Half Portion	230	5	8
Cobia, Half Portion	400	26	6
Cod, Half Portion	170	2	8
Corvina, Half Portion	180	2	7
Flounder, Half Portion	200	2	8
Grouper, Half Portion	210	2	6
Haddock, Half Portion	180	2	6
Lake Whitefish, Half Portion	210	2	6
Mahi-Mahi, Half Portion	200	3	6
Monchong, Half Portion	190	2	7
New Orleans Shrimp, Half Portion	250	19	3
Opah, Half Portion	280	12	8
Perch, Half Portion	170	2	6
Pompano, Half Portion	240	8	6
Red Rockfish, Half Portion	170	3	6
• Rock Island Stuffed Tilapia, Half Portion	410	16	22
Salmon, Half Portion	270	9	6
Seabass, Half Portion	230	6	6
Shrimp Bruschetta, Half Portion	140	7	6
Snapper, Half Portion	210	2	8
• Sole, Half Portion	140	2	6
Tilapia, Half Portion	210	3	9
Trout, Rainbow, Half Portion	220	10	6
Tuna, Half Portion	200	1	7
Wahoo, Half Portion	220	3	8
Walleye, Half Portion	170	2	7

▶ RED ROBIN			
Appetizers			
Chili Chili Con Queso, 445 g	1374	88	109
Creamy Spinach & Artichoke Dip, 522 g	1117	60	101
Guacamole & Salsa with Chips, 346 g	814	47	88
• Jump Starter Cheese Sticks, 238 g	603	33	48
Jump Starter Onion Rings, 221 g	653	38	71
Jumps Starter Jalapeño Coins, 207 g	773	61	49
Just-in-quesadilla Vegetarian, 461 g	872	48	68

▶ RED ROBIN (cont.)

	Cal	Fat	Cbs
Just-in-quesadilla, 574 g	1071	55	69
• Nacho Ordinary Chili Nachos w/ Chkn, 772 g	2084	134	132
Nacho Ordinary Chili Nachos, 673 g	1954	132	130
RR's Buzzard Wings, 449 g	1076	84	4
Towering Onion Rings, 546 g	1773	112	171

Bottomless Beverages

	Cal	Fat	Cbs
• Freckled Lemonade Light, 356 g	68	0	17
Freckled Lemonade, 356 g	126	0	32
Peach Iced Tea, 395 g	103	0	26
Peachberry Fruit Cooler, 284 g	260	0	61
Pomegranate Iced Tea, 395 g	96	0	23
Raspberry Iced Tea, 395 g	103	0	26
Very Berry Raspberry Limeade, 397 g	205	0	51

Chicken Sandwiches

	Cal	Fat	Cbs
Blackened Chicken Sandwich, 331 g	694	34	52
Bruschetta Chicken Sandwich, 362 g	682	31	55
California Chicken Sandwich, 397 g	836	44	52
Chicken Caprese Sandwich, 353 g	676	29	52
Crispy Chicken Sandwich, 364 g	909	54	70
• Simply Grilled Chicken Sandwich, 279 g	420	8	51
Teriyaki Chicken Sandwich, 412 g	905	48	64
• Whiskey River BBQ Chicken, 386 g	965	52	72

Chillin Concoctions

	Cal	Fat	Cbs
• Groovy Smoothie, 422 g	314	2	76
Hawaiian Heart Throb Smoothie, 420 g	431	3	100
• Root Beer Float, 791 g	456	9	101

Desserts

	Cal	Fat	Cbs
• Birthday Sundae, 146 g	376	18	49
Hot Apple Crisp, 497 g	784	13	165
Hot Fudge Sundae, 303 g	800	36	111
Kid Sundae, 146 g	376	18	49
• Mountain High Mudd Pie, 453 g	1373	63	184

Entrees

	Cal	Fat	Cbs
Arctic Cod Fish & Chips, 475 g	1118	67	83
• Buffalo Clucks & Fries, 579 g	1696	121	100
Classic Creamy Mac 'n' Cheese, 680 g	1230	73	91
Clucks & Fries, 460 g	1452	92	100
Ensenada Chicken Platter, 552 g	757	41	26
• Grilled Chicken alla Caprese, 583 g	686	34	51
Jumbo Shrimp & Slaw Platter, 682 g	1256	56	148
Prime Rip Dip, 627 g	1008	55	74
Red Veggie Rice Bowl, 795 g	714	8	150
Red's Rice Bowl, 801 g	830	10	137
Red's Salmon Rice Bowl, 824 g	741	7	129
Shrimps & Cod Duo, 720 g	1435	84	133
Steak Sliders Entrée (2 Sliders), 359 g	795	42	65

• MOST HEALTHY   • LEAST HEALTHY

RED ROBIN (cont.)

	Cal	Fat	Cbs
Gourmet Burger			
A.1. Peppercorn Burger, 361 g	1025	59	70
• All American Patty Melt, 416 g	1315	98	60
Bleu Ribbon Burger, 386 g	999	57	70
Burnin Love Burger, 390 g	936	60	55
Chili Chili Cheeseburger, 406 g	923	50	59
Gourmet Cheeseburger, 364 g	931	60	53
Guacamole Bacon Burger, 394 g	1046	64	54
• Natural Burger, 284 g	569	24	51
Pub Burger, 387 g	957	55	54
Red Robin Bacon Cheeseburger, 344 g	1030	69	51
Royal Red Robin Burger, 410 g	1196	83	52
Sauted Shroom Burger, 442 g	961	56	58
The Banzai Burger, 398 g	1033	62	68
Whiskey River BBQ Burger, 390 g	1114	68	72
Kid Beverages			
Banana Milkshakes, 318 g	378	15	59
Chocolate Milkshake, 307 g	437	16	71
Groovy Smoothie, 293 g	207	2	49
Hawaiian Heart Throb Smoothie, 302 g	300	2	69
Mint Brownie Shake, 30 g	479	24	66
Peach Milkshakes, 317 g	378	15	59
Raspberry Milkshakes, 307 g	505	15	89
• Rocky Magic Milk Shake, 320 g	586	27	83
Root Beer Float, 301 g	138	3	30
• Strawberry Milkshakes, 305 g	334	15	48
• Strawberry Smoothie, 290 g	122	0	30
Vanilla Milk Shake, 263 g	323	15	45
Kids Entrees			
Carnival Corn Dog, 112 g	295	12	36
Cheesy Mac n Cheesy, 255 g	420	22	42
Chick N Cheese Quesadilla, 220 g	568	26	33
Chick Chick Chicken fingers, 114 g	372	22	19
• Chick on a stick, 107 g	152	4	0
Grilled Cheesewich, 157 g	440	29	30
Parmesan Noodles, 200 g	427	24	43
Rad Chicken Burger, 159 g	302	6	28
Rad Garden Burger, 151 g	282	6	40
Rad Robin Burger, 102 g	286	12	28
Rad Turkey Burger, 133 g	403	22	29
Rad Vegan Boca Burger, 194 g	289	4	39
Red Cheese Pizza, 261 g	605	27	58
• Red Pizzeria Pizza, 278 g	690	35	58
Red Robbinetti Spaghetti, 297 g	297	2	56
Kid's Sides			
Apple Slices, 57 g	20	0	8

RED ROBIN (cont.)

	Cal	Fat	Cbs
Melon Wedge, 180 g	61	0	15
Mandarin Oranges, 57 g	28	0	7
• Side Baby Carrots, 122 g	300	30	6
• Side Broccoli, 57 g	20	0	4
Side Salad, 117 g	38	1	7
Steak Fries, 85 g	217	9	30
Steamed Veggies, 184 g	55	0	12

Milkshakes & Malts

	Cal	Fat	Cbs
Monster Malt Banana, 626 g	815	30	129
Monster Malt Chocolate, 610 g	904	31	148
Monster Malt Peach, 624 g	815	30	129
• Monster Malt Raspberry, 610 g	1105	30	168
Monster Malt Strawberry, 606 g	749	30	113
Monster Malt Vanilla, 572 g	757	31	113
Monster Shake Banana, 583 g	646	27	99
Monster Shake Chocolate, 566 g	735	28	118
Monster Shake Mint Brownie, 571 g	848	42	120
Monster Shake Peach, 581 g	646	27	99
Monster Shake Raspberry, 566 g	936	27	138
• Monster Shake Strawberry, 563 g	579	27	83
Monster Shake Vanilla, 528 g	588	28	83
Rookie Magic, 550 g	883	40	127

Other Favorite

	Cal	Fat	Cbs
Crispy Arctic Cod Sandwich, 312 g	605	29	61
Garden Burger, 299 g	561	23	73
• Grilled Salmon Sandwich, 366 g	855	50	53
Grilled Turkey Burger, 254 g	641	37	50
• Lettuce Wrap your burger, 306 g	422	42	8
Vegan Boca Burger, 342 g	546	21	61

Salads

	Cal	Fat	Cbs
Apple Harvest Chicken Salad, 577 g	812	44	64
Asian Chicken Salad, 627 g	458	10	54
• Fajita Fiesta Pollo Salad, 605 g	959	54	57
Mighty Caesar W/ Blackened, 526 g	790	48	43

Sandwiches & Wraps

	Cal	Fat	Cbs
BLTA Croissant, 571 g	759	41	72
Caesar's Chicken Wraps, 620 g	892	43	85
Crispy Arctic Cod Sandwich, 312 g	605	29	61
Garden Burger, 299 g	561	23	73
Grilled Salmon Sandwich, 366 g	855	50	53
Grilled Turkey Burger, 254 g	641	37	50
• Lettuce Wrap your burger, 306 g	422	42	8
Vegan Boca Burger, 342 g	546	21	61
• Whiskey River BBQ Chkn Wrap, 686 g	1152	62	100

Side Salads

	Cal	Fat	Cbs
• House Salad, 117 g	38	1	7

• MOST HEALTHY   • LEAST HEALTHY

RED ROBIN (cont.)

	Cal	Fat	Cbs
• Side Caesar Salads, 186 g	313	21	21
Side Salads, 117 g	38	1	7

Sides

	Cal	Fat	Cbs
Apple Slices, 113 g	40	0	16
• Celery, 68 g	11	0	2
Chipotle Beans, 113 g	111	1	21
Coleslaw, 226 g	252	18	23
Melon Wedges, 180 g	61	0	29
• Onion Rings, 212 g	724	54	62
Red Robin Steak Fries, 170 g	434	18	60
Side Focaccia Bread, 113 g	300	6	48
Texas Toast, 43 g	65	0	14

Soups (Cup)

	Cal	Fat	Cbs
• Chicken Tortilla Soup, 198 g	207	10	16
• Clamdigger's Clam Chowder, 210 g	346	20	26
French Onion Soup, 246 g	254	13	22
Red Housemade Chili, 181 g	276	16	13

RITA'S

Additional Items

	Cal	Fat	Cbs
Ritaccino® Cafe & Mocha	780	13	146

Cones & Toppings

	Cal	Fat	Cbs
• Cake Cone (1)	10	0	2
Hot Caramel	90	1	20
Hot Fudge	90	3	15
• M&M's® Minis®	140	4	19
Nilla® Wafers	120	2	22
Oreo® Cookies	140	2	20
Snyder's® Pretzel Snaps	110	0	24
Sprinkles (per 1 tbsp)	35	1	5
Waffle Cone (1)	40	0	8

Custard & Soft-Serve (Regular Cup)

	Cal	Fat	Cbs
All Custard flavors, 5 3/4 oz.	330	11	39
• Hot Fudge Sundae w/ M&M's® Mini's®	560	18	74
Hot Fudge Sundae w/ M&M's® Mini's®-Slenderita™	460	7	84
• Slenderita™ Fat-Free Soft-Serve, 5 3/4 oz.	230	0	49

Gelati

	Cal	Fat	Cbs
• Chocolate Custard Regular w/ SF Ice	305	7	53
Coffee Custard Regular w/ Sugar-Free Ice	290	8	50
Orange Cream Custard Reg w/ SF Ice	290	8	49
• Slenderita™ FF Soft-Serve Reg w/ SF Ice	220	0	57
Strawberry Custard Regular w/ SF Ice	295	7	51
Vanilla Custard Regular w/ SF Ice	290	8	49

Italian Ice (Regular)

	Cal	Fat	Cbs
Cream Ice, 12 oz.	385	4	109
Italian Ice, 12 oz.	320	0	66

• MOST HEALTHY • LEAST HEALTHY

RITA'S (cont.)

	Cal	Fat	Cbs
M&M's® Mini 's®			
• Choco Custard - Blendini™ w/ SF Ice	540	14	81
Coffee Custard - Blendini™ w/ SF Ice	530	16	76
Orange Crm Custard - Blendini™ w/ SF Ice	520	16	74
• Slenderita™ FF Soft-Serve - Blendini™ w/ SF Ice	420	4	86
Strwbry Custard - Blendini™ w/ SF Ice	530	15	78
Vanilla Custard - Blendini™ w/ SF Ice	530	16	74
Misto® (Regular)			
Chocolate Misto® w/ Sugar-Free Ice	290	5	68
Vanilla Misto® w/ Sugar-Free Ice	285	5	66
Nilla® Wafers			
• Choco Custard - Blendini™ w/ SF Ice	520	12	84
Coffee Custard - Blendini™ w/ SF Ice	510	13	79
Orange Cream Custard - Blendini™ w/ SF Ice	510	13	77
• Slenderita™ FF Soft-Serve - Blendini™ w/ SF Ice	410	2	89
Strwbry Custard - Blendini™ w/ SF Ice	510	13	81
Vanilla Custard - Blendini™ w/ SF Ice	510	13	77
Oreo® Cookies			
• Choco Custard - Blendini™ w/ SF Ice	540	12	81
Coffee Custard - Blendini™ w/ SF Ice	520	13	77
Orange Crm Custard - Blendini™ w/ SF Ice	520	13	74
• Slenderita™ FF Soft-Serve - Blendini™ w/ SF Ice	420	2	86
Strwbry Custard - Blendini™ w/ SF Ice	520	13	78
Vanilla Custard - Blendini™ w/ SF Ice	520	13	74
Snyder 's® Pretzels			
• Choco Custard - Blendini™ w/ SF Ice	510	10	85
Coffee Custard - Blendini™ w/ SF Ice	500	12	80
Orange Crm Custard - Blendini™ w/ SF Ice	500	12	79
• Slenderita™ FF Soft-Serve - Blendini™ w/ SF Ice	400	0	90
Strwbry Custard - Blendini™ w/ SF Ice	500	11	82
Vanilla Custard - Blendini™ w/ SF Ice	500	12	78

ROBEKS

	Cal	Fat	Cbs
Bowls			
Acai Especial, 14 oz.	385	5	87
Fresh Juices			
ABC, 12 oz.	150	0	33
Apple, 12 oz.	180	0	45
Carrot, 12 oz.	98	0	22
• Green-V, 12 oz.	96	1	19
G-Snap, 12 oz.	120	1	24
• Monkey C, 12 oz.	186	1	44
Orange, 12 oz.	168	1	39
Raspberry Lemonade, 12 oz.	164	0	40
Frozen Yogurt			
1 or 2 Flavors (Average), 12 oz.	250	0	58

• MOST HEALTHY   • LEAST HEALTHY

▶ ROBEKS (cont.)

	Cal	Fat	Cbs
Gourmet Pretzels			
• Apple Cinnamon	470	25	78
Spinach Feta	430	9	70
• Tomato Parmesan	420	10	67
Muffins			
Banana	310	11	43
Blueberry	300	10	42
• Chocolate	320	11	45
• Pumpkin Muffin (Seasonal)	270	5	57
Naturally Light			
Banana Mango	162	0	42
• Pineapple Mango	172	0	44
Raspberry Banana	161	0	42
• Strawberry Pineapple	131	0	33
Power Cookies			
• Breakfast Bar	230	10	33
Chocolate Chip with Walnuts	404	12	60
Lemon Poppyseed	371	7	63
Oatmeal Raisin Walnut	375	7	64
Peanut Butter	426	14	59
Shakes & Freezes			
• 800 lb. Gorilla, 12 oz.	434	9	58
• Bananasplit Shake, 12 oz.	274	0	56
Lemon Freeze, 12 oz.	282	2	66
Orange Freeze, 12 oz.	290	1	63
P-Nut Power Shake, 12 oz.	362	16	39
Smoothies			
Acai Energizer, 12 oz.	161	1	33
• Awesome Acai, 12 oz.	146	1	32
Banzai Blueberry, 12 oz.	172	1	29
Berry Brilliance, 12 oz.	192	1	45
Big Wednesday, 12 oz.	201	1	49
Cardio Cooler, 12 oz.	244	1	45
Citrus Stinger, 12 oz.	198	1	44
Cranberry Quest, 12 oz.	208	1	49
Dr. Robeks, 12 oz.	186	1	42
Green Tea Sensation, 12 oz.	199	2	37
Guava Lava, 12 oz.	206	1	50
Hummingbird, 12 oz.	211	1	50
Infinite Orange, 12 oz.	182	1	42
Mahalo Mango, 12 oz.	201	1	50
Malibu Peach, 12 oz.	181	0	44
Outrageous Raspberry, 12 oz.	182	1	44
Passionfruit Cove, 12 oz.	193	1	46
Pina Koolada, 12 oz.	212	1	50
Polar Pineapple, 12 oz.	183	1	45

• MOST HEALTHY • LEAST HEALTHY

ROBEKS (cont.)	Cal	Fat	Cbs
Pomegranate Passion, 12 oz.	190	0	46
Pomegranate Power, 12 oz.	217	1	50
• Pro Arobek, 12 oz.	260	1	52
Raspberry Romance, 12 oz.	209	0	50
Robeks Rejuvenator, 12 oz.	221	1	51
South Pacific Squeeze, 12 oz.	200	1	47
Strawnana Berry, 12 oz.	188	0	44
Venice Burner, 12 oz.	227	1	48
Zen Berry, 12 oz.	217	1	51

ROCKFISH SEAFOOD GRILL

Choose a Fresh Fish

	Cal	Fat	Cbs
Ahi Tuna	248	N/A	N/A
Alaskan Flounder	255	N/A	N/A
• Chicken	188	N/A	N/A
North Atlantic Salmon	356	N/A	N/A
Shrimp	325	N/A	N/A
Tilapia	341	N/A	N/A
Trophy Rainbow Trout	355	N/A	N/A
• U.S. Farm-Raised Catfish	488	N/A	N/A

Choose a Sauce

	Cal	Fat	Cbs
Ancho Cream	102	N/A	N/A
• Lemon-Butter	244	N/A	N/A
Maple Glaze	106	N/A	N/A
Pontchartrain	115	N/A	N/A
Roasted Red Pepper	34	N/A	N/A
• Tomatillo Salsa	18	N/A	N/A

Choose a Side

	Cal	Fat	Cbs
• Mixed Veggies	17	N/A	N/A
• New Potatoes	152	N/A	N/A
Steamed Spinach	17	N/A	N/A
Wild Rice	100	N/A	N/A

Salads

	Cal	Fat	Cbs
Pacific Cove Crab Salad	423	18	33
• Roaring River Salmon Salad	462	19	30
Seared Ahi Tuna Salad	335	14	10
• Small Southwest Caesar Salad	251	34	17

Starters

	Cal	Fat	Cbs
• Maryland Crab Cakes	522	34	13
Mexican Shrimp Martini	271	5	17
• Shrimp Cocktail	178	2	8

Stream

	Cal	Fat	Cbs
Ahi Tuna Ciabatta	516	17	41
Baked & Stuffed Shrimp	493	34	19
• Louisiana Gumbo	445	16	54
• Santa Fe Fish Tacos	564	18	101

ROCKFISH SEAFOOD GRILL (cont.)	Cal	Fat	Cbs
Tilapia In The Bag	501	18	31
Tilapia Pontchartrain	493	24	9

ROCKY ROCOCO

Bread
	Cal	Fat	Cbs
• Breadsticks w/ Jalapeño Chz Sc, 6, 8 oz.	531	18	72
Breadsticks w/ Marinara Sauce, 6, 8 oz.	420	7	72
• Wheat muffin, 1 muffin	200	4	38

Pasta (Regular)
Can't Decide, 14 oz.	464	9	77
• Fettuccine w/ Alfredo Sauce, 14 oz.	459	14	66
• Spaghetti w/ Meatballs, 15 oz.	628	16	89
Spaghetti w/ Tomato Sauce, 14 oz.	470	4	87

Pizza (Regular Slice)
• Cheese Pizza, 6 oz.	380	9	54
Garden Pizza, 8 oz.	391	10	56
Pepperoni Pizza, 6 oz.	427	13	54
• Sausage Mushroom Pizza, 8 oz.	499	19	55
Sausage Pizza, 7 oz.	495	19	54

ROLY POLY

Chicken
Basil Cashew Chicken	298	10	30
Buffalo Chicken	335	9	28
Buffalo Slim On Wheat	271	5	28
Catalina Chicken	315	11	28
Chicken Caesar	309	11	30
Chicken Cordon Bleu	308	11	26
Chicken Fajita	316	9	28
Chicken Popper	284	8	29
• Cobb Salad	256	12	27
Delhi Chicken	326	12	33
• Hickory Chicken	348	10	25
Oriental Chicken	269	4	29
Pesto Chicken	322	9	28
Santa Fe Chicken	304	11	28

Classic Soups
Baja Chicken Enchilada, 6 oz.	210	14	12
Broccoli Cheddar, 6 oz.	160	11	10
Clam Chowder, 6 oz.	150	5	12
Classic Chili, 6 oz.	160	5	18
Harvest Mushroom Bisque, 6 oz.	90	5	11
Loaded Baked Potato, 6 oz.	170	11	15
Mexican Style Chicken Tortilla, 6 oz.	130	3	18
• Old Fashioned Chicken Noodle, 6 oz.	70	2	11
Roasted Garlic Tomato, 6 oz.	160	11	12

• MOST HEALTHY   • LEAST HEALTHY

ROLY POLY (cont.)

	Cal	Fat	Cbs
• Seafood Bisque, 6 oz.	217	14	12
Classic Vegetable Soups			
Corn & Green Chile Bisque, 6 oz.	130	7	14
• Garden Vegetable, 6 oz.	60	0	12
• Spring Asparagus, 6 oz.	130	9	10
Ham and Smoked Pork			
Italian Classic	334	12	32
Key West Cuban	328	9	44
• Peachtree Melt	309	11	27
Pork Melt	310	11	26
Porky's Nightmare	319	12	28
• Southside Club	367	17	30
Otis Spunkmeyer			
Chocolate Chip Cookie, 3 oz.	380	17	53
• Oatmeal Raisin Cookie, 3 oz.	350	15	52
• White Choco Macadamia Nut Cookie, 3 oz.	390	20	50
Roast Beef and Steak			
• Chipotle Cheesesteak	345	15	27
Pepper Steak	268	10	28
Philly Melt	278	11	25
Ranch Roast	321	15	28
• Russian Beef	259	9	26
Santa Fe Steak	327	13	27
Steak Fajita	316	12	27
Roly Poly Salad			
Alpine Chef Salad	317	16	13
Buffalo Chicken Salad	504	25	13
Buffalo Cobb Salad	457	22	10
Chipotle Caesar Salad	521	25	21
Cobb Salad	517	27	12
• Frisco Chicken Salad	527	25	20
Greek Salad	168	10	14
• Just Veggies Salad	95	0	19
Las Olas Salad	254	11	15
Roly Chef Salad	340	19	12
Spa Salad	255	15	26
Spicy Caesar Salad	507	19	33
Walnut Spinach Salad	420	33	14
Roly Poly Sauces and Dressing			
Asian Tahini Dressing, 1 Tbsp	61	5	3
Basil Mayo, 1 Tbsp	87	9	0
Chipotle Ranch, 1 Tbsp	75	8	1
Cranberry Honey Mustard, 1 Tbsp	53	4	4
Curry Sauce, 1 Tbsp	101	11	0
• Dill Dressing, 1 Tbsp	106	11	0
Dill Horseradish Sauce, 1 Tbsp	54	5	1

ROLY POLY (cont.)

	Cal	Fat	Cbs
Fajita Sauce, 1 Tbsp	76	8	1
Fat Free Apple Ranch Dressing, 1 Tbsp	23	0	5
Fat Free Creole Sauce, 1 Tbsp	15	0	3
Fat Free Curried Mayonnaise, 1 Tbsp	11	0	2
Fat Free Horsey Ranch, 1 Tbsp	27	0	5
Fat Free Sundried Tomato Bas, 1 Tbsp	24	0	5
Lite Dill Dressing, 1 Tbsp	17	1	2
Oriental Sesame Dressing, 1 Tbsp	65	0	3
• Peach Salsa, 1 Tbsp	9	0	2
Peaches & Pepper Relish, 1 Tbsp	71	0	16
Pesto Mayonnaise, 1 Tbsp	104	11	0
Roasted Red Pepper Mayonnaise, 1 Tbsp	23	2	0
Roasted Red Pepper Hummus, 1 Tbsp	84	3	10
Spicy Cajun Mayonnaise, 1 Tbsp	35	3	0
Tarragon Mayonnaise, 1 Tbsp	100	11	0

Roly Poly Specials

	Cal	Fat	Cbs
Alpine Chicken Melt on Wheat	415	16	30
BBQ Steak	302	11	27
BBQ Veggie Ranchero on Wheat	230	4	38
Black And Bleu Club	309	13	25
Cajun Chicken Melt	385	14	33
Cajun Club	341	15	35
Caribbean Mix	399	18	28
Carnita Chicken	401	14	37
Carnita Steak	362	14	37
Carolina Shrimp Melt	262	10	30
• Cherry Pecan Chicken Club	591	31	47
Chicken Bruschetta	342	9	35
Chicken Pizza	397	15	34
Chipotle Chicken	391	16	27
Christo Melt	340	16	30
Coney Island Melt	441	28	31
Cranberry Hummer	324	17	34
Creole Chicken on Wheat	231	5	30
Extreme Veggie on Wheat	251	9	35
Ginger Shrimp on Wheat	222	3	37
Grand Central	408	20	38
Guilt Free Gobbler on Wheat	292	5	38
• Harvest Melt on Wheat	190	4	31
Hawaiian Chicken on Wheat	280	6	35
Holiday Meltdown	390	18	36
Indian Chicken Melt on Wheat	292	6	32
Jalapeño BBQ	313	12	29
Longhorn Melt	420	20	32
Mandarin Tuna on Wheat	260	5	34
Monster Fajita	371	15	34

• MOST HEALTHY   • LEAST HEALTHY

ROLY POLY (cont.)

	Cal	Fat	Cbs
Monterey Chicken	417	18	37
Moroccan Tofu on Wheat	246	9	31
Nantucket Lobster	309	15	36
New Orleans Melt	283	10	32
New Yorker	299	12	33
Nutty Avocado	276	12	35
Orange County Smoked Turkey	492	27	37
Original Jack	242	10	28
Palm Beach Tuna on Wheat	305	11	32
Peking Chicken on Wheat	229	5	31
Pesto Club	352	15	35
Pig Roast	302	10	34
Pineapple Jack	291	13	34
Ranchero Chicken	362	11	38
Ranchero Steak	357	13	37
Roly Poly Pounder	424	19	35
Roly Polynesian	371	15	34
Roly Reuben	349	18	29
Roma Chicken on Wheat	333	9	33
Salmon Club	282	11	28
Salmon Roll	298	14	29
Sesame Mix	245	10	29
Shrimp Club	311	15	31
Spinach Popper	192	7	27
Spinach Salad	255	11	28
Steak & Bearnaise	351	15	31
Teriyaki Tuna	391	18	34
Thai Peanut Chicken on Wheat	395	16	30
Thai Peanut Tofu on Wheat	236	9	31
Tofu Tahini on Wheat	238	9	30
Tuna Club	377	18	31
Turkey Saga	331	15	35
Westport Club on Wheat	363	17	32
Wild Scallion	291	16	30

Roly Polys Kids, Eggs

	Cal	Fat	Cbs
• All American Egg Roly on White	405	20	24
Huevos Rancheros on White	359	16	35
Kids Cheese Dog on White	240	11	24
• Kids Chicken Melt on White	191	6	24
Kids Grilled Cheese on White	215	8	23
Kids Meat And Cheese on White	205	5	24
Kids Peanut Butter And Jelly on White	252	9	51
Steak And Eggs on White	306	12	31
Veggie Scramble Egg Roly on White	294	14	32
Western Egg Roly on White	308	14	32

• MOST HEALTHY   • LEAST HEALTHY

ROLY POLY (cont.)

	Cal	Fat	Cbs
Tuna Salad			
• Classic Tuna Melt	338	17	26
• Popeye's Tuna on Wheat	303	4	31
Texas Tuna	309	12	30
Thai Hot Tuna	338	11	30
Tuna Luau	324	14	34
Turkey			
California Turkey	328	12	30
Cider House Melt on Wheat	243	5	26
Greek Turkey on Wheat	268	8	33
Hickory Cristo	291	9	25
Hot Honey	299	8	25
Italian Turkey	329	11	36
• Pesto Turkey Club	376	19	28
Smokehouse Turkey	323	10	27
Thanksgiving	285	7	36
Turkey Applejack	319	12	30
• Tuscan Turkey	219	2	31
Wild Turkey	278	11	31
Veggie and Cheese			
California Hummer	305	13	32
French Twist	254	9	27
Italian Veggie	255	8	33
Monster Veggie	285	9	27
• Nut & Honey	341	17	35
Spinach Stuffer	232	8	32
• Ultimate Veggie	180	1	33
Veggie Fajita	239	8	27

ROUND TABLE PIZZA

	Cal	Fat	Cbs
Appetizers			
Buffalo Wings, 1 wing	70	2	1
Caesar Salad (Individual), 4 oz.	60	1	5
Garden Salad (Individual), 7 oz.	45	0	7
Garlic Bread, 1 roll	360	9	72
• Garlic Bread with Cheese, 1 roll	540	13	72
Garlic Parmesan Twists, 1 twist	170	2	26
Honey BBQ Wings, 1 wing	80	2	2
• Pizza Sauce Dipping Sauce, 2 oz.	30	0	6
Side of Grilled Chicken, 2 oz.	100	1	0
Dessert			
Dessert Pizza, 1 Slice	210	2	32
Gourmet Classic Sandwiches			
• Chicken Club, 1 oz.	700	14	77
Ham Club, 1 oz.	640	14	78
• Lay's Classic Potato Chips, 1 oz.	150	1	15

ROUND TABLE PIZZA (cont.)

	Cal	Fat	Cbs
RT Veggie Sandwich, 1 oz.	530	11	83
Turkey Club, 1 oz.	620	14	77
Turkey Pesto, 1 oz.	610	14	74
Turkey Santa Fe, 1 oz.	630	14	75
Pizza Dessert (1 serving = 1 slice) (Original Crust)			
Cheese, 8	250	5	27
Chicken & Garlic Gourmet, 8	270	5	27
Gourmet Veggie, 8	260	5	29
• Guinevere's Garden Delight, 8	240	4	28
Hawaiian, 8	240	5	29
Italian Garlic Supreme, 8	300	6	27
King Arthur Supreme, 8	300	6	28
Maui Zaui (Polynesian Sauce), 8	280	5	32
Maui Zaui (Zesty Red Sauce), 8	270	5	29
• Montague's All Meat Marvel, 8	330	7	27
Smokehouse Combo: Chicken, 8	300	6	29
Smokehouse Combo: Pepperoni, 8	310	7	29
Ulti-Meat, 8	330	7	27
Wombo Combo, 8	300	7	29
Pizza Dessert (1 serving = 1 slice) Pan Crust			
Cheese, 8	330	6	41
Chicken & Garlic Gourmet, 8	360	6	42
Gourmet Veggie, 8	350	6	43
• Guinevere's Garden Delight, 8	320	5	42
Hawaiian, 8	330	5	43
Italian Garlic Supreme, 8	390	7	42
King Arthur Supreme, 8	360	7	42
Maui Zaui (Polynesian Sauce), 8	370	6	46
Maui Zaui (Zesty Red Sauce), 8	360	6	44
Montague's All Meat Marvel, 8	380	7	41
Smokehouse Combo: Chicken, 8	380	7	43
Smokehouse Combo: Pepperoni, 8	390	7	43
• Ulti-Meat, 8	410	8	41
Wombo Combo, 8	390	7	43
Pizza Dessert (1 serving = 1 slice) Skinny Crust			
Cheese, 8	210	5	19
Chicken & Garlic Gourmet, 8	230	5	20
Gourmet Veggie, 8	220	5	21
• Guinevere's Garden Delight, 8	200	4	21
Hawaiian, 8	210	5	22
Italian Garlic Supreme, 8	260	6	20
King Arthur Supreme, 8	260	6	21
Maui Zaui (Polynesian Sauce), 8	240	5	24
Maui Zaui (Zesty Red Sauce), 8	230	5	22
• Montague's All Meat Marvel, 8	290	7	20
Smokehouse Combo: Chicken, 8	260	5	21

• MOST HEALTHY   • LEAST HEALTHY

ROUND TABLE PIZZA (cont.)

	Cal	Fat	Cbs
Smokehouse Combo: Pepperoni, 8	270	7	21
Ulti-Meat, 8	290	7	20
Wombo Combo, 8	270	6	21

RUBIO'S

Burritos

	Cal	Fat	Cbs
Baja Grill Burrito Chicken, 371 g	630	28	55
Baja Grill Burrito Steak, 371 g	720	38	56
Bean & Cheese Burrito, 371 g	760	37	78
Big Burrito Especial Chicken, 521 g	820	31	102
• Big Burrito Especial Steak, 521 g	900	38	102
Blackened Mahi Mahi Burrito, 309 g	640	31	60
Carnitas Rajas Burrito, 414 g	790	33	77
Chicken Rajas Burrito, 408 g	750	27	76
Chile Lime Salmon Burrito, 309 g	670	37	61
Fish Burrito, 368 g	750	41	75
Grilled Mesquite Shrimp Burrito, 363 g	730	34	75
Grilled Veggie Burrito, 348 g	680	27	75
HealthMex Chicken Burrito, 354 g	520	14	69
HealthMex Mahi Mahi Burrito, 343 g	560	20	67
• HealthMex Veggie Burrito, 377 g	500	15	74
Mahi Mahi Burrito, 309 g	650	34	59
Steak Rajas Burrito, 408 g	830	34	76

Desserts

	Cal	Fat	Cbs
Brownie, 85 g	430	22	57
Churro, 45 g	170	8	22

Dressings

	Cal	Fat	Cbs
• Chipotle, 28 g	110	11	1
Chopped, 71 g	120	11	3
• Surfside Citrus, 57 g	250	23	10

Enchiladas (single)

	Cal	Fat	Cbs
• Carnitas, 199 g	380	23	24
• Cheese, 168 g	340	21	23
Chicken, 203 g	370	21	23

Grilled Gourmet Tacos

	Cal	Fat	Cbs
Garlic Herb Shrimp, 163 g	340	19	24
Grilled Chicken, 163 g	320	17	24
• Grilled Portobello & Poblano, 177 g	290	17	26
• Grilled Steak, 163 g	350	21	24

Kid's Meal

	Cal	Fat	Cbs
• Bean & Cheese Burrito, 252 g	580	27	66
Cheese Quesadilla, 167 g	560	31	46
Chicken Taquitos (2), 116 g	230	10	21
• Mini Churro, 23 g	80	4	11

Other Favorites

	Cal	Fat	Cbs
Cheese Quesadilla, 385 g	1120	70	87

• MOST HEALTHY   • LEAST HEALTHY

RUBIO'S (cont.)

	Cal	Fat	Cbs
Chicken Quesadilla, 470 g	1200	70	89
• Chicken Taquitos (3), 211 g	270	8	83
Nachos Grande Chicken, 544 g	1340	78	114
• Nachos Grande Steak, 544 g	1430	87	114
Nachos Grande, 459 g	1270	78	112
Steak Quesadilla, 470 g	1270	78	89

Salads, Wrap Saladas & Bowls (dressing/sauce incl)

	Cal	Fat	Cbs
Blackened Mahi Mahi Surfside Citrus Salad, 439 g	520	32	33
• Blackened Mahi Mahi Surfside Citrus Wrapsalada, 453 g	820	44	72
Chkn Balsamic & Roasted Veggie Salad, 408 g	340	12	29
Chkn Balsamic & Rst Veg Wrapsalada, 422 g	630	25	69
Chicken Chipotle Ranch Salad, 434 g	480	32	23
Chkn Chipotle Ranch Wrapsalada, 448 g	770	45	62
Chicken Chopped Salad Wrapsalada, 428 g	780	38	72
Chicken Chopped Salad, 471 g	500	25	37
Chicken Grilled Grande Bowl, 527 g	630	27	62
Chicken Surfside Citrus Salad, 434 g	500	30	34
Chkn Surfside Citrus Wrapsalada, 448 g	800	43	73
• Side Salad, 145 g	90	3	13

Salads, Wrapsaladas & Bowls (No Dressing)

	Cal	Fat	Cbs
Blackened Mahi Mahi Surfside Citrus Salad, 383 g	270	8	23
Blackened Mahi Mahi Surfside Citrus Wrapsalada, 397 g	570	21	63
Chkn Balsamic & Roasted Veggie Salad, 352 g	250	7	21
Chkn Balsamic & Rst Veg Wrapsalada, 365 g	540	20	60
Chicken Chipotle Ranch Salad, 378 g	260	11	20
Chkn Chipotle Ranch Wrapsalada, 392 g	560	24	59
• Chkn Chopped Salad Wrapsalada, 357 g	660	27	69
Chicken Chopped Salad, 400 g	380	14	33
Chicken Grilled Grande Bowl, 499 g	550	18	61
Chicken Surfside Citrus Salad, 377 g	250	7	24
Chkn Surfside Citrus Wrapsalada, 391 g	550	20	63
• Side Salad, 116 g	45	0	8

Salsas

	Cal	Fat	Cbs
• Salsa Picante, 28 g	20	1	2
• Salsa Regular, 28 g	5	0	1
Salsa Roasted Chipotle, 28 g	5	0	1
Salsa Verde, 28 g	5	0	1

Sides

	Cal	Fat	Cbs
• Black Beans, regular, 116 g	100	1	17
Chips, regular, 51 g	260	13	33
• Guacamole & Chips, 266 g	790	49	85
Pinto Beans, regular, 116 g	110	2	22
Rice, regular, 85 g	120	1	25

Street Tacos

	Cal	Fat	Cbs
Carnitas, 67 g	100	5	9
• Chicken, 70 g	90	3	9

• MOST HEALTHY   • LEAST HEALTHY

▶ RUBIO'S (cont.)	Cal	Fat	Cbs
• Steak, 70 g	120	6	9
Tacos			
Blackened Mahi Mahi Taco, 149 g	240	9	26
Chile Lime Salmon Taco, 149 g	250	12	26
• Fish Taco Especial, 177 g	320	18	31
Grilled Chicken Taco, 158 g	250	12	23
Grilled Mahi Mahi Taco, 149 g	250	11	25
Grilled Mesquite Shrimp Taco, 132 g	220	10	23
Grilled Steak Taco, 143 g	220	10	22
• HealthMex Chicken Taco, 141 g	130	1	22
HealthMex Mahi Mahi Taco, 143 g	170	4	21
World Famous Fish Taco, 149 g	270	13	30

▶ RUBY TUESDAY			
Appetizers (4 servings per item)			
Asian Dumplings	114	5	11
Asian Sesame Wings	190	10	5
Beef Queso Dip	378	24	28
Boston Barbecue Wings	167	7	6
Buffalo Shrimp	126	6	11
Cheddar Fries	335	20	25
Chicken Strips - Boston Barbecue	169	8	14
Chicken Strips - Buffalo	168	9	10
Chicken Strips - Thai Phoon	233	16	10
Chicken Strips - Traditional	148	8	9
• Dip Trio	467	33	27
Fire Wings	159	9	1
Four Way Sampler	354	20	20
Fresh Guacamole Dip	359	24	20
Fried Mozzarella	182	11	11
• Jumbo Lump Crab Cake	68	4	3
Pimento Cheese Dip	284	20	16
Queso Dip	317	20	26
Southwestern Spring Rolls	173	10	14
Spinach Artichoke Dip	310	19	23
Thai Phoon Shrimp	191	13	11
Wing Sampler	232	12	6
Brunch Menu			
Bacon Slices (5 each)	200	18	0
Berry Good Yogurt Parfait	162	3	26
Chocolate Chip Mini Cookies (2 each)	160	8	20
Cranapple Crepes	1251	41	196
• Grapes	52	0	13
Homestyle Biscuits	140	5	20
Kids Eggscellent Combo	170	12	1
Kids Patty Cakes	511	27	52

• MOST HEALTHY • LEAST HEALTHY

▶ RUBY TUESDAY (cont.)

	Cal	Fat	Cbs
Mini Benedicts - Crab Cake	625	38	38
Mini Benedicts - Crispy Southern Chkn	614	31	41
Mini Benedicts - Salmon Cake	674	43	35
Mini Benedicts - Steak	482	25	28
Mini Benedicts Trio	875	48	54
Pancake Syrup (1 oz vol)	109	0	27
Pancakes	891	41	104
Seasoned Potatoes	420	24	40
Spinach & Mushroom Omelet	496	33	7
Steak & Eggs	1342	53	121
Sunrise Quesadilla - Bacon Avocado	1589	114	43
Sunrise Quesadilla - California Club	1704	115	44
• Sunrise Quesadilla - Cheeseburger	1835	126	63
Western Omelet	628	45	5

Combinations

	Cal	Fat	Cbs
Broccoli & Cheese Soup	302	22	15
Buffalo Chicken Minis	623	23	64
Clam Chowder	318	20	17
Crab Cake Minis	616	27	60
Pimento Cheese Sandwich Minis	670	40	53
• Pimento Cheeseburger Minis	880	58	49
Ruby Minis	755	47	48
Salmon Cake Minis	665	33	57
Turkey Minis	567	28	50
Veggie Minis	690	27	92
• White Bean Chicken Chili	233	8	21

Desserts

	Cal	Fat	Cbs
Berry Good Yogurt Parfait	162	3	26
Blondie for One	625	27	86
• Chocolate Chip Cookie - Mini	80	4	10
Double Chocolate Cake	897	40	124
• Italian Cream Cake	990	56	108
New York Cheesecake	736	60	82
Tiramisu	545	29	66
White Choco Macadamia Nut Cookie - Mini	85	5	10

Dressings & Sauces (per ounce)

	Cal	Fat	Cbs
Asian BBQ Sauce	60	3	7
Asian Sesame Sauce	83	5	8
Boston BBQ Sauce	42	0	10
Caramel Sauce	100	0	25
Chocolate Sauce	120	3	21
Lemon Butter Sauce	88	9	1
Marinara Sauce	17	1	1
Orange Peanut Sauce	88	4	11
Parmesan Cream Sauce	64	6	2
• Salsa	10	0	1

RUBY TUESDAY (cont.)

	Cal	Fat	Cbs
Signature Parmesan Dressing	150	16	1
Spicy Southwestern Ranch Dressing	111	12	1
• Sweet Chile Sauce	170	17	2
Feature Menu			
Asian Salmon & Shrimp	682	48	9
Chesapeake Catch	499	30	8
Crispy Shrimp Sampler	894	48	68
Jumbo Lump Crab Cake	273	17	11
• Lobster Carbonara	1605	101	100
• Lobster Tails entrée	225	7	0
New Orleans Seafood	439	27	3
Steak & Lobster Mac 'n Cheese	986	55	34
Steak (7 oz.) & Lobster Tail	461	21	1
Fork-Tender Ribs			
Asian Sesame Glazed Half-Rack	542	32	18
Classic Barbecue Half-Rack	485	24	26
• Memphis Dry Rub Half-Rack	460	29	6
Ribs & Louisiana Fried Shrimp	908	41	64
Ribs, Wings & Shrimp	1034	50	53
• Triple Play	1051	50	67
Handcrafted Burgers			
Alpine Swiss Burger	1251	82	65
Bacon Cheeseburger	1252	86	61
• Bison Bacon Cheeseburger	1032	61	61
Boston Blue Burger	1446	96	80
Brewmaster Burger	1244	82	70
Classic Cheeseburger	1192	81	61
Pimento Cheese Burger	1282	89	61
Ruby's Classic Burger	1122	75	60
• Smokehouse Burger	1461	97	83
Three Cheese Burger	1352	94	61
Handcrafted Steaks			
Cowboy Sirloin	650	31	21
Peppercorn Mushroom Sirloin	490	20	12
• Petite Sirloin	349	18	1
• Rib Eye	1141	99	1
Shrimp Scampi & Steak	942	58	39
Steak (7 oz.) & Lobster Tail	461	21	1
Top Sirloin	419	20	1
Kids' Menu			
• Beef Minis	719	43	47
Butter Pasta	681	31	80
• Chicken Breast	134	2	1
Chicken Tenders	355	18	22
Chop Steak	384	32	1
Fried Shrimp	211	9	19

• MOST HEALTHY   • LEAST HEALTHY

▶ RUBY TUESDAY (cont.)

	Cal	Fat	Cbs
Grilled Cheese	440	20	48
Mac & Cheese	680	37	58
Mini Cookies	320	15	40
Pasta Marinara	583	14	88
Sundae	574	29	70
Turkey Minis	552	27	47
Premium Sandwiches			
• Avocado Turkey Burger	1234	81	62
Bella Turkey Burger	1126	69	67
Buffalo Chicken Burger	1127	67	74
Chicken BLT	1137	66	74
The Ultimate Chicken	1222	67	60
• Turkey Burger	997	61	62
Premium Seafood			
Asian Glazed Salmon	599	41	9
Chesapeake Catch	499	30	8
• Crab Cake Dinner	271	17	10
Creole Catch	277	13	2
Herb Crusted Tilapia	402	24	9
Lobster Ravioli	883	55	57
New Orleans Seafood	439	27	3
• Parmesan Shrimp Pasta	1314	80	94
Salmon Florentine	776	56	9
Prime Burgers			
Triple Prime Bacon Cheddar Burger	1445	115	45
• Triple Prime Burger	1225	96	45
Triple Prime Cheddar Burger	1385	110	45
• Triple Prime Havarti Burger	1465	116	45
Quesadillas			
Buffalo Shrimp Quesadilla	1465	89	87
California Club Quesadilla	1364	91	42
Cheeseburger Quesadilla	1495	102	61
Chicken Quesadilla	1089	70	41
• Fresh Avocado Quesadilla	1065	75	46
• Southwestern Quesadilla	1574	107	68
Salad Sensations			
Asian Salmon Spinach Salad	638	29	35
• Avocado Shrimp Salad	610	41	28
• Carolina Chicken Salad	1151	70	48
Club House Salad	921	59	21
Santa Fe Chicken Salad	675	35	30
Southwestern Beef Salad	1133	81	48
Signature Sides			
Baked Potato - Plain	282	2	46
Baked Potato - with butter & sour cream	441	17	48
Brown-Rice Pilaf	226	7	33

• MOST HEALTHY   • LEAST HEALTHY

RUBY TUESDAY (cont.)

	Cal	Fat	Cbs
Creamy Mashed Cauliflower	136	8	9
Entrée Bread	140	7	14
• Fresh Steamed Broccoli	84	6	3
• Loaded Baked Potato	591	29	48
Onion Straws	298	21	20
Piping-Hot Fries	396	18	50
Sauteed Baby Portabella Mushrooms	98	4	10
Succotash	249	16	13
Sugar Snap Peas	113	6	6
White Cheddar Mashed Potatoes	169	10	19

Smart Eating Choices

	Cal	Fat	Cbs
Baked Potato - Plain	282	2	46
Brown-Rice Pilaf	226	7	33
Chicken Bella	417	14	9
Creamy Mashed Cauliflower	136	8	9
Creole Catch	277	13	2
• Fresh Steamed Broccoli	84	6	3
Grilled Chicken Salad	503	27	5
Grilled Chicken Wrap	443	16	40
New Orleans Seafood	439	27	3
Plain Grilled Chicken	260	3	0
Plain Grilled Petite Sirloin	248	7	0
Plain Grilled Salmon	420	26	0
Plain Grilled Top Sirloin	319	10	0
Sauteed Baby Portabella Mushrooms	98	4	10
Sugar Snap Peas	113	6	6
• Turkey Burger Wrap	658	33	45
White Bean Chicken Chili	233	8	21
White Cheddar Mashed Potatoes	169	10	19

Soda Shop

	Cal	Fat	Cbs
• Berry Fusion	148	0	28
Classic Coke Float	384	14	64
Dream Cream Soda - Orange Creamsicle	202	7	33
Dream Cream Soda - Peaches 'n Cream	244	7	44
Dream Cream Soda - Strawberry	245	7	44
• Ruby's Root Beer Float	399	14	68

Specialties

	Cal	Fat	Cbs
• Barbecue Grilled Chicken	310	3	11
Chicken & Broccoli Pasta	1628	103	95
Chicken Bella	417	14	9
Chicken Florentine	520	22	9
Chicken Fresco	437	18	9
• Chicken Piccata	1673	101	113
Chicken Tender Dinner	591	31	36
Louisiana Fried Shrimp	423	17	38
Parmesan Chicken Pasta	1628	93	113

• MOST HEALTHY   • LEAST HEALTHY

RUBY TUESDAY (cont.)

	Cal	Fat	Cbs
Zero Proof Beverages			
Freshly Made Lemonade - Blackberry	190	0	46
Freshly Made Lemonade - Mixed Berry	190	0	46
Freshly Made Lemonade - Raspberry	185	0	46
• Freshly Made Lemonade -Pomegranate	235	0	59
Freshly Made Lemonade -Strawberry	192	0	48
Handcrafted Fruit Tea - Blackberry	162	0	39
• Handcrafted Fruit Tea - Mango	104	0	26
Handcrafted Fruit Tea - Mixed Berry	162	0	39
Handcrafted Fruit Tea - Peach	162	0	41
Handcrafted Fruit Tea - Raspberry	162	0	39
Peach Splash	157	0	38
POM Tea	114	0	29
RT Palmer	125	0	31
Tropical Sunrise	193	0	45

RUNZA

	Cal	Fat	Cbs
Chicken Sandwiches			
• BBQ Chkn Snd - Crispy, 196 g	520	19	56
BBQ Chkn Snd - Grilled, 192 g	390	9	46
Buffalo Chkn Snd - Crispy, 241 g	450	21	47
Buffalo Chkn Snd - Grilled, 273 g	440	13	36
Deluxe Chkn Snd - Crispy, 201 g	480	19	51
• Deluxe Chkn Snd - Grilled, 207 g	380	12	40
Smothered Chkn Snd - Crispy, 213 g	500	19	52
Smothered Chkn Snd - Grilled, 207 g	380	10	41
Desserts			
Blue Rspbry Runza® Slushie™ - med, 519 g	300	0	76
Cake Cone w/ Choco Ice Cream, 146 g	250	7	38
Cake Cone w/ Swirl Ice Cream, 146 g	250	7	38
Cake Cone w/ Vanilla Ice Cream, 146 g	250	7	38
Cappuccino Shake - regular, 314 g	470	18	65
Cherry Runza® Slushie™ - med, 519 g	300	0	76
Chocolate Chip Cookie, 85 g	310	16	34
Choco Ice Cream Dish - medium, 140 g	230	7	33
• Chocolate Shake - regular, 341 g	510	16	80
Chocolate Sundae, 168 g	300	7	51
Cookie Dough Sundae, 176 g	360	11	57
Grape Runza® Slushie™ - med, 519 g	310	0	78
Pepsi® Runza® Slushie™ - med, 519 g	220	0	60
• Raspberry Smoothie	220	0	54
Strawberry Shake - regular, 314 g	470	16	72
Swirl Ice Cream Dish - medium, 140 g	230	7	33
Turtle Sundae, 170 g	330	12	48
Vanilla Ice Cream Dish - medium, 140 g	230	7	33
Vanilla Shake - regular, 327 g	470	16	69

• MOST HEALTHY   • LEAST HEALTHY

▶ RUNZA (cont.)

	Cal	Fat	Cbs
Dressings & Sauces			
Dorothy Lynch, 70 g	260	14	29
Jalapeño Ranch, 65 g	280	28	2
• Poppyseed, 74 g	390	36	18
• Raspberry Vinaigrette, 58 g	25	0	6
Drinks			
Coffee, 290 g	0	0	0
• Iced Tea - medium, 638 g	0	0	0
• Smoothie - Banana, 220 g	220	0	54
Smoothie - Mango	220	0	54
Smoothie - Strawberry	220	0	54
Fries & Onion Rings			
French Fries - medium, 129 g	410	23	46
• Frings®, 180 g	540	28	64
• Onion Ring Dip, 59 g	90	6	4
Onion Rings- medium, 115 g	370	20	41
Garden Fresh Salads			
Asian Grilled Chicken Salad	380	7	58
Aztec Grilled Chicken Salad	390	5	40
Kids Meals			
• Chicken Strips, 167 g	460	25	42
Kids Runza® Sandwich, 195 g	530	24	64
• Mini Corn Dogs, 166 g	550	32	56
Small Hamburger (plain), 168 g	500	24	55
Other			
American Cheese, 19 g	60	4	1
• Bacon, 20 g	120	11	0
• Mushrooms, 38 g	5	0	1
Swiss Cheese, 19 g	70	5	0
The Runza® Way, 68 g	25	0	5
Other Sandwiches/Variety			
• 2 piece Chicken Strips, 80 g	190	10	11
• Fish Sandwich, 178 g	490	24	50
Mini Corn Dogs (5), 79 g	280	17	25
Polish Dog, 138 g	420	26	30
Runza® Burgers			
BBQ, Bacon & Swiss Burger, 216 g	560	27	40
Runza® Legendary Hamburgers			
1/2 lb. Double Chzburger (The Runza® Way), 295 g	640	32	37
1/4 lb. Bacon Cheeseburger, 193 g	510	29	36
1/4 lb. Chzburger (The Runza® Way), 207 g	430	21	32
1/4 lb. French Onion Burger, 236 g	550	34	28
1/4 lb. Jalapeño Burger, 268 g	720	50	34
1/4 lb. Kansas City Burger, 216 g	560	27	40
• 1/4 lb. Legend Supreme, 203 g	770	37	62
1/4 lb. Swiss Chz Mshr Burger, 174 g	450	25	36

● MOST HEALTHY ● LEAST HEALTHY

RUNZA (cont.)

	Cal	Fat	Cbs
Junior Cheeseburger, 133 g	330	17	28
• Junior Chzburger (The Runza® Way), 149 g	310	14	30
Junior Swiss Mushroom Burger, 149 g	380	21	26

Runza® Mini Chicken Wraps

	Cal	Fat	Cbs
Buffalo Mini Chicken Wrap	340	17	35
Ranch Mini Chicken Wrap	340	17	34

Runza® Sandwiches

	Cal	Fat	Cbs
Cheese Runza® Sandwich, 234 g	560	21	66
• Italian Runza® Sandwich, 220 g	730	19	116
• Original Runza® Sandwich, 215 g	500	17	65
Swiss Chz Mshr Runza® Snd, 275 g	590	25	68

Salads

	Cal	Fat	Cbs
Asian Grilled Chkn (incl Asian dressing)	380	7	58
Chicken Caesar with croutons, 350 g	300	13	14
• Side Salad, 129 g	30	1	4
Southwest Chicken with salsa, 317 g	440	23	35
Sweet Berry Chicken, 312 g	410	16	20
• Tossed Salad with Crispy Chkn, 360 g	440	27	29
Tossed Salad with croutons, 302 g	290	15	25
Tossed Salad with Grilled Chicken, 336 g	280	13	13

Soups (Bowl)

	Cal	Fat	Cbs
Boston Clam Chowder, 276 g	320	23	33
Broccoli Cheese, 310 g	360	27	35
Cauliflower Cheese, 287 g	330	26	32
Chicken Noodle, 305 g	170	5	21
Homemade Chili, 334 g	310	10	26
Potato with Bacon, 296 g	310	20	40
• Vegetable Beef, 270 g	110	3	13
Vegetable Cheese, 296 g	330	22	28
• Wisconsin Cheese, 299 g	430	35	36

SAMMY'S WOODFIRED PIZZA

	Cal	Fat	Cbs
Chinese Chicken Salad	450	12	47
Chopped Chicken Salad	425	11	30
• Fresh Tomato Basil Soup	110	5	10
Oak Roasted Salmon on Ponzu Salad	470	19	21
Roast Chicken Pesto Wrap	480	20	22
• Tomato Angel Hair Pasta	700	18	115

SAMURAI SAM'S TERIYAKI GRILL

Individual Items (Regular)

	Cal	Fat	Cbs
Brown Rice, 227 g	250	2	53
Dark Chicken, 99 g	190	9	2
Salmon, 113 g	100	2	1
Shrimp, 71 g	70	1	0
Steak, 99 g	170	7	1

• MOST HEALTHY   • LEAST HEALTHY

SAMURAI SAM'S TERIYAKI (cont.)	Cal	Fat	Cbs
• Veggies, 71 g	20	0	4
White Chicken, 99 g	170	4	2
White Rice, 227 g	290	0	65
• Yakisoba Noodles, 227 g	370	5	85

Kid's Teriyaki Rice Bowls

	Cal	Fat	Cbs
• Dark Chicken, Brown Rice, 198 g	280	6	37
Steak, Brown Rice, 198 g	270	5	36
• White Chicken, Brown Rice, 198 g	260	3	37

Other Bowls (Regular)

	Cal	Fat	Cbs
• Orange Peel Dark Chkn, Brown Rice, 425 g	520	11	72
Orange Peel White Chkn, Brown Rice, 425 g	490	5	73
• Riceless White Chkn (no sauce, on side), 326 g	230	4	16
Sweet and Sour Dark Chkn, Brown Rice, 425 g	510	11	71
Sweet and Sour White Chkn, Brown Rice, 425 g	480	5	71

Salads

	Cal	Fat	Cbs
• Oriental Chicken Salad, 326 g	340	12	26
Sesame Garden Noodle Salad, 369 g	270	5	27
• Side Salad, 71 g	10	0	2

Sauces/Dressings

	Cal	Fat	Cbs
• Chinese Salad Dressing, 43 g	130	8	14
Orange Peel Sauce, 30 g	60	0	14
Oriental Vinaigrette, 43 g	50	4	5
Spicy Teriyaki Sauce, 30 g	50	0	13
• Sweet and Sour Sauce, 30 g	35	0	9
Teriyaki Sauce, 30 g	40	0	9

Sides

	Cal	Fat	Cbs
• California Roll (1 roll), 170 g	260	1	46
Crab Rangoon (3 pieces), 85 g	210	12	20
• Grilled Chkn & Veg Eggroll (1 ea), 85 g	140	5	17

Teriyaki Rice Bowls (Regular)

	Cal	Fat	Cbs
Dark Chkn & Shrimp, Brown Rice, 425 g	460	7	68
Dark Chkn & Steak, Brown Rice, 425 g	500	10	68
Dark Chicken, Brown Rice, 425 g	500	11	69
Dark Chicken, White Rice Spicy, 425 g	560	10	84
Salmon, Brown Rice, 617 g	590	5	105
Shrimp, Brown Rice, 397 g	380	3	66
Spicy Steak & Broccoli, Brown Rice, 427 g	500	9	71
Steak, Brown Rice, 425 g	490	9	67
Sumo Bowl, Brown Rice, 808 g	1020	23	111
• Veggie, Brown Rice, 369 g	320	2	69
White Chkn & Shrimp, Brown Rice, 425 g	440	4	68
White Chkn & Steak, Brown Rice, 425 g	480	7	68
White Chicken, Brown Rice, 425 g	480	5	69
White Chicken, White Rice Spicy, 425 g	530	4	84

• MOST HEALTHY • LEAST HEALTHY

SAMURAI SAM'S TERIYAKI (cont.)

	Cal	Fat	Cbs
Teriyaki Wraps (includes veggies)			
Dark Chicken, Brown Rice, 391 g	650	17	90
• Dark Chicken, White Rice - Spicy, 391 g	680	16	99
Steak, Brown Rice, 391 g	630	15	89
• Veggie, Brown Rice, 420 g	530	9	100
White Chicken, Brown Rice, 391 g	620	12	90
White Chkn, White Rice - Spicy, 391 g	660	11	99
Teriyaki Yakisoba Noodle Bowls (includes veggies)			
Dark Chicken, 483 g	640	13	112
• Dark Chicken - Spicy, 483 g	680	13	119
Dark Chicken & Steak, 483 g	640	12	111
Salmon, 511 g	590	7	111
Shrimp, 483 g	570	6	110
Steak, 483 g	640	11	111
Steak - Spicy, 483 g	660	11	118
• Veggie, 454 g	500	6	114
White Chicken, 483 g	630	8	112
White Chicken - Spicy, 483 g	650	8	119
White Chicken & Steak, 483 g	630	10	112

SCHLOTZSKY'S

	Cal	Fat	Cbs
Chips			
• Barbeque	220	12	25
Cracked Pepper	220	12	25
Jalapeño	220	12	25
Mesquite BBQ Baked Crisps	140	4	24
• Original Baked Crisps	140	3	26
Original Kettle Chips	190	11	18
Regular (Plain)	220	12	25
Salt & Vinegar	220	12	25
Sour Cream & Onion	220	12	25
Desserts			
Brownie	417	22	54
• Carrot Cake	717	42	80
Chocolate Chip Cookie	160	8	22
Fudge Chocolate Chip Cookie	160	8	22
New York-Style Cheesecake	350	23	30
• Oatmeal Raisin Cookie	150	6	22
Sugar Cookie	160	7	22
White Chocolate Macadamia Cookie	170	9	21
Kids			
Cheese Pizza	479	13	73
Cheese Sandwich	394	15	48
Ham & Cheese Sandwich	424	16	49
• Pepperoni Pizza	523	17	73
• Turkey Sandwich	300	5	49

SCHLOTZSKY'S (cont.)

	Cal	Fat	Cbs
Panini			
Classic Swiss & Tomato	624	26	63
Grilled Chicken Romano	570	16	62
• Mozzarella & Portobello	485	15	63
• Panini Italiano	736	32	67
Smoked Ham Crostini	644	23	67
Smoked Turkey & Guacamole	602	21	69
Pizza			
• Baby Spinach Salad	454	7	80
Bacon Tomato & Portobello	619	23	75
BBQ Chicken & Jalapeño	715	16	99
Combination Special	639	25	76
Double Cheese	597	21	74
Fresh Tomato & Pesto	556	19	73
Grilled Chicken & Pesto	683	22	75
Mediterranean	560	20	74
Pepperoni & Double Cheese	685	30	74
Smoked Turkey & Jalapeño	653	21	78
• Thai Chicken	724	23	85
Vegetarian Special	540	17	74
Salads			
Baby Spinach & Feta	113	7	6
Caesar	103	5	10
Chicken Salad	292	15	12
Garden	51	1	12
Greek	137	8	13
Grilled Chicken Caesar	221	8	12
Ham & Turkey Chef	254	13	14
Pasta Salad	68	3	12
Potato Salad	242	13	29
• Side Salad	26	1	7
• Turkey Chef	309	18	14
Sandwiches (Medium)			
• Albuquerque Turkey	974	51	81
Angus Beef & Provolone	762	29	81
Angus Corned Beef	581	13	78
Angus Corned Beef Reuben	909	40	80
Angus Pastrami & Swiss	904	36	83
Angus Pastrami Reuben	909	39	80
Angus Roast Beef & Cheese	784	32	75
BLT	559	21	74
Cheese Original-Style	791	38	76
Chicken & Pesto	568	14	73
Chicken Breast	513	6	78
Chipotle Chicken	551	14	68
Deluxe Original-Style	956	46	80

● MOST HEALTHY ● LEAST HEALTHY

SCHLOTZSKY'S (cont.)

	Cal	Fat	Cbs
Dijon Chicken	576	11	79
• Fresh Veggie	484	12	77
Ham & Cheese Original-Style	733	27	80
Homestyle Tuna	563	16	73
Santa Fe Chicken	622	15	76
Smoked Turkey Breast	519	9	77
Smoked Turkey Reuben	895	38	84
Texas Schlotzsky's	756	31	73
The Original	771	34	78
Turkey & Guacamole	563	13	82
Turkey Bacon Club	787	32	77
Turkey Original-Style	831	35	80

Soups

	Cal	Fat	Cbs
• Boston Clam Chowder, Cup	175	11	20
Broccoli Cheese Soup, Cup	172	14	12
Chicken Tortilla Soup, Cup	143	6	15
• Hearty Vegetable Beef Soup, Cup	60	3	7
Old Fashioned Chicken Noodle Soup, Cup	83	2	12
Potato with Bacon Soup, Cup	177	10	22
Timberline Chile, Cup	275	9	31
Tomato Basil Soup, Cup	200	5	30
Vegetarian Vegetable Soup, Cup	98	1	22
Wisconsin Cheese Soup, Cup	263	20	20

Wraps

	Cal	Fat	Cbs
Asian Chicken	537	12	80
Feta & Portobello	618	39	55
• Grilled Chicken & Guacamole	689	36	60
• Homestyle Tuna	457	17	55
Parmesan Chicken Caesar	556	21	61

SHEETZ

Breakfast

	Cal	Fat	Cbs
Bagel, 115 g	250	3	49
BEC Burrito, 128 g	250	10	28
Biscuit, 81 g	259	11	35
Breakfast Sausage Dipper, 109 g	354	22	27
Chicken Biscuit, 138 g	378	15	46
Egg and Cheese Croissant, 112 g	272	20	27
Egg and Cheese Meltz, 155 g	421	20	46
Egg and Cheese Shmagel, 165 g	331	10	50
• Egg and Cheese Shmiscuit, 159 g	450	27	36
Egg and Cheese Shmuffin, 135 g	320	17	26
Hashbrowns, 64 g	130	8	14
• Muffin, 57 g	129	1	25
Sausage Biscuit, 124 g	434	28	35
Sausage Breakfast Burrito, 128 g	300	16	29

• MOST HEALTHY • LEAST HEALTHY

SHEETZ (cont.)

	Cal	Fat	Cbs
Western Burrito, 128 g	250	10	27
Burgers			
• Double Burgerz, 83 g	230	11	22
• Gourmet Burger, 198 g	602	31	49
Jr. Burgerz, 83 g	230	11	22
Burrito			
Chicken Burrito, 317 g	639	20	77
• Plain Burrito, 235 g	522	16	77
• Steak Burrito, 317 g	705	24	78
Chicken Sandwich			
• Grilled Chicken Sandwich, 198 g	391	6	50
Homestyle Crispy Chkn Snd, 198 g	472	13	64
• Spicy Crispy Chicken Sandwich, 198 g	492	14	64
Ciabatta Sandwich			
• Chicken Salad Ciabatta, 197 g	481	25	51
Deli Ciabatta, 156 g	373	15	44
Ham ciabatta, 156 g	302	6	45
• Italian Ciabatta, 99 g	231	4	42
Roast Beef Ciabatta, 99 g	231	4	42
Tuna Ciabatta, 197 g	445	20	51
Turkey Ciabatta, 156 g	282	6	44
Coffeez®			
Breakfast Blend, 12 g	8	0	2
Colombian, 12 g	8	0	2
Decaf House Blend, 12 g	8	0	2
House Blend, 12 g	8	0	2
Serious Dark Roast, 12 g	8	0	2
Vanilla Nut Cream, 12 g	8	0	2
Coffeez® Extras			
Amaretto Creamer, 1	40	2	7
Cinnamon Hazelnut Creamer, 1	40	2	7
• Equal Packets, 1	0	0	0
• French Vanilla Creamer, 1	45	2	6
Half & Half Creamer, 1	15	1	0
Mocha Creamer, 1	40	2	6
Splenda Packet, 1	0	0	0
Sugar Packet, 1	15	0	4
Sweet'N Low Packet, 1	0	0	0
Cold Subz			
BLT Sub, 273 g	887	40	96
• Cheese Sub, 198 g	484	5	90
• Chicken Salad Sub, 451 g	983	48	108
Club Sub, 311 g	585	9	94
Deli Sub, 311 g	767	27	94
Ham Sub, 311 g	626	9	96
Italian Sub, 311 g	727	21	94

• MOST HEALTHY   • LEAST HEALTHY

▶ SHEETZ (cont.)

	Cal	Fat	Cbs
Roast Beef Sub, 311 g	565	8	92
Tuna Salad Sub, 394 g	912	37	108
Turkey Sub, 311 g	585	9	94
Crispy Chicken Strips			
Regular (3) Chicken Strips, 128 g	242	8	23
Cupo'ccino® / Hot Chocolate			
Almond-Honey, 12 g	195	5	38
• Butterscotch Krimpet, 12 g	225	8	38
Candy Cane Cupo'ccino, 12 g	210	8	36
Choc. Covered Pretzel, 12 g	195	5	38
Cotton Candy, 12 g	210	5	39
Creme Brulee Cupo'ccino, 12 g	210	6	38
• Fat Free French Vanilla Cupo'ccino, 12 g	105	0	26
French Vanilla Cupo'ccino, 12 g	213	8	38
Harvest Spice Cupo'ccino, 12 g	209	8	38
Hot Chocolate, 12 g	186	3	39
Sugar Free Caramel Pecan, 12 g	168	5	30
Vanilla Chai Cupo'ccino, 12 g	208	6	38
Drink Shmart			
• Shmart Frozen Java Latte, 16 g	336	2	46
• Shmart Frozen Mocha, 16 g	366	2	52
Shmart Smoothie, 16 g	360	2	52
Flatbread Sandwichez			
• California Turkey Flatbread, 292 g	717	39	65
Cuban Flatbread, 235 g	478	15	60
• Grilled Cheese Flatbread, 173 g	447	15	55
Italian Flatbread, 257 g	621	29	62
Mozz.and Tomato Flatbread, 279 g	622	30	59
Fried Appetizerz			
• Appetizer Sampler, 192 g	508	21	59
Cup of Onion Rings, 162 g	338	16	43
• Jalapeño Poppers, 103 g	310	10	44
Mac n' Cheese Bites, 103 g	341	17	38
Mozzarella Sticks, 177 g	367	15	37
Frozen Drinks			
Frozen Plain Latte (No Flavor), 16 g	268	10	44
• Frozen Plain Mocha (No Flavor), 16 g	348	10	68
Frozen Vanilla Cream, 16 g	244	14	28
Fruit Smoothie			
Chocolate Covered Strawberry, 16 g	329	0	80
• MTO Froozie, 16 g	278	0	67
OrangeCrm, 16 g	318	8	61
Strawberry Banana Smoothie, 16 g	288	0	71
Strawberry Lemonade Smoothie, 16 g	288	0	71
• Wildberry Banana Smoothie, 16 g	349	0	83
Wildberry Lemonade Smoothie, 16 g	349	0	83

• MOST HEALTHY   • LEAST HEALTHY

SHEETZ (cont.)

Fry & Sides	Cal	Fat	Cbs
3 Cheese Mac and Cheese, 204 g	180	10	15
Cheese Fryz, 408 g	672	32	81
• Chili Mac and Cheese, 190 g	129	6	14
Coleslaw, 142 g	198	9	28
Cup of Fryz, 145 g	258	10	36
Garlic Fryz, 323 g	554	49	102
Grande Fryz, 295 g	526	21	74
Mac and Cheese, 190 g	129	6	14
Nachoz and Cheese - Small, 88 g	282	14	34
• Smokehouse Fryz, 436 g	983	53	103

Hot Dogs	Cal	Fat	Cbs
Hot Dogz, 91 g	260	15	24

Hot Drinks	Cal	Fat	Cbs
• Hot Chocolate Plain (No Flavor), 16 g	312	7	55
• Hot Plain Latte (No Flavor), 16 g	133	5	14
Hot Plain Mocha (No Flavor), 16 g	213	5	38
Steamer, 16 g	192	7	67

Hot Subz	Cal	Fat	Cbs
• Chicken Sub, 362 g	719	13	90
Meatball Sub, 525 g	863	28	125
• Pepperoni Sub, 283 g	879	41	90
Steak Sub, 361 g	851	21	93

Iced Drinks	Cal	Fat	Cbs
Iced Plain Latte (No Flavor), 16 g	212	4	35
Iced Plain Mocha (No Flavor), 16 g	292	4	59

Melt	Cal	Fat	Cbs
• Bacon Melt, 150 g	552	22	70
Club Melt, 170 g	402	7	69
Ham Melt, 170 g	422	7	70
• Roast Beef Melt, 113 g	351	5	67
Turkey Melt, 170 g	402	7	69

Nacho & Quesadilla	Cal	Fat	Cbs
Cheese Quesadilla, 308 g	848	44	57
Nachos Bueno, 136 g	513	23	65

Pizza	Cal	Fat	Cbs
Pizza Slice, 145 g	350	15	37

Pretzel	Cal	Fat	Cbs
Cheddar Cheese Pretzel, 177 g	510	15	78
• Cinnamon Sugar Pretzel, 171 g	570	105	102
Jalapeño Pretzel, 177 g	480	12	75
• Plain Pretzel, 171 g	450	2	93
Pumpkin Pretzel, 177 g	470	6	93
Salted Pretzel, 171 g	540	12	93

Salad	Cal	Fat	Cbs
Chef Salad, 268 g	149	4	12

• MOST HEALTHY • LEAST HEALTHY

▶ SHEETZ (cont.)

	Cal	Fat	Cbs
Crispy Chicken Salad, 282 g	269	8	30
• Garden Salad, 154 g	27	0	7
• Grilled Chicken Caesar Salad, 145 g	365	29	4
Grilled Chicken Salad, 236 g	144	4	7
Steak Salad, 236 g	211	8	8
Taco Salad, 199 g	254	10	38

Sandwich
	Cal	Fat	Cbs
• Chicken Salad Sandwich, 143 g	363	23	30
Deli Sandwich, 120 g	302	17	24
Ham and Cheese Sandwich, 190 g	344	6	53
Italian Sandwich, 120 g	275	13	24
Roast Beef Sandwich, 120 g	167	4	22
Tuna Salad Sandwich, 143 g	327	18	30
• Turkey Sandwich, 102 g	164	4	23

Shweetz® Cinnamon Rolls
	Cal	Fat	Cbs
• Cinnamon Roll (Cream Cheese Icing), 1	460	18	66
• Cinnamon Roll (Glazed), 1	380	14	58
Cinnamon Roll (Peanut Butter Icing), 1	440	16	68
Cinnamon Roll (Vanilla Icing), 1	440	16	68

Shweetz® Cookies
	Cal	Fat	Cbs
Chocolate Chunk Cookie, 1	210	10	28
• Chocolate No Bakes, 1	180	8	24
Oatmeal Raisin Cookie, 1	200	9	27
Peanut Butter Cookie, 1	230	14	23
Peanut Butter No Bakes, 1	180	8	24
• Pink Iced Cookie, 1	270	12	37
Raisin Filled Cookie, 1	220	8	35

Shweetz® Doughnuts
	Cal	Fat	Cbs
Apple Fritter, 1	450	25	49
Chocolate Iced Custard Filled, 1	380	17	51
Chocolate Iced Glazed Ring, 1	350	16	47
Choco Iced Glazed Ring w/ Sprinkles, 1	370	17	49
Cream Filled Chocolate Iced, 1	420	20	57
Cream Filled Glazed, 1	360	17	47
• Glazed Ring, 1	290	14	35
• Old Fashion Chocolate Cake, 1	530	33	54
Old Fashion Vanilla Cake, 1	480	26	57
Raspberry Filled Glazed, 1	330	14	46
Vanilla Iced Glazed Ring w/ Sprinkles, 1	360	16	49

Shweetz® Muffins and Cupcakes
	Cal	Fat	Cbs
• Blueberry Muffin, 1	440	24	50
Carrot Cake Muffin, 1	440	20	60
• Chocolate Iced Cupcake, 1	390	15	63
Vanilla Iced Cupcake, 1	420	19	59

Wraps
	Cal	Fat	Cbs
• Grilled Chicken Caesar Wrap, 239 g	470	25	32

• MOST HEALTHY　　• LEAST HEALTHY

SHEETZ (cont.)	Cal	Fat	Cbs
Grilled Chicken Wrap, 150 g	259	7	23
Steak Wrap, 150 g	326	11	24
• Turkey Wrap, 166 g	213	6	27

SHONEY'S

	Cal	Fat	Cbs
All Star Breakfast			
• Pancake Platter - w/bacon	665	11	110
Pancake Platter w/sausage patties	776	21	110
Sunrise Special	1472	62	191
Burgers			
• All American	1160	93	40
• BBQ Bacon Cheeseburger	1470	117	45
Classic Burger	1360	111	40
Mushroom Swiss Burger	1195	89	42
Chicken			
• Blackened Chicken Sandwich	722	36	40
• Chicken Salad Croissant	644	33	39
Grilled Chicken Sandwich	722	36	40
Classic Sandwiches			
• BLT Croissant	580	48	26
Philly Cheese Steak Sandwich	1139	74	61
Reuben	837	45	44
Slim Jim Sandwich	695	36	57
• Turkey Club Sandwich	1250	83	60
Country Fried Steak & Eggs			
Bacon Egg Cheddar Croissant (only)	792	57	30
• Big Biscuit Skillet	981	56	93
Ham Egg White & Swiss	679	44	27
• Sirloin Steak & Eggs only	580	36	3
Country Fried Steak Skillet			
Fiesta Skillet	1028	76	42
Desserts			
Apple Crisp	810	38	81
Banana Split Sundae	543	21	93
Hot Fudge Cake	709	30	101
Hot Fudge Sundae	536	25	68
• Key Lime Cheesecake	830	58	74
Peach Sundae	370	17	46
Peanut Butter Pie	570	35	57
• Strawberry Pie Slice	349	13	53
Strawberry Sundae	373	17	47
Entrée Skillets			
• Artichoke & Pulled Crabmeat Casserole	1411	80	134
Lemon Chkn w/Mushrooms & Wild Rice	1221	277	92
• Slow-Cooked Pot Roast	833	45	58

• MOST HEALTHY   • LEAST HEALTHY

SHONEY'S (cont.)

	Cal	Fat	Cbs
Entrees			
10 oz. Ribeye Steak	1485	90	97
12 oz. T-Bone Steak	1725	110	100
• 16 oz. Porterhouse Steak	2168	136	97
8 oz. Steakhouse Sirloin	1379	83	97
Blackened Chicken w/BBQ Sauce	584	18	39
Blackened Chicken w/Honey Mustard	786	44	33
Chicken Strips	1320	88	91
• Grilled Chicken w/BBQ Sauce	448	20	14
Grilled Chicken w/Honey Mustard	650	46	22
Grilled Salmon	516	34	27
Half-O-Pound	1323	103	62
Pan-Blackened Catfish Fry	914	60	66
Smothered Liver & Onions	776	46	48
Southern Catfish Fry	1464	78	137
Entrees Salads			
• Fried Chicken Salad	1097	70	93
Grilled Chicken Salad	1059	56	70
• Salmon Salad	869	60	49
Kids Menu			
Cheeseburger	788	56	41
Fish Wrap	491	32	25
• Grilled Cheese	448	32	24
• Mac & Cheese	966	54	83
Spaghetti	772	34	85
Perfect Pastas			
Baked Spaghetti	1459	54	145
Lasagna (Full Portion)	1138	65	93
Pile O Shrimp Basket			
Fish n Chips Basket	1312	74	102
Fish Sandwich	1190	63	105
Sides			
Baked Potato - plain	225	0	51
Biscuit (1)	190	9	23
• Chili Cheese Fries	681	42	61
French Fries	518	30	56
• Fruit Bowl	62	0	15
Garlic Grecian Bread	330	24	23
Grits	395	2	86
Homefries	119	6	15
Loaded Potato Mix	113	13	8
Mashed Potatoes	238	11	31
Onion Rings	490	35	51
Toast	128	2	23
Wild Rice	149	4	25

• MOST HEALTHY   • LEAST HEALTHY

SHONEY'S (cont.)

	Cal	Fat	Cbs
Starters			
Angus Steak Chili	621	37	50
• Chicken Enchilada Soup	444	22	50
• Chicken Strips	1269	84	87
Onion Rings Jumbo Order	980	69	102

SILVER MINE SUBS

	Cal	Fat	Cbs
Breads and Tortilla Wraps			
• 10" White Flour Tortilla Wrap, 71 g	210	5	36
• Wheat- medium (8"), 112 g	280	4	52
White - medium (8"), 112 g	280	2	52
Cheeses (Medium)			
• Cheddar Chz - med or double small, 30 g	118	10	1
• Provolone Chz - med or double small, 30 g	107	9	1
Cold Sub Sandwiches (Medium)			
California Gulch, 8", 363 g	736	36	66
Caribou, 8", 350 g	704	34	59
Comstock, 8", 352 g	657	28	55
• Dodge City, 8", 362 g	1011	69	57
Georgetown, 8", 331 g	660	29	59
King Bullion, 8", 352 g	636	26	55
Lawless Leadville, 8", 352 g	629	26	55
Mother Lode, 8", 500 g	999	56	58
Silver City, 8", 380 g	870	53	58
• Tombstone, 8", 362 g	617	24	55
Virginia City, 8", 352 g	645	28	58
Desserts			
Chocolate Chunk Cookie, 85 g	387	15	59
Deluxe Fudge Brownie, 85 g	409	21	54
Hot Sub Sandwiches (Medium)			
• Boomtown, 8", 295 g	809	46	55
• Coeur D'Alene, 8", 280 g	490	10	52
Cripple Creek, 8", 337 g	708	31	58
Frontier, 8", 321 g	679	23	67
Homestake, 8", 344 g	547	15	61
Silver Plume, 8", 358 g	710	30	58
Steam Engine, 8", 387 g	804	43	61
Kid's			
• Fruit Snacks, 25 g	80	0	19
Goldfish Crackers, 21 g	100	4	14
• Ham & Cheddar Cheese, 50 g	113	8	1
Ham & Provolone Cheese, 45 g	88	6	1
Turkey & Cheddar Cheese, 50 g	105	7	1
Turkey & Provolone Cheese, 45 g	80	5	1
Lowfat Sub Sandwiches (Medium)			
Caribou, 8", 276 g	380	4	58

• MOST HEALTHY   • LEAST HEALTHY

SILVER MINE SUBS (cont.)

	Cal	Fat	Cbs
Comstock, 8", 308 g	440	7	54
Homestake, 8", 314 g	440	7	60
King Bullion, 8", 308 g	419	5	54
Lawless Leadville, 8", 308 g	412	5	56
• Pikes Peak Or Bust, 8", 216 g	327	4	58
• Silver Plume, 8", 314 g	493	9	58
Tombstone, 8", 318 g	400	3	55
Virginia City, 8", 308 g	428	7	57

Meats

	Cal	Fat	Cbs
Bacon - 9 strips (Med Boomtown), 63 g	302	23	0
Grilled Chkn - Grilled Chkn Salad, 84 g	135	5	2
Grilled Chkn - Med Silver Plume, 126 g	203	7	3
Grilled Chkn - Sm Silver Plume, 84 g	135	5	2
Ham - Medium, 120 g	138	5	3
Meatballs - Medium, 140 g	383	32	2
Pepperoni - Medium, 84 g	420	39	0
Philly Cheesesteak - Medium, 126 g	150	5	6
Roast Beef - Medium cold, 120 g	150	5	0
Roast Beef - Medium hot, 168 g	210	8	0
• Salami - Medium, 120 g	493	45	0
Tuna Salad - Medium, 134 g	336	26	11
• Turkey - Medium, 120 g	107	1	0

Other Sandwich Items & Extras

	Cal	Fat	Cbs
Au Jus Sauce - side of, 140 g	9	0	0
• Cholula Hot sauce, 7 g	0	0	0
Lemon Packet, 4 g	0	0	0
• Marinara Sauce - medium, 42 g	17	0	3

Salads & Salad Related Items

	Cal	Fat	Cbs
Chef Salad, 208 g	82	2	6
Croutons - 1 package, 14 g	35	0	4
• Cucumbers - Grld Chkn, Chef, Garden, 22 g	3	0	1
Garden Salad, 148 g	21	0	5
Grape Tom Grld Chix, Chef, Garden, 28 g	8	0	2
• Grilled Chicken Salad, 232 g	156	5	7
Romaine Lettuce Mix - Grld Chix, Chef, Garden, 98 g	10	0	2
Side Salad, 81 g	11	0	3

Sandwich Dressings (Medium)

	Cal	Fat	Cbs
Avocado, 18 g	34	2	3
• Oil, 5 g	40	5	0
• Oregano, 0 g	0	0	0
Vinegar, 5 g	0	0	0

Sides

	Cal	Fat	Cbs
Baked Lays (1.13 oz.), 32 g	130	2	26
BBQ Lays (1.5 oz.), 42 g	230	15	23
Cool Ranch Doritos (1.75 oz.), 49 g	250	13	32

SILVER MINE SUBS (cont.)

	Cal	Fat	Cbs
Fruit Cup, 113 g	80	0	19
Harvest Cheddar Sun Chips (1.5 oz.), 42 g	210	9	29
Lays Potato Chips (1.5 oz.), 42 g	230	15	23
Nacho Cheese Doritos (1.75 oz.), 49 g	250	13	30
• Potato Salad, 156 g	270	15	33
• Whole Dill Pickle, 168 g	5	0	0

Soup & Chili & Related Items

	Cal	Fat	Cbs
Broccoli Cheese (8 oz cup), 250 g	160	8	17
• Chili (8 oz cup), 250 g	280	13	26
• Oyster crackers (1 package), 14 g	60	2	10
Side of Wheat Bread, 75 g	187	3	35
Side of White Bread, 75 g	186	1	35

Veggie Sub Sandwiches (Medium)

	Cal	Fat	Cbs
Pikes Peak Or Bust, 8", 290 g	651	33	59

Veggies (Medium)

	Cal	Fat	Cbs
• Black Olives, 44 g	69	7	3
Cucumbers, 28 g	4	0	1
Green Peppers, 22 g	5	0	1
Hot Banana Peppers, 18 g	3	0	1
Jalapeños, 20 g	3	0	1
Lettuce, 42 g	4	0	1
Mushrooms, 22 g	5	0	1
Onion, 18 g	8	0	2
• Pickle Slices, 44 g	0	0	1
Sprouts, 10 g	3	0	0
Tomato, 34 g	6	0	1

SKYLINE CHILI

Bowls

	Cal	Fat	Cbs
• Chili Bean Bowl	270	12	17
Chili Bowl	270	16	6
Chili Cheese Bowl	440	30	6
• Coney Bowl	870	69	9
Loaded Chili Bowl	580	40	18
Vegetarian Black Beans and Rice Bowl	320	9	46

Burritos

	Cal	Fat	Cbs
All Chili Burrito	560	30	37
All Chili Burrito Deluxe	650	35	45
Black Bean Burrito	600	25	67
Black Bean Burrito Deluxe	690	30	75
Chili Bean Mix Burrito	610	30	54
• Chili Bean Mix Burrito Deluxe	700	36	62
• Chili Cheese Melt	350	16	33

Chili Spaghetti Dishes (Regular)

	Cal	Fat	Cbs
3-Way	760	44	43
4-Way Bean	850	45	59

SKYLINE CHILI (cont.)

	Cal	Fat	Cbs
4-Way Onion	770	44	46
5-Way	840	45	58
Black Bean & Rice 3-Way	800	40	74
Black Bean & Rice 4-Way	810	40	77
• Black Bean & Rice 5-Way	880	40	89
Black Bean & Rice Spaghetti	490	12	79
• Chili Spaghetti	450	18	43
Coneys			
• Cheese Coney	340	22	17
Chili Cheese Sandwich	290	17	17
• Regular Chili Sandwich	180	7	17
Regular Coney	220	12	17
Dressings			
Chili Ranch Dressing	275	29	0
Greek Salad Dressing	250	28	1
Fresh Selects Salads			
Buffalo Chicken Salad	150	7	7
Classic Chicken Salad	150	7	8
Garden Salad	80	5	6
Greek Chicken Salad	170	8	9
• Greek Salad	60	4	5
• Southwest Chicken Salad	460	16	18
Fresh Selects Wraps			
Buffalo Chicken Wrap	520	21	55
Classic Chicken Wrap	510	21	55
• Greek Chicken Wrap	510	21	54
• Southwest Chicken Wrap	670	30	65
Kids Meals			
• Kids 3-Way Special	380	22	22
Kids Coney Special without cheese	210	12	15
Kids Double Wiener Hot Doggy Special w/o chz	250	17	15
Kids P'sghetti Special	280	16	19
• Kids Single Wiener Hot Doggy Special w/o chz	160	9	14
Sides			
• Bowl of Crackers	100	3	20
Cheddar Bread Half	260	20	16
• French Fries	630	33	79
Garlic Bread Half	200	15	16
Side of Cheese	230	19	1
Side of Chili	130	8	3
Steamed Potatoes			
3-Way Potato	870	49	75
4-Way Potato	890	49	78
• 5-Way Potato	950	50	90
Cheddar Potato	740	41	72
Chili Potato	440	8	74

• MOST HEALTHY   • LEAST HEALTHY

SMOOTHIE KING

• Plain Potato	310	0	72
Sour Cream Potato	570	27	72
Build Up			
• Gladiator®5 varies w/fruit choice	180	0	1
High Protein Smoothie - Almond Mocha	366	9	42
High Protein Smoothie - Banana	322	9	32
High Protein Smoothie - Chocolate	366	9	42
High Protein Smoothie - Lemon	372	9	44
High Protein Smoothie - Pineapple	320	9	29
The Activator® - Chocolate	404	1	83
The Activator® - Strawberry	556	1	121
The Activator® - Vanilla	406	1	83
The Hulk™ - Chocolate	876	31	124
• The Hulk™ - Strawberry	1035	32	161
The Hulk™ - Vanilla	872	32	121
Get Energy			
Acai Adventure®	435	5	92
Coffee - Caramel	340	1	66
• Coffee - Mocha	260	2	43
Coffee - Vanilla	347	1	69
Go Goji™	433	0	104
Green Tea Tango® varies w/fruit choice	282	3	52
Instant Vigor™	366	0	86
Pep Upper®	411	0	97
• Power Punch Plus®	500	1	113
Power Punch®	428	1	101
Super Punch Plus®	459	0	117
Super Punch™	395	0	100
Indulge			
Banana Boat®	524	12	97
Coconut Surprise®	460	7	90
Malts	680	33	83
Mo'Cuccino™ - Caramel	570	12	102
Mo'Cuccino™ - Mocha	444	12	73
Mo'Cuccino™ - Vanilla	525	12	92
Peanut Power ®	549	22	74
Peanut Power Plus™ Chocolate	717	27	98
• Peanut Power Plus™ Grape	749	22	122
Peanut Power Plus™ Strawberry	699	22	112
Pina Colada Island ®	600	10	110
Shakes	670	33	81
• Yogurt Delight® varies w/fruit choice	333	4	59
Kids Kups			
• Berry Interesting™	277	0	69
Choc-A-Laka™	245	3	44
CW Jr.™	270	0	68

▶ SMOOTHIE KING (cont.)

	Cal	Fat	Cbs
Gimme Grape™	265	0	64
Lil' Angel™	223	0	56
• Smarti Tarti™	200	0	49
Snack Right			
Banana Berry Treat®	364	0	86
Berry Punch™	360	0	91
Caribbean Way®	395	0	97
Cherry Picker ®	439	1	103
• Fruit Fusion®	355	1	76
Grape Expectations®	398	0	95
• Grape Expectations®	548	0	133
Lemon Twist® Banana	358	0	87
Lemon Twist® Strawberry	438	0	107
Light & Fluffy®	395	0	99
Peach Slice Plus®	464	0	110
Pineapple Surf ®	461	1	104
Strawberry X-Treme®	366	0	92
Stay Healthy			
• Blueberry Heaven®	325	1	73
Cranberry Cooler™	496	0	120
• Cranberry Supreme™	554	1	130
Hearty Apple®	405	1	86
Immune Builder®	380	1	89
Kiwi Island Treat®	498	1	116
Mangosteen Madness™	383	0	94
Orange Ka-BAM®	465	0	117
Pomegranate Punch™	464	0	110
Yerba Mate - Mango™	372	0	92
Yerba Mate - Mixed Berry™	348	0	84
Yerba Mate - Pomegranate™	372	0	91
Trim Down			
Angel Food™	354	0	84
Blackberry Dream™	365	1	88
Celestial Cherry High™	341	0	83
Island Impact®	311	0	73
Island Treat®	333	0	82
Low Carb Smoothie6	268	9	7
Mangofest™	285	0	72
Muscle Punch Plus™	366	1	84
Muscle Punch®	364	1	84
• Passion Passport®	395	0	96
Peach Slice®	314	0	72
Pineapple Pleasure®	280	0	67
Raspberry Collider™	338	0	86
Raspberry Sunrise™	392	0	95
Slim-N-Trim™ - Chocolate	297	2	57

• MOST HEALTHY   • LEAST HEALTHY

SMOOTHIE KING (cont.)

	Cal	Fat	Cbs
• Slim-N-Trim™ - Orange-Vanilla	215	1	46
Slim-N-Trim™ - Strawberry	375	1	84
Slim-N-Trim™ - Vanilla	253	1	53
Strawberry Kiwi Breeze®	376	0	90
The Shredder™ - Chocolate	311	3	36
The Shredder™ - Strawberry	356	1	56
The Shredder™ - Vanilla	283	2	30
Youth Fountain™	253	0	61

SONIC DRIVE-IN

Add-in Flavors & Toppings (Medium)

	Cal	Fat	Cbs
Blue Coconut, 18 g	35	0	9
Bubble Gum, 19 g	40	0	9
Cherry, 23 g	50	0	14
• Chocolate Topping Add-In, 38 g	100	0	23
Fresh Lemon Add-In, 18 g	5	0	2
• Fresh Lime Add-In, 14 g	5	0	1
Grape, 19 g	40	0	9
Green Apple, 20 g	60	0	15
Lo-Cal Diet Cherry+, 19 g	10	0	2
Orange, 18 g	40	0	10
Pineapple Topping, 35 g	60	0	14
Strawberry Topping, 35 g	70	0	17
Vanilla, 19 g	40	0	11
Watermelon, 19 g	45	0	12

Breakfast Items

	Cal	Fat	Cbs
Brkfst Burrito Bacon, Egg & Chz, 159 g	450	27	38
Brkfst Burrito Ham, Egg & Chz, 183 g	440	23	37
Brkfst Burrito Ssge, Egg & Chz, 169 g	480	31	38
Brkfst Toaster® Bacon, Egg & Chz, 167 g	530	32	40
Brkfst Toaster® Ham, Egg & Chz, 186 g	490	26	40
Brkfst Toaster® - Ssge, Egg & Chz, 194 g	620	42	40
CroisSONIC® Brkfst Snd - Bacon, 150 g	510	36	29
CroisSONIC® Brkfst Snd - Ssge, 177 g	600	46	29
French Toast Sticks (4), 120 g	500	31	49
• Jr. Breakfast Burrito, 116 g	330	21	25
• Ssge Biscuit Dippers w/ Gravy (3), 260 g	690	44	57
Steak and Egg Breakfast Burrito, 246 g	590	34	47
SuperSONIC® Breakfast Burrito, 239 g	570	36	48

Burgers

	Cal	Fat	Cbs
California Cheeseburger, 266 g	690	39	57
Chili Cheeseburger, 226 g	660	35	56
Green Chili Cheeseburger, 287 g	630	31	56
Hickory Cheeseburger, 236 g	640	31	61
Jalapeño Burger, 218 g	550	26	53
Jalapeño Cheeseburger, 236 g	620	31	54

• MOST HEALTHY   • LEAST HEALTHY

▶ SONIC DRIVE-IN (cont.)

	Cal	Fat	Cbs
Jr. Bacon Cheeseburger, 142 g	410	23	31
• Jr. Burger, 117 g	310	15	30
Jr. Deluxe Burger, 134 g	350	20	28
Jr. Double Cheeseburger, 190 g	570	35	33
SONIC® Bacon Chzburger w/ Mayo, 279 g	780	48	57
SONIC® Burger w/ Mayo, 248 g	650	37	55
SONIC® Cheeseburger w/ Mayo, 266 g	720	42	56
• SuperSONIC® Chzburger w/ Mayo, 343 g	980	64	58
SuperSONIC® Jalapeño Chzburger, 313 g	890	53	56
Thousand Island Burger, 248 g	610	32	56
Chicken			
• Chicken Strip Dinner (4), 385 g	930	43	100
Crispy Chicken Bacon Ranch, 255 g	610	34	48
Crispy Chicken Sandwich, 224 g	550	32	46
Grilled Chicken Bacon Ranch, 253 g	470	22	35
Grilled Chicken Sandwich, 222 g	400	19	32
• Jumbo Popcorn Chkn®- Small (4 oz.), 113 g	380	22	27
Condiments			
• French Fry Sauce, 14 g	25	0	7
Marinara Sauce, 28 g	15	0	3
• Picante Sauce, 14 g	5	0	1
Cones & Dishes			
Vanilla Cone, 133 g	180	6	30
Vanilla Dish, 184 g	240	9	36
Coneys			
• Corn Dog, 74 g	210	11	23
• Ex-Long Chili Cheese Coney, 258 g	660	39	55
Regular Coney, 149 g	390	23	32
Cream Pie Shakes (Regular)			
Banana Cream Pie Shake, 470 g	590	19	98
• Chocolate Cream Pie Shake, 475 g	660	19	114
• Coconut Cream Pie Shake, 450 g	580	20	93
Strawberry Cream Pie Shake, 464 g	620	19	106
CreamSlush® Treat (Regular)			
• Blue Coconut CreamSlush® Treat, 437 g	430	13	76
Cherry CreamSlush® Treat, 437 g	440	13	77
Grape CreamSlush® Treat, 437 g	430	13	76
Lemon CreamSlush® Treat, 446 g	430	13	77
• Lemon-Berry CreamSlush® Treat, 450 g	460	12	85
Lime CreamSlush® Treat, 444 g	430	13	77
Orange CreamSlush® Treat, 437 g	430	13	77
Strawberry CreamSlush® Treat, 441 g	450	12	84
Watermelon CreamSlush® Treat, 437 g	440	13	77
Desserts			
Banana Fudge Sundae, 282 g	440	16	70
Banana Split, 309 g	420	9	80

• MOST HEALTHY   • LEAST HEALTHY

SONIC DRIVE-IN (cont.)

	Cal	Fat	Cbs
Everyday Value Menu			
• Chicken Strip Sandwich, 145 g	420	22	39
Jr. Butterfinger® Sundae, 90 g	170	6	26
Jr. FRITOS® Chili Cheese Wrap, 116 g	330	17	34
Jr. M&Ms® Sundae, 91 g	180	7	26
• Jr. Oreo® Sundae, 85 g	150	5	22
• Jr. Reese's PB Cups® Sundae, 90 g	160	5	27
Famous Slushes (Medium)			
Blue Coconut Slush, 559 g	290	0	76
• Bubble Gum Slush, 560 g	290	0	76
Cherry Slush, 560 g	290	0	78
Grape Slush, 560 g	290	0	76
• Green Apple Slush, 561 g	310	0	81
Minute Maid® Crnbry Juice Slush, 560 g	290	0	77
Orange Slush, 559 g	290	0	77
Watermelon Slush, 560 g	290	0	78
Floats/Blended Floats (Regular)			
Barq's® Root Beer Float/Blended Float, 356 g	300	8	56
Coca-Cola® Float/Blended Float, 355 g	290	8	54
• Diet Coke® Float/Blended Float, 348 g	220	8	33
• Dr Pepper® Float/Blended Float, 407 g	310	8	58
Sprite Zero™ Float/Blended Float, 348 g	220	8	33
Sprite® Float/Blended Float, 355 g	290	8	53
Fruit Smoothies (Regular)			
• Strawberry Fruit Smoothie, 420 g	500	0	124
Strawberry-Banana Fruit Smoothie, 435 g	460	0	113
• Tropical Fruit Smoothie, 415 g	440	0	108
Iced Tea (Medium)			
Cranberry Tea, 416 g	40	0	11
• Diet Green Tea, 384 g	5	0	0
Iced Tea, 414 g	5	0	1
Peach Iced Tea, 414 g	5	0	.1
Raspberry Iced Tea, 414 g	5	0	2
• Sweet Iced Tea, 431 g	180	0	48
Kids' Meal			
• Apple Slices, 68 g	35	0	9
w/ FF Caramel Dipping Sauce, 96 g	120	0	27
Chicken Strips (2), 70 g	200	11	10
Corn Dog, 74 g	210	11	23
Fresh Banana, 120 g	110	0	27
• Grilled Cheese, 110 g	380	20	39
Limeades (Medium)			
Cherry Limeade, 453 g	220	0	59
Limeade, 445 g	170	0	47
Lo-Cal Diet Cherry+ Limeade, 432 g	15	0	3

• MOST HEALTHY   • LEAST HEALTHY

SONIC DRIVE-IN (cont.)

	Cal	Fat	Cbs
• Lo-Cal Diet Lime Limeade, 428 g	10	0	1
Minute Maid® Cranberry Limeade, 445 g	200	0	53
• Strawberry Limeade, 449 g	230	0	60

Limited Time Only Products

	Cal	Fat	Cbs
• Ched R Pepper SuperSONIC® Chzburger, 419 g	1250	80	74
Cranberry Limeade Chiller, 14 oz., 465 g	680	27	107
Pineapple Limeade Chiller, 14 oz., 490 g	710	27	113

Malts (Regular)

	Cal	Fat	Cbs
Banana Malt, 442 g	490	17	1
Caramel Malt, 439 g	550	18	1
Chocolate Malt, 439 g	550	17	1
Hot Fudge Malt, 437 g	580	22	1
Peanut Butter Fudge Malt, 436 g	620	29	1
• Peanut Butter Malt, 434 g	670	36	1
Pineapple Malt, 436 g	510	17	1
Strawberry Malt, 436 g	520	17	1
• Vanilla Malt, 422 g	480	18	1

Ocean Water® (Medium)

	Cal	Fat	Cbs
Ocean Water®, 433 g	200	0	53

Powerade® Drinks & Slushes (Medium)

	Cal	Fat	Cbs
Powerade® Mountain Blast®, 425 g	110	0	30
Powerade® Mountain Blast® Slush, 561 g	290	0	78

Premium Roast Coffees

	Cal	Fat	Cbs
• Coffee, 415 g	10	0	2
Iced Latté, Caramel, 352 g	260	8	44
Iced Latté, Caramel/Hazelnut, 351 g	260	8	44
• Iced Latté, Chocolate /Caramel, 351 g	260	8	45
Iced Latté, Chocolate /Hazelnut, 351 g	250	7	45
Iced Latté, Chocolate, 351 g	260	7	45
Iced Latté, Hazelnut, 351 g	260	7	44

Real Fruit Slushes (Medium)

	Cal	Fat	Cbs
• Lemon Real Fruit Slush, 577 g	290	0	78
• Lemon-Berry Real Fruit Slush, 580 g	310	0	83
Lime Real Fruit Slush, 573 g	290	0	78
Strawberry Real Fruit Slush, 562 g	310	0	82

Salads

	Cal	Fat	Cbs
Crispy Chicken Salad, 326 g	340	19	24
Grilled Chicken Salad, 338 g	250	10	12

Shakes (Regular)

	Cal	Fat	Cbs
• Banana Shake, 439 g	470	16	76
Chocolate Shake, 436 g	540	16	89
Hot Fudge Shake, 434 g	570	21	85
Peanut Butter Fudge Shake, 433 g	610	28	81
• Peanut Butter Shake, 429 g	640	34	75
Pineapple Shake, 433 g	500	16	80
Strawberry Shake, 433 g	510	16	83

• MOST HEALTHY   • LEAST HEALTHY

▶ SONIC DRIVE-IN (cont.)

	Cal	Fat	Cbs
Vanilla Shake, 419 g	470	17	71
Single Topping Sundaes			
Carmel, 248 g	390	13	64
Chocolate, 255 g	410	13	67
• Hot Fudge, 253 g	440	18	63
Jr. Butterfinger® Sundae, 90 g	170	6	26
Jr. M&Ms® Sundae, 91 g	180	7	26
Jr. Oreo® Sundae, 85 g	150	5	22
Jr. Reeses PB Cups® Sundae, 90 g	160	5	27
• Nuts Add-On, 4 g	20	2	1
Pineapple, 252 g	370	13	58
Strawbery, 252 g	380	13	61
Snacks & Sides			
Breaded Pork Fritter Sandwich, 242 g	640	0	66
Ched 'R' Bites® (12), 84 g	280	0	22
Ched 'R' Peppers® (4), 120 g	330	1	36
• Fish Sandwich, 246 g	650	0	71
French Fries - Medium, 113 g	330	0	48
FRITOS® Chili Pie - Medium, 138 g	470	0	36
Mozzarella Sticks, 140 g	440	1	40
Onion Rings - Medium, 156 g	440	0	55
Pickle-O's®, 113 g	310	0	36
• Tots - Medium, 70 g	200	0	20
SONIC Blast® (Regular)			
Butterfinger® SONIC Blast®, 373 g	580	22	88
M&M's® SONIC Blast®, 374 g	600	24	88
• Oreo® SONIC Blast®, 363 g	540	21	80
Reese's PB Cups® SONIC Blast®, 372 g	560	19	89
SONIC Chillers™			
Cherry Limeade Chiller, 365 g	410	9	82
• Java Chiller, Caramel, 424 g	540	18	86
Java Chiller, Caramel/Hazelnut, 424 g	530	18	85
Java Chiller, Chocolate, 423 g	540	18	87
Java Chiller, Chocolate/Caramel, 424 g	540	18	85
Java Chiller, Chocolate/Hazelnut, 424 g	540	18	86
Java Chiller, Hazelnut, 424 g	530	18	86
• Limeade Chiller, 351 g	380	9	75
Strawberry Limeade Chiller, 408 g	490	9	101
TOASTER® Sandwiches			
Bacon Chzburger TOASTER® Snd, 243 g	670	39	52
• BLT TOASTER® Sandwich, 149 g	500	29	45
• Chkn Club TOASTER® Snd, 257 g	740	46	55
Country Fried Steak TOASTER® Snd, 243 g	670	37	71
Upgrades			
• Bacon, 13 g	70	5	0
Cheese, 18 g	60	5	2

SONIC DRIVE-IN (cont.)

	Cal	Fat	Cbs
Chili, 33 g	50	4	2
• Green Chiles, 28 g	5	0	1
Grilled Onions, 28 g	25	2	2
Jalapeño, 21 g	5	0	1
Slaw, 28 g	45	3	4
Wraps			
Crispy Chicken Wrap, 234 g	490	23	49
• FRITOS® Chili Cheese Wrap, 241 g	670	39	66
• Grilled Chicken Wrap, 250 g	390	14	39

SOUPER SALAD

	Cal	Fat	Cbs
Beverage			
Lemonade, Mango, 20 oz.	184	0	42
• Lemonade, Premium, 20 oz.	160	0	40
Lemonade, Strawberry, 20 oz.	184	0	42
• Smoothie, Mango, 20 oz.	350	0	89
Smoothie, Strawberry, 20 oz.	320	0	84
Breads			
Blueberry Bread, 1	110	2	22
• Cheese Drop Biscuits, 1	70	3	8
Cheese Pizza, 1	70	3	8
Cornbread, 1	130	4	23
Garlic Breadsticks, 1	130	5	18
Gingerbread, 1	130	5	22
• Green Chili Cornbread, 1	150	4	24
Mushroom Pizza, 1	80	3	9
Pepperoni Pizza, 1	90	4	8
Sausage Pizza, 1	80	4	9
Vegetable Pizza, 1	80	3	9
Condiments			
• Cholula Hot Sauce, 1/4 tsp	0	0	0
Crackers, Gold, Waverly, 1	30	1	4
• Melba Toast, 1	45	1	8
Red Pepper, Crushed, 1/4 tsp	0	0	0
Romano -Parmesan Blend, 1 Tbl	20	1	2
Desserts			
Chocolate Pudding, 1/2 Cup	150	5	28
Cottage Cheese, 1/2 Cup	90	2	5
• Jell-O, sugar free, 1/2 Cup	10	0	0
Shortcake, 4	80	2	14
Sliced Peaches, 1/2 Cup	70	0	17
Strawberry Topping, 1/2 Cup	150	0	38
• Vanilla Pudding, 1/2 Cup	160	5	28
Whipped Topping, 1/2 Cup	100	8	8
Dressings			
• Chipotle Ranch, 2 oz.	280	28	8

SOUPER SALAD (cont.)	Cal	Fat	Cbs
• Fat Free Cranberry, 2 oz.	100	0	24
House Vinaigrette, 2 oz.	220	22	4
Dry Toppings			
Bacon Bits, Imitation, 2 Tbl	50	2	4
Croutons, 1/4 Cup	40	2	6
• Goldfish Crackers, 10	25	1	4
Peanuts, Hot N Spicy, 2 Tbl	100	8	4
Raisins, 2 Tbl	60	0	14
• Sunflower Seeds, 2 Tbl	110	10	3
Vanilla Wafers, 4	70	2	13
Potato Bar			
Bacon Bits, Real, 2 Tbl	80	7	0
Baked Potato, 1	200	0	46
Colby, Shredded, 2 oz.	110	9	1
• Green Onion, 1 Tbl	2	0	0
Picante Sauce, 2 Tbl	10	0	0
• Sweet Potato, 1	200	0	48
Texas Style Chili, 2 oz.	70	3	5
Prepared Salads			
Broccoli Cauliflower Coleslaw, 1/3 Cup	80	6	6
California Chicken Salad, 1/3 Cup	80	6	4
Chickpea Salad, 1/3 Cup	110	6	11
Fettuccine Pasta Salad, 1/3 Cup	100	5	11
Fisherman's Kettle, 1/3 Cup	120	8	9
Gazpacho Salad, 1/3 Cup	30	3	3
• Ham & Macaroni Salad, 1/3 Cup	190	13	15
Italian Macaroni Salad, 1/3 Cup	170	11	14
Jalapeño Chicken & Wild Rice, 1/3 Cup	60	5	4
Loaded Potato Salad, 1/3 Cup	110	6	12
Marinated Mushrooms, 1/3 Cup	60	7	1
Mediterranean Pasta Salad, 1/3 Cup	100	6	10
Mustard Potato Salad, 1/3 Cup	80	5	7
Pasta de Garden, 1/3 Cup	80	5	8
Red Potato Salad, 1/3 Cup	50	4	5
• Roasted Vegetables, 1/3 Cup	20	2	2
Santa Fe Corn Salad, 1/3 Cup	100	4	13
Sweet Garden Slaw, 1/3 Cup	35	2	4
Tuna Skroodle Pasta Salad, 1/3 Cup	130	9	10
Salad Bar			
Beets, 1/4 Cup	20	0	4
Black Olives, 1/4 Cup	60	5	0
Broccoli, 2	5	0	1
Carrots, 1/4 Cup	10	0	3
Cauliflower, 2	5	0	1
Celery, 1/4 Cup	5	0	1
Cheddar Cheese (Imitation), 1/4 Cup	60	4	7

• MOST HEALTHY   • LEAST HEALTHY

SOUPER SALAD (cont.)

	Cal	Fat	Cbs
Eggs, 1/4 Cup	70	5	0
Garbanzo Beans, 1/4 Cup	60	2	10
Green Bell Peppers, 1/4 Cup	10	0	2
Green Olives, 1/4 Cup	30	3	0
Green Peas, 1/4 Cup	25	0	4
Iceberg Lettuce, 1 Cup	10	0	2
Jalapeño, 1/4 Cup	15	0	4
Mushrooms, 1/4 Cup	5	0	1
Pepperoncini, 1	5	0	1
Pepperoni, 4	40	4	0
Radishes, 1/4 Cup	5	0	1
• Red Kidney Beans, 1/4 Cup	80	0	14
Red Onions, 3	5	0	1
Roma Tomatoes, 1/4 Cup	10	0	2
• Romaine Lettuce, 1 Cup	5	0	1
Spinach, 1 Cup	10	0	3
Turkey Ham, 1/4 Cup	50	4	0
Zucchini, 1/4 Cup	5	0	1
Soft Serve			
Carmel Dessert Topping, 1 Tbl	50	1	11
Chocolate Syrup, 1 Tbl	50	0	12
Oreo Crumbles, 1 Tbl	30	1	4
Peanuts, Granulated, 2 Tbl	100	9	4
• Rainbow Sprinkles, 1 Tbl	25	1	4
• Soft Serve Cone, 1	120	3	22
Soft Serve, Vanilla, 1/2 cup	100	3	19
Soups			
Adobe Rice and Chicken, 5 oz. bowl	120	6	10
Beef Mushroom Barley, 5 oz. bowl	80	2	11
Beef Noodle, 5 oz. bowl	70	2	8
Beef Shellini, 5 oz. bowl	90	3	11
Beef Stroganoff, 5 oz. bowl	110	5	9
Black Bean, 5 oz. bowl	80	2	20
Broccoli Cheese, 5 oz. bowl	70	3	10
Cherokee Joe's Cornbread, 5 oz. bowl	70	2	13
Chicken Creole, 5 oz. bowl	100	4	12
• Chicken Enchilada, 5 oz. bowl	180	12	13
Chicken Gumbo, 5 oz. bowl	90	4	10
Chicken Mushroom Barley, 5 oz. bowl	80	3	9
Chicken Noodle with Stars, 5 oz. bowl	40	3	2
Chicken Tetrazzini, 5 oz. bowl	120	5	9
Chicken Tortilla, 5 oz. bowl	60	2	7
Cream of Broccoli, 5 oz. bowl	60	2	9
Cream of Cauliflower, 5 oz. bowl	60	2	10
Cream of Chicken, 5 oz. bowl	100	5	9
Cream of Mushroom, 5 oz. bowl	80	4	10

SOUPER SALAD (cont.)	Cal	Fat	Cbs
Cream of Spinach, 5 oz. bowl	70	3	10
• French Onion, 5 oz. bowl	40	1	6
German Potato, 5 oz. bowl	110	5	13
Holiday Harvest, 5 oz. bowl	90	6	5
Hungarian Mushroom, 5 oz. bowl	110	7	10
Mama Mia Chicken, 5 oz. bowl	80	3	8
Mexican Corn Cheddar, 5 oz. bowl	80	3	14
Minestrone, 5 oz. bowl	70	1	13
Mushroom Barley, 5 oz. bowl	70	2	12
New England Clam Chowder, 5 oz. bowl	100	4	14
Pasta e Fagioli, 5 oz. bowl	80	2	14
Pasta Tortellini Soup, 5 oz. bowl	100	4	13
Potato Corn Chowder, 5 oz. bowl	120	5	16
Potato Leek, 5 oz. bowl	100	3	16
Pumpkin Bisque, 5 oz. bowl	70	3	9
Red Beans, Rice & Sausage, 5 oz. bowl	90	2	19
Santa Fe Chicken Soup, 5 oz. bowl	110	5	11
Seafood Bisque, 5 oz. bowl	120	8	8
Seafood Gumbo, 5 oz. bowl	110	5	13
Shrimp Creole, 5 oz. bowl	90	2	13
Southwest Chicken, 5 oz. bowl	90	2	16
Tamale Soup, 5 oz. bowl	110	4	12
Tomato Basil, 5 oz. bowl	70	3	9
Twice Baked Potato, 5 oz. bowl	110	6	12
Vegan Split Pea, 5 oz. bowl	90	1	16
Vegetable Beef, 5 oz. bowl	80	3	11
Vegetable Lentil, 5 oz. bowl	70	0	16
Vegetable, 5 oz. bowl	50	1	11
Vegetarian Butter Bean, 5 oz. bowl	70	0	21
Vegetarian Vegetable, 5 oz. bowl	50	1	11
White Bean Chicken Chili Stew, 5 oz. bowl	70	3	9
Zucchini Chicken, 5 oz. bowl	80	3	9
Taco Bar			
Beef Lasagna, 1/2 Cup	180	8	13
Corn Taco Shells, 1	50	2	7
Flour Tortilla, 1	90	3	16
Macaroni & Cheese, 1/2 Cup	163	8	15
• Marinara, 2 Tbl	10	0	2
Meaty Marinara Sauce, 2 Tbl	20	1	2
Nacho Cheese Sauce, 2 oz.	45	2	6
Pico de Gallo, 2 oz.	15	0	4
Spaghetti, 1/2 Cup	120	3	21
• Taco Beef, 2 oz.	200	13	2
Vegetable Lasagna, 1/2 Cup	120	4	14
Tossed Salads			
Apple Candied Walnut Salad, 1 Cup	130	11	7

• MOST HEALTHY   • LEAST HEALTHY

SOUPER SALAD (cont.)

	Cal	Fat	Cbs
Caesar Salad, 1 Cup	50	4	4
California Strawberry Salad, 1 Cup	60	3	8
Chicago Chopped Salad, 1 Cup	120	10	3
Chicken Caesar Salad, 1 Cup	90	6	5
• Chicken Chipotle Ranch Salad, 1 Cup	170	13	7
Cobb Salad, 1 Cup	100	8	2
Italian Salad, 1 Cup	50	2	8
Mango Berry Salad, 1 Cup	110	6	13
• Mediterranean Greek Salad, 1 Cup	35	2	3
Shrimp and Crab Louie, 1 Cup	130	10	5
Zesty Feta & Seafood Salad, 1 Cup	60	2	8

SOUPLANTATION

Breads Muffins

	Cal	Fat	Cbs
Apple Cinnamon Bran Muffin (96% FF), 1 pc	130	1	30
Apple Raisin Muffin, 1 piece	150	7	22
Banana Crunch Muffin Top (NSA), 1 piece	120	5	19
Banana Nut Muffin, 1 piece	170	7	22
BBQ Chkn Focaccia on Honey Wheat Crust, 1 pc	200	8	23
Black Forest Muffin, 1 piece	230	9	36
Bruschetta Focaccia, 1 piece	140	7	15
Buffalo Chkn Focaccia on Honey Wheat Crust, 1 pc	170	7	20
Buttermilk Biscuits, 1 biscuit	190	8	25
Buttermilk Cornbread (Low-Fat), 1 piece	140	2	27
Cappuccino Chip Muffin, 1 piece	190	6	31
Caribbean Key Lime Muffin, 1 piece	170	6	28
Carrot Pineapple Muffin w/ Oat Bran, 1 pc	150	6	23
Cherry Nut Muffin, 1 piece	150	7	22
Chile Corn Muffin (Low-Fat), 1 piece	140	3	27
Chipotle Lime Butter, 1 Tbsp.	90	10	0
Chocolate Brownie Muffin, 1 piece	180	8	26
Chocolate Chip Muffin, 1 piece	170	8	22
Choco Peanut Butter Chip Muffin, 1 piece	220	10	31
Country Blackberry Muffin, 1 piece	170	6	27
Cran Orange Bran Muffin (96% FF), 1 pc	130	1	30
Date N' Honey Bran, 1 piece	150	6	24
• French Quarter Praline Muffin, 1 piece	250	10	35
Fruit Medley Bran Muffin (96% FF), 1 pc	130	1	29
Garlic Asiago Focaccia, 1 piece	160	8	19
Georgia Peach Poppyseed Muffin, 1 piece	150	6	20
Grilled Cheese Focaccia, 1 piece	190	10	18
Indian Grain Bread (Low-Fat), 1 piece	200	2	35
Irish Soda Bread, 1 piece	180	5	29
Lemon Vanilla Butter, 1 Tbsp.	90	8	3
Mango Tropics Muffin w/ Coconut, 1 pc	180	7	28
Maple Walnut Muffin, 1 piece	230	10	32

• MOST HEALTHY   • LEAST HEALTHY

▶ SOUPLANTATION (cont.)

	Cal	Fat	Cbs
Old World Greek Focaccia, 1 piece	190	9	24
Pauline's Apple Walnut Cake, 1 piece	220	12	24
Pepperoni Focaccia, 1 piece	190	9	21
Pesto & Sun-Dried Tomato Focaccia, 1 pc	170	8	20
Pineapple Marshmallow Whip, 1/4 cup	240	13	33
Pumpkin Raisin Muffin, 1 piece	150	6	25
Quattro Formaggio Focaccia, 1 piece	140	5	20
Ragin Cajun Veg Focaccia (Veg), 1 piece	160	7	19
Roasted Potato Focaccia, 1 piece	150	6	17
Rst Red Pepper w/ Honeywheat Focaccia, 1 pc	170	8	20
Sauteed Vegetable Focaccia, 1 piece	180	9	19
Sourdough Bread (Low-Fat), 1 piece	150	1	27
Southwest Chipotle Focaccia, 1 piece	160	5	19
Spiced Pumpkin Muffin w/ Cran, 1 piece	180	7	29
Strawberry Buttermilk Muffin, 1 piece	140	6	21
• Sweet Cherry Butter, 1 Tbsp.	80	7	4
Sweet Orange & Cranberry Muffin, 1 pc	200	7	33
Sweet Strawberry Butter, 1 Tbsp.	80	7	4
Taffy Apple Muffin, 1 piece	160	6	25
Tangy Lemon Muffin, 1 piece	140	4	24
Thai Chicken Focaccia w/ Peanuts, 1 piece	170	7	20
Whole Wheat Buttermilk Biscuits, 1 piece	180	6	31
Wildly Blue Blueberry Muffin, 1 piece	140	5	22
Wowie Maui Focaccia w/ Ham, 1 piece	170	7	21
Zucchini Nut Muffin, 1 piece	150	7	22

Breakfast

	Cal	Fat	Cbs
Belgian Waffles, 1 piece	90	0	16
Blueberry Sauce / Blbry Stir-In, 2 Tbsp.	60	0	15
Country Ham & Egg Brkfst Burrito	210	10	21
Egg Scramble Focaccia w/ Bacon, 1 piece	180	8	20
French Toast (Plain), 1 piece	150	4	25
Homemade Oatmeal (Plain), 3/4 cup	110	2	19
Mediterranean Sunrise Pasta, 1 cup	210	12	19
Potatoes O'Brien, 1/2 cup	140	6	19
Scrambled Eggs, 1/2 cup	135	8	2
• Sticky Granola Clusters w/ Almonds, 1/4 cup	270	14	30
• Strawberry Sauce/ Strwbry Stir-In, 2 Tbsp.	45	0	11
Sweet Cinn Biscuits w/ Frosting, 1 piece	270	13	37
Sweet Maple Buttermilk Biscuit, 1 piece	290	9	39
Sweet Pepper & Ssge Egg Brkfast Burrito	210	11	20
Sweet Strwbry Buttermilk Biscuit, 1 piece	250	9	40
Tom's Country Gravy, 2 Tbsp.	90	5	8
Warm Marion Blackberry Sauce, 1/4 cup	80	0	19
Zucchini Fritatta, 1 piece	160	6	22

Desserts

	Cal	Fat	Cbs
Apple Cobbler, 1/2 cup	360	10	67

• MOST HEALTHY   • LEAST HEALTHY

SOUPLANTATION (cont.)

	Cal	Fat	Cbs
Apple Medley (Fat-Free), 1/2 cup	70	0	18
Banana Pudding, 1/2 cup	160	4	27
Banana Royale (Fat-Free), 1/2 cup	80	0	20
Butterscotch Pudding (Low-Fat), 1/2 cup	140	3	24
Candy Sprinkles (Low-Fat), 1 Tbsp.	70	3	11
• Caramel Apple Cobbler, 1/2 cup	390	12	68
Caramel Syrup, 2 Tbsp.	130	1	30
Carrot & Cream Chz Lava Cake, 1 piece	320	15	40
Cherry Apple Cobbler, 1/2 cup	330	10	57
Choco Chip Cookie - 1 Small, 1 cookie	75	3	10
Chocolate Frozen Yogurt (NF), 1/3 cup	110	0	22
Chocolate Lava Cake, 1/2 cup	330	8	62
Choco PntBtr Cookie Bars, 1 piece	270	12	37
Choco Peanut Butter Cookie Cups, 1 pc	140	6	18
Chocolate Pudding (Low-Fat), 1/2 cup	150	3	25
Choco Pudding (Low-Fat, NSA), 1/2 cup	90	2	21
Cranberry Apple Cobbler, 1/2 cup	370	10	58
Cran-Raspberry Gelatin (Fat-Free), 1/2 cup	100	0	26
Deep Choco Winter Mint Lava Cake, 1/2 cup	330	8	58
Gelatin (Fat-Free), 1/2 cup	80	0	20
• Gelatin (Sugar Free, Fat-Free), 1/2 cup	10	0	0
Gooey Caramel Pumpkin Cake, 1/2 cup	280	9	45
Granola Topping, 2 Tbsp.	110	4	16
Green Tea Mousse, 1/2 cup	190	8	29
Holiday Cookies w/ Sprinkles, Sm, 1 cookie	80	4	12
Hot Lemon Lava Cake, 1/2 cup	320	11	51
Nutty Waldorf Salad (Low-Fat), 1/2 cup	90	3	14
Oatmeal Raisin Cookie - 1 small, 1 cookie	120	5	16
Orange Creamsicle Lava Cake, 1/2 Cup	310	11	50
Pineapple Gelatin (Fat-Free), 1/2 cup	120	0	29
Pineapple Upside-Down Cake, 1/2 cup	270	10	42
Raspberry Apple Cobbler, 1/2 cup	380	11	67
Rice Pudding (Low-Fat), 1/2 cup	110	2	20
Shortcake, 1 piece	220	7	36
Strawberry Apple Cobbler, 1/2 cup	340	10	67
Sugar-Free Cherry Choco Mousse, 1/2 cup	40	3	3
Sugar-free Chocolate Mousse, 1/2 cup	40	3	3
Sugar-free Lemon Mousse, 1/2 cup	40	3	4
Sugar-free Raspberry Mousse, 1/2 Cup	40	3	4
Sugar-free Strawberry Mousse, 1/2 cup	40	3	4
Tapioca Pudding (Low-Fat), 1/2 cup	140	3	24
Vanilla Frozen Yogurt (Nonfat), 1/3 cup	100	0	21
Vanilla Pudding, 1/2 cup	150	4	27

Dressings

Avocado Ranch Dressing, 2 Tbsp.	150	14	4
Bacon Dressing, 2 Tbsp.	110	11	7

• MOST HEALTHY   • LEAST HEALTHY

▶ SOUPLANTATION (cont.)

	Cal	Fat	Cbs
Basil Vinaigrette, 2 Tbsp.	160	17	1
Chow Mein Noodles, 1/4 Cup	70	1	15
Cran Orange Vinaigrette (LF), 2 Tbsp.	80	2	15
Creamy Sesame Soy Dressing, 2 Tbsp.	170	17	5
Cucumber Drss (Reduced Calorie), 2 Tbsp.	70	7	3
Garlic Parm Seasoned Croutons, 5 pieces	80	5	6
Green Chili Ranch Dressing, 2 Tbsp.	150	14	4
Honey Lime Cilantro Vinaigrette, 2 Tbsp.	100	6	15
Honey Mint Lemonade, 2 Tbsp.	130	7	19
Italian Vinaigrette w/ Basil & Romano Chz, 2 Tbsp.	150	15	1
Kahlena French Dressing, 2 Tbsp.	120	9	10
Lemon Greek Vinaigrette, 2 Tbsp.	150	15	2
Monterey Blue Salad Dressing, 2 Tbsp.	120	11	5
Parmesan Pepper Cream Drss, 2 Tbsp.	140	16	1
Pineapple Vinaigrette, 2 Tbsp.	110	11	5
• Poppy Seed Orange Vinaigrette (LF), 2 Tbsp	45	2	7
Roasted Garlic Dressing, 2 Tbsp.	100	10	3
Smoky BBQ Vinaigrette, 2 Tbsp.	110	10	5
Spicy Buffalo Ranch Dressing, 2 Tbsp.	130	14	2
• Spicy Southwest Chipotle, 2 Tbsp.	190	20	2
Strawberry Balsamic Vinaigrette, 2 Tbsp.	130	13	2
Sweet Maple Dressing, 2 Tbsp.	180	17	6
Tomato Basil Croutons, 5 pieces	70	5	5
Warm Bacon Dressing, 2 Tbsp.	110	10	5

Hot Pastas Kitchen Favorites

	Cal	Fat	Cbs
100% Whole Wheat Jalapeño & Salsa pasta (Veg), 1 cup	250	6	46
4 Cheese Alfredo (Vegetarian), 1 cup	390	13	50
Arizona Marinara (Vegetarian), 1 cup	360	11	47
Beefy Meatball Stroganoff, 1 cup	340	21	28
Broccoli Alfredo w/ Basil (Veg), 1 cup	380	17	45
Broccoli Chz Baked Potato Topper (Veg), 1 cup	120	7	10
Bruschetta (Vegetarian), 1 cup	260	4	41
Carbonara Pasta w/ Bacon, 1 cup	290	10	43
Chzy Scalloped Potatoes w/ Bacon, 1 cup	240	17	15
• Chicken Tetrazzini, 1 cup	480	23	47
Cilantro Lime Pesto (Vegetarian), 1 cup	370	21	36
Creamy Bruschetta (Vegetarian), 1 cup	360	16	43
Creamy Herb Chicken, 1 cup	310	17	32
Curried Pineapple & Ginger (LF, Non-Veg), 1 cup	200	2	40
Fettuccine Alfredo (Vegetarian), 1 cup	390	18	41
Fire-Rst Tomato Basil Alfredo (Veg), 1 cup	370	14	44
Garden Veg w/ Italian Sausage, 1 cup	300	10	42
Garden Vegetable w/ Meatballs, 1 cup	310	10	44
Greek Mediterranean (Vegetarian), 1 cup	290	8	45
Hand-Crafted Mexican Beans (LF, Veg), 1 cup	260	2	47
Italian Ssge w/ Red Pepper Puree, 1 cup	250	10	35

● MOST HEALTHY   ● LEAST HEALTHY

SOUPLANTATION (cont.)

	Cal	Fat	Cbs
Italian Vegetable Beef, 1 cup	290	9	43
Lemon Cream w/ Capers (Non-Veg), 1 cup	390	21	44
Linguini w/ Clam Sauce, 1 cup	380	10	56
Macaroni & Cheese (Vegetarian), 1 cup	330	15	40
Nutty Mushroom (Vegetarian), 1 cup	390	20	42
Oriental Noodle & Green Bean (LF, Veg), 1 cup	240	3	45
Pasta Florentine (Vegetarian), 1 cup	360	10	54
Penne Arrabbiatta (Vegetarian), 1 cup	340	10	43
Ragin Cajun w/ Andouille Sausage, 1 cup	370	22	33
Roasted Eggplant Marinara (Veg), 1 cup	340	10	43
Rst Garlic & Asiago Alfredo (Veg), 1 cup	330	11	45
Rst Mshr Alfredo w/ Rosemary (Veg), 1 cup	380	14	44
• Salsa de Lupe (Fat-Free, Vegan), 1/4 cup	30	0	6
Sautéed Balsamic Vegs (Vegan), 1/2 cup	100	6	11
Smoked Salmon & Dill, 1 cup	360	16	41
Smoky BBQ Baked Beans (LF, Non-Veg), 1 cup	320	3	61
Spicy Italian Sausage & Peppers, 1 cup	360	11	43
Steamed Vegs w/ Lemon Herb Butter (Veg), 1/2 cup	130	9	10
Stuffing (Non-Vegetarian), 1/2 cup	210	12	20
Tom Spinach Whole Wheat (Veg), 1 cup	250	10	33
Tuscany Ssge w/Capers & Olives, 1 cup	240	10	29
Vegetable Ragu (Vegetarian), 1 cup	250	6	41
Vegetarian Marinara w/ Basil (Veg), 1 cup	260	4	44
Walnut Pesto (Vegetarian), 1 cup	310	9	42

Prepared Salads

	Cal	Fat	Cbs
100% Whole Wheat Arugula Citrus (Vegan), 1/2 cup	210	10	29
• 100% Whole Wheat Crm Chipotle Salad (Veg), 1/2 cup	350	25	31
100% Whole Wheat Sicilian Penne w/ Feta & Pepp, 1/2 cup	250	14	30
100% Whole Wheat Spicy Asian Pnt Salad (Vegan), 1/2 cup	260	14	32
Ambrosia w/ Coconut (Veg), 1/2 cup	190	9	30
Artichoke Rice (Vegetarian), 1/2 cup	190	12	19
• Aunt Doris' Red Pepper Slaw (FF, Vegan), 1/2 cup	70	0	18
Baja Bean & Cilantro (Low-Fat, Vegan), 1/2 cup	180	3	29
BBQ Potato (Vegetarian), 1/2 cup	170	9	21
Bistro Potato (Vegetarian), 1/2 cup	290	19	27
Buffalo Blue Potato Salad (Veg), 1/2 Cup	190	13	16
Carrot Raisin (Low-Fat, Veg), 1/2 cup	90	3	17
Chinese Krab (Vegetarian), 1/2 cup	160	8	19
Citrus Noodles w/ Snow Peas (Veg), 1/2 cup	140	5	19
Confetti Avocado Slaw (Veg), 1/2 cup	140	9	12
Dijon Potato w/ Garlic Dill Vinaigrette (Vegan), 1/2 cup	150	12	9
Field Corn & Very Wild Rice (Veg), 1/2 cup	170	9	19
German Potato, 1/2 cup	150	6	23
Greek Couscous w/ Feta Chz & Pinenuts (Veg), 1/2 cup	210	14	25
Italian White Bean (Vegan), 1/2 cup	140	5	19
Jalapeño Potato (Vegetarian), 1/2 cup	170	9	21

• MOST HEALTHY • LEAST HEALTHY

SOUPLANTATION (cont.)

	Cal	Fat	Cbs
Joan's Broccoli Madness (Non-Veg), 1/2 Cup	180	14	11
Lemon Linguini w/ Toasted Pinenuts, 1/2 Cup	230	13	26
Lemon Rice w/ Cashews (Vegan), 1/2 cup	160	7	23
Mandarin Noodles w/ Broccoli (LF, Vegan), 1/2 cup	170	3	31
Mandarin Shells w/ Almonds (LF, Vegan), 1/2 cup	120	3	19
Old Fashioned Macaroni w/ Ham, 1/2 cup	200	13	18
Oriental Ginger Slaw w/ Krab (Low-Fat), 1/2 cup	70	3	8
Penne Pasta w/ Chkn in Citrus Vinaigrette (LF), 1/2 cup	130	3	20
Pesto Pasta (Vegetarian), 1/2 cup	180	9	21
Picnic Potato (Vegetarian), 1/2 cup	190	14	17
Pineapple Coconut Slaw (Veg), 1/2 cup	150	10	14
Poppyseed Coleslaw (Veg), 1/2 cup	120	9	9
Provencal Green Bean & Potato (Vegan), 1/2 cup	220	14	25
Red Potato & Tomato (Veg), 1/2 cup	170	11	17
Red, White, & Blue Potato Salad (w/ bacon), 1/2 Cup	190	13	15
Rst Potato w/ Chipotle Chile Vinaigrette (Vegan), 1/2 cup	140	6	18
San Francisco Herb Rice (Non-Veg), 1/2 cup	180	6	27
Shrimp & Seafood Shells, 1/2 cup	210	13	20
Smoky Ham & Cheddar Broccoli Slaw, 1/2 cup	260	18	21
Southern Black-Eyed Pea (Veg), 1/2 cup	130	6	18
Southern Dill Potato (LF, Veg), 1/2 cup	120	3	20
SW Rice & Beans (Low-Fat, Veg), 1/2 cup	90	3	15
Spicy Cajun Shells (Vegetarian), 1/2 cup	300	13	40
Spicy SW Pasta (Low-Fat, Veg), 1/2 cup	130	3	21
Summer Barley w/ Black Beans (LF, Vegan), 1/2 cup	110	3	19
Sweet & Sour Broccoli Slaw (LF, Vegan), 1/2 cup	150	3	28
Sweet Marinated Vegs (FF, Vegan), 1/2 cup	80	0	19
Sweet Tomato, Basil & Mozz. (Veg), 1/2 cup	170	6	23
Tabouli (Vegan), 1/2 cup	200	10	24
Thai Citrus & Brown Rice (Vegan), 1/2 cup	220	12	26
Thai Noodle w/ Chkn & Peanut Sc, 1/2 cup	190	10	19
Three Bean Marinade (Vegan), 1/2 cup	170	6	27
Tom Cucumber Marinade (Vegan), 1/2 cup	80	5	8
Tuna Tarragon, 1/2 cup	250	15	21
Turkey Chutney Pasta, 1/2 cup	240	12	20
Wheat Berry & Curry (Vegetarian), 1/2 cup	210	5	36
Whole Grain Fiesta Couscous (Veg), 1/2 cup	280	11	39
Wild Rice & Chicken, 1/2 cup	300	21	21
Zesty Tortellini (Vegetarian), 1/2 cup	230	15	20

Soups

	Cal	Fat	Cbs
8 Vegetable Chicken Stew, 1 cup	160	7	17
Albondigas Locas (Meatball Soup), 1 cup	210	11	19
• Asian Ginger Broth (Low-Fat, Veg), 1 cup	50	2	6
Basmati Lentil Soup, 1 cup	210	7	29
Beef & Barley Stew, 1 cup	240	10	19
Better Than Mom's Beef Stew, 1 cup	270	17	19

SOUPLANTATION (cont.)

	Cal	Fat	Cbs
Big Chunk Chkn Noodle (Low-Fat), 1 cup	170	3	19
Border Black Bean & Chorizo Soup, 1 cup	240	10	27
Broccoli Cheese (Vegetarian), 1 cup	270	19	17
• Canadian Cheese w/ Smoked Ham, 1 cup	350	26	22
Chz Stuffed Cappelletti (Non-Veg), 1 cup	250	11	31
Cheesy Corn Chowder w/ Bacon, 1 Cup	220	11	25
Chesapeake Corn Chowder (Non-Veg), 1 cup	290	17	30
Chicken & Rice, 1 cup	160	5	18
Chicken Dijon (Reduced Sodium), 1 cup	210	13	18
Chicken Divan, 1 Cup	240	15	18
Chicken Fajitas & Black Bean, 1 cup	280	7	37
Chicken Pot Pie Stew, 1 cup	310	21	21
Chkn Tortilla w/ Jalapeño Chiles & Tom (LF), 1 cup	100	3	11
Chili Cheeseburger, 1 cup	290	12	29
Chunky Potato Chz w/ Thyme (Veg), 1 cup	240	11	25
Clss Creamy Tom Soup (Non-Veg), 1 cup	200	13	19
Classic French Onion (Non-Veg), 1 cup	150	6	21
Classic Shrimp Bisque, 1 cup	240	16	15
Clss Minestrone (LF, Vegan), 1 cup	120	2	20
Continental Lentil & Spinach (LF, Veg), 1 cup	160	2	18
Corned Beef & Cabbage, 1 cup	220	6	17
Country Corn & Red Potato Chowder (Non-Veg), 1 cup	220	8	35
Cream of Broccoli (Vegetarian), 1 cup	260	19	19
Cream of Chicken, 1 cup	290	21	16
Cream of Mshr (Non-Vegetarian), 1 cup	290	24	15
Crm of Rosemary Potato (Non-Veg), 1 cup	320	22	26
Creamy Herbed Turkey, 1 cup	320	22	18
Crm Pumpkin Bisque w/ Pine Nuts, 1 cup	190	7	31
Creamy Vegetable Chowder (Veg), 1 cup	270	14	26
Curried Yellow Split Pea (LF, Veg), 1 cup	230	2	40
Deep Kettle House Chili (Non-Veg), 1 cup	230	3	26
Deep Kettle House Chili w/ 33% more meat!, 1 cup	250	8	26
Deep Kettle House Chili w/ 50% more meat!, 1 cup	290	11	29
El Paso Lime & Chicken, 1 cup	160	4	24
Cauliflower w/ Proud to be American Chz (Veg), 1 cup	280	21	19
Sweet Tomato Basil (Veg), 1 cup	220	15	20
Fire-Rst Green Chile & Corn Chowder w/ Bacon, 1 cup	240	15	21
Garden Fresh Vegetable (LF, Veg), 1 cup	150	2	27
Garden of Eatin' (Low-Fat, Veg), 1 cup	150	3	25
Golden Yam Bisque (Vegetarian), 1 cup	220	8	28
Green Chile Stew w/ Pork, 1 cup	170	6	18
Indian Lentil (Low-Fat, Vegan), 1 cup	160	3	25
Irish Potato Leek (Vegetarian), 1 cup	260	16	23
Lemon Chicken Orzo, 1 cup	220	9	21
Ld Baked Potato & Chz w/ Bacon, 1 cup	290	18	24
Longhorn Beef Chili, 1 cup	190	6	25

• MOST HEALTHY   • LEAST HEALTHY

SOUPLANTATION (cont.)

	Cal	Fat	Cbs
Marvelous Minestrone w/ Bacon, 1 cup	220	8	31
Minestrone w/ Italian Sausage, 1 cup	220	12	17
Moroccan Garbanzo & Lentil Bean (LF, Veg), 1 cup	230	2	40
Mulligatawny (Non-Vegetarian), 1 cup	240	14	17
Neighbor Joe's Gumbo (Non-Veg), 1 cup	210	10	20
New Mexican Corn Tortilla w/ Chkn, 1 cup	200	10	19
New Orleans Jambalaya (Non-Veg), 1 cup	210	11	18
Old Fashion Veg (Low-Fat, Veg), 1 cup	100	2	18
Pinto Bean & Basil Barley (LF, Veg), 1 cup	160	2	29
Posole w/ Pork, 1 cup	150	6	8
Potato Tomato & Spinach (LF, Veg), 1 cup	150	2	28
Ratatouille Provencale (FF, Vegan), 1 cup	110	0	25
Roasted Mshr w/ Sage (Non-Veg), 1 cup	320	26	19
Rustic Tuscan Stew (LF, Non-Veg), 1 cup	140	2	25
Santa Fe Black Bean Chili (LF, Vegan), 1 cup	190	3	26
Savory Turkey Harvest, 1 cup	220	12	18
Smoky Pinto & Brown Rice (LF, Veg), 1 cup	150	2	28
Southwest Tomato Cream (Veg), 1 cup	130	7	14
Southwest Tkey Chowder w/ Bacon, 1 cup	240	15	21
Spicy Navajo Veg Soup (FF, Vegan), 1 cup	110	0	26
Spicy Sausage & Pasta, 1 cup	300	12	34
Spicy Tamale Chili, 1 cup	190	8	24
Split Pea & Potato Barley (LF, Veg), 1 cup	200	2	37
Split Pea w/ Ham, 1 cup	290	10	36
Sweet Potato Corn Chowder w/ Ham, 1 cup	220	7	36
Sweet Tomato Onion (Vegan), 1 cup	90	3	13
Texas Red Chili (Non-Veg), 1 cup	190	7	24
Three Cheese Tortellini (Veg), 1 cup	180	6	28
Three-Bean Turkey Chili (Low-Fat), 1 cup	170	3	24
Tomato Chipotle Bisque (Non-Veg), 1 cup	250	17	20
Tomato Parm & Veg (LF, Veg), 1 cup	120	3	18
Turkey Cassoulet w/ Bacon, 1 cup	240	12	17
Tkey Noodle Soup w/ 100% Whole Wheat Noodles, 1 cup	160	4	24
Turkey Vegetable, 1 cup	210	12	15
U.S. Senate Bean w/ Smoked Ham, 1 cup	150	4	20
Veg Bean & Barley Stew (LF, Veg), 1 cup	150	2	28
Vegetable Medley (Low-Fat, Veg), 1 cup	90	1	14
Vegetarian Harvest (Vegan), 1 cup	200	10	23
White Bean & Lime Chicken Chili, 1 cup	220	5	29
X-treme Spice Veg Chili w/ Energy Boost (LF, Vegl), 1 cup	100	1	17
Yankee Clipper Clam Chowder w/ Bacon, 1 cup	310	20	21
Tossed Salads			
Azteca Taco w/ Turkey, 1 cup	130	9	7
Bartlett Pear & Caramel Walnut, 1 cup	180	12	13
BBQ Julienne Chopped w/ Chkn, 1 cup	210	11	23
• BBQ Smokehouse w/ Bacon & Peanuts, 1 cup	290	17	25

● MOST HEALTHY   ● LEAST HEALTHY

SOUPLANTATION (cont.)

	Cal	Fat	Cbs
Buffalo Chicken, 1 cup	180	14	10
Caesar Salad Asiago (Non-Veg), 1 cup	270	22	10
California Cobb w/ Bacon, 1 cup	190	15	7
Cambay Curry w/ Almonds & Coconut (Veg), 1 cup	220	17	17
Cape Cod Spinach w/ Walnuts & Bacon, 1 cup	170	14	6
Cherry Chipotle Spinach (Veg), 1 cup	160	8	20
Chicken Tortilla, 1 cup	180	10	16
Classic Antipasto, 1 cup	280	21	18
• Classic Greek (Vegetarian), 1 cup	120	9	4
Club Blue BLT w/ Bacon, 1 cup	270	17	20
Country French w/ Bacon, 1 cup	210	18	7
Crunchy Island Pineapple (Veg), 1 cup	160	8	20
Field of Greens: Citrus Vinaigrette (Vegan), 1 cup	150	12	10
Field of Greens: Sweet Maple (Veg), 1 cup	180	15	10
Green Chile Ranch w/ Spicy Tortilla Chips (Veg), 1 cup	260	16	24
Honey Minted Fruit Toss (Veg), 1 cup	140	6	20
Mandarin Spinach w/ Caramel Walnuts (Vegan), 1 cup	170	11	14
Mediterranean Bistro Potato, 1 cup	230	11	26
Monterey Blue w/ Peanuts (Veg), 1 cup	270	17	25
Outrageous Orange w/ Cashews (Veg), 1 cup	210	15	16
Ragin' Cajun w/ Chicken, 1 cup	220	14	15
Ranch House BLT w/ Tkey & Bacon, 1 cup	190	13	11
Rst Veg w/ Feta & Olives (Veg), 1 cup	190	15	12
San Marino Spinach w/ Pumpkin Seeds & Cran (Veg), 1 cup	200	13	13
Sedona Green Chile & Chipotle (Non-Veg), 1 cup	220	16	15
Smkd Tkey & Spinach w/ Almonds, 1 cup	190	10	20
Sonoma Spinach w/ Honey Dijon Vinaigrette (Veg), 1 cup	210	14	11
Spiced Pecan & Rst Veg w/ Bacon, 1 cup	200	13	15
Spinach Gorgonzola w/ Spiced Pecans & Bacon, 1 cup	230	19	9
Strwbry Fields w/ Carmel Walnuts (Vegan), 1 cup	130	8	15
Summer Lemon w/ Spiced Pecans (Veg), 1 cup	220	17	16
Thai Peanut & Red Pepper (Vegan), 1 cup	220	11	23
Thai Udon & Peanut (Vegan), 1 cup	220	13	19
Traditional Spinach w/ Bacon, 1 cup	190	13	11
Won Ton Chicken Happiness, 1 cup	170	5	11

SOUTHERN TSUNAMI

	Cal	Fat	Cbs
California Roll, 270 g	628	5	129
Classic Miso Roll, 306 g	758	9	13
Cream Cheese Roll, 280 g	794	19	123
Crunchy Shrimp Roll, 273 g	773	18	129
Dragon Roll (FW Eel), 288 g	785	18	130
Eel Roll (FW Eel), 281 g	770	16	125
• Red Chili Roll, 255 g	600	13	89
Spicy Roll (Baby Shrimp), 286 g	710	8	133
Spicy Roll (Salmon), 279 g	745	14	121

SOUTHERN TSUNAMI (cont.)

	Cal	Fat	Cbs
Spicy Roll (Tuna), 285 g	731	9	125
• Stardust Combo, 352 g	981	9	200
Tempura Roll, 315 g	806	11	146
Tsunami Roll, 260 g	734	12	133
Vegetable Combo (12 pcs.), 267 g	618	6	128
Condiments			
• Green Horseradish, 4 g	7	0	1
Pickled Ginger, 13 g	9	0	24
• Soy Sauce, 7 g	16	0	2
Salads			
• Edamame Salad, 113 g	124	7	9
Edamame (Soybean), 75 g	90	5	3
• Seabreeze Salad, 113 g	13	3	23

STARBUCKS

Bakery			
8-Grain Roll	350	8	67
Apple Bran Muffin	350	9	64
Apple Fritter	420	20	59
Asiago Bagel	310	5	54
Blueberry Oat Bar	370	14	47
Blueberry Scone	460	22	61
Blueberry Streusel Muffin	360	11	59
Butter Croissant	310	18	32
Cheese Danish	420	25	39
Chocolate Bloom Cupcake	420	27	42
Chocolate Chunk Cookie	360	17	50
Chocolate Croissant	300	17	34
• Chocolate Mini Sparkle Doughnut	120	6	16
Chocolate Old-Fashioned Doughnut	420	21	57
Chonga Bagel	310	5	52
Cinnamon Chip Scone	480	18	70
Cranberry Orange Scone	490	18	73
Double Chocolate Brownie	410	24	46
Double Iced Cinnamon Roll	490	20	70
Hawaiian Bagel	360	8	60
Iced Lemon Pound Cake	490	23	68
Lowfat Red Raspberry Muffin	340	6	65
Mallorca Sweet Bread	420	25	42
Maple Oat Pecan Scone	440	18	59
Marble Pound Cake	350	13	53
Marshmallow Dream Bar	210	4	43
Morning Bun	350	16	45
Multigrain Bagel	320	4	62
Old-Fashioned Glazed Doughnut	420	21	57
Outrageous Oatmeal Cookie	370	14	56

• MOST HEALTHY   • LEAST HEALTHY

STARBUCKS (cont.)

	Cal	Fat	Cbs
Petite Vanilla Bean Scone	140	5	21
Plain Bagel	300	1	64
Pumpkin Bread	390	15	60
Pumpkin Scone	480	17	78
• Raspberry Scone	500	26	59
Red.Fat Banana Choco Chip Coffee Cake	390	7	79
Red.Fat Cinnamon Swirl Coffee Cake	340	9	62
Reduced-Fat Very Berry Coffee Cake	350	10	58
Rich Toffee Pecan Bar	380	22	42
Starbucks® Classic Coffee Cake	440	19	63
Starbucks® Indulgent Chocolate Cookie	320	19	40
Vanilla Buttercream Cupcake	400	23	46
Vanilla Mini Sparkle Doughnut	120	6	16
Zucchini Walnut Muffin	490	28	52

Brewed Coffee

	Cal	Fat	Cbs
Clover® Brewed Coffee	5	0	0
Decaf Pike Place™ Roast	5	0	0
Pike Place™ Roast	5	0	0

Chocolate Beverages

	Cal	Fat	Cbs
Hot Chocolate	300	9	47
White Hot Chocolate	410	12	61

Espresso Beverages

	Cal	Fat	Cbs
Caffè Latte	190	7	18
Caffè Mocha	260	8	41
Cappuccino	120	4	12
Caramel Macchiato	240	7	34
Cinnamon Dolce Latte	260	6	40
Dark Cherry Mocha	320	8	57
Flavored Latte	250	6	36
Iced Caffè Latte	130	5	13
Iced Caffè Mocha	200	6	35
Iced Caramel Macchiato	230	6	33
Iced Cinnamon Dolce Latte	200	4	34
Iced Dark Cherry Mocha	250	5	51
Iced Flavored Latte	250	6	36
Iced Peppermint Mocha	260	6	52
Iced Peppermint White Choco Mocha	400	9	72
• Iced Skinny Flavored Latte	110	4	12
Iced White Chocolate Mocha	340	9	55
Peppermint Mocha	330	8	58
• Peppermint White Chocolate Mocha	470	12	78
Skinny Cinnamon Dolce Latte	180	6	18
Skinny Flavored Latte	180	6	18
White Chocolate Mocha	400	11	61

Frappuccino® Blended Beverages

	Cal	Fat	Cbs
Caffè Vanilla Frappuccino® Blended Coffee	310	3	67

• MOST HEALTHY • LEAST HEALTHY

STARBUCKS (cont.)

	Cal	Fat	Cbs
Caffè Vanilla Frappuccino® Light Blended Coffee	190	1	42
Caramel Frappuccino® Blended Coffee	270	4	53
Caramel Frappuccino® Light Blended Coffee	160	2	30
Chai Frappuccino® Blended Crème	330	2	67
Cinn Dolce Frappuccino® Blended Coffee	260	3	52
Cinn Dolce Frappuccino® Blended Crème	320	2	64
Cinn Dolce Frappuccino® Light Blended Coffee	140	1	29
Coffee Frappuccino® Blended Coffee	240	3	48
• Coffee Frappuccino® Light Blended Coffee	130	1	25
Double Choco Chip Frappuccino® Blended Crème	400	8	75
Espresso Frappuccino® Blended Coffee	190	3	38
Green Tea Frappuccino® Blended Crème	380	3	78
Java Chip Frappuccino® Blended Coffee	340	8	64
Java Chip Frappuccino® Light Blended Coffee	200	5	36
Mocha Frappuccino® Blended Coffee	260	4	54
Mocha Frappuccino® Light Blended Coffee	140	1	29
Strwbry & Crème Frappuccino® Blended Crème	360	3	74
Vanilla Bean Frappuccino® Blended Crème	350	3	72
• White Choco Frappuccino® Blended Crème	480	0	89
White Choco Mocha Frappuccino® Blended Coffee	300	5	59

Fruit & Snack Plates
Fruit & Cheese Plate	380	21	37
Protein Plate	370	17	39

Hot Breakfast
Bacon, Gouda Chz & Egg Frittata on Artisan Roll	380	20	31
Black Forest Ham, Parm Frittata & Chdr on Artisan Roll	370	16	32
• Brown Sugar Top for Starbucks® Perfect Oatmeal	50	0	13
Dried Fruit Top for Starbucks® Perfect Oatmeal	100	0	24
Egg White, Spinach & Feta Wrap	280	10	33
Huevos Rancheros Wrap	330	15	35
Nut Medley Top for Starbucks® Perfect Oatmeal	100	9	2
Red.Fat Tkey Bacon w/ Egg Whites on English Muffin	340	10	47
• Ssge, Egg & Chz on English Muffin	500	29	42
Starbucks® Perfect Oatmeal	140	3	25

Kids' Drinks & Others
Flavored Steamed Milk	200	6	28

Salads
Couscous Salad with Curried Chicken	360	7	59
Deluxe Fruit Blend	90	0	23

Sandwiches, Panini & Wraps
• Chicken & Vegetable Wrap	290	9	36
Chicken Santa Fe	380	10	47
• Egg Salad Sandwich	490	22	54
Ham & Swiss Sandwich	360	9	43
Roma Tomato & Mozzarella Sandwich	380	18	40

● MOST HEALTHY   • LEAST HEALTHY

STARBUCKS (cont.)

	Cal	Fat	Cbs
Tarragon Chicken Salad Sandwich	480	11	62
Tuna Melt Panini	390	12	49
Turkey & Swiss Sandwich	390	13	36

Tazo® Teas

	Cal	Fat	Cbs
• Tazo® Awake™ Brewed Tea	0	0	0
Tazo® Black Shaken Iced Tea	80	0	21
• Tazo® Black Shaken Iced Tea Lemonade	130	0	33
• Tazo® Calm™ Brewed Tea	0	0	0
Tazo® China Green Tips Brewed Tea	0	0	0
Tazo® Earl Grey Brewed Tea	0	0	0
Tazo® Full Leaf Chai Tea	0	0	0
Tazo® Orange Blossom Brewed Tea	0	0	0
Tazo® Passion™ Brewed Tea	0	0	0
• Tazo® Refresh™ Brewed Tea	0	0	0
Tazo® Shaken Iced Green Tea	80	0	21
Tazo® Shaken Iced Green Tea Lemonade	130	0	33
Tazo® Shaken Iced Passion Tea	80	0	21
Tazo® Shaken Iced Passion Tea Lemonade	130	0	33

Vivanno™ Smoothies

	Cal	Fat	Cbs
Chocolate Vivanno™ Smoothie	270	5	48
• Orange Mango Vivanno™ Smoothie	260	2	51
• Strawberry Vivanno™ Smoothie	280	2	56

Yogurt Parfaits

	Cal	Fat	Cbs
• Dark Cherry Yogurt Parfait	310	4	61
• Greek Yogurt Honey Parfait	290	12	43
Strawberry & Blueberry Yogurt Parfait	300	4	60

STEAK ESCAPE

7" Sandwiches

	Cal	Fat	Cbs
Cajun Chicken, 245 g	408	5	58
• Capicola Portion, 28 g	31	1	0
Chicken Portion, 112 g	120	4	0
• Classic Italian Sub, 238 g	471	11	60
Ham Portion, 84 g	75	1	3
Salami Portion, 28 g	105	9	0
Steak Portion, 112 g	130	5	0
Turkey Club, 224 g	380	2	62
Turkey Portion, 84 g	75	1	3
Vegetarian, 252 g	311	1	65
Wild West BBQ, 273 g	455	6	60

Fresh-Cut Fries

	Cal	Fat	Cbs
12 oz. cup, 168 g	498	26	67

Grilled Salads

	Cal	Fat	Cbs
• Side Salad, 168 g	40	1	8
Side Salad with Chicken, 316 g	177	5	11
Side Salad with Ham, 302 g	132	2	8

• MOST HEALTHY   • LEAST HEALTHY

STEAK ESCAPE (cont.)

	Cal	Fat	Cbs
• Side Salad with Steak, 316 g	187	6	11
Side Salad with Turkey, 302 g	132	2	8
Kids Chicken Tenders			
All White Meat Chkn Tenders (2), 109 g	240	11	21
Kids Sandwiches			
Chicken, 110 g	205	7	29
• Ham, 106 g	183	1	31
• Steak, 110 g	210	3	29
Turkey, 106 g	183	1	31
Loaded Fries			
Bacon & Cheddar, 308 g	905	44	88
Ranch & Bacon, 308 g	1044	71	84
Loaded Smashed Potatoes			
Bacon & Cheddar, 476 g	636	26	91
Ranch & Bacon, 476 g	692	34	87
Smashed Potatoes			
• Plain, 392 g	246	0	53
Potatoes with Chicken, 568 g	383	4	56
Potatoes with Ham, 554 g	338	2	59
• Potatoes with Steak, 568 g	393	5	56
Potatoes with Turkey, 554 g	338	2	59
Toppings			
Bacon (1 oz.), 28 g	32	3	2
Black Olives, 42 g	11	0	2
• Cheddar, 28 g	116	8	1
Jalapeño Peppers, 42 g	11	N/A	N/A
• Lettuce, 28 g	2	0	0
Mild Peppers, 42 g	11	0	4
Parmesan, 7 g	30	2	0
Provolone, 21 g	80	6	0
Tomatoes, 56 g	24	0	2
White American (1 oz.), 28 g	101	9	3

SUB STATION II

Sandwiches

Bologna & Cheese	658	47	44
Corned Beef & Cheese	613	39	40
Genoa Salami, Pepperoni & Cheese	791	58	43
Ham & Cheese	582	36	48
Ham, Bologna & Cheese	645	44	42
Ham, Bologna, Cappicola & Cheese	624	42	41
• Ham, Bologna, Genoa Salami, Pepp, Cappicola, Tkey & Chz	823	57	43
• Ham, Cappicola & Cheese	580	36	42
Ham, Genoa Salami & Cheese	679	45	45
Ham, Genoa Salami, Pepperoni & Cheese	789	55	48
Ham, Pepperoni & Cheese	720	49	48

• MOST HEALTHY   • LEAST HEALTHY

STEAK ESCAPE (cont.)

	Cal	Fat	Cbs
Ham, Turkey & Cheese	606	37	49
Provolone, Swiss & American Cheese	700	49	40
Roast Beef & Cheese	631	40	44
Roast Beef, Ham & Cheese	608	38	42
Roast Beef, Ham, Turkey & Cheese	628	39	39
Roast Beef, Turkey & Cheese	603	38	41
Turkey & Cheese	601	37	48

SUBMARINA

Subs

	Cal	Fat	Cbs
• Albacure Tuna, 6"	757	54	48
ARB, 6"	490	24	49
ATC, 6"	495	22	46
• Bacon, 6"	338	12	42
Baja, 6"	663	31	58
BLT, 6"	473	25	47
Cali, 6"	655	30	60
California Sub, 6"	545	26	46
Chicken Breast Filet, 6"	395	13	44
Chicken Caesar, 6"	535	24	42
Club Sub, 6"	483	20	45
Combo Cheese, 6"	730	45	45
East Coast Sub, 6"	604	33	47
Ham & Salami, 6"	538	28	46
Ham & Turkey, 6"	403	15	45
Ham, 6"	423	17	46
Hot Pastrami, 6"	366	16	44
Italian Sub, 6"	604	34	46
Meatball, 6"	380	14	53
Monterey Chicken, 6"	570	24	56
Oven Roasted Chicken, 6"	395	13	44
Pepper Fiesta, 6"	410	12	45
Peppered Garden, 6"	575	26	45
Peppered Ranch, 6"	460	19	45
Pepperoni & Salami, 6"	668	41	47
Pepperoni, 6"	650	40	47
Proscuitto, 6"	420	21	45
Roast Beef & Ham, 6"	438	17	45
Roast Beef & Turkey, 6"	428	15	45
Roast Beef, 6"	440	17	45
Salami, 6"	620	36	47
Santa Fe, 6"	523	23	47
Triple Play, 6"	438	16	45
Turkey, 6"	395	13	44
Veggie, 6"	470	27	48

• MOST HEALTHY   • LEAST HEALTHY

SUBMARINA (cont.)

	Cal	Fat	Cbs
Sub Salads			
• Albacore Tuna	593	50	11
• Garden Salad	35	0	5
Grilled Chicken Caesar	430	30	9
Santa Fe Salad	338	20	10

SUBWAY

	Cal	Fat	Cbs
6" Egg Omelet Sandwich (with Egg White)			
Black Forest Ham, Egg (White) & Chz, 203 g	350	9	46
Double Bacon, Egg (White) & Chz, 193 g	420	15	46
• Egg (White) & Cheese, 174 g	320	8	45
• Mega, 240 g	610	35	46
Sausage, Egg (White) & Cheese, 231 g	570	31	45
Steak, Egg (White) & Cheese, 217 g	390	10	47
Western (Egg White) with Cheese, 212 g	360	11	47
6" Limited Time Offer/Regional Subs			
• Barbecue Chicken, 240 g	310	5	54
Barbecue Rib Patty, 247 g	430	18	48
Buffalo Chkn (w/ reg Ranch drss), 276 g	420	15	48
Chkn Pizziola (includes chz), 298 g	460	15	51
LF Buffalo Chkn (w/ light Ranch), 276 g	370	7	55
• Pastrami, Big (includes cheese), 270 g	590	29	49
Subway Seafood Sensation® w/ chz, 252 g	460	22	53
Tkey Bacon Avocado w/ chz, 275 g	420	15	51
Tuscan Chkn (includes chz), 275 g	390	9	52
Veggie Patty, 254 g	390	7	57
6" Low Fat Sandwiches			
Black Forest Ham, 226 g	290	5	48
Oven Roasted Chicken, 240 g	320	5	49
Roast Beef, 240 g	310	5	46
Subway Club®, 247 g	320	5	48
• Sweet Onion Chicken Teriyaki, 283 g	380	5	60
Tkey Breast & Black Forest Ham, 236 g	300	4	48
Turkey Breast, 226 g	280	4	48
• Veggie Delite®, 169 g	230	3	45
6" Omelet Sandwiches (w/ Regular Egg)			
Black Forest Ham, Egg & Cheese, 217 g	450	19	47
Double Bacon, Egg & Cheese, 207 g	520	25	47
Egg & Cheese, 189 g	420	18	46
• Mega, 255 g	710	45	46
Sausage, Egg & Cheese, 245 g	670	41	46
Steak, Egg & Cheese, 231 g	490	20	48
Western, Egg & Cheese, 226 g	450	19	47
6" Sandwiches			
Big Philly Cheesesteak, 311 g	520	18	54
• BLT, 164 g	360	13	45

SUBWAY (cont.)

	Cal	Fat	Cbs
6" Chicken & Bacon Ranch, 299 g	570	28	49
Cold Cut Combo, 252 g	410	16	48
Italian B.M.T.®, 245 g	450	20	48
• Meatball Marinara, 379 g	580	23	71
Spicy Italian, 240 g	520	28	48
Subway Melt®, 256 g	380	11	49
The Feast, 331 g	540	22	51
Tuna, 252 g	530	30	46
8" Pizza			
• Cheese, 293 g	680	22	96
Cheese & Veggies, 381 g	740	25	100
Pepperoni, 323 g	790	32	96
• Sausage, 336 g	820	34	97
Breads			
9-Grain Wheat Bread, 78 g	210	2	41
Hearty Italian Bread, 75 g	220	2	41
Honey Oat, 89 g	260	3	49
Italian (White) Bread, 71 g	200	2	38
Italian Herbs & Cheese, 82 g	250	5	41
Monterey Cheddar, 82 g	240	5	39
Parmesan Oregano Bread, 75 g	220	3	41
Roasted Garlic, 82 g	230	3	45
Flatbread, 94 g	240	5	41
• Light Wheat English Muffin, 57 g	90	1	16
• Wrap, 103 g	310	8	51
Breakfast Sides			
Hash Browns (4 pc), 74 g	150	9	17
Cheese			
American, Processed, 11 g	40	4	1
Monterey Cheddar, Shredded, 14 g	50	5	1
• Mozzarella, Shredded, 14 g	40	3	0
• Natural Cheddar, 15 g	60	5	0
Pepperjack, 14 g	50	4	0
Provolone, 14 g	50	4	0
Swiss, 14 g	50	5	0
Chips			
Baked Lay's® Sour Cream & Onion, 32 g	140	4	24
• Baked Lay's®, 32 g	130	2	23
• Chips (all varieties), 1 bag, 25-57 g	207	11	25
Doritos Nacho, 50 g	250	13	30
Lays® Classic, 43 g	230	15	23
Sunchips Harvest Cheddar, 43 g	210	9	29
Cookies & Desserts			
• Apple Pie, 71 g	250	10	37
• Apple Slices - 1 package, 71 g	35	0	9
Chocolate Chip, 45 g	210	10	30

• MOST HEALTHY   • LEAST HEALTHY

SUBWAY (cont.)

	Cal	Fat	Cbs
Chocolate Chunk, 45 g	220	10	30
Double Chocolate Chip, 45 g	210	10	30
M & M®, 45 g	210	10	32
Oatmeal Raisin, 45 g	200	8	30
Peanut Butter, 45 g	220	12	26
Sugar, 45 g	220	12	28
White Chip Macadamia Nut, 45 g	220	11	29
Yogurt Dannon Light & Fit®, 170 g	80	0	16

Egg Muffin Melts (w/ Egg White)

	Cal	Fat	Cbs
Black Forest Ham, Egg & Chz, 119 g	160	4	18
Double Bacon, Egg & Chz, 115 g	190	7	18
• Egg & Cheese, 105 g	140	4	18
• Mega, 138 g	290	17	18
Sausage, Egg & Cheese, 134 g	270	15	18
Steak, Egg & Cheese, 122 g	170	5	19
Western Egg with Cheese, 124 g	160	4	19

Egg Muffin Melts (w/ Regular Egg)

	Cal	Fat	Cbs
Black Forest Ham, Egg & Cheese, 119 g	180	7	18
Double Bacon, Egg & Cheese, 115 g	220	10	18
• Egg & Cheese, 105 g	170	18	18
• Mega, 138 g	310	20	18
Sausage, Egg & Cheese, 134 g	290	18	19
Steak, Egg & Cheese, 122 g	190	7	19
Western, Egg & Cheese, 124 g	180	7	N/A

Flatbread Sandwiches

	Cal	Fat	Cbs
Black Forest Ham on Flatbread, 242 g	320	7	47
Oven Roasted Chkn on Flatbread, 256 g	350	8	49
Roast Beef on Flatbread, 256 g	340	8	46
Subway Club® on Flatbread, 272 g	350	8	47
• Sweet Onion Chkn Teriyaki on Flatbread, 298 g	410	7	60
Tkey Breast & Black Forest Ham on Flatbread, 251 g	330	7	48
Turkey Breast on Flatbread, 242 g	310	6	47
• Veggie Delite® on Flatbread, 185 g	260	5	45

Individual Meats

	Cal	Fat	Cbs
Chicken Patty, Roasted, 71 g	90	3	4
Chicken Strips, 71 g	80	2	0
Cold Cut Combo Meats, 71 g	140	11	2
Egg Patty, Regular, 85 g	110	8	3
Egg White Patty, 85 g	70	2	3
Ham, 57 g	60	2	2
Italian BMT® Meats, 64 g	180	14	2
• Meatballs, 198 g	310	17	25
Roast Beef, 71 g	80	3	1
Seafood Sensation, 71 g	190	16	7
Spicy Italian Meats, 59 g	250	22	2
Steak (no cheese), 71 g	112	4	4

• MOST HEALTHY   • LEAST HEALTHY

SUBWAY (cont.)

	Cal	Fat	Cbs
Subway Club® Meats, 78 g	90	3	2
Tuna, 71 g	260	24	0
• Turkey Breast, 57 g	50	1	2
Veggie Patty, 85 g	160	5	12
Kids Meals Sandwiches			
• Roast Beef, 138 g	200	3	30
• Veggie Delite®, 101 g	150	2	30
Low Fat Footlong Sandwiches			
Footlong Black Forest Ham, 452 g	570	9	95
Footlong Oven Roasted Chicken, 481 g	640	9	98
Footlong Roast Beef, 481 g	630	9	92
Footlong Subway Club®, 495 g	640	10	96
• Footlong Sweet Onion Chkn Teriyaki, 566 g	760	9	121
Footlong Turkey Breast & Black Forest Ham, 471 g	590	8	96
Footlong Turkey Breast, 452 g	570	7	95
• Footlong Veggie Delite®, 339 g	460	5	91
Salads			
Black Forest Ham, 356 g	110	3	12
Oven Roasted Chicken (Strips), 371 g	130	3	10
Roast Beef, 371 g	140	4	10
Subway Club®, 387 g	140	4	12
• Sweet Onion Chicken Teriyaki, 413 g	200	3	25
Turkey Breast & Ham, 366 g	120	3	12
Turkey Breast, 356 g	110	2	12
• Veggie Delite®, 300 g	50	1	10
Sandwich Condiments			
Bacon, 2 strips, 9 g	45	4	0
• Chipotle Southwest Sauce, 21 g	100	10	1
Olive Oil Blend, 1 tsp, 5 g	45	5	0
Red Wine Vinaigrette, Fat Free, 21 g	30	0	6
Sweet Onion Sauce, Fat Free, 21 g	40	0	9
• Vinegar, 1 tsp, 8 g	0	0	0
Soup (Bowl)			
Chicken & Dumpling, 10 oz.	170	5	23
Chicken Tortilla, 10 oz.	110	2	11
• Chili Con Carne, 10 oz.	340	11	35
Chipotle Chicken Corn Chowder, 10 oz.	140	3	22
Cream of Potato with Bacon, 10 oz.	240	13	26
Fire-Roasted Tomato Orzo, 10 oz.	130	1	24
Golden Broccoli & Cheese, 10 oz.	180	11	16
Minestrone, 10 oz.	90	1	17
New England Style Clam Chowder, 10 oz.	150	5	20
• Roasted Chicken Noodle, 10 oz.	80	2	12
Rosemary Chicken and Dumpling, 10 oz.	90	2	14
Spanish Style Chkn & Rice w/ Pork, 10 oz.	110	3	16

• MOST HEALTHY   • LEAST HEALTHY

SUBWAY (cont.)

	Cal	Fat	Cbs
Tomato Garden Vegetable w/ Rotini, 10 oz.	90	1	20
Vegetable Beef, 10 oz.	100	2	17
Wild Rice with Chicken, 10 oz.	230	11	26

Vegetables

	Cal	Fat	Cbs
Banana Peppers, 3 rings, 4 g	0	0	0
Cucumbers, 3 slices, 17 g	5	0	1
• Green Peppers, 3 strips, 7 g	0	0	0
Jalapeño Peppers, 3 rings, 4 g	5	0	0
Lettuce, 21 g	5	0	0
Olives, 3 rings, 3 g	5	0	0
Onions, 14 g	5	0	1
• Tomatoes, 3 wheels, 34 g	5	0	2

SWEET TOMATOES

Breads Muffins

	Cal	Fat	Cbs
Apple Cinn Bran Muffin (96% FF), 1 pc	130	1	30
Apple Raisin Muffin, 1 piece	150	7	22
Banana Crunch Muffin Top (NSA), 1 piece	120	5	19
Banana Nut Muffin, 1 piece	150	7	22
BBQ Chkn Focaccia on Honey Wheat Crust, 1 pc	200	8	23
Black Forest Muffin, 1 piece	230	9	36
Bruschetta Focaccia, 1 piece	140	7	15
Buffalo Chkn Focaccia on Honey Wheat Crust, 1 pc	170	7	20
Buttermilk Biscuits, 1 biscuit	190	8	25
Buttermilk Cornbread (Low-Fat), 1 piece	140	2	27
Cappuccino Chip Muffin, 1 piece	190	6	31
Caribbean Key Lime Muffin, 1 piece	170	6	28
Carrot Pineapple Muffin w/ Oat Bran, 1 pc	150	6	23
Cherry Nut Muffin, 1 piece	150	7	22
Chile Corn Muffin (Low-Fat), 1 piece	140	3	27
Chipotle Lime Butter, 1 Tbsp.	90	10	0
Chocolate Brownie Muffin, 1 piece	180	8	26
Chocolate Chip Muffin, 1 piece	170	8	24
Choco Peanut Butter Chip Muffin, 1 piece	220	10	31
Country Blackberry Muffin, 1 piece	170	6	27
Cran Orange Bran Muffin (96% FF), 1 pc	130	1	30
Date N' Honey Bran, 1 piece	150	6	24
• French Quarter Praline Muffin, 1 piece	250	10	35
Fruit Medley Bran Muffin (96% FF), 1 pc	130	1	29
Garlic Asiago Focaccia, 1 piece	160	8	19
Georgia Peach Poppyseed Muffin, 1 piece	160	6	20
Grilled Cheese Focaccia, 1 piece	190	10	18
Indian Grain Bread (Low-Fat), 1 piece	200	2	35
Irish Soda Bread, 1 piece	180	5	29
Lemon Vanilla Butter, 1 Tbsp.	90	8	3
Mango Tropics Muffin w/ Coconut, 1 pc	180	7	28

• MOST HEALTHY   • LEAST HEALTHY

SWEET TOMATOES (cont.)	Cal	Fat	Cbs
Maple Walnut Muffin, 1 piece	230	10	32
Old World Greek Focaccia, 1 piece	190	9	24
Pauline's Apple Walnut Cake, 1 piece	220	12	24
Pepperoni Focaccia, 1 piece	190	9	21
Pesto & Sun-Dried Tomato Focaccia, 1 pc	170	8	20
Pineapple Marshmallow Whip, 1/4 cup	240	13	33
Pumpkin Raisin Muffin, 1 piece	150	6	25
Quattro Formaggio Focaccia, 1 piece	140	5	20
Ragin Cajun Veg Focaccia (Veg), 1 pc	160	7	19
Roasted Potato Focaccia, 1 piece	150	6	17
Rst Red Pepper w/ Honeywheat Focaccia, 1 pc	170	8	20
Sauteed Vegetable Focaccia, 1 piece	180	9	19
Sourdough Bread (Low-Fat), 1 piece	150	1	27
Southwest Chipotle Focaccia, 1 piece	160	8	19
Spiced Pumpkin Muffin w/ Cran, 1 pc	180	7	29
Strawberry Buttermilk Muffin, 1 piece	140	6	21
• Sweet Cherry Butter, 1 Tbsp.	80	7	4
Sweet Orange & Cranberry Muffin, 1 pc	200	7	33
Sweet Strawberry Butter, 1 Tbsp.	80	7	4
Taffy Apple Muffin, 1 piece	160	6	25
Tangy Lemon Muffin, 1 piece	140	4	24
Thai Chkn Focaccia w/ Peanuts, 1 piece	170	7	20
Whole Wheat Buttermilk Biscuits, 1 piece	180	6	31
Wildly Blue Blueberry Muffin, 1 piece	140	5	22
Wowie Maui Focaccia w/ Ham, 1 piece	170	7	21
Zucchini Nut Muffin, 1 piece	150	7	22

Breakfast

	Cal	Fat	Cbs
Belgian Waffles, 1 piece	90	0	16
Blueberry Sauce / Blueberry Stir-In, 2 Tbsp.	60	0	15
Country Ham & Egg Breakfast Burrito	210	10	21
Egg Scramble Focaccia w/ Bacon, 1 piece	180	8	20
French Toast (Plain), 1 piece	150	4	25
Homemade Oatmeal (Plain), 3/4 cup	110	2	19
Mediterranean Sunrise Pasta, 1 cup	210	12	19
Potatoes O'Brien, 1/2 cup	140	6	19
Scrambled Eggs, 1/2 cup	135	8	2
• Sticky Granola Clusters w/ Almonds, 1/4 cup	270	14	30
• Strawberry Sauce/ Strwbry Stir-In, 2 Tbsp.	45	0	11
Sweet Cinn Biscuits w/ Frosting oz. 1 pc	270	13	37
Sweet Maple Buttermilk Biscuit, 1 piece	240	9	39
Sweet Pepper & Ssge Egg Brkfst Burrito	210	11	20
Sweet Strawberry Buttermilk Biscuit, 1 pc	250	9	40
Tom's Country Gravy, 2 Tbsp.	90	5	8
Warm Marion Blackberry Sauce, 1/4 cup	80	0	20
Zucchini Fritatta, 1 piece	160	6	22

SWEET TOMATOES (cont.)

Desserts

	Cal	Fat	Cbs
Apple Cobbler, 1/2 cup	360	10	67
Apple Medley (Fat-Free), 1/2 cup	70	0	18
Banana Pudding, 1/2 cup	160	4	27
Banana Royale (Fat-Free), 1/2 cup	80	0	20
Butterscotch Pudding (Low-Fat), 1/2 cup	140	3	24
Candy Sprinkles (Low-Fat), 1 Tbsp.	70	3	11
• Caramel Apple Cobbler, 1/2 cup	390	12	68
Caramel Syrup, 2 Tbsp.	130	1	30
Carrot & Crm Chz Lava Cake oz. 1 piece	320	15	40
Cherry Apple Cobbler, 1/2 cup	330	10	57
Chocolate Chip Cookie - 1 Small, 1 cookie	75	3	10
Chocolate Frozen Yogurt (Nonfat), 1/3cup	110	0	22
Chocolate Lava Cake, 1/2 cup	330	8	62
Choco PntBtr Cookie Bars, 1 piece	270	12	37
Choco PntBtr Cookie Cups, 1 piece	140	6	18
Chocolate Pudding (Low-Fat), 1/2 cup	150	3	25
Choco Pudding (Low-Fat, NSA), 1/2 cup	90	2	21
Chocolate Syrup oz. 2 Tbsp.	110	3	20
Cranberry Apple Cobbler, 1/2 cup	370	10	58
Cran-Raspberry Gelatin (FF), 1/2 cup	100	0	26
Deep Choco Winter Mint Lava Cake, 1/2 cup	330	8	58
Gelatin (Fat-Free), 1/2 cup	80	0	20
• Gelatin (Sugar Free, Fat-Free), 1/2 cup	10	0	0
Gooey Caramel Pumpkin Cake, 1/2 cup	280	9	45
Granola Topping, 2 Tbsp.	110	4	16
Green Tea Mousse, 1/2 cup	190	8	29
Holiday Cookies w/ Sprinkles, Sm, 1 cookie	80	4	12
Hot Lemon Lava Cake, 1/2 cup	320	11	51
Nutty Waldorf Salad (Low-Fat), 1/2 cup	90	3	14
Oatmeal Raisin Cookie - 1 small, 1 cookie	120	5	16
Orange Creamsicle Lava Cake, 1/2 Cup	310	11	50
Pineapple Gelatin (Fat-Free), 1/2 cup	120	0	29
Pineapple Upside-Down Cake, 1/2 cup	270	10	42
Raspberry Apple Cobbler, 1/2 cup	380	11	67
Rice Pudding (Low-Fat), 1/2 cup	110	2	20
Shortcake, 1 piece	220	7	36
Strawberry Apple Cobbler, 1/2 cup	340	10	67
Sugar-Free Cherry Choco Mousse, 1/2 cup	40	3	3
Sugar-free Chocolate Mousse, 1/2 cup	40	3	3
Sugar-free Lemon Mousse, 1/2 cup	40	3	4
Sugar-free Raspberry Mousse, 1/2 Cup	40	3	4
Sugar-free Strawberry Mousse, 1/2 cup	40	3	4
Tapioca Pudding (Low-Fat), 1/2 cup	140	3	24
Vanilla Frozen Yogurt (Nonfat), 1/3 cup	100	0	21
Vanilla Pudding, 1/2 cup	150	4	27

● MOST HEALTHY   • LEAST HEALTHY

SWEET TOMATOES (cont.)

	Cal	Fat	Cbs
Dressings			
Bacon Dressing, 2 Tbsp.	110	11	7
Basil Vinaigrette, 2 Tbsp.	160	17	1
Chow Mein Noodles, 1/4 Cup	70	1	15
Cran Orange Vinaigrette (Low-Fat), 2 Tbsp.	80	2	15
Creamy Sesame Soy Dressing, 2 Tbsp.	170	17	5
Cucumber Drss (Reduced Calorie), 2 Tbsp.	70	7	3
Green Chili Ranch Dressing, 2 Tbsp.	150	14	4
Honey Lime Cilantro Vinaigrette, 2 Tbsp.	100	6	15
Honey Mint Lemonade, 2 Tbsp.	130	7	19
Italian Vinaigrette w/ Basil & Romano Chz, 2 Tbsp.	150	15	1
Kahlena French Dressing, 2 Tbsp.	90	9	10
Lemon Greek Vinaigrette, 2 Tbsp.	150	15	2
Monterey Blue Salad Drss oz. 2 Tbsp.	120	11	5
Parmesan Pepper Cream Drss oz. 2 Tbsp.	140	16	1
Pineapple Vinaigrette, 2 Tbsp.	120	11	5
• Poppy Seed Orange Vinaigrette (LF), 2 Tbsp.	45	2	7
Roasted Garlic Dressing, 2 Tbsp.	100	10	3
Smoky BBQ Vinaigrette, 2 Tbsp.	110	10	5
• Spicy Southwest Chipotle, 2 Tbsp.	190	20	2
Strawberry Balsamic Vinaigrette, 2 Tbsp.	130	13	2
Sweet Maple Dressing, 2 Tbsp.	180	17	6
Warm Bacon Dressing, 2 Tbsp.	110	10	5
Hot Pastas Kitchen Favorites			
100% Whole Wheat Jalapeño & Salsa pasta (Veg), 1 cup	250	6	46
4 Cheese Alfredo (Vegetarian), 1 cup	390	13	50
Arizona Marinara (Vegetarian), 1 cup	360	11	47
Beefy Meatball Stroganoff, 1 cup	340	21	28
Broccoli Alfredo w/ Basil (Veg), 1 cup	380	17	45
Broccoli Chz Baked Potato Topper (Veg), 1 cup	120	7	10
Bruschetta (Vegetarian), 1 cup	260	4	41
Carbonara Pasta w/ Bacon, 1 cup	290	10	43
Chzy Scalloped Potatoes w/ Bacon, 1 cup	240	17	15
• Chicken Tetrazzini, 1 cup	480	23	47
Cilantro Lime Pesto (Vegetarian), 1 cup	370	21	36
Creamy Bruschetta (Vegetarian), 1 cup	360	16	43
Creamy Herb Chicken, 1 cup	310	17	32
Curried Pineapple & Ginger (LF), 1 cup	200	2	40
Fettuccine Alfredo (Vegetarian), 1 cup	390	18	41
Fire-RstTomato Basil Alfredo (Veg), 1 cup	370	14	44
Garden Vegetable w/ Italian Ssge, 1 cup	300	10	42
Garden Vegetable w/ Meatballs, 1 cup	310	10	44
Greek Mediterranean (Vegetarian), 1 cup	290	8	45
Hand-Crafted Mexican Beans (LF, Veg), 1 cup	260	2	47
Italian Ssg w/ Red Pepper Puree, 1 cup	250	10	35
Italian Vegetable Beef, 1 cup	290	9	43

SWEET TOMATOES (cont.)

	Cal	Fat	Cbs
Lemon Cream w/ Capers (Non-Veg), 1 cup	390	21	44
Linguini w/ Clam Sauce, 1 cup	380	10	56
Macaroni & Cheese (Vegetarian), 1 cup	330	15	40
Nutty Mushroom (Vegetarian), 1 cup	390	20	42
Oriental Noodle & Green Bean (LF, Veg), 1 cup	240	3	45
Pasta Florentine (Vegetarian), 1 cup	360	10	54
Penne Arrabbiatta (Vegetarian), 1 cup	340	5	43
Ragin Cajun w/ Andouille Sausage, 1 cup	370	22	33
Roasted Eggplant Marinara (Veg), 1 cup	340	10	43
Rst Garlic & Asiago Alfredo (Veg), 1 cup	330	11	45
Rst Mshr Alfredo w/ Rosemary (Veg), 1 cup	380	14	44
• Salsa de Lupe (Fat-Free, Vegan), 1/4 cup	30	0	6
Sautéed Balsamic Veg (Vegan), 1/2 cup	100	6	11
Smoked Salmon & Dill, 1 cup	360	16	41
Smoky BBQ Baked Beans (LF), 1 cup	320	3	61
Spicy Italian Sausage & Peppers, 1 cup	360	11	43
Stm Veg w/ Lemon Herb Butter (Veg), 1/2 cup	130	9	10
Stuffing (Non-Vegetarian), 1/2 cup	210	12	20
Tom Spinach Whole Wheat (Veg), 1 cup	250	10	33
Tuscany Ssge w/Capers & Olives, 1 cup	240	13	29
Vegetable Ragu (Vegetarian), 1 cup	250	6	41
Vegetarian Marinara w/ Basil (Veg), 1 cup	260	4	44
Walnut Pesto (Vegetarian), 1 cup	310	9	42

Prepared Salads

	Cal	Fat	Cbs
100% Whole Wheat Arugula Citrus (Vegan), 1/2 cup	210	10	29
• 100% Whole Wheat Crm Chipotle Salad (Veg), 1/2 cup	350	25	31
100% Whole Wheat Sicilian Penne w/ Feta & Pep, 1/2 cup	250	14	30
100% Whole Wheat Spicy Asian Peanut Salad (Vegan), 1/2 cup	260	14	32
Ambrosia w/ Coconut (Vegetarian), 1/2 cup	190	9	30
Artichoke Rice (Vegetarian), 1/2 cup	190	12	16
• Aunt Doris' Red Pepper Slaw (FF, Vegan), 1/2 cup	70	0	18
Baja Bean & Cilantro (LF, Vegan), 1/2 cup	180	3	29
BBQ Potato (Vegetarian), 1/2 cup	170	9	21
Bistro Potato (Vegetarian), 1/2 cup	290	19	27
Buffalo Blue Potato Salad (Veg), 1/2 Cup	190	13	16
Carrot Raisin (Low-Fat, Veg), 1/2 cup	90	3	17
Chinese Krab, 1/2 cup	160	8	19
Citrus Noodles w/ Snow Peas (Veg), 1/2 cup	140	6	19
Confetti Avocado Slaw (Veg), 1/2 cup	140	9	12
Dijon Potato w/ Garlic Dill Vinaigrette (Vegan), 1/2 cup	150	12	9
Field Corn & Very Wild Rice (Veg), 1/2 cup	170	9	19
German Potato oz. 1/2 cup	150	6	23
Greek Couscous w/ Feta Chz & Pinenuts (Veg), 1/2 cup	210	10	25
Italian White Bean (Vegan), 1/2 cup	140	5	19
Jalapeño Potato (Vegetarian), 1/2 cup	170	9	21
Joan's Broccoli Madness, 1/2 cup	180	14	11

• MOST HEALTHY   • LEAST HEALTHY

SWEET TOMATOES (cont.)

	Cal	Fat	Cbs
Lemon Linguini w/Tst Pinenuts oz. 1/2 Cup	230	13	26
Lemon Rice w/ Cashews (Vegan), 1/2 Cup	160	7	23
Mandarin Noodles w/ Broccoli (LF, Vegan), 1/2 cup	170	3	31
Mandarin Shells w/ Almonds (LF, Vegan), 1/2 cup	120	3	19
Old Fashioned Macaroni w/ Ham, 1/2 cup	200	13	18
Oriental Ginger Slaw w/ Krab (Low-Fat), 1/2 cup	70	3	8
Penne Pasta w/ Chkn in Citrus Vinaigrette (LF), 1/2 cup	130	3	20
Pesto Pasta (Vegetarian), 1/2 cup	180	9	21
Picnic Potato (Vegetarian), 1/2 cup	190	14	17
Pineapple Coconut Slaw (Veg), 1/2 cup	150	10	14
Poppyseed Coleslaw (Veg), 1/2 cup	120	9	9
Provencal Green Bean & Potato (Vegan), 1/2 cup	220	14	25
Red Potato & Tomato (Veg), 1/2 cup	170	11	17
Red, White, & Blue Potato Salad (w/ bacon), 1/2 cup	190	13	15
Rst Potato w/ Chipotle Chile Vinaigrette (Veg), 1/2 cup	140	6	18
San Francisco Herb Rice (Non-Veg), 1/2 cup	180	6	27
Shrimp & Seafood Shells, 1/2 cup	210	13	20
Smoky Ham & Cheddar Broccoli Slaw oz. 1/2 cup	260	18	21
Southern Black-Eyed Pea (Veg), 1/2 cup	130	6	18
Southern Dill Potato (LF, Veg), 1/2 cup	120	3	20
SW Rice & Beans (Low-Fat, Veg), 1/2 cup	90	3	15
Spicy Cajun Shells (Vegetarian), 1/2 cup	300	13	40
Spicy SW Pasta (LF, Vegan), 1/2 cup	130	3	21
Summer Barley w/ Black Beans (LF, Vegan), 1/2 cup	110	3	19
Sweet & Sour Broccoli Slaw (LF, Vegan), 1/2 cup	150	3	28
Sweet Marinated Veg (FF, Vegan), 1/2 cup	80	0	19
Sweet Tomato, Basil & Mozz. (Veg), 1/2 cup	170	6	25
Tabouli (Vegan), 1/2 cup	200	10	24
Thai Citrus & Brown Rice (Vegan), 1/2 cup	220	12	26
Thai Noodle w/ Chkn & Peanut Sauce, 1/2 cup	190	10	19
Three Bean Marinade (Vegan), 1/2 cup	170	6	27
Tomato Cucumber Marinade (Vegan), 1/2 cup	80	5	8
Tuna Tarragon, 1/2 cup	250	15	21
Turkey Chutney Pasta oz. 1/2 cup	240	12	20
Wheat Berry & Curry (Veg), 1/2 cup	210	5	36
Whole Grain Fiesta Couscous (Veg), 1/2 cup	280	11	39
Wild Rice & Chicken, 1/2 cup	300	21	21
Zesty Tortellini (Vegetarian), 1/2 cup	230	15	20
Soups			
8 Vegetable Chicken Stew, 1 cup	160	7	17
Albondigas Locas (A Meatball Soup), 1 cup	210	11	19
• Asian Ginger Broth (Low-Fat, Veg), 1 cup	50	2	6
Basmati Lentil Soup, 1 cup	210	7	29
Beef & Barley Stew, 1 cup	240	10	19
Better Than Mom's Beef Stew, 1 cup	270	17	19
Big Chunk Chkn Noodle (Low-Fat), 1 cup	170	3	19

SWEET TOMATOES (cont.)

	Cal	Fat	Cbs
Border Black Bean & Chorizo Soup, 1 cup	240	10	27
Broccoli Cheese (Vegetarian), 1 cup	270	19	17
• Canadian Chz w/ Smoked Ham, 1 cup	350	26	22
Chze Stuffed Cappelletti (Non-Veg), 1 cup	250	11	31
Cheesy Corn Chowder w/ Bacon, 1 cup	220	11	25
Chesapeake Corn Chowder (Non-Veg), 1 cup	290	17	30
Chicken & Rice, 1 cup	160	5	18
Chicken Dijon (Reduced Sodium), 1 Cup	210	13	18
Chicken Divan, 1 cup	240	15	18
Chicken Fajitas & Black Bean, 1 cup	280	7	37
Chicken Pot Pie Stew, 1 cup	310	21	21
Chkn Tortilla w/ Jalapeño Chiles & Tom (LF) 1 cup	100	3	11
Chili Cheeseburger, 1 cup	290	12	29
Chunky Potato Chz w/ Thyme (Veg), 1 cup	240	11	25
Classic Creamy Tomato Soup, 1 cup	200	13	19
Classic French Onion oz. 1 cup	150	6	21
Classic Shrimp Bisque, 1 cup	240	16	15
Classical Minestrone (LF, Vegan), 1 cup	120	2	20
Continental Lentil & Spinach (LF, Veg), 1 cup	160	2	28
Corned Beef & Cabbage, 1 cup	150	6	17
Country Corn & Red Potato Chowder, 1 cup	220	8	35
Cream of Broccoli (Vegetarian), 1 cup	260	19	19
Cream of Chicken, 1 cup	290	21	16
Cream of Mushroom, 1 cup	290	24	15
Cream of Rosemary Potato, 1 cup	320	22	26
Creamy Herbed Turkey, 1 cup	320	22	18
Creamy Pumpkin Bisque w/ Pine Nuts, 1 cup	190	7	31
Creamy Vegetable Chowder (Veg), 1 cup	270	14	26
Curried Yellow Split Pea (LF, Veg), 1 cup	230	2	40
Deep Kettle House Chili (Low-Fat), 1 cup	230	3	26
El Paso Lime & Chicken, 1 cup	160	4	24
Sweet Tomato Basil (Veg), 1 cup	220	15	20
w/ - Cauliflower w/ Proud to be American Chz (Veg), 1 cup	280	21	19
Fire-Rst Green Chile & Corn Chowder w/ Bacon, 1 cup	240	15	21
Garden Fresh Vegetable (Low-Fat, Veg), 1 cup	150	2	27
Garden of Eatin' (Low-Fat, Veg), 1 cup	150	3	25
Golden Yam Bisque (Vegetarian), 1 cup	220	8	28
Green Chile Stew w/ Pork, 1 cup	170	6	18
Indian Lentil (Low-Fat, Vegan), 1 cup	160	3	25
Irish Potato Leek (Vegetarian), 1 cup	260	16	23
Lemon Chicken Orzo oz. 1 cup	220	9	21
Ld Baked Potato & Chz w/ Bacon, 1 cup	290	18	24
Longhorn Beef Chili, 1 cup	190	6	25
Marvelous Minestrone w/ Bacon, 1 cup	220	8	31
Minestrone w/ Italian Sausage, 1 cup	220	12	17
Moroccan Garbanzo & Lentil Bean (LF, Veg), 1 cup	230	2	40

• MOST HEALTHY   • LEAST HEALTHY

SWEET TOMATOES (cont.)

	Cal	Fat	Cbs
Mulligatawny, 1 cup	240	14	17
Neighbor Joe's Gumbo oz. 1 cup	210	10	20
New Mexican Corn Tortilla w/ Chkn, 1 cup	200	10	19
New Orleans Jambalaya, 1 cup	210	11	18
Old Fashion Vegetable (LF, Veg), 1 cup	100	2	18
Pinto Bean & Basil Barley (LF, Veg), 1 cup	160	2	29
Posole w/ Pork, 1 cup	150	6	8
Potato Tomato & Spinach (LF, Veg), 1 cup	150	2	28
Ratatouille Provencale (FF, Vegan), 1 cup	110	0	25
Roasted Mushroom w/ Sage, 1 cup	320	26	19
Rustic Tuscan Stew (LF, Non-Veg), 1 cup	140	2	25
Santa Fe Black Bean Chili (LF, Vegan), 1 cup	190	3	26
Savory Turkey Harvest, 1 cup	220	12	18
Smoky Pinto & Brown Rice (LF, Veg), 1 cup	150	2	28
Southwest Tomato Cream (Veg), 1 cup	130	7	14
SW Turkey Chowder w/ Bacon, 1 cup	240	15	21
Spicy Navajo Veg Soup (FF, Veg), 1 cup	110	0	26
Spicy Sausage & Pasta, 1 cup	300	12	34
Spicy Tamale Chili, 1 cup	190	8	24
Split Pea & Potato Barley (LF, Veg), 1 cup	200	2	37
Split Pea w/ Ham, 1 cup	290	10	36
Sweet Potato Corn Chowder w/ Ham, 1 cup	220	7	36
Sweet Tomato Onion (LF, Vegan), 1 cup	90	3	13
Texas Red Chili (Non-Vegetarian), 1 cup	190	7	24
Three Cheese Tortellini oz. 1 cup	180	6	28
Three-Bean Turkey Chili (Low-Fat), 1 cup	170	3	24
Tomato Chipotle Bisque, 1 cup	250	17	20
Tomato Parm & Veg (Low-Fat, Veg), 1 cup	120	3	18
Turkey Cassoulet w/ Bacon, 1 cup	240	12	17
Tkey Noodle Soup w/ 100% Whole Wheat Noodles, 1 cup	160	4	24
Turkey Vegetable, 1 cup	210	12	15
U.S. Senate Bean w/ Smkd Ham, 1 cup	150	4	20
Vegetable Bean & Barley Stew (LF, Veg), 1 cup	150	2	28
Vegetable Medley (Low-Fat, Veg), 1 cup	90	1	14
Vegetarian Harvest (Vegan), 1 cup	200	10	23
White Bean & Lime Chicken Chili, 1 cup	220	5	29
X-treme Spice Veg Chili w/ Energy Boost (LF, Veg), 1 cup	100	1	17
Yankee Clipper Clam Chowder w/ Bacon, 1 cup	310	20	21

Tossed Salads

	Cal	Fat	Cbs
Azteca Taco w/ Turkey oz. 1 cup	130	9	7
Bartlett Pear & Caramel Walnut (Veg) oz. 1 cup	180	12	13
BBQ Julienne Chopped w/ Chkn oz. 1 cup	210	11	23
• BBQ Smokehouse w/ Bacon & Peanuts oz. 1 cup	290	17	25
Buffalo Chicken oz. 1 cup	180	14	10
Caesar Salad Asiago (Non-Veg) oz. 1 cup	270	22	10
California Cobb w/ Bacon oz. 1 cup	190	15	7

• MOST HEALTHY   • LEAST HEALTHY

SWEET TOMATOES (cont.)

	Cal	Fat	Cbs
Cambay Curry w/ Almonds & Coconut (Veg) oz. 1 cup	220	17	17
Cape Cod Spinach w/Walnuts & Bacon oz. 1 cup	170	14	6
Cherry Chipotle Spinach (Veg) oz. 1 cup	160	8	20
Chicken Tortilla oz. 1 cup	180	10	16
Classic Antipasto oz. 1 cup	280	21	18
• Classic Greek (Vegetarian) oz. 1 cup	120	9	4
Club Blue BLT w/ Bacon oz. 1 cup	270	17	20
Country French w/ Bacon oz. 1 cup	210	18	7
Crunchy Island Pineapple (Veg) oz. 1 cup	160	8	20
Citrus Vinaigrette (Vegan) oz. 1 cup	150	12	10
Sweet Maple (Veg) oz. 1 cup	180	15	10
Green Chile Ranch w/ Spicy Tortilla Chips (Veg) oz. 1 cup	260	16	24
Honey Minted Fruit Toss (Veg) oz. 1 cup	140	6	20
Mandarin Spinach w/ Caramel Walnuts (Vegan) oz. 1 cup	170	11	14
Mediterranean Bistro Potato oz. 1 cup	230	11	26
Monterey Blue w/ Peanuts (Veg) oz. 1 cup	270	17	25
Outrageous Orange w/ Cashews (Veg) oz. 1 cup	210	15	16
Ragin' Cajun w/ Chicken oz. 1 cup	220	14	15
Ranch House BLT w/Turkey & Bacon oz. 1 cup	190	13	11
Rst Vegetables w/ Feta & Olives (Veg) oz. 1 cup	190	15	12
San Marino Spinach w/ Pumpkin Seeds & Cran (Veg) oz. 1 cup	200	15	11
Sedona Green Chile & Chipotle (Non-Veg) oz. 1 cup	220	16	15
Smkd Tkey & Spinach w/ Almonds oz. 1 cup	190	10	20
Sonoma Spinach w/ Honey Dijon Vinaigrette (Veg) 1 cup	210	14	16
Spiced Pecan & Rst Veg w/ Spinach oz. 1 cup	200	13	15
Spinach Gorgonzola w/ Spiced Pecans & Bacon oz. 1 cup	230	19	9
Strwbry Fields w/ Carmel Walnuts (Vegan) oz. 1 cup	130	8	15
Summer Lemon w/ Spiced Pecans oz. 1 cup	220	17	16
Thai Peanut & Red Pepper (Vegan) oz. 1 cup	220	11	23
Thai Udon & Peanut (Vegan) oz. 1 cup	220	13	19
Traditional Spinach w/ Bacon oz. 1 cup	190	13	11
Won Ton Chicken Happiness oz. 1 cup	170	5	15

SWISS CHALET

Entrée Salads & Stir-Frys

Bacon Ranch Salad, 437 g	530	57	22
Chalet Chopped Salad, 489 g	440	42	29
Chicken Stir Fry, Without w/ Rice, 367 g	430	40	26
• Crispy Tortilla Strips, 26 g	150	15	13
Fish & Chips (Fish Only), 178 g	450	42	29
Fresh Vegetable Stir Fry w/o Rice, 255 g	320	37	26
Grilled Chicken Caesar Salad, 407 g	680	63	42
Spinach Chicken Salad, 353 g	170	3	14

From the Grill

Half Rack BBQ Ribs, 226 g	650	65	6

● MOST HEALTHY   ● LEAST HEALTHY

SWISS CHALET (cont.)

	Cal	Fat	Cbs
Rotisserie Chicken			
Chicken Pot Pie, 428 g	550	52	63
• Classic Double Leg (With Skin), 278 g	630	62	4
Classic Half Chicken (With Skin), 298 g	610	49	5
• Classic 1/4 Chkn Breast (Skinless), 124 g	180	5	0
Classic 1/4 Chkn Leg (Skinless), 116 g	220	15	0
Health Check Classic 1/4 Chkn, 368 g	360	18	14
Side Selections			
Creamy Coleslaw, 180 g	200	22	15
• Fresh, Hand-Cut Fries, 168 g	530	42	64
Gravy, 113 g	45	2	7
Mashed Potatoes, 140 g	150	6	27
Oven-Baked Potato, 284 g	220	0	48
Ramekin of Creamy Coleslaw, 64 g	70	8	5
Seasoned Rice, 170 g	240	5	48
Side Caesar Salad with Dressing, 108 g	210	29	9
• Side Garden Salad, 110 g	20	0	5
Side Greek Salad, 129 g	45	4	5
Sweet Kernel Corn, 170 g	140	2	30
Starters			
Caesar Salad, 161 g	420	57	16
Chalet Chicken Soup, Bowl, 340 ml	170	6	17
Chalet Chicken Wings, 198 g	N/A	52	23
Cheese Perogies, 7 Pieces, 196 g	550	15	69
Chicken Spring Rolls, 4 Pieces, 168 g	400	25	45
• Crispy Dry Ribs, 400 g	920	98	4
• Garden Salad, 199 g	40	0	9
Garlic Cheese Loaf, 276 g	860	82	77
Garlic Loaf, 219 g	420	54	74
Greek Salad, 179 g	80	8	6
Wraps, Sandwiches & Burgers			
• Chargrilled Bacon Cheese Burger, 298 g	890	83	46
Chargrilled Bacon Cheese Burger, 213 g	680	80	4
Chargrilled Hamburger, 250 g	710	60	43
Chargrilled Hamburger, 165 g	490	58	1
Chargrilled Veggie Burger, 198 g	330	18	52
• Chargrilled Veggie Burger, 113 g	110	17	10
Chicken Caesar Wrap, 338 g	890	77	62
Chicken on a Kaiser (Dark Meat), 241 g	510	22	42
Chicken on a Kaiser (White Meat), 241 g	440	9	42
Chipotle Chicken Sandwich, 227 g	490	12	72
Classic Hot Chkn Snd (Dark Meat), 386 g	450	23	29
Classic Hot Chkn Snd (White Meat), 386 g	380	9	29
Rotisserie Chicken Club Wrap, 355 g	820	62	58
Rotisserie Chicken Quesadilla, 312 g	620	35	72

• MOST HEALTHY • LEAST HEALTHY

T.J. CINNAMONS

	Cal	Fat	Cbs
• Cinnamon Roll, 149 g	2026	42	292
Cinnamon Twist, 71 g	260	14	33
Cream Cheese Icing, 28 g	117	5	18
Mocha Chill, 340 g	264	4	46
Original Gourmet Cinnamon Roll®, 149 g	507	10	73
Pecan Sticky Bun, 184 g	688	22	91
Sticky Bun Smear w/ pecans, 35 g	181	12	18
TJ Cinnamons Mocha Chill®, 354 g	306	7	48
TJ Icing, 28 g	117	5	18
• Whipped Cream, 14 g	43	3	1

TACO BELL

Beverages

	Cal	Fat	Cbs
Mango Strwbry Frutista Freeze®, 479 g	250	0	62
Strawberry Frutista Freeze®, 479 g	230	0	57

Burritos

	Cal	Fat	Cbs
1/2 lb Cheesy Potato Burrito, 248 g	530	25	57
1/2 lb Combo Burrito, 241 g	450	18	52
1/2 lb Nacho Crunch Burrito, 234 g	520	25	54
7 Layer Burrito, 283 g	510	18	68
Burrito Supreme® - Beef, 248 g	420	15	52
Burrito Supreme® - Chicken, 248 g	390	12	51
• Burrito Supreme® - Steak, 248 g	380	12	51
Cheesy Bean & Rice Burrito, 227 g	480	21	60
Cheesy Double Beef Burrito, 227 g	470	20	54
• Grilled Stuft Burrito - Beef, 325 g	700	30	79
Grilled Stuft Burrito - Chicken, 325 g	650	24	77
Grilled Stuft Burrito - Steak, 325 g	640	24	76

Chalupas

	Cal	Fat	Cbs
• Chalupa Baja - Beef, 153 g	410	26	31
Chalupa Baja - Chicken, 153 g	390	23	29
Chalupa Baja - Steak, 153 g	380	23	29
Chalupa Nacho Cheese - Beef, 153 g	370	22	31
Chalupa Nacho Cheese - Chicken, 153 g	340	18	30
• Chalupa Nacho Cheese - Steak, 153 g	330	19	30
Chalupa Supreme - Beef, 153 g	370	21	31
Chalupa Supreme - Chicken, 153 g	350	18	30
Chalupa Supreme - Steak, 153 g	340	18	29

Fresco Menu

	Cal	Fat	Cbs
Fresco Bean Burrito, 128 g	160	5	21
• Fresco Burrito Supreme® - Chkn, 241 g	340	8	50
• Fresco Crunchy Taco, 92 g	150	7	13
Fresco Grilled Steak Soft Taco, 135 g	170	4	22
Fresco Ranchero Chkn Soft Taco, 241 g	330	8	49
Fresco Soft Taco - Beef, 113 g	180	7	22

• MOST HEALTHY • LEAST HEALTHY

TACO BELL (cont.)

	Cal	Fat	Cbs
Fully Loaded Taco Salads			
• Chicken Ranch Taco Salad, 420 g	910	54	71
Chipotle Steak Taco Salad, 420 g	900	57	70
Fiesta Taco Salad, 463 g	770	41	75
• Fiesta Taco Salad w/o Shell, 404 g	460	24	41
Gorditas			
• Gordita Baja® - Beef, 153 g	340	18	30
Gordita Baja® - Chicken, 153 g	320	15	29
Gordita Baja® - Steak, 153 g	310	15	28
Gordita Nacho Cheese - Beef, 153 g	290	14	31
Gordita Nacho Cheese - Chicken, 153 g	270	10	30
• Gordita Nacho Cheese - Steak, 153 g	260	11	29
Gordita Supreme® - Beef, 153 g	300	13	31
Gordita Supreme® - Chicken, 153 g	270	10	29
Gordita Supreme® - Steak, 153 g	270	11	29
Nachos and Sides			
Cheesy Fiesta Potatoes, 135 g	270	16	28
• Mexican Rice, 85 g	130	4	21
• Nachos BellGrande®, 305 g	770	42	78
Nachos Supreme, 191 g	440	24	42
Nachos, 99 g	330	21	31
Pintos 'n Cheese, 128 g	180	7	19
Regional Menu Items			
• Cheese Quesadilla, 142 g	470	26	40
Chili Cheese Burrito, 156 g	370	16	40
• Tostada, 170 g	250	10	29
Specialties			
Chicken Quesadilla, 184 g	520	28	41
Chicken Taquitos, 128 g	320	11	37
Crunchwrap Supreme®, 254 g	540	21	71
Enchirito® - Beef, 213 g	370	17	35
Enchirito® - Chicken, 213 g	350	14	34
Enchirito® - Steak, 213 g	340	14	33
• Express Taco Salad, 447 g	660	34	67
Guacamole Side, 21 g	35	3	2
Mexican Pizza, 213 g	540	30	47
MexiMelt®, 128 g	280	14	23
• Salsa Side, 21 g	5	0	1
Steak Quesadilla, 184 g	510	28	40
Steak Taquitos, 128 g	310	11	37
Tacos			
• Crunchy Taco Supreme®, 113 g	200	12	15
• Double Decker® Taco Supreme®, 191 g	360	15	41
Double Decker® Taco, 156 g	330	13	38
Grilled Steak Soft Taco, 128 g	250	14	20
Ranchero Chicken Soft Taco, 135 g	270	14	21

• MOST HEALTHY   • LEAST HEALTHY

TACO BELL (cont.)	Cal	Fat	Cbs
Soft Taco Supreme® - Beef, 135 g	240	11	24
Volcano Menu			
Volcano Burrito, 303 g	800	42	81
• Volcano Nachos, 354 g	1000	62	89
• Volcano Taco, 92 g	240	17	14
Why Pay More®!			
Bean Burrito, 198 g	370	10	55
• Beefy 5 Layer Burrito, 248 g	550	22	69
Caramel Apple Empanada, 85 g	310	15	39
Cheese Roll-Up, 64 g	200	10	19
Chicken Burrito, 177 g	440	20	48
Chicken Soft Taco, 99 g	200	8	19
• Cinnamon Twists, 35 g	170	7	26
Crispy Potato Soft Taco, 106 g	260	13	31
Crunchy Taco, 78 g	170	10	12
Soft Taco - Beef, 99 g	210	9	21
Triple Layer Nachos, 142 g	350	18	39
TACO CABANA			
Bowls and Salads			
Beef Enchilada (each)	225	12	13
Bowl with Black Beans	910	45	103
Bowl with Borracho Beans	970	48	109
• Bowl with Refried Beans	1090	58	113
Cheese Enchilada (each)	320	23	13
Shrimp Enchilada (each)	190	8	19
• Sour Cream Chicken Enchilada (each)	170	6	20
Breakfast Burritos			
Bacon & Egg Burrito	410	18	41
• Barbacoa Burrito	510	25	40
• Chorizo & Egg Burrito	400	18	42
Potato & Egg Burrito	440	21	48
Breakfast Platters			
• Eggs Mexicana Platter	900	51	69
Huevos Rancheros - Fried Eggs	850	48	66
• Huevos Rancheros - Scrambled Eggs	720	35	66
Steak Fajitas & Fried Eggs	880	47	68
Steak Fajitas & Scrambled Eggs	750	33	69
Breakfast Tacos			
• Bacon & Egg Taco	200	9	20
• Barbacoa Taco	250	12	19
Chorizo & Egg Taco	200	9	20
Potato & Egg Taco	220	11	23
Burritos			
Bean & Cheese Burrito	730	35	77
Beef Burrito - taco meat	710	30	71

• MOST HEALTHY   • LEAST HEALTHY

TACO CABANA (cont.)

	Cal	Fat	Cbs
• Beef Burrito Ultimo - taco meat	800	38	74
• Black Bean Burrito	450	8	82
Chicken Burrito - stewed chicken	660	25	73
Chicken Burrito Ultimo - stewed chicken	760	33	76
Chicken Fajita (dark) Burrito	620	25	64
Chicken Fajita (white) Burrito	630	24	65
Steak Fajita Burrito	650	27	65
Cabana Bowls			
Beef - taco meat	1160	62	114
Beef - taco meat w/o shell	770	35	81
Chicken - stewed chicken	1140	60	116
• Chicken - stewed chicken w/o shell	750	33	83
Chicken (breast) Fajita	1190	60	115
Chicken (breast) Fajita w/o shell	790	33	82
Chicken (thigh) Fajita	1180	61	114
Chicken (thigh) Fajita w/o shell	780	34	82
• Steak Fajita	1200	63	115
Steak Fajita w/o shell	810	37	82
Chalupas			
Bean & Cheese Chalupa	290	17	23
Beef Chalupa	310	16	24
• Chicken Chalupa	290	14	26
• Guacamole Chalupa	340	21	30
Chips and Queso			
Chips & Queso, personal or w/ combo meal	380	31	42
Chips & Queso, regular	900	72	87
Crispy Tacos			
Beef Taco - taco meat	180	10	11
Chicken Taco - stewed chicken	160	7	13
Dinners: Super Tex-Mex Dinner			
• Carne Guisada Dinner	840	28	93
Chicken Fajita Taco Dinner (dark)	900	25	125
Chicken Fajita Taco Dinner (white)	920	24	126
Enchilada Dinner	1270	66	115
Mexican Dinner	1130	53	113
Steak Fajita Taco Dinner	940	28	126
• Super Tex-Mex Dinner	1490	76	141
Taco Dinner	990	40	112
Drinks			
Kid's Chips & Queso side	380	31	42
• Kid's Quesadilla	520	29	39
• Kid's Refried Beans & Rice side	190	8	25
Slushie - Banana	260	0	64
Slushie - Mango	260	0	66
Slushie - Strawberry	250	0	60
Smoothie - Banana	380	0	88

• MOST HEALTHY   • LEAST HEALTHY

TACO CABANA (cont.)

	Cal	Fat	Cbs
Smoothie - Mango	380	0	91
Smoothie - Strawberry	370	0	85
Fajita Taco Salads			
Chicken (dark) Fajita	710	47	44
• Chicken (dark) Fajita - without shell	320	20	11
Chicken (white) Fajita	720	46	45
Chicken (white) Fajita - without shell	330	19	12
• Steak Fajita	740	49	45
Steak Fajita - without shell	350	22	12
Flameante Chicken			
• 1/2 Flameante Chicken Dinner	1220	54	83
1/4 Dark Flameante Chicken Dinner	920	41	82
• 1/4 White Flameante Chicken Dinner	770	22	81
Flautas			
Chicken Flauta	100	4	10
Personal Nachos: Queso			
Bean & Cheese (Queso)	510	37	54
Beef Nachos (Queso)	460	35	43
Chicken (dark) Fajita Nachos (Queso)	520	40	46
Chicken (white) Fajita Nachos (Queso)	530	39	46
• Chicken Nachos (Queso)	440	32	45
Steak Fajita Nachos (Queso)	540	41	46
• Super Beef Nachos (Queso)	680	49	59
Super Chicken Nachos (Queso)	660	47	60
Personal Nachos: Shredded Cheese			
Bean & Cheese (Shredded) Nachos	580	45	50
Beef Nachos (Shredded)	540	42	39
Chicken (dark) Fajita Nachos (Shredded)	600	47	42
Chicken (white) Fajita Nachos (Shredded)	600	47	42
• Chicken Nachos (Shredded)	520	40	41
Steak Fajita Nachos (Shredded)	610	49	42
• Super Beef Nachos (Shredded)	760	57	55
Super Chicken Nachos (Shredded)	730	54	56
Personal Quesadillas			
• Cheese Quesadilla	710	39	61
Chicken Fajita Quesadilla, (dark)	760	40	62
Chicken Fajita Quesadilla, (white)	760	40	62
• Steak Fajita Quesadilla	770	42	62
Regular Nachos: Queso			
Bean & Cheese Nachos	1020	75	108
Beef Nachos	930	69	87
Chicken (dark) Fajita Nachos	1050	80	92
Chicken (white) Fajita Nachos	1060	79	93
• Chicken Nachos	880	64	89
Steak Fajita Nachos	1080	82	93
• Super Beef Nachos	1370	98	117

TACO CABANA (cont.)

	Cal	Fat	Cbs
Super Chicken Nachos	1320	93	120
Regular Nachos: Shredded Cheese			
Bean & Cheese Nachos	1170	90	100
Beef Nachos	1080	84	78
Chicken (dark) Fajita Nachos	1200	95	84
Chicken (white) Fajita Nachos	1200	94	85
• Chicken Nachos	1030	79	81
Steak Fajita Nachos	1220	97	85
• Super Beef Nachos	1520	113	109
Super Chicken Nachos	1470	108	112
Regular Quesadillas			
• Cheese Quesadilla	1250	73	93
Chicken Fajita Quesadilla, (dark)	1340	76	95
Chicken Fajita Quesadilla, (white)	1350	75	96
• Steak Fajita Quesadilla	1370	79	96
Shrimp			
• Shrimp Enchilada	190	8	19
Shrimp Tampico Quesadilla, personal	850	46	62
• Shrimp Tampico Quesadilla, regular	1450	83	94
Sides and Add-Ons			
Bacon	40	3	0
Beef Enchilada	225	12	13
Black beans	80	0	14
Borracho beans	110	3	16
• Cheese Enchilada	320	23	13
Corn Tortilla - each	70	1	15
Flour Tortilla - each	120	3	19
Guacamole (3 oz.)	110	9	7
Queso (3 oz.)	200	15	5
Refried beans	250	13	24
Rice	120	1	25
• Salsa Fuego (1 oz.)	5	0	1
Salsa Ranch (1 oz.)	35	4	1
Salsa Roja (1 oz.)	5	0	1
Salsa Verde (1 oz.)	10	0	1
Scrambled Egg	60	4	0
Shredded Cheese (1 oz.)	110	9	0
Sour Cream (3 oz.)	160	14	3
Sour Cream Chicken Enchilada	170	6	20
Southwest Ranch Dressing (1 oz.)	112	11	2
Sizzling Fajitas: Personal			
• Chicken Fajita (dark)	700	21	92
Chicken Fajita (white)	710	20	93
• Steak Fajita	730	24	93
Sizzling Fajitas: Regular Platter			
• Chicken Fajita (dark)	1590	53	200

• MOST HEALTHY   • LEAST HEALTHY

TACO CABANA (cont.)

	Cal	Fat	Cbs
Chicken Fajita (white)	1610	51	202
• Steak Fajita	1640	57	202

Soft Tacos

	Cal	Fat	Cbs
• Bean & Cheese Taco	300	14	31
Beef Taco - taco meat	230	9	21
Black Bean Taco	200	4	34
Carne Guisada Taco	190	5	20
• Chicken Fajita Taco (dark)	180	5	20
Chicken Fajita Taco (white)	190	4	21
Chicken Taco	210	7	23
Steak Fajita Taco	200	6	21

Taco Salads

	Cal	Fat	Cbs
• Beef - taco meat	1030	65	69
Beef - taco meat - w/o shell	640	38	37
Chicken - stewed chicken	990	60	72
• Chicken - stewed chicken - w/o shell	600	33	39

TACO DEL MAR

Baja Bowls

	Cal	Fat	Cbs
Beef, refried, 574 g	830	35	81
• Chicken, refried, 574 g	790	31	79
• Fish, refried, 638 g	880	41	95
Pork, refried, 574 g	790	33	81

Breakfast Menu

	Cal	Fat	Cbs
Breakfast taco, flour, refried, 116 g	260	15	18
Egg & cheese burrito, refried, 285 g	490	19	59
Egg & cheese taco, flour, refried, 95 g	200	10	17
Eggs, 57 g	90	7	1
Hash Browns, 56 g	110	6	13
Mondito brkfst burrito, refried, 354 g	640	31	62
• Mondo brkfst burrito, refried, 587 g	1080	50	105
• Potatoes Diced, 50 g	60	1	11
Sausage, 35 g	100	8	1

Desserts

	Cal	Fat	Cbs
• Brownie, Oreo, 92 g	400	17	59
• Cookie, Butter, 71 g	220	10	31
Cookie, Choc Chip, 71 g	240	12	34
Cookie, Choc Chip/Nut, 71 g	240	13	30
Cookie, Milk Choc, 71 g	240	12	31
Cookie, Oat/Rsn/Wnut, 71 g	240	11	35
Cookie, Peanut Butter, 71 g	240	13	27
Cookie, Triple Choc, 71 g	230	12	31
Cookie, White Ch Mac, 71 g	270	16	30

Enchiladas

	Cal	Fat	Cbs
• Beef, 662 g	1030	37	115
• Cheese, 562 g	820	27	112

• MOST HEALTHY   • LEAST HEALTHY

TACO DEL MAR (cont.)

	Cal	Fat	Cbs
Chicken, 662 g	990	33	113
Pork, 662 g	990	35	114
Kids Menu			
• Kids bean & cheese burrito & chips, 271 g	760	31	95
Kids bean & cheese burrito, 214 g	480	17	58
Kids chips & cheese, 85 g	400	22	38
Kids quesadilla & chips, 150 g	600	27	71
Kids quesadilla, 93 g	320	14	34
Kids taco, beef, 85 g	270	15	16
• Kids taco, chicken, 85 g	250	13	15
Kids taco, pork, 85 g	250	14	16
Mondito Burritos			
• Beef, refried, 313 g	555	19	71
• Cheese, refried, 277 g	460	13	69
Chicken, refried, 313 g	545	17	70
Fish, refried, 288 g	505	21	61
Pork, refried, 313 g	545	18	71
Mondo Burritos			
• Beef, refried, 615 g	1070	36	134
Cheese, refried, 544 g	870	24	130
Chicken, refried, 615 g	1030	32	131
• Fish, refried, 551 g	840	30	110
Pork, refried, 615 g	920	24	132
Nachos & Chips			
Chips & salsa, 198 g	590	27	78
Nachos, refried, 475 g	1190	65	110
Quesadillas			
• Beef, 353 g	800	37	66
• Cheese, 282 g	710	35	63
Chicken, 353 g	770	33	64
Pork, 353 g	770	35	65
Sauces			
Enchilada Sauce, 85 g	35	0	7
• Green Sauce, 28 g	5	0	1
Guacamole, 35 g	40	4	2
Habanero Sauce, 28 g	10	0	1
Queso, 57 g	80	6	2
Red Sauce, 28 g	5	0	1
Salsa, 85 g	15	0	4
• White Sauce, 28 g	120	13	1
Sides			
Beans, black, 120 g	140	2	24
Beans, refried, 120 g	160	4	24
• Beans, whole pinto, 120 g	90	0	20
Beef, 99 g	200	11	4
Cheese, 28 g	110	9	1

• MOST HEALTHY   • LEAST HEALTHY

TACO DEL MAR (cont.)

	Cal	Fat	Cbs
Chicken, 99 g	170	7	1
Cod, 78 g	120	4	13
Pork, 99 g	170	8	3
• Rice, 170 g	230	3	45
Taco Salads			
Beef, refried, 595 g	930	49	75
• Chicken, refried, 595 g	900	45	73
• Fish, refried, 617 g	1040	61	89
Pork, refried, 595 g	900	46	74
Tacos			
Hard, beef, 135 g	270	15	17
Hard, chicken, 135 g	260	13	16
Hard, fish, 131 g	270	15	23
Hard, pork, 135 g	260	14	17
Soft, beef, 165 g	280	11	28
• Soft, chicken, 165 g	260	9	27
Soft, fish, 162 g	270	11	34
Soft, pork, 165 g	260	10	28
• Soft, veggie, 215 g	310	8	49
Tortillas			
Corn Tortillas, 52 g	120	2	24
Flour Tortilla 10", 65 g	210	5	33
• Spinach Tortilla 13", 112 g	350	10	56
Taco Salad Shell, 59 g	280	16	29
• Taco Shell, 22 g	110	5	14
Tomato Tortilla 13", 112 g	350	10	56
Whole Wheat Tortilla 13", 114 g	300	5	54
Vegan Mondo			
Mondito, refried, 299 g	430	11	70
Mondo, refried, 580 g	800	19	133

TACO JOHN'S

10g or Less of Fat	Cal	Fat	Cbs
• Bean Burrito, 173 g	310	5	56
Chicken Softshell Taco, 113 g	190	6	19
• Chili, 213 g	160	6	17
Crispy Taco, 92 g	180	10	13
Mexican Rice, 170 g	250	6	45
Refried Beans, 269 g	260	2	50
Softshell Taco, 106 g	190	8	20
Taco Burger, 135 g	250	9	28
Breakfast Menu			
Breakfast Burrito – Bacon, 217 g	550	25	56
Breakfast Burrito – Sausage, 246 g	640	35	56
Breakfast Egg Burrito – Bacon, 201 g	500	24	43
Breakfast Egg Burrito – Sausage, 232 g	590	34	44

• MOST HEALTHY   • LEAST HEALTHY

TACO JOHN'S (cont.)

	Cal	Fat	Cbs
Breakfast Egg Burrito, 187 g	420	19	42
• Breakfast Taco – Bacon, 106 g	270	13	25
Breakfast Taco – Sausage, 120 g	310	18	25
Potato Olés® Scrambler – Regr Bacon, 439 g	1030	67	72
• Potato Olés® Scrambler – Reg Ssge, 475 g	1140	79	72
Scrambler Burrito – Bacon, 246 g	550	25	58
Scrambler Burrito – Sausage, 274 g	640	32	58

Burritos

	Cal	Fat	Cbs
• Bean Burrito, 187 g	360	9	56
• Beef Grilled Burrito, 233 g	600	32	52
Beefy Burrito, 187 g	440	20	45
Chicken & Potato Burrito, 237 g	470	19	56
Chicken Grilled Burrito, 233 g	590	29	50
Combination Burrito, 187 g	400	14	50
Crunchy Chicken & Potato Burrito, 251 g	600	28	65
Meat & Potato Burrito, 237 g	500	23	58
Super Burrito, 251 g	450	18	54

Condiments

	Cal	Fat	Cbs
• Bacon Ranch Dressing – 1.5 oz portion, 43 g	130	10	10
Guacamole – 2 oz. portion, 57 g	90	6	8
• Hot Sauce – 1 oz. portion, 28 g	10	0	1
Mild Sauce – 1 oz. portion, 28 g	10	0	1
Nacho Cheese – 3 oz portion, 85 g	120	9	5
Pico de Gallo – 1 oz. portion, 28 g	10	0	1
Salsa – 2 oz portion, 57 g	20	0	4
Super Hot Sauce – 1 oz. portion, 28 g	10	0	1

Current Promotions

	Cal	Fat	Cbs
Chili Fritos® Bowl, 163 g	310	18	26
Chili Fritos® Burrito, 239 g	600	29	64

Desserts

	Cal	Fat	Cbs
Apple Grande, 96 g	270	12	39
• Choco Taco, 113 g	390	20	48
Churro, 55 g	190	7	15
• Giant Goldfish® Grahams, 14 g	70	2	11

Local Favorites

	Cal	Fat	Cbs
• Chili Cheese Potato Olés®, 305 g	590	36	55
Chili Enchilada, 216 g	310	16	24
Chilito, 130 g	360	15	40
• Mexi Rolls® -2 Piece w/o Nacho Chz, 54 g	130	5	14
Ranch Burrito – Beef, 201 g	440	22	45
Ranch Burrito – Chicken, 201 g	400	17	44
Smothered Burrito, 322 g	510	20	60

Sides

	Cal	Fat	Cbs
• Chili w/o Crackers & Cheese, 213 g	160	6	17
Mexican Rice, 170 g	250	6	45
Nachos, 142 g	380	23	38

• MOST HEALTHY • LEAST HEALTHY

TACO JOHN'S (cont.)

	Cal	Fat	Cbs
• Potato Olés® - Medium, 201 g	600	36	62
Refried Beans w/o Cheese, 255 g	260	2	47

Snacks

	Cal	Fat	Cbs
Chips & Queso, 191 g	430	25	43
Cini-Sopapilla Bites®, 74 g	210	5	37

Specialties

	Cal	Fat	Cbs
Chicken Taco Salad w/o Dressing, 361 g	480	27	35
Crunchy Chkn Taco Salad w/o Drss, 383 g	660	40	47
Crunchy Chicken w/o Sauce, 143 g	450	27	24
• Quesadilla Melt – Cheesy, 161 g	440	22	43
Quesadilla Melt – Fajita Beef, 246 g	540	28	49
Quesadilla Melt – Fajita Chicken, 246 g	510	23	47
Super Nachos – Regular, 358 g	810	48	74
• Super Potato Olés® -Regular, 478 g	1030	65	87
Taco Salad w/o Dressing, 361 g	520	33	37

Tacos

	Cal	Fat	Cbs
Chicken Softshell Taco, 113 g	190	6	19
• Crispy Taco, 92 g	180	10	13
Softshell Taco, 113 g	220	11	21
• Stuffed Grilled Taco, 211 g	560	25	63
Taco Bravo®, 184 g	340	13	40
Taco Burger, 142 g	270	12	28

TACO MAYO

Burritos

	Cal	Fat	Cbs
Bean Burrito	496	16	71
Beef & Bean Burrito	494	19	56
Beef Burrito	492	23	41
Dbl Smothered Dbl Queso Burrito - Chkn	883	32	101
Double Smothered Chkn Burrito - Chili Queso	879	32	99
• Double Smothered Chili Queso Burrito	955	40	100
Double Smothered Chili Queso Burrito - Steak	905	34	99
Double Smothered Double Queso Burrito - Steak	910	34	101
Double Smothered Verde Queso Burrito - Chkn	856	31	101
Double Smothered Verde Queso Burrito - Steak	883	32	101
Fajita Grilled Burrito - Chicken	492	23	42
Fajita Grilled Burrito - Steak	519	25	42
Kids Meal - Bean Burrito	874	40	106
SalsaLITA Beef & Bean Burrito	455	15	58
SalsaLITA Beef Grilled Burrito	411	13	55
• SalsaLITA Chicken Burrito	325	8	40
SalsaLITA Chicken Grilled Burrito	387	8	54
SalsaLITA Steak Burrito	351	9	40
SalsaLITA Steak Grilled Burrito	413	10	54
Super Burrito - Beef	539	23	57
Super Burrito - Chicken	407	16	39

⯈ TACO MAYO (cont.)

	Cal	Fat	Cbs
Super Burrito - Steak	434	18	39
Drinks			
Pina Colada Chiller	479	25	59
Strawberry Chiller	378	7	79
Favorites			
Choco Taco	290	15	36
• Cinnamon Crisps	114	6	14
Crispy Beef Taco	161	9	10
Kids Meal - Cheese Quesadilla	582	35	51
Kids Meal - Crispy Beef Taco	540	33	45
Kids Meal - Soft Beef Taco	606	35	52
• Loco Melt	814	57	56
SalsaLITA Chicken Soft Taco	167	4	18
SalsaLITA Steak Soft Taco	187	5	18
Soft Beef Taco	228	11	17
Soft Chicken Taco	184	6	16
Soft Steak Taco	204	7	16
Taco Burger	303	13	28
Tostada	295	13	37
Tostada Melt	524	32	35
Fresh Grilled			
3-Cheese Quesadilla Beef	645	36	43
• 3-Cheese Quesadilla Chicken	569	28	42
3-Cheese Quesadilla Steak	595	29	42
Mexicali Bowl - Chicken	1152	59	115
• Mexicali Bowl - Steak	1158	60	115
Mexicali Grilled Burrito - Chicken	607	30	54
Mexicali Grilled Burrito - Steak	633	32	54
Mexicali Queso Bowl - Chicken	967	36	117
Mexicali Queso Bowl - Steak	974	37	117
Quesadilla - Cheese	596	35	45
Quesadilla - Chicken	676	37	46
Quesadilla - Fajita Chicken	698	39	47
Quesadilla - Fajita Steak	725	40	47
Quesadilla - Steak	703	39	46
Tamale Melt (Seasonal)	617	34	50
Tamale Platter (seasonal)	714	31	78
Tamales - 6 Pack w/Chili (LTO)	677	37	49
Nachos			
3-Cheese Nachos - Beef Supreme	793	42	68
3-Cheese Nachos - Cheese	458	26	43
3-Cheese Nachos - Chicken Supreme	717	34	67
3-Cheese Nachos - Steak Supreme	566	28	47
Classic Nachos - Beef Supreme	719	37	70
• Classic Nachos - Cheese	377	19	45
Classic Nachos - Chicken Supreme	643	29	69

• MOST HEALTHY   • LEAST HEALTHY

TACO MAYO (cont.)

	Cal	Fat	Cbs
Classic Nachos - Steak Supreme	669	31	69
• Ultimate Grande' Nacho	1040	55	98

Salads

	Cal	Fat	Cbs
Acapulco Salad - Chicken	678	50	35
• Acapulco Salad - Steak	705	51	35
• SalsaLITA Chicken Salad	278	6	33
SalsaLITA Steak Salad	305	8	33
Taco Salad - Beef	705	38	57
Taco Salad - Chicken	438	23	30
Taco Salad - Steak	444	25	30

Sides

	Cal	Fat	Cbs
Guac -N- Chips	399	22	45
• Mexicali Rice	160	1	36
• Potato Locos (large)	586	37	55
Queso -N- Chips	449	22	49
Refried Beans	294	9	43

TACO TIME

Burritos

	Cal	Fat	Cbs
Beef, Bean & Cheese, 9 oz.	490	17	55
Big Juan, Chicken, 12 oz.	580	16	70
Big Juan, Ground Beef, 12 oz.	630	23	73
Casita, Chicken, 11 oz.	490	17	42
Casita, Ground Beef, 11 oz.	540	24	46
Chicken & Black Bean, 10 oz.	490	16	54
• Chicken B.L.T., 10 oz.	690	39	43
Crisp Chicken, 5 oz.	380	17	33
Crisp Ground Beef, 5 oz.	430	21	36
• Crisp Pinto Bean, 5 oz.	360	14	47
Crispy Chicken Ranchero, 12 oz.	600	31	51
Soft Ground Beef, 7 oz.	430	16	43
Soft Pinto Bean, 7 oz.	370	10	54
Soft Veggie, 10 oz.	520	17	73

Desserts

	Cal	Fat	Cbs
Churro with cinnamon & sugar, 2 oz.	250	16	27
• Churro, plain, 2 oz.	210	16	17
• Crustos, 4 oz.	290	6	58
Empanada, Apple, 4 oz.	230	7	40
Empanada, Bavarian Crème, 4 oz.	240	9	36
Empanada, Cherry, 4 oz.	240	7	41
Empanada, Pumpkin, 4 oz.	260	8	42

Fries and Sides

	Cal	Fat	Cbs
Chips, Taco, 2 oz.	150	4	27
• Fries, Cheddar, Medium, 7 oz.	500	35	39
Fries, Mexi, Medium, 6 oz.	390	26	38
Fries, Stuffed, Medium, 7 oz.	460	28	42

• MOST HEALTHY   • LEAST HEALTHY

TACO TIME (cont.)

	Cal	Fat	Cbs
• Mexi-Rice, 4 oz.	80	1	17
Refritos, 7 oz.	210	6	26

Individual Items

	Cal	Fat	Cbs
10" Flour Tortilla, 3 oz.	210	5	37
• 11" Wheat Tortilla, 3 oz.	260	6	44
Crispy Chicken Strips, 3 oz.	110	4	1
Crispy Taco Shells (each), 1 oz.	100	7	8
Fajita Chicken Strips, 3 oz.	90	0	1
Ground Beef, 3 oz.	140	7	4
Guacamole, 1 oz.	50	5	2
Salsa, Salsa Fresca, 1 oz.	10	0	2
Salsa, Salsa Nuevo, 1 oz.	10	0	2
• Salsa, Salsa Verde, 1 oz.	5	0	2
Shredded Cheddar Cheese, 1 oz.	60	5	0
Tortilla Salad Bowl, 8", 2 oz.	150	9	17

Other Favorites

	Cal	Fat	Cbs
Cheddar Melt, 3 oz.	250	12	25
Chimichanga, Chicken, 13 oz.	610	20	63
Chimichanga, Ground Beef, 13 oz.	650	27	63
• Enchilada, Chicken, 7 oz.	230	5	17
Enchilada, Ground Beef, 7 oz.	290	12	21
• Nachos, Grande, 17 oz.	930	43	96
Street Tacos, Pork, 7 oz.	270	9	29
Taco Burger, 8 oz.	460	26	31
Tostada, Bean, 4 oz.	230	13	21
Tostada, Chicken, 7 oz.	320	13	22
Tostada, Ground Beef, 7 oz.	380	20	25

Salads

	Cal	Fat	Cbs
• Taco, Regular - Chicken, 10 oz.	310	13	22
Taco, Regular - Ground Beef, 9 oz.	370	20	24
Tostada Delight, Chicken, 9 oz.	450	19	35
• Tostada Delight, Ground Beef, 9 oz.	490	26	36

Tacos

	Cal	Fat	Cbs
• Crisp Ground Beef, 4 oz.	260	17	12
Crisp, Ground Beef w/ Sour Cream, 5 oz.	290	19	12
Soft, Chicken, 7 oz.	360	9	40
Soft, Ground Beef, 7 oz.	420	16	43
Soft, Junior, 5 oz.	310	13	28
Super Soft, Chkn - Wheat Tortilla, 11 oz.	530	16	60
Super Soft, Chicken, 11 oz.	530	16	59
• Super Soft, Ground Beef - Wheat Tortilla, 11 oz.	590	23	63
Super Soft, Ground Beef, 11 oz.	590	23	62

TACONE

Breakfast Wraps

	Cal	Fat	Cbs
El Grande Wrap, 149 g	280	16	20

• MOST HEALTHY   • LEAST HEALTHY

▶ TACONE (cont.)

	Cal	Fat	Cbs
Venice Beach Wrap, 354 g	630	31	46
Desserts			
Fresh Fruit Salad, 227 g	80	0	21
Farm Fresh Salads			
• Caesar, 307 g	500	46	18
Fiesta, 310 g	340	19	18
T.J. Cobb, 272 g	430	30	6
Flavor Sides			
• Grilled Veggies + Feta, 113 g	170	14	6
Spa Salad, 225 g	190	9	22
• Sweet Potato Fries, 109 g	190	9	23
Global Grill Platter			
Empire Steak, 468 g	380	21	14
Napa Valley Chicken, 355 g	320	15	10
Rotisserie Chicken, 595 g	830	37	37
• Tradewind Shrimp, 457 g	250	12	14
Gourmet Wraps			
Baja, 215 g	370	11	54
Baja Wrap with Chicken, 238 g	420	13	47
• Buffalo Kickin' Chicken Wrap	460	12	43
Campfire, 213 g	340	12	41
Kickin' Fried Chicken, 151 g	280	11	22
Kingston	320	10	41
Malibu Melt, 173 g	360	17	25
Mambo, 146 g	220	7	26
Perfect Ten Wrap	360	17	43
Pilgrim, 158 g	260	14	21
• Spa, 136 g	200	9	26
Thai Cone, 177 g	300	9	35
Grilled Sandwiches			
• Angus Khan Burger, 411 g	1150	69	56
Chick-a-Boom, 256 g	570	38	25
Great Gobbler, 237 g	470	24	40
United Steak of America, 196 g	560	40	23
• Veggie Caprese, 115 g	310	18	29
Kids			
• Grilled Cheese, 68 g	220	11	20
Kickin' Fried Chicken Jr., 142 g	250	24	7
• Quesadilla Jr., 122 g	420	22	35
Quesadillas			
• 4 Cheese, 85 g	210	11	18
• Apollonia, 225 g	640	39	39
BBQ Chicken, 136 g	300	13	28
Smoothies & Desserts			
Bikini Blast, 617 g	410	2	94
Blue Voodoo, 583 g	400	1	93

• MOST HEALTHY   • LEAST HEALTHY

TACONE (cont.)

	Cal	Fat	Cbs
• Orangabang, 539 g	360	1	84
Palm Peach, 834 g	500	2	116
• Pink Flamingo, 658 g	520	1	125

Tacone® Sides

	Cal	Fat	Cbs
Black Beans + Jack Cheese, 128 g	210	5	27
Down-Home Coleslaw, 113 g	35	1	7
• Homemade Tortilla Chips + Salsa, 142 g	300	12	42
Seasoned French Fries, 108 g	200	9	29
Seasoned Potato Chips, 86 g	160	8	21
Tacone® Rice, 170 g	240	1	51
Tacone® Side Salad, 100 g	140	11	9
• Thai Cucumber Salad, 122 g	20	0	5

TASTEE-FREEZ

For Tastee-Freez desserts please see page 461

TCBY

Hand-Scooped Frozen Yogurt (Medium)

Blueberry and Cream, 170 g	300	6	48
Butter Pecan, 170 g	360	17	42
Chocolate Chocolate, 170 g	280	8	45
Choco Chunk Cookie Dough, 170 g	360	13	55
Cookies & Cream, 170 g	320	10	50
Cotton Candy, 170 g	270	8	44
Mint Chocolate Chunk, 170 g	330	12	49
Mocha Almond, 170 g	340	12	50
NSA Choco Choco Swirl, 170 g	200	1	49
NSA Vanilla Fudge Brownie 170 g	240	5	51
Peaches and Cream, 170 g	260	6	44
• Peanut Butter Delight, 170 g	400	18	51
Pralines & Cream, 170 g	330	11	52
• Psychedelic Sorbet, 170 g	200	0	51
Rainbow Cream, 170 g	270	8	43
Rocky Road, 170 g	400	17	53
Strawberries and Cream, 170 g	260	6	45
Vanilla Bean, 170 g	270	8	43
Vanilla Chocolate Chip, 170 g	330	12	48

Soft Serve Frozen Yogurt

Cake Batter, 95 g	110	2	23
Cheesecake, 95 g	120	2	23
Chocolate, 95 g	110	2	23
Classic Tart, 95 g	90	0	21
Coffee, 95 g	120	2	23
Fat Free Dutch Chocolate, 95 g	110	0	24
Golden Vanilla, 95 g	120	2	23
Mango Sorbet, 95 g	110	0	26

• MOST HEALTHY   • LEAST HEALTHY

▶ TCBY (cont.)

	Cal	Fat	Cbs
• NSA Fat Free Chocolate, 95 g	80	0	23
NSA Fat Free Mountain Blackberry, 95 g	90	0	24
NSA Fat Free Peach, 95 g	90	0	24
NSA Fat Free Strawberry, 95 g	90	0	24
NSA Fat Free Vanilla, 95 g	90	0	25
NSA White Chocolate Macadamia, 95 g	90	0	24
Old Fashioned Vanilla (Fat Free), 95 g	110	0	23
Orange Sorbet, 95 g	100	0	24
• Peanut Butter, 95 g	130	2	26
Raspberry Sorbet, 95 g	100	0	25
Strawberry Kiwi Sorbet, 95 g	100	0	24
Strawberry, 95 g	110	2	23
White Chocolate Mousse, 95 g	120	2	23

Smoothies

	Cal	Fat	Cbs
Beriyo Berrilicious, 16 fl.oz.	260	2	N/A
Beriyo Black' N Blue, 16 fl.oz.	260	2	N/A
Beriyo Mango Tango, 16 fl.oz.	310	2	N/A
Beriyo Mangolada, 16 fl.oz.	310	5	N/A
Beriyo Mondo Mango, 16 fl.oz.	280	1	N/A
Beriyo Peach Palm, 16 fl.oz.	300	4	N/A
• Beriyo Pina Paradise, 16 fl.oz.	320	10	N/A
Beriyo Pink Pineapple, 16 fl.oz.	310	7	N/A
• Beriyo Purely Peach, 16 fl.oz.	260	1	N/A
Beriyo Straight-Up Strawberry, 16 fl.oz.	260	2	N/A
Beriyo Strawberry Bananza, 16 fl.oz.	300	2	N/A
Beriyo Strawberry Fling, 16 fl.oz.	320	2	N/A

▶ THE COFFEE BEAN

Coffee Ice Blended® Drinks (Regular)

	Cal	Fat	Cbs
Black Forest Ice Blended®	500	7	91
Black Forest Ice Blended® NSA Powder	270	2	47
• Caramel Ice Blended®	540	9	99
Caramel Ice Blended® NSA Powder	300	2	57
Hazelnut Ice Blended®	440	18	66
Mocha Ice Blended®	370	6	68
• Mocha Ice Blended® NSA Powder	140	0	24
Ultimate Mocha Ice Blended®	420	7	75
Ultimate Mocha Ice Blended® NSA Powder	190	2	31
Ultimate Vanilla Ice Blended®	440	10	73
Ultimate Vanilla Ice Blended® NSA Powder	200	3	32
Vanilla Ice Blended®	390	8	67
Vanilla Ice Blended® NSA Powder	150	1	25
White Chocolate Ice Blended®	470	15	76

Coffee-free Ice Blended® Drinks (Regular)

	Cal	Fat	Cbs
• Banana Caramel Ice Blended®	570	9	110
Banana Caramel Ice Blended® NSA Powder	330	2	69

• MOST HEALTHY   • LEAST HEALTHY

THE COFFEE BEAN (cont.)

	Cal	Fat	Cbs
Chai Mate Ice Blended®	410	8	74
Chai Mate Ice Blended® NSA Powder	170	1	33
Green Tea Ice Blended®	410	8	69
Malibu Dream Ice Blended®	440	8	82
Malibu Dream Ice Blended® NSA Powder	200	1	41
Pomegranate Blueberry Ice Blended®	460	1	87
Pom Blbry Ice Blended® NSA Powder	220	1	46
Pure Chocolate Ice Blended®	390	6	72
• Pure Choco Ice Blended® NSA Powder	160	1	28
Pure Vanilla Ice Blended®	410	8	70
Pure Vanilla Ice Blended® NSA Powder	170	1	29

Fru Tea Ice Blended® Drinks (Regular)

	Cal	Fat	Cbs
• Frozen Lemonade FruTea®	320	0	83
Mucho Mango FruTea®	240	0	60
• Pomegranate FruTea®	210	0	58

Iced Espresso & Coffee Drinks (Regular)

	Cal	Fat	Cbs
Cappuccino Over Ice	110	4	10
• Caramel Latte Over Ice	350	3	64
Caramel Latte Over Ice NSA Powder	290	2	54
Hazelnut Latte Over Ice	310	9	46
Iced Coffee	10	0	1
• Iced Tea	0	0	1
Latte Over Ice	190	6	16
Mocha Latte Over Ice	270	3	46
Mocha Latte Over Ice NSA Powder	160	0	25
Tea Latte Over Ice Chocolate Powder	160	3	31
Tea Latte Over Ice NSA Choco Powder	50	0	9
Tea Latte Over Ice NSA Vanilla Powder	60	0	10
Tea Latte Over Ice Vanilla Powder	180	4	31
Vanilla Latte Over Ice	280	4	46
Vanilla Latte Over Ice NSA Powder	170	0	26
White Chocolate Latte Over Ice	320	8	49

THE GREAT AMERICAN BAGEL

Bagels

	Cal	Fat	Cbs
4-Grain Honey, 5 oz.	390	4	80
Apple Cinnamon Oat Bran, 5 oz.	370	4	73
Apple Cinnamon Sugar, 5 oz.	390	4	78
Apple Crumb, 9 oz.	620	11	118
Asiago, 6 oz.	520	16	72
Asiago with Black & Green Olives, 7 oz.	540	20	70
Banana Nut, 5 oz.	410	9	69
Blueberry Crumb, 9 oz.	630	10	122
Blueberry, 5 oz.	370	4	75
Cheddar Bacon, 7 oz.	600	23	71
Cheddar Herb, 5 oz.	390	8	66

• MOST HEALTHY   • LEAST HEALTHY

THE GREAT AMERICAN (cont.)

	Cal	Fat	Cbs
Cheddar Onion, 6 oz.	500	13	75
Cheddar Salsa, 7 oz.	500	17	68
• Cheddar Twist, 9 oz.	800	27	107
Chocolate Chip, 5 oz.	420	8	78
Cinnamon Delight, 7 oz.	640	18	108
Cinnamon Raisin, 5 oz.	380	4	76
Egg, 5 oz.	370	5	70
Everything, 5 oz.	380	5	73
French Toast, 5 oz.	430	8	77
Garlic, 5 oz.	390	4	75
Harvest 10-Grain, 5 oz.	410	8	73
Hot Tomazzor, 8 oz.	520	13	77
Jalapeño Cheddar, 5 oz.	370	7	63
Onion, 5 oz.	380	4	74
Peanut Butter Chocolate Chip, 5 oz.	420	8	76
Pesto, 5 oz.	360	5	67
Plain, 5 oz.	360	4	71
Poppy, 5 oz.	390	6	72
Provolone, 6 oz.	460	11	72
Pumpernickel, 5 oz.	360	4	71
Salt, 5 oz.	360	4	71
Sesame, 5 oz.	390	6	72
Sourdough Baguette, 4 oz.	300	4	56
Spinach Herb, 5 oz.	350	4	70
Strawberry Crumb, 9 oz.	630	10	123
Strawberry, 5 oz.	380	4	76
Stuffed Pepperoni, 9 oz.	570	17	78
Stuffed Spinach, 9 oz.	640	20	86
Sun-Dried Tomato Basil, 5 oz.	390	4	74
Swiss Cheese, 6 oz.	470	12	72
Tomazzor, 8 oz.	520	13	77
Veggie, 5 oz.	310	4	61
• Whole Wheat Baguette, 4 oz.	290	4	56
Whole Wheat, 5 oz.	370	4	74

TIM HORTON'S

Bagels

	Cal	Fat	Cbs
• 12 Grain, 114 g	330	9	52
Blueberry, 114 g	270	1	55
Cinnamon Raisin, 114 g	270	1	55
Everything, 114 g	280	2	53
Onion, 114 g	260	2	53
• Plain, 114 g	260	2	52
Poppy Seed, 114 g	270	2	53
Sesame Seed, 114 g	270	3	53
Wheat 'N Honey, 114 g	300	3	60

• MOST HEALTHY   • LEAST HEALTHY

▶ TIM HORTON'S (cont.)

	Cal	Fat	Cbs
Beverages			
Café Mocha, 10 oz.	160	7	25
Coffee (1 cream, 1 sugar), 10 oz.	75	4	9
Decaffeinated Coffee (1 cream, 1 sugar), 10 oz.	75	4	9
English Toffee, 10 oz.	220	6	40
• Flavor Shot, 1 ml	5	0	1
French Vanilla, 10 oz.	240	7	39
Hot Chocolate, 10 oz.	240	6	45
Hot Smoothee, 10 oz.	260	10	39
Iced Cappuccino- Milk, 12 oz.	180	2	39
• Iced Cappuccino, 12 oz.	300	15	41
Steeped Tea (1 cream, 1 sugar), 10 oz.	50	1	10
Breakfast			
Bagel BELT, 266 g	450	14	58
Hashbrown, 47 g	100	5	12
Breakfast Sandwiches			
Bacon, Egg, Cheese, 159 g	420	23	34
• Egg, Cheese, 149 g	370	19	34
• Sausage, Egg, Cheese, 191 g	540	35	35
Cake Donuts			
• Chocolate Glazed, 75 g	260	10	39
• Old Fashion Glazed, 75 g	320	19	35
Old Fashion Plain, 58 g	260	19	20
Sour Cream Glazed, 58 g	270	17	27
Cake Timbits			
• Chocolate Glazed, 19 g	70	3	10
• Old Fashion Plain, 16 g	70	5	5
• Sour Cream Glazed, 19 g	90	5	12
Cookies			
Caramel Chocolate Pecan, 52 g	230	11	32
Chocolate Chunk, 52 g	230	9	35
• Oatmeal Raisin Spice, 52 g	220	8	35
• Peanut Butter, 52 g	280	16	27
Triple Chocolate, 52 g	250	13	31
White Chocolate Macadamia Nut, 52 g	240	12	31
Cream Cheese			
• Garlic and Herb, 1.5 oz.	140	13	2
• Light Plain, 1.5 oz.	85	6	3
Light Strawberry, 1.5 oz.	100	6	8
Plain, 1.5 oz.	130	12	2
Filled Donuts			
• Angel Cream, 89 g	310	13	46
• Blueberry, 78 g	230	8	36
Boston Cream, 89 g	250	9	38
Canadian Maple, 89 g	260	9	41
Strawberry, 78 g	230	8	36

• MOST HEALTHY   • LEAST HEALTHY

TIM HORTON'S (cont.)	Cal	Fat	Cbs
Filled Timbits			
• Banana Cream, 21 g	60	2	9
• Blueberry, 21 g	60	2	10
Lemon, 21 g	60	2	9
Strawberry, 21 g	60	2	10
Muffins			
Blueberry Bran, 128 g	300	10	53
Blueberry, 128 g	330	11	55
• Chocolate Chip, 128 g	430	16	69
Cranberry Blueberry Bran, 128 g	290	10	51
Cranberry Fruit, 128 g	350	12	59
Fruit Explosion, 128 g	360	11	61
• Low fat Blueberry, 128 g	290	3	62
Low Fat Cranberry, 128 g	290	3	62
Raisin Bran, 128 g	360	10	65
Strawberry Sensation, 128 g	350	11	61
Wheat Carrot, 128 g	400	19	55
Whole Grain Raspberry, 128 g	400	17	58
Other			
Honey Cruller, 80 g	320	19	37
Walnut Crunch, 80 g	360	23	35
Sandwiches Country Buns			
White, 92 g	240	1	49
Whole wheat, 92 g	230	1	46
Soups & Chili			
Beef Stew, 10 oz.	236	8	25
Chicken Noodle, 10 oz.	120	2	18
• Chili, 10 oz.	300	16	18
Cream of Broccoli, 10 oz.	160	9	16
Creamy Field Mushroom, 10 oz.	150	3	28
Hearty Potato Bacon, 10 oz.	250	13	23
• Hearty Vegetable, 10 oz.	70	0	14
Minestrone, 10 oz.	120	4	24
Split Pea with Ham, 10 oz.	150	3	27
Turkey and Wild Rice, 10 oz.	120	2	21
Vegetable Beef Barley, 10 oz.	110	2	21
Specialty Baked Goods			
Cheese Croissant, 66 g	230	14	19
Cherry Cheese Danish, 85 g	230	10	27
Chocolate Danish, 94 g	340	16	42
• Cinnamon Roll- Frosted, 119 g	470	25	57
Cinnamon Roll- Glazed, 108 g	420	23	50
Maple Pecan Danish, 93 g	290	12	37
• Plain Croissant, 59 g	200	11	21
Plain Tea Biscuit, 100 g	250	9	35
Raisin Tea Biscuit, 100 g	290	10	45

• MOST HEALTHY   • LEAST HEALTHY

TIM HORTON'S (cont.)

	Cal	Fat	Cbs
'Tim's Own® Sandwiches			
BLT, 207 g	450	18	53
• Chicken Salad, 265 g	380	9	55
Egg Salad, 208 g	390	13	52
Ham & Swiss, 270 g	440	12	56
• Toasted Chicken Club, 244 g	460	7	70
Turkey Bacon Club, 276 g	440	8	63
Yeast Donuts			
Apple Fritter, 95 g	300	11	49
• Blueberry Fritter, 110 g	330	10	55
Chocolate Dip, 62 g	210	9	30
Honey Dip, 62 g	210	8	33
• Maple Dip, 62 g	210	8	31
Yeast Timbits			
Apple Fritter, 17 g	50	15	9
Honey Dip, 17 g	60	15	9
Yogurt & Berries			
Creamy Vanilla, 6 oz.	180	3	32
Strawberry, 6 oz.	150	3	28

TOPZ

	Cal	Fat	Cbs
Aero Fries, Rings & Nuggets			
Aero Fries, 158 g	380	14	58
• Aero Onion Rings, 166 g	298	11	46
Chili Cheese Fries, 301 g	589	27	66
Dessertz			
Brownie, 105 g	350	5	67
• Chocolate Chip Cookie, 105 g	385	9	67
• Low Fat Ice Cream w/Choc. Syrup, 162 g	255	7	43
Oatmeal Raisin Cookie, 105 g	385	9	67
Fresh Gourmet Salads			
• Chinese Chicken Salad, 392 g	322	14	17
Dijon Deli Chopped Salad, 382 g	229	13	9
Ginger Grilled Ahi Salad, 392 g	312	15	10
• Small Dijon Deli Salad, 21 g	101	6	3
Fruit Shakez			
• Chocolate Banana Shake, 472 g	460	8	80
Chocolate Shake, 372 g	360	9	55
Raspberry Shake, 427 g	404	9	64
• Strawberry Shake, 427 g	356	9	54
Gourmet Hot Dogs			
• Beef Chili Dog, 269 g	485	24	49
Double Turkey Dog, 242 g	390	8	60
Hebrew National Beef Dog, 230 g	450	21	52
• Turkey Chili Dog, 255 g	355	9	53

• MOST HEALTHY   • LEAST HEALTHY

TOPZ (cont.)

	Cal	Fat	Cbs
Gourmet Lean Burgers			
• 1/4 lb. Black Angus Burger, 301 g	507	25	40
1/4 lb. Black Angus Chili Burger, 318 g	489	21	42
• Garden Burger, 228 g	355	12	46
Turkey Burger, 301 g	449	19	40
Kidz Mealz			
• Kids Grilled Cheese, 62 g	207	9	24
Kidz Beef Dog, 145 g	405	21	40
• Kidz Burger, 184 g	408	19	33
Kidz Turkey Dog, 131 g	275	7	44
Signature Chili			
Signature Chili, 291 g	329	17	17
Signature Lean Sandwich			
Classic Grilled Cheese Sandwich, 123 g	414	18	47
• Ginger Grilled Ahi Sandwich, 268 g	384	11	37
• Grilled Chz & Tomato Sandwich, 144 g	418	18	48
Grilled Chkn Breast Sandwich, 290 g	396	10	39

TROPICAL SMOOTHIE

	Cal	Fat	Cbs
Bistro Sandwiches			
• Cranberry Walnut Chicken Salad™	737	40	71
Hummus Veggie™	668	26	84
The Italian™	462	16	38
Turkey Bacon Ranch™	429	13	37
Turkey Guacamole™	593	14	75
Ultimate Club™	524	19	43
• Wasabi Roast Beef™	374	11	33
Breakfast Wraps			
• All American	558	23	53
Early Bird™	617	24	68
Salsa Sunrise™	568	23	54
• Western	636	28	57
Cheeses			
American	50	5	0
• Cheddar (1/3 cup)	177	15	1
Low Fat Mozzarella (1/3 cup)	115	7	1
• Parmesan (1/8 cup)	48	3	0
Pepper Jack	56	4	0
Provolone	74	6	0
Swiss	78	6	0
Coffee Smoothies			
• Caramel Cream™	591	11	117
• Cinn City™	326	8	56
Coffee Nut™	343	11	52
Mocha Madness™ °	445	12	76

• MOST HEALTHY   • LEAST HEALTHY

TROPICAL SMOOTHIE (cont.)

	Cal	Fat	Cbs
Gourmet Salads			
Chicken Caesar™	487	39	10
Cranberry Walnut Chicken Salad™	476	38	20
• Sesame Chicken™	580	19	73
Southwest Chicken™	474	27	34
Thai Chicken™	501	11	74
• TSC Signature™	349	13	37
Grilled Flatbreads			
Baja Chicken™	455	16	48
Caribbean Luau™	452	12	57
Chicken Pesto™	456	17	45
• Honey Ham & Swiss™	411	12	53
Mediterranean Veggie™	468	17	61
• Peanut Butter Banana Crunch™	613	21	91
Kid's Smoothies (12 oz.)			
Awesome Orange™	188	3	39
• Banana Mania™	199	1	45
Chocolate Chimp™	156	3	31
• Jetty Junior™	79	0	18
Kids Food Items			
Cheese Pizza	368	13	45
Cheese Quesadilla	491	23	52
• Cheese Quesadilla add Chicken	542	24	53
Grilled Cheese Flatbread	425	22	40
• Ham & American Flatbread	332	10	41
Turkey & Provolone Flatbread	361	10	41
Low Fat Smoothies			
Blimey Limey™	211	0	52
• Blue Lagoon™	130	1	30
Hawaiian Breeze™	179	0	42
Island Fever™	222	0	53
Jetty Punch™	168	1	39
Kiwi Quencher™	215	0	51
Mango Magic™	199	0	46
Paradise Point™	249	1	58
Peaches' N Silk™	163	0	39
Pineapple Delight™	227	0	55
Rockin' Raspberry™	201	1	47
Strawberry Beach™	137	0	31
• Sunny Day™	290	1	70
Sunrise Sunset™	210	0	50
Sauces & Dressings (1 oz.)			
• Bistro Sauce	121	7	14
Buffalo Sauce	8	0	2
Guacamole	53	4	3

• MOST HEALTHY   • LEAST HEALTHY

▶ TROPICAL SMOOTHIE (cont.)	Cal	Fat	Cbs
Jamaican Jerk Sauce	40	0	9
Pesto	97	9	1
• Salsa	4	0	1
Sesame	75	4	9
Thai Peanut	74	3	10
TSC Signature™	40	2	5
Simply Indulgent Smoothies			
Bahama Mama™	345	8	67
Beach Bum™	364	5	75
Chocolate Chiller™	354	7	67
• Peanut Butter Cup	520	21	73
Tropi-Colada™	312	5	65
Supercharged Smoothies- Power Up			
Health Nut™	328	7	42
Immune Blast™	241	1	57
Kiwi Citrus Green Tea™	276	0	65
Lean Machine™	161	1	37
Muscle Blaster™	284	3	41
• Peanut Paradise™	490	18	49
Stress Defender™	264	0	62
• Very Berry Green Tea™	160	1	36
Supercharged Smoothies-Super Fruit			
• Acai Berry Boost™	231	2	53
Get-Up-and-Goji™	232	0	55
• Pomegranate Plunge™	274	0	67
Toasted Wraps			
Buffalo Chicken™	623	26	60
Cordon Bleu™	688	32	55
Jamaican Jerk Chicken™	624	17	79
King Caesar™	604	29	56
Popeye's Favorite™	623	25	60
• Sesame Chicken™	803	23	113
Southwest Chicken™	563	20	69
Thai Chicken™	722	15	113
Totally Turkey™	617	25	55
• Veggie Veggie™	508	17	72
Toasted Wraps (Junior)			
All American	352	15	37
• Early Bird™	396	15	45
Salsa Sunrise™	362	14	38
• Western	344	13	39
Tropical Tradition Smoothies			
Cranberry Truffle™	447	5	97
Peppermint Mocha (at select locations)™	530	9	104

• MOST HEALTHY   • LEAST HEALTHY

TUBBY'S

Burger Subs (Regular)	Cal	Fat	Cbs
All American Cheeseburger	810	48	56
• Big Tub	671	56	55
Burger Special	898	59	59
Cheeseburger	911	60	59
Mushroom Burger	868	59	53
• Pizza Burger	929	60	62
Taco	827	47	67

Chicken Subs (Regular)

	Cal	Fat	Cbs
Chicken & Broccoli	552	23	56
Chicken & Cheddar	543	23	54
• Chicken Club	705	41	53
Chicken Fajita	445	12	57
Chicken Parmesan	426	14	51
• Grilled Chicken	346	5	52

Deli Subs (Regular)

	Cal	Fat	Cbs
Club Sub	705	41	53
Famous	004	35	55
• Ham & Cheese	568	30	54
Turkey & Cheese	626	32	51
• Turkey Club	850	39	83

Specialty Subs (Regular)

	Cal	Fat	Cbs
BLT	636	42	50
Cold Veggie	462	14	66
• Italian Sausage	729	45	56
• Tuna	417	18	47
Veggie Stir Fry	652	27	89

Steak Subs (Regular)

	Cal	Fat	Cbs
Mushroom Steak	833	26	52
Pepper Steak	709	46	52
• Philly Cheesesteak	685	40	49
• Pizza Steak	986	57	85
Portabella Mushroom	801	48	54
Steak & Cheddar	833	56	52
Steak & Cheese	823	56	51
Steak Special	746	46	58

UNA MAS

Burritos	Cal	Fat	Cbs
Foghead Burrito	874	35	99
Grilled Fajita Burrito, Chicken	666	28	70
Pineapple Thai Burrito	660	19	66
• Roasted Pasilla Veggie Burrito	480	20	59
San Lucas Fish Burrito	645	29	63
• Una Mas Carnitas Burrito	1199	77	49

• MOST HEALTHY   • LEAST HEALTHY

UNA MAS (cont.)

	Cal	Fat	Cbs
Nachos and Chips			
Chips and Guacamole	820	48	96
• Chips and Salsa	580	24	86
• Mas Nachos	1780	92	188
Quesadillas			
Monterey & Shrimp Quesadilla	310	8	51
The Monterey	310	8	51
Rice and Beans			
Frijoles Negros	140	1	24
• Mexican Fried Rice	90	4	10
Pinto Beans	150	2	26
• Rice and Beans	240	6	36
Salad Dressings			
Lime Jalapeño Vinaigrette	260	30	1
Tangy Lime Vinaigrette	300	35	1
Salads			
Margarita Salad	45	0	10
Soups			
Tortilla Soup - Small	60	2	8
Specialties			
• Crispy Taco	290	13	30
• Enchiladas Rojas	240	8	33
Taquitos	280	14	31
Specialty Drinks (Small)			
Aqua Fresca Melon	130	0	32
Aqua Fresca Sandia	140	0	34
Aqua Fresca Strawberry	120	0	31
Aqua Fresca Strawberry Banana	190	0	47
• Horchata	480	4	96
• Strawberry Lemonade	70	0	19
Tacos			
San Lucas Fish Taco - Cabo Style	320	19	26
Taqueria Taco	100	4	20
Una Mas Carnitas Taco	190	3	30
Una Mas Taco	190	4	30
VILLAGE INN			
3-Course Sirloin Steak	640	22	70
Chicken Caesar Salad	380	16	25
• Chicken Noodle Soup	80	2	10
• Chicken Stir-Fry Dinner Skillet	710	24	83
Cinnamon Raisin French Toast	370	11	57
Fruit & Nut Multigrain Pancakes	490	10	91
Garden Grand Salad	350	20	25
Grilled Chicken Sandwich	460	16	46
Grilled Tilapia	630	20	64

• MOST HEALTHY   • LEAST HEALTHY

VILLAGE INN (cont.)

	Cal	Fat	Cbs
Half Sandwich & Soup	290	9	27
Minestrone Soup	100	2	17
Vegetable Beef Soup	140	7	12
Veggie Omelette	490	16	69

WAHOO'S FISH TACO

A la Carte

	Cal	Fat	Cbs
Banzai Veggie, 1	152	4	25
Blackened Chicken, 1	186	5	22
Blackened Fish, 1	208	7	23
Carne Asada, 1	181	5	22
Carnitas, 1	233	8	23
Charbroiled Chicken, 1	203	5	26
Charbroiled Fish, 1	209	7	23
• Cheese, 1	329	20	16
Mushroom, 1	148	4	23
• Shrimp, 1	146	4	23
Tofu, 1	193	6	24
Veggie, Brown Rice, Black Beans, 1	211	4	36
Veggie, Brown Rice, White Beans, 1	198	4	34
Veggie, White Rice, Black Beans, 1	215	4	36
Veggie, White Rice, White Beans, 1	202	4	34

Baja Roll

	Cal	Fat	Cbs
Baja Roll w/ brown rice, white beans, 1	444	9	78
Wet Baja Roll Combo w/ brown rice, white beans, 1	723	27	90

Banzai Bowl

	Cal	Fat	Cbs
• #12 Shrimp Bowl, Brown Rice, White Beans, 1	591	12	105
#14 Tofu Bowl, Brown Rice, White Beans, 1	734	19	110
Blackened Chkn, Brown Rice, White Beans, 1	728	14	115
Blackened Fish, Brown Rice, White Beans, 1	773	18	115
Carne Asada, Brown Rice, White Beans, 1	713	14	116
• Carnitas, Brown Rice, White Beans, 1	837	20	117
Charbroiled Chkn, Brown Rice, White Beans, 1	727	14	115
Charbroiled Fish, Brown Rice, White Beans, 1	775	18	115
Shrimp, Brown Rice, White Beans, 1	628	12	115
Tofu, Brown Rice, White Beans, 1	724	16	117

Banzai Burrito

	Cal	Fat	Cbs
Blackened Chkn, Brown Rice, White Beans, 1	576	16	77
Blackened Fish, Brown Rice, White Beans, 1	621	21	77
Blackened Mshr, Brown Rice, White Beans, 1	488	14	81
Carne Asada, Brown Rice, White Beans, 1	563	17	79
• Carnitas, Brown Rice, White Beans, 1	684	23	79
Charbroiled Chkn, Brown Rice, White Beans, 1	575	16	77
Charbroiled Fish, Brown Rice, White Beans, 1	622	21	77
• Shrimp, Brown Rice, White Beans, 1	476	14	77
Tofu, Brown Rice, White Beans, 1	573	19	80

• MOST HEALTHY   • LEAST HEALTHY

WAHOO'S FISH TACO (cont.)

	Cal	Fat	Cbs
Vegetarian, Brown Rice, White Beans, 1	485	14	82

Chopped Salad

	Cal	Fat	Cbs
Banzai Veggie, Brown Rice, White Beans, 1	231	3	45
Blackened Chkn, Brown Rice, White Beans, 1	310	6	38
Blackened Fish, Brown Rice, White Beans, 1	355	10	38
Blackened Mshr, Brown Rice, White Beans, 1	222	3	42
Carne Asada, Brown Rice, White Beans, 1	298	6	39
• Carnitas, Brown Rice, White Beans, 1	419	12	40
Charbroiled Chkn, Brown Rice, White Beans, 1	309	5	38
Charbroiled Fish, Brown Rice, White Beans, 1	357	10	38
• Shrimp, Brown Rice, White Beans, 1	210	4	38
Vegetarian, Brown Rice, White Beans, 1	313	5	60

Cookies

	Cal	Fat	Cbs
Oatmeal Raisin, 2	240	9	36
White Chocolate Macadamia Nut, 2	270	12	37

Desserts

	Cal	Fat	Cbs
Brownie with Walnuts, 2	250	12	33
Chocolate Chip Cookie, 2	260	10	39

Kid's Menu

	Cal	Fat	Cbs
Black Bean & Cheese Burrito, 1	674	29	75
Kid Nachos, 1	561	35	40

Mini Quesadilla

	Cal	Fat	Cbs
• Mini Quesadilla W/ Brown Rice, White Beans, 1	625	24	81
Banzai Veggie, Brown Rice, White Beans, 1	280	5	53
Blackened Chkn, Brown Rice, White Beans, 1	315	6	49
Blackened Fish, Brown Rice, White Beans, 1	334	8	49
Blackened Mshr, Brown Rice, White Beans, 1	276	5	51
Carne Asada, Brown Rice, White Beans, 1	310	6	50
Carnitas, Brown Rice, White Beans, 1	362	9	50
Charbroiled Chkn, Brown Rice, White Beans, 1	314	6	49
Charbroiled Fish, Brown Rice, White Beans, 1	335	8	49
• Shrimp, Brown Rice, White Beans, 1	272	5	50
Tofu, Brown Rice, White Beans, 1	315	7	51
White Bean & Cheese Burrito, 1	622	29	66

Nachos

	Cal	Fat	Cbs
Carne Asada, 4	285	17	18
• Cheese, 4	263	16	17
• Chicken, 4	288	17	17
Shrimp, 4	266	17	16

Quesadilla

	Cal	Fat	Cbs
Banzai Veggie, 3	223	12	18
Carne Asada, 3	243	13	17
• Cheese, 3	213	12	16
Chicken, 3	246	13	16
• Fish, 3	260	14	16
Shrimp, 3	218	12	16

• MOST HEALTHY   • LEAST HEALTHY

WAHOO'S FISH TACO (cont.)

	Cal	Fat	Cbs
Salad dressings			
Roasted Pepper Cilantro -3 Oz., 1	39	0	8
Side Kicks			
1/2 Bean & 1/2 Rice, Brown Rice, Black Beans, 1	359	5	66
1/2 Bean & 1/2 Rice, Brown Rice, White Beans, 1	294	5	55
1/2 Bean & 1/2 Rice, White Rice, Black Beans, 1	378	5	70
1/2 Bean & 1/2 Rice, White Rice, White Beans, 1	313	5	58
• Side Black Beans, 1	442	3	82
Side Brown Rice, 1	350	7	64
Side Corn Tortillas -3 Ea., 1	144	2	29
Side Flour Tortilla -1 Ea., 1	300	11	46
Side Green Sauce -3 Oz., 1	39	0	8
Side Guacamole -3 Oz., 1	108	10	5
Side Mr. Lee Chili Sauce -0.5 Oz., 1	43	3	3
• Side Salsa -3 Oz., 1	18	0	4
Side White Beans, 1	286	3	54
Side White Rice, 1	389	8	71
Soups, Salads & Sandwiches			
Chicken Tortilla Soup, 1	54	1	5
Garden Salad, 1	38	0	8
Starters			
• Baja Rolls, 3	168	8	17
Jumbo French Fries, 4	130	4	20
• Maui Onion Rings, 4	128	5	18
Taquitos (3 per order)			
Carne Asada, 1	326	10	42
• Carnitas, 1	417	15	42
Chicken, 1	334	9	41
• Chips (Basket), 2	243	12	33
Fish, 1	384	15	41
Wahoo Bowls			
# 6 Carne Asada Bowl, Brown Rice, White Beans, 1	716	16	106
# 6 Maui Bowl, Brown Rice, White Beans, 1	718	15	107
# 8 Blackened Fish Bowl, Brown Rice, White Beans, 1	802	21	105
• # 8 Shrimp Bowl, Brown Rice, White Beans, 1	591	12	105
# 8 Teriyaki Fish Bowl, Brown Rice, White Beans, 1	808	22	105
# 9 Veggie Bowl, Brown Rice, White Beans, 1	637	11	119
#10 Carnitas Bowl, Brown Rice, White Beans, 1	897	25	108
• #10 Kahlua Pig Bowl, Brown Rice, White Beans, 1	901	25	109
7 Teriyaki Chkn Bowl, Brown Rice, White Beans, 1	737	15	105
8 Charbroiled Fish Bowl, Brown Rice, White Beans, 1	804	22	105
Blackened Chkn Bowl, Brown Rice, White Beans, 1	734	15	105
Charbroiled Chkn Bowl, Brown Rice, White Beans, 1	733	15	104
Wahoo's Salad			
Banzai Veggie, 1	297	18	24
Blackened Chicken, 1	417	22	14

• MOST HEALTHY   • LEAST HEALTHY

WAHOO'S FISH TACO (cont.)

	Cal	Fat	Cbs
Blackened Fish, 1	484	28	14
Carne Asada, 1	399	23	16
• Carnitas, 1	580	32	18
Charbroiled Chicken, 1	416	21	14
Charbroiled Fish, 1	487	29	14
• Shrimp, 1	274	19	15
Veggie, Brown Rice, White Beans, 1	422	20	47

Wahoo's Sandwich

	Cal	Fat	Cbs
Blackened Chicken, 1	512	18	51
Blackened Fish, 1	552	22	51
Carne Asada, 1	502	19	52
• Carnitas, 1	607	24	53
Charbroiled Chicken, 1	512	18	51
Charbroiled Fish, 1	553	22	51
• Sandwich Side Fries, 1	331	11	50
Sandwich Side Onion Rings, 1	340	14	48
Shrimp, 1	425	16	51

Wet Banzai Burritos Green Sauce

	Cal	Fat	Cbs
Blackened Chkn, Brown Rice, White Beans, 1	893	33	97
Blackened Fish, Brown Rice, White Beans, 1	912	38	92
Blackened Mshr, Brown Rice, White Beans, 1	806	31	101
Carne Asada, Brown Rice, White Beans, 1	880	34	98
• Carnitas, Brown Rice, White Beans, 1	1002	40	99
Charbroiled Chkn, Brown Rice, White Beans, 1	892	33	97
Charbroiled Fish, Brown Rice, White Beans, 1	914	38	92
• Shrimp, Brown Rice, White Beans, 1	793	31	97
Tofu, Brown Rice, White Beans, 1	891	36	100
Vegetarian, Brown Rice, White Beans, 1	802	31	101

Wet Banzai Burritos Red Sauce

	Cal	Fat	Cbs
Blackened Chkn, Brown Rice, White Beans, 1	841	34	86
Blackened Fish, Brown Rice, White Beans, 1	886	39	86
Blackened Mshr, Brown Rice, White Beans, 1	754	32	90
Carne Asada, Brown Rice, White Beans, 1	829	35	87
• Carnitas, Brown Rice, White Beans, 1	950	41	88
Charbroiled Chkn, Brown Rice, White Beans, 1	840	34	86
Charbroiled Fish, Brown Rice, White Beans, 1	888	39	86
• Shrimp, Brown Rice, White Beans, 1	741	32	86
Tofu, Brown Rice, White Beans, 1	839	37	89
Vegetarian, Brown Rice, White Beans, 1	750	32	91

Wet Classic Burritos Green Sauce

	Cal	Fat	Cbs
Blackened Chicken, 1	786	36	66
Blackened Fish, 1	836	40	68
Blackened Mushroom, 1	698	33	70
Carne Asada, 1	774	36	67
Carnitas, 1	894	42	69
Charbroiled Chicken, 1	785	36	66

• MOST HEALTHY   • LEAST HEALTHY

► WAHOO'S FISH TACO (cont.)

	Cal	Fat	Cbs
Charbroiled Fish, 1	838	40	68
• Shrimp, 1	691	34	68
Tofu, 1	785	38	70
• Veggie, Brown Rice, Black Beans, 1	911	36	111
Veggie, Brown Rice, White Beans, 1	872	36	104
Veggie, White Rice, Black Beans, 1	869	32	113
Veggie, White Rice, White Beans, 1	886	36	106

Wet Classic Burritos Red Sauce

	Cal	Fat	Cbs
Blackened Chicken, 1	760	37	60
Blackened Fish, 1	818	40	64
Blackened Mushroom, 1	672	34	64
Carne Asada, 1	748	37	61
Carnitas, 1	868	43	63
Charbroiled Chicken, 1	759	36	60
Charbroiled Fish, 1	812	41	62
• Shrimp, 1	665	34	62
Tofu, 1	759	39	64
• Veggie, Brown Rice, Black Beans, 1	885	37	105
Veggie, Brown Rice, White Beans, 1	847	37	98
Veggie, White Rice, Black Beans, 1	843	33	107
Veggie, White Rice, White Beans, 1	860	37	100

► WE'RE ROLLING PRETZEL CO.

Pretzels

	Cal	Fat	Cbs
Cinnamon Sugar Pretzel	492	5	102
Garlic Pretzel	448	10	78
• Plain Pretzel	368	1	78
• Pretzel Rods, 10 pack	641	8	125
Pretzel w/Butter & Salt	401	5	78
Raisin Pretzel	473	5	97

Sandwiches and Salads

	Cal	Fat	Cbs
• Chicken Salad	574	20	70
Classic Italian	573	17	69
Ham & Swiss	491	10	69
• Turkey & Swiss	439	6	71

► WENDY'S

Boneless Wings & Crispy Chicken Nuggets

	Cal	Fat	Cbs
5 Piece Chicken Nuggets	230	14	13
• Barbecue Nugget Sauce	45	0	11
Spicy Chipotle Boneless Wings	500	20	48
Sweet & Sour Nugget Sauce	50	0	12
• Sweet & Spicy Asian Boneless Wings	540	18	62

Frosty™ Treats

	Cal	Fat	Cbs
• Chocolate Frosty Small	310	8	52
Chocolate Fudge Frosty Shake, Small	410	11	69

• MOST HEALTHY   • LEAST HEALTHY

WENDY'S (cont.)

	Cal	Fat	Cbs
Coffee Toffee Twisted Frosty, Vanilla	540	20	83
Coffee Toffee Twisted Frosty, Chocolate	540	20	83
Frosty™-cino, Small	380	11	63
• M&M's Twisted Frosty, Vanilla	560	19	87
M&M's® Twisted Frosty, Chocolate	550	19	86
Oreo Twisted Frosty, Vanilla	440	14	72
Oreo® Twisted Frosty, Chocolate	440	14	72
Strawberry Frosty Shake, Small	390	11	66
Twisted Frosty, Chocolate	480	16	77
Twisted Frosty, Vanilla	480	16	77
Vanilla Bean Frosty Shake, Small	380	11	64
Vanilla Frosty Float with Coca-Cola®*	390	7	75
Vanilla Frosty Small	310	8	52

Garden Sensations® Salads

	Cal	Fat	Cbs
Ancho Chipotle Ranch Dressing	90	8	3
Buttery Best Spread	50	5	0
Caesar Side Salad	70	4	4
Cheddar Cheese, shredded	70	6	1
• Chicken BLT Salad	470	27	23
Chicken Caesar Salad	180	4	8
Crispy Noodles	70	3	10
Homestyle Garlic Croutons	70	3	9
• Hot Chili Seasoning Packet	5	0	1
Italian Vinaigrette	130	11	8
Mandarin Chicken® Salad	180	2	17
Mandarin Orange Cup	90	0	21
Medium French Fries	410	19	56
Oriental Sesame Dressing	170	10	19
Plain Baked Potato, 10 oz.	270	0	61
Roasted Almonds	130	11	4
Saltine Crackers	25	1	5
Seasoned Tortilla Strips	110	5	13
Side Salad	35	0	8
Small Chili	220	7	22
Sour Cream & Chives Baked Potato	320	4	63
Southwest Taco Salad	440	23	29

Sandwiches

	Cal	Fat	Cbs
1/4 lb. Hamburger Patty	220	15	0
American Cheese	70	5	1
American Cheese Jr.	40	4	0
Applewood Smoked Bacon – 1 strip	30	3	1
Bacon Deluxe Single	650	37	46
Bacon Jr. – 1 strip	15	1	0
Baconator® Single	610	34	43
Cheeseburger, Kids' Meal	260	11	26
Chicken Club Sandwich	630	30	56

WENDY'S (cont.)

	Cal	Fat	Cbs
Crispy Chicken Patty	200	12	13
Crispy Chicken Sandwich	350	15	38
Double Stack™	360	18	27
Double w/Everything and Cheese	750	42	44
Grilled Chicken Go Wrap	250	10	24
Hamburger, Kids' Meal	220	8	26
Homestyle Chicken Fillet	230	11	14
Homestyle Chicken Fillet Sandwich	460	16	53
Homestyle Chicken Go Wrap	310	15	29
• Iceberg Lettuce Leaf	0	0	0
Jr. Bacon Cheeseburger	310	16	26
Jr. Cheeseburger	270	11	27
Jr. Cheeseburger Deluxe	300	14	29
Jr. Hamburger	230	8	26
Jr. Hamburger Patty	90	6	0
Natural Swiss Cheese	70	6	0
Onion – 4 rings	5	0	1
Premium Bun	190	2	36
Sandwich Bun	120	1	24
Single w/Everything	470	21	43
Spicy Chicken Fillet	240	10	16
Spicy Chicken Fillet Sandwich	470	16	55
Spicy Chicken Go Wrap	320	15	30
Tomato – 1 slice	5	0	1
Tortilla	130	4	21
• Triple w/Everything and Cheese	1030	62	44
Ultimate Chicken Grill Fillet	110	2	1
Ultimate Chicken Grill Sandwich	340	7	41

WETZEL'S PRETZELS

Pretzel

	Cal	Fat	Cbs
Wetzel's Original with Butter, 1	384	4	NA
Wetzel's Original without Butter, 1	336	1	NA

WHATABURGER

Breakfast

	Cal	Fat	Cbs
Biscuit and Gravy, 149 g	560	33	54
Biscuit Snd w/ bacon, egg & chz, 163 g	500	32	33
Biscuit Sandwich with egg & chz, 154 g	450	28	33
Biscuit Snd w/ sausage, egg & chz, 225 g	690	49	33
Biscuit with bacon, 97 g	350	20	32
Biscuit with sausage, 159 g	540	37	32
• Biscuit, 88 g	300	17	32
Breakfast On A Bun® with bacon, 128 g	360	21	25
Breakfast On A Bun® with Ssge, 190 g	550	38	25
Breakfast Platter with bacon, 278 g	730	45	93

WHATABURGER (cont.)

	Cal	Fat	Cbs
• Breakfast Platter with sausage, 340 g	920	63	93
Egg Sandwich, 119 g	310	17	25
Honey Butter Chicken Biscuit, 167 g	560	34	50
Pancakes with bacon, 158 g	580	11	104
Pancakes with sausage, 220 g	780	28	104
Pancakes, plain, 149 g	540	7	104
Taquito with bacon & egg, 153 g	380	21	27
Taquito with bacon, egg, & chz, 166 g	420	24	27
Taquito with potato & egg, 176 g	430	23	57
Taquito with potato, egg & chz, 189 g	470	27	57
Taquito with sausage & egg, 166 g	410	24	27
Taquito with sausage, egg, & chz, 179 g	450	28	27

Burgers

	Cal	Fat	Cbs
• Justaburger®, 124 g	290	15	26
Whataburger Jr.®, 168 g	300	15	28
Whataburger® with bacon & chz, 361 g	780	43	59
Whataburger®, 323 g	620	30	58
Whataburger®, Double Meat, 407 g	870	49	58
• Whataburger®, Triple Meat, 492 g	1120	68	58

Chicken & Fish

	Cal	Fat	Cbs
• Chicken Strip, 1 piece, 58 g	150	8	11
Grilled Chicken Sandwich, 268 g	470	19	49
• Whatacatch® Dinner (2 piece), 1104 g	1630	89	181
Whatacatch® Sandwich, 182 g	450	24	44
Whatachick'n® Sandwich, 282 g	550	27	57

Desserts

	Cal	Fat	Cbs
• Cinnamon Roll, 128 g	390	9	71
Cookie, Chocolate Chunk, 51 g	230	11	31
• Cookie, Sugar, 51 g	210	9	31
Hot Apple Pie, 86 g	250	12	31

Drinks (Medium)

	Cal	Fat	Cbs
• Coffee Decaf, Colombian, 473 g	10	0	2
Coffee, Colombian, 473 g	10	0	2
• Malt, chocolate, 716 g	1050	25	188
Malt, strawberry, 716 g	1040	24	188
Malt, vanilla, 716 g	940	27	155
Shake, chocolate, 716 g	1000	26	171
Shake, strawberry, 716 g	990	26	171
Shake, vanilla, 716 g	890	28	139

Kid's Menu

	Cal	Fat	Cbs
Kid's Meal Chicken Strips, 114 g	300	16	22
Kid's Meal Justaburger®, 117 g	290	15	25

Salads

	Cal	Fat	Cbs
• Chicken Strips, 352 g	350	16	33
Garden, 238 g	50	0	11
Grilled Chicken, 337 g	220	7	18

• MOST HEALTHY • LEAST HEALTHY

WHATABURGER (cont.)

	Cal	Fat	Cbs
• Side Salad, 120 g	25	0	5
Sides			
• French Fries, Medium, 128 g	480	27	55
• Fruit Chew, 26 g	80	0	19
Gravy, White Peppered, 16 g	80	4	9
Hash Brown Sticks, 4 each, 65 g	200	12	60
Onion Rings, Medium, 121 g	400	25	37
Texas Toast, 1 slice, 46 g	150	7	20

WHITE CASTLE

Breakfast Condiments

	Cal	Fat	Cbs
• Butter, 5 g	30	4	0
Cream Cheese, 28 g	100	10	0
Grape Jelly - 1 Container, 14 g	35	0	9
• Maple Syrup- 1 Container, 43 g	120	0	31
Strawberry Jam - 1 container, 14 g	40	0	10

Breakfast Sandwich Alterations

	Cal	Fat	Cbs
Bologna - Louisville & Nashville regions, 28 g	150	12	2
Egg, 50 g	70	5	0
Hamburger meat (100% beef), 25 g	70	6	0
• Hashbrown, 83 g	310	28	14
Sausage, 37 g	150	14	0
• Strip of Bacon, 5 g	30	3	0
Wheat Toast (select regions), 50 g	130	2	24
White Toast (select regions), 50 g	130	2	25

Breakfast Sides

	Cal	Fat	Cbs
Apple Danish (Cincinnati, Detroit regions), 113 g	450	24	52
• Chz Danish (Cincinnati, Detroit regions), 127 g	490	25	62
Choco Frosted Donuts (Twin Pack), 113 g	460	24	120
Cinnamon Danish, 113 g	490	25	60
Cinn Roll (Cincinnati, Detroit regions), 106 g	420	20	56
French Twist Donuts (Twin Pack), 113 g	460	24	58
Plain Old Fashion Donut (Single), 99 g	385	21	51
• Spud Bites Single (select regions), 119 g	360	28	25
Strwbry Danish (Cincinnati region), 127 g	480	21	67

Coffee, Teas & Hot Chocolate (Medium)

	Cal	Fat	Cbs
Coffee Decaffeinated, 16 g	0	0	0
Coffee, 16 g	5	0	0
Gold Peak Iced Tea, Black Sweet (select regions), 30 g	220	0	59
• Gold Peak Iced Tea, Black Unsweet (select regions), 30 g	0	0	0
• Gold Peak Iced Tea, Southern Style (select regions), 30 g	270	0	76
Gold Peak Iced Tea, White Citrus (select regions), 30 g	240	0	62
Hot Chocolate, 16 g	240	6	41

Condiments

	Cal	Fat	Cbs
Hot Sauce - 1 Packet, 7 g	5	0	1
Lemon Juice - 1 Packet, 4 g	5	0	1

• MOST HEALTHY   • LEAST HEALTHY

▶ WHITE CASTLE (cont.)

	Cal	Fat	Cbs
Condiments on Sandwiches			
Hamburger Sauce, 1 1/2 tsp - Detroit region, 7 g	0	0	0
Spicy Hamburger Sauce, 1 1/2 tsp - Chicago region, 7 g	0	0	1
Crave Coolers			
Crave Cooler Coke, 30 g	140	0	39
Crave Cooker Fanta Wild Cherry, 30 g	140	0	39
Desserts			
Choco Chunk Cookie (select regions), 38 g	170	8	23
• Oatmeal Raisin Cookie (select regions), 38 g	160	6	23
• White Choco Macadamia Cookie (select regions), 38 g	180	9	22
Milk Shakes			
• Chocolate Shake, 30 g	780	14	152
Strawberry Shake, 30 g	780	12	148
• Vanilla Shake, 30 g	670	12	122
Sandwich Alterations			
American Cheese slice, 8 g	30	2	0
Bacon, 5 g	30	3	0
Jalapeño Cheese slice, 8 g	20	3	1
• Traditional Bun, 25 g	70	1	12
Sandwiches Doubles			
Double Bacon Cheeseburger, 117 g	350	22	21
Double Cheeseburger, 113 g	300	17	20
• Double Fish with cheese, 164 g	610	48	25
Double Fish without cheese, 149 g	550	43	24
Double Garlic Chz & Mshr Burger (select regions), 146 g	300	17	23
Double Jalapeño Cheeseburger, 107 g	280	17	21
• Double White Castle, 98 g	240	12	21
Sandwiches on a Bun			
• Bacon, 36 g	130	6	12
Bacon, Cheese, 43 g	150	9	12
Bacon, Egg, 86 g	200	11	12
Bacon, Egg, Cheese, 88 g	190	11	13
Bologna, Chz - Louisville & Nashville regions, 61 g	240	15	14
Bologna, Egg - Louisville & Nashville regions, 103 g	290	18	14
Bologna, Egg, Chz - Louisville & Nashville regions, 111 g	310	20	15
Egg, 75 g	140	6	12
Egg, Cheese, 83 g	160	8	13
Hamburger, Cheese, 58 g	160	9	12
Hamburger, Egg, 100 g	200	11	12
Hamburger, Egg, Cheese, 108 g	230	14	13
Sausage, 62 g	220	15	12
Sausage, Cheese, 70 g	250	17	13
Sausage, Egg, 112 g	290	20	13
• Sausage, Egg, Cheese, 120 g	320	22	13
Sandwiches Singles			
Bacon Cheeseburger, 65 g	190	11	13

● MOST HEALTHY　　● LEAST HEALTHY

WHITE CASTLE (cont.)

	Cal	Fat	Cbs
Bacon Jalapeño Cheeseburger, 65 g	190	12	14
Cheeseburger, 67 g	170	9	15
Chicken Breast Sandwich, 102 g	360	26	20
Chkn Breast Sandwich w/Cheese, 110 g	390	28	20
Chicken Ring Sandwich, 84 g	350	28	16
Chicken Ring Sandwich w/Cheese, 92 g	380	30	16
Chkn Supreme - Detroit & Cincinnati regions, 115 g	420	31	20
Fish Sandwich, 87 g	310	22	18
Fish w/Cheese, 95 g	340	24	18
Garlic Chz & Mshr Burger (select regions), 79 g	170	9	14
Jalapeño Cheeseburger, 60 g	160	9	14
Pulled Pork BBQ Sandwich, 82 g	170	5	25
Surf & Turf, 153 g	480	33	26
• Surf & Turf with cheese, 169 g	540	38	27
• Traditional Bun with Cheese, 33 g	90	3	12
White Castle, 55 g	140	6	13

Side Sauces

	Cal	Fat	Cbs
Cheese Sauce (Nacho), 47 g	50	4	3
Cinnamon Sauce - 1 Container, 28 g	110	4	20
• Marinara Sauce - 1 Container, 28 g	15	0	4
Seafood Sauce - 1 Container, 28 g	30	0	7
Tartar Sauce - 1 Container, 28 g	90	8	4
• White Castle Zesty Zing Sauce - 1 Container, 28 g	120	11	4

Sides (Regular)

	Cal	Fat	Cbs
Buffalo Chicken Rings, 6 Rings, 146 g	146	48	14
Chicken Rings, 6 Rings, 143 g	530	47	12
• Clam Strips, 128 g	128	17	5
Fish Nibblers, 141 g	141	16	28
French Fries, 159 g	370	25	33
Homestyle Onion Rings, 141 g	480	33	40
Mozzarella Cheese Sticks, 5 Sticks, 183 g	183	55	36
• Onion Chips Regular, 173 g	670	50	46
Onion Rings Regular, 112 g	340	22	33
Ranch Chicken Rings, 6 Rings, 146 g	146	48	14

WIENERSCHNITZEL

Breakfast

	Cal	Fat	Cbs
Biscuit & Gravy, 138 g	350	17	42
Biscuit with Bacon, 97 g	330	17	35
Biscuit with Egg & Bacon, 154 g	390	21	36
Biscuit with Egg & Sausage, 181 g	490	30	40
Biscuit with Egg, 138 g	320	15	36
Biscuit with Egg, Bacon & Chz, 168 g	440	25	36
Biscuit with Egg, Sausage & Chz, 195 g	540	34	40
Biscuit with Sausage, 124 g	430	26	39
Biscuit, 81 g	260	11	35

• MOST HEALTHY   • LEAST HEALTHY

WIENERSCHNITZEL (cont.)

	Cal	Fat	Cbs
Breakfast Platter with Bacon, 267 g	600	40	40
• Breakfast Platter with Sausage, 293 g	700	49	44
Burrito w/ Egg, Bacon & Chz, 156 g	360	19	29
Burrito w/ Egg, Bacon, Ssge & Chz, 186 g	470	25	39
Burrito w/ Egg, Chorizo Ssge & Chz, 182 g	540	35	29
Burrito with Egg, Sausage & Chz, 182 g	460	28	33
Chili Cheese Egg Burrito, 156 g	310	13	31
Chorizo Breakfast Burrito, 256 g	670	41	38
Country Breakfast, 294 g	640	40	47
Croissant w/ Egg, Bacon & Chz, 172 g	520	31	40
Croissant w/ Egg, Sausage & Chz, 199 g	620	40	44
French Toast Sticks, 148 g	490	29	49
Hash Browns, 80 g	290	25	14
Sandwich w/ Egg, Bacon & Chz, 144 g	300	15	26
Snd w/ Egg, Sausage & Chz, 171 g	400	24	30
• Syrup, 31 g	120	0	31

Burgers & Specialty

	Cal	Fat	Cbs
1/3 lb Spicy Polish Sausage Dog, 274 g	650	34	62
Chicken Deluxe Sandwich, 200 g	430	21	37
Chili Burger, 145 g	310	9	29
Chili Cheese Fries Burrito, 139 g	350	16	39
Chili Cheeseburger, 159 g	350	13	29
Chipotle Ranch Pupsters, 147 g	440	24	43
• Corn Dog, 82 g	250	17	15
Deluxe Cheeseburger, 235 g	450	23	33
Deluxe Hamburger, 221 g	400	19	33
Double Chili Cheeseburger, 260 g	560	24	35
• Fish & Chips, 278 g	710	52	50
Fish Wrap, 145 g	450	28	38
Italian Sausage Sandwich, 156 g	350	17	31
Mini Corn Dogs (6-pack), 99 g	320	22	22
Original Burger, 150 g	290	9	29
Pastrami Burger, 202 g	510	26	30
Pastrami Sandwich, 221 g	580	34	36
Polish Sausage Sandwich, 208 g	490	29	39
Sea Dog, 143 g	350	17	38

Fries & Sides

	Cal	Fat	Cbs
• Chili Cheese Fries, 231 g	540	38	39
Jalapeño Poppers (3 pack), 65 g	210	11	21
Regular Fries, 99 g	300	22	25
• Side Salad, 91 g	70	5	2

Hot Dogs

	Cal	Fat	Cbs
Angus All Beef BBQ Bacon Dog, pretzel bun, 219 g	650	35	61
Angus All Beef BBQ Bacon Dog, seeded bun, 199 g	570	34	42
Angus All Beef Chicago Dog, pretzel bun, 344 g	600	27	69
Angus All Beef Chicago Dog, seeded bun, 324 g	520	27	50

• MOST HEALTHY   • LEAST HEALTHY

WIENERSCHNITZEL (cont.)

	Cal	Fat	Cbs
Angus All Beef Chili Chz Dog, pretzel bun, 227 g	620	32	59
Angus All Beef Chili Chz Dog, seeded bun, 208 g	540	32	40
Angus All Beef Chili Dog, pretzel bun, 213 g	570	28	58
Angus All Beef Chili Dog, seeded bun, 193 g	490	27	39
Angus All Beef Coney Island Dog, pretzel bun, 227 g	570	28	59
Angus All Beef Coney Island Dog, seeded bun, 208 g	490	27	40
Angus All Beef Deluxe Dog, pretzel bun, 253 g	550	27	58
Angus All Beef Deluxe Dog, seeded bun, 234 g	470	26	39
Angus All Beef Kraut Dog, pretzel bun, 214 g	540	27	56
Angus All Beef Kraut Dog, seeded bun, 195 g	460	26	37
Angus All Beef Mustard Dog, pretzel bun, 187 g	530	27	55
Angus All Beef Mustard Dog, seeded bun, 168 g	450	26	36
• Angus All Beef Pastrami Dog, pretzel bun, 260 g	680	38	57
Angus All Beef Pastrami Dog, seeded bun, 241 g	600	38	38
Angus All Beef Plain Hot Dog, pretzel bun, 183 g	530	27	55
Angus All Beef Plain Hot Dog, seeded bun, 163 g	450	26	36
Angus All Beef Relish Dog, pretzel bun, 207 g	540	27	57
Angus All Beef Relish Dog, seeded bun, 199 g	460	26	39
Angus All Beef Stadium Dog, pretzel bun, 211 g	550	27	58
Angus All Beef Stadium Dog, seeded bun, 191 g	470	26	39
Original BBQ Bacon Dog, pretzel bun, 169 g	510	23	59
Original BBQ Bacon Dog, standard bun, 132 g	380	21	33
Original Chicago Dog, pretzel bun, 294 g	460	15	67
Original Chicago Dog, standard bun, 257 g	330	13	41
Original Chili Chz Dog, pretzel bun, 179 g	480	20	57
Original Chili Chz Dog, standard bun, 142 g	350	18	31
Original Chili Dog, pretzel bun, 165 g	430	16	57
Original Chili Dog, standard bun, 128 g	300	14	31
Original Coney Island Dog, pretzel bun, 177 g	430	16	57
Original Coney Island Dog, standard bun, 141 g	300	14	31
Original Deluxe Dog, pretzel bun, 203 g	410	15	56
Original Deluxe Dog, standard bun, 167 g	280	13	30
Original Kraut Dog, pretzel bun, 166 g	400	15	54
Original Kraut Dog, standard bun, 129 g	270	13	28
Original Mustard Dog, pretzel bun, 137 g	400	15	53
Original Mustard Dog, standard bun, 101 g	270	13	27
Original Pastrami Dog, pretzel bun, 210 g	550	26	55
Original Pastrami Dog, standard bun, 174 g	420	24	30
Original Plain Dog, pretzel bun, 133 g	400	15	53
Original Plain Hot Dog, standard bun, 96 g	270	13	27
Original Relish Dog, pretzel bun, 157 g	410	15	56
Original Relish Dog, standard bun, 121 g	280	13	30
Original Stadium Dog, pretzel bun, 161 g	410	15	54
Original Stadium Dog, standard bun, 124 g	280	13	30
Turkey BBQ Bacon Dog, pretzel bun, 173 g	500	21	60
Turkey BBQ Bacon Dog, standard bun, 136 g	370	19	34

• MOST HEALTHY   • LEAST HEALTHY

WIENERSCHNITZEL (cont.)

	Cal	Fat	Cbs
Turkey Chicago Dog, pretzel bun, 298 g	450	13	68
Turkey Chicago Dog, standard bun, 261 g	320	11	42
Turkey Chili Cheese Dog, pretzel bun, 183 g	470	18	58
Turkey Chili Chz Dog, standard bun, 146 g	340	16	32
Turkey Chili Dog, pretzel bun, 169 g	420	14	58
Turkey Chili Dog, standard bun, 132 g	290	12	32
Turkey Coney Island Dog, pretzel bun, 181 g	420	14	58
Turkey Coney Island Dog, standard bun, 145 g	290	12	32
Turkey Deluxe Dog, pretzel bun, 207 g	400	13	57
Turkey Deluxe Dog, standard bun, 171 g	270	11	31
Turkey Kraut Dog, pretzel bun, 170 g	390	13	55
Turkey Kraut Dog, standard bun, 133 g	260	11	29
Turkey Mustard Dog, pretzel bun, 141 g	390	13	54
• Turkey Mustard Dog, standard bun, 105 g	260	11	28
Turkey Pastrami Dog, pretzel bun, 214 g	540	24	56
Turkey Pastrami Dog, standard bun, 178 g	410	22	30
Turkey Plain Dog, pretzel bun, 137 g	390	13	54
Turkey Plain Dog, standard bun, 100 g	260	11	28
Turkey Relish Dog, pretzel bun, 161 g	400	13	57
Turkey Relish Dog, standard bun, 125 g	270	11	31
Turkey Stadium Dog, pretzel bun, 165 g	400	13	57
Turkey Stadium Dog, standard bun, 128 g	270	11	31

Tastee-Freez Desserts

	Cal	Fat	Cbs
• Banana Split, 450 g	820	24	149
Cone, 4 oz Kids Choco Dipped, 122 g	400	25	43
• Cone, 4 oz Kids Plain, 94 g	210	7	34
Freezee, Butterfinger, 279 g	620	24	100
Freezee, M&M, 279 g	630	25	99
Freezee, Oreo, 279 g	630	25	99
Freezee, Reese's PntBtr Cup, 279 g	630	26	97
Mini Sundae, Chocolate, 107 g	230	7	42
Mini Sundae, Hot Fudge, 107 g	250	9	40
Mini Sundae, Strawberry, 107 g	210	7	37
Old Fashion Sundae, Caramel, 181 g	400	14	66
Old Fashion Sundae, Chocolate, 181 g	390	14	64
Old Fashion Sundae, Hot Fudge, 181 g	400	16	63
Old Fashion Sundae, Pineapple, 181 g	370	14	59
Old Fashion Sundae, Strawberry, 181 g	370	14	59
Shake, Chocolate, 311 g	650	23	110
Shake, Strawberry, 312 g	650	23	111
Shake, Vanilla, 312 g	650	23	110
Tastee Float, Mountain Dew, 422 g	440	12	85
Tastee Float, Mug Root Beer, 422 g	440	12	83
Tastee Float, Tropicana Strwbry Lemonade, 421 g	450	12	82

WINCHELL'S	Cal	Fat	Cbs
Bagels			
Blueberry Bagel, 113 g	280	1	60
Blueberry Bagel w/ Cream Chz, 143 g	380	11	61
• Blueberry Bagel w/ Butter, 127 g	380	12	60
Cinnamon Raisin Bagel, 113 g	280	1	59
Cinn Raisin Bagel w/ Cream Chz, 142 g	380	11	60
Cinnamon Raisin Bagel w/Butter, 127 g	380	12	59
Egg Bagel, 113 g	280	1	57
Egg Bagel w/ Cream Cheese, 142 g	370	11	58
Egg Bagel w/Butter, 127 g	380	12	57
• Jalapeño Bagel, 113 g	250	1	51
Jalapeño Bagel w/ Cream Chz, 142 g	350	11	52
Jalapeño Bagel w/Butter, 127 g	350	12	51
Onion Bagel, 113 g	270	2	55
Onion Bagel w/ Cream Cheese, 142 g	370	11	56
Onion Bagel w/Butter, 127 g	370	12	55
Plain Bagel, 113 g	280	1	57
Plain Bagel w/ Cream Cheese, 142 g	380	11	58
Plain Bagel w/Butter, 127 g	380	12	57
Whole Wheat Bagel, 113 g	260	1	55
Whole Wheat Bagel w/ Cream Chz, 142 g	360	11	56
Whole Wheat Bagel w/Butter, 127 g	360	12	55
Bakery			
Apple Spice Muffins, 154 g	490	19	77
Banana Nut Bread, 111 g	430	25	45
Banana Nut Muffins, 160 g	610	33	67
Blueberry Bread, 132 g	430	18	63
Blueberry Muffins, 132 g	430	18	63
Bran Muffin, 164 g	450	16	74
Carrot Cake, 228 g	670	29	98
Chocolate Chip Bread, 137 g	540	25	77
Chocolate Chip Muffin, 144 g	580	27	82
Cinnamon Buns, 143 g	460	18	68
Cinnamon Rolls-Glazed, 155 g	630	31	80
Cranberry Nut Bread, 134 g	430	23	49
• Cranberry Nut Muffins, 205 g	670	37	74
Cranberry Orange Bread, 124 g	310	12	49
Cran Orange Muffins w/o crystal sugar, 186 g	470	18	73
Cream Cheese Bread, 188 g	410	18	54
Cream Cheese Muffins, 177 g	610	27	81
Croissant, 126 g	510	26	58
Double Chocolate Muffins, 174 g	640	29	91
Lemon Poppy Seed Bread, 100 g	330	13	48
Lemon Poppy Seed Muffins, 135 g	470	20	68
Pineapple Coconut Bread, 119 g	390	17	54
Pineapple Coconut Muffing, 182 g	600	27	83

• MOST HEALTHY   • LEAST HEALTHY

WINCHELL'S (cont.)

	Cal	Fat	Cbs
Pineapple Cream Cheese Muffins, 196 g	620	27	83
Pineapple Upsidedown Muffins, 177 g	470	17	75
• Puffies w/ Vanilla Cream Filling, 50 g	150	8	16
Pumpkin Nut Bread, 107 g	370	19	44
Pumpkin Nut Muffing, 164 g	580	31	66
Quesadilla Bread, 161 g	610	33	69
Sticky Buns, 117 g	400	20	47

Donuts

	Cal	Fat	Cbs
Apple w/ Cinnamon Crumb Filled Jelly Donut, 146 g	450	18	65
• Bear Claw, 184 g	700	33	89
Buttermilk Bar, 74 g	300	18	32
Cherry Iced French Donut, 72 g	270	14	32
Cherry Iced w/Rainbow Sprinkles White Cake, 94 g	340	14	51
Cherry Iced White Cake, 88 g	310	14	46
Choc Cake Choc Iced w/ Choco Sprinkles, 80 g	260	11	42
Choc Cake Choc Iced w/ Rainbow Sprinkles, 80 g	260	11	42
Chocolate Cake, 60 g	190	10	25
Chocolate Ice Bar, 91 g	380	19	44
Chocolate Iced Buttermilk Bar, 109 g	420	19	61
Chocolate Iced Chocolate Cake, 74 g	240	10	36
Chocolate Iced French Donut, 72 g	270	15	31
Chocolate Iced Raised Round, 66 g	220	9	31
Chocolate Iced Twist, 98 g	400	19	48
Choco Iced w/ Coconut Choco Cake, 85 g	290	14	41
Choco Iced w/ Peanuts Choco Cake, 81 g	280	13	38
Chocolate Iced White Cake, 88 g	320	14	45
Donut Holes w/ Cinn Crumb Topping, 90 g	340	17	46
Donut Holes w/ Cinn Sugar Topping, 90 g	350	13	55
Donut Holes w/ Coconut Topping, 90 g	370	21	44
Donut Holes w/ Donut Sugar, 90 g	370	16	54
Donut Holes w/ Sprinkles, 90 g	360	15	55
Donut Sugar White Cake, 80 g	300	14	40
• French Donut, 51 g	150	12	8
Glaze Donut Holes, 69 g	270	13	36
Glazed Apple Fritters, 176 g	600	23	93
Glazed Blueberry Fritters, 169 g	540	23	75
Glazed Butterfly, 136 g	530	23	74
Glazed Buttermilk Bar, 109 g	420	18	61
Glazed French Donut, 72 g	270	14	32
Glazed Pineapple Fritters, 181 g	680	34	81
Glazed Raised Round, 66 g	220	9	31
Glazed Twist, 98 g	390	19	48
Glazed Wheat & Spice, 86 g	310	15	42
Lemon Iced White Cake, 88 g	310	14	46
Lemon w/ Donut Sugar Filled Jelly Donut, 139 g	430	16	62
Maple Iced Bar, 91 g	380	19	44

• MOST HEALTHY   • LEAST HEALTHY

WINCHELL'S (cont.)

	Cal	Fat	Cbs
Maple Iced Buttermilk Bar, 109 g	420	19	62
Maple Iced French Donut, 72 g	270	14	32
Maple Iced White Cake, 88 g	320	14	46
Old Fashioned Chocolate Iced, 110 g	420	18	59
Old Fashioned Glazed, 110 g	410	17	60
Old Fashioned Maple Iced, 110 g	410	18	60
Old Fashioned Plain, 74 g	300	17	31
Orange Iced Cake, 88 g	310	14	46
Rspbry w/ Glaze Filled Jelly Donut, 153 g	480	15	78
Rspbry w/ PntBtr Filled Jelly Donut, 146 g	480	18	70
Strawberry w/ PntBtr Filled Jelly Donut, 146 g	480	18	69
Strwbry w/ Sugar Filled Jelly Donut, 146 g	460	15	74
Sugared Raised Round, 66 g	230	9	34
Sugared Twist, 105 g	430	19	58
Vanilla Cream w/ Choco Icing Filled Donut, 139 g	410	16	59
Vanilla Iced French Donut, 72 g	270	14	32
Vanilla Iced w/ Choco Sprinkles White Cake, 94 g	340	14	51
Vanilla Iced w/ Peanuts White Cake, 94 g	360	17	47
Vanilla Iced w/ Rainbow Sprinkles White Cake, 94 g	340	14	51
Vanilla Iced White Cake, 88 g	320	14	46
Wheat & Spice w/ Cinn Crumb Topping, 107 g	390	19	52
White Cake, 66 g	240	13	28
White Cake - Vanilla Iced w/ Coconut, 99 g	370	18	50
White Cake w/Cinnamon Crumb, 95 g	340	16	46

Drinks (Medium)

	Cal	Fat	Cbs
Chai Chilla (20 oz.), 540 g	780	30	116
French Vanilla Cappuccino Chilla (20 oz.), 542 g	810	37	107
• French Vanilla Caramel Cappuccino Chilla (20 oz.), 609 g	980	37	147
Hot Chai Tea (20 oz.), 592 g	470	15	81
• Hot Cocoa (20 oz.), 592 g	440	14	77
Hot French Vanilla Cappuccino (20 oz.), 592 g	490	16	80
Hot Mocha Cappuccino (20 oz.), 592 g	470	15	78
Mocha Cappuccino Chilla (20 oz.), 542 g	740	25	115
Mocha Caramel Cappuccino Chilla (20 oz.), 567 g	840	23	145
Strawberry Banana Chilla (20 oz.), 567 g	500	11	98

Sandwiches

	Cal	Fat	Cbs
Bacon and Cheddar on Croissant, 164 g	670	39	58
• Bacon & Cheddar on Plain Bagel, 151 g	440	14	57
Chipotle Sandwich on Croissant, 312 g	900	57	63
Chipotle Snd on Plain Bagel, 299 g	660	31	63
• Chorizo Sandwich on Croissant, 373 g	1270	92	67
Chorizo Sandwich on Plain Bagel, 360 g	1040	67	67
Egg and Cheese on Croissant, 298 g	1010	68	64
Egg and Cheese on Plain Bagel, 285 g	780	43	64
Ham and Cheese on Croissant, 224 g	750	43	63
Ham and Cheese on Plain Bagel, 225 g	610	28	62

• MOST HEALTHY   • LEAST HEALTHY

▌WINCHELL'S (cont.)

	Cal	Fat	Cbs
Ham, Egg, Cheese on Croissant, 340 g	1060	70	65
Ham, Egg, Chz on Plain Bagel, 327 g	830	45	65
Ranchero on Croissant, 396 g	1080	70	67
Ranchero on Plain Bagel, 383 g	850	45	66

▌WINGSTREET

12" Fit 'n Delicious® Pizza

	Cal	Fat	Cbs
Chkn, Mushrooms & Jalapeño, 93 g	170	5	22
• Chkn, Red Onion & Green Pepper, 95 g	180	5	23
• Diced Red Tom, Mshr & Jalapeño, 87 g	150	4	23
Green Pepper, Red Onion & Diced Red Tom, 89 g	150	4	24
Ham, Pineapple & Diced Red Tom, 84 g	160	5	24
Ham, Red Onion & Mushroom, 84 g	160	5	23

12" Medium Hand-Tossed Style Pizza

	Cal	Fat	Cbs
Cheese Only, 84 g	220	8	26
Dan's Original, 103 g	260	12	26
Ham & Pineapple, 91 g	200	7	27
Hawaiian Luau, 98 g	240	10	27
Italian Sausage & Red Onion, 99 g	240	11	27
• Meat Lover's®, 105 g	300	16	25
Pepperoni & Mushroom, 91 g	210	8	26
Pepperoni, 83 g	230	10	25
Spicy Sicilian, 99 g	250	11	26
Supreme, 98 g	260	12	26
Triple Meat Italiano, 96 g	260	12	25
• Veggie Lover's®, 102 g	200	7	27

12" Medium Pan Pizza

	Cal	Fat	Cbs
Cheese Only, 91 g	240	11	27
Dan's Original, 110 g	280	14	27
Ham & Pineapple, 97 g	230	9	28
Hawaiian Luau, 104 g	260	12	28
Italian Sausage & Red Onion, 106 g	270	13	28
• Meat Lover's®, 113 g	330	18	27
Pepperoni & Mushroom, 97 g	240	10	27
Pepperoni, 90 g	250	12	26
Spicy Sicilian, 106 g	270	13	27
Supreme, 112 g	290	14	27
Triple Meat Italiano, 103 g	290	15	27
• Veggie Lover's®, 107 g	230	9	28

12" Medium Thin 'N Crispy® Pizza

	Cal	Fat	Cbs
Cheese Only, 65 g	190	9	22
Dan's Original, 85 g	240	12	22
Ham & Pineapple, 73 g	180	6	23
Hawaiian Luau, 81 g	220	10	24
Italian Sausage & Red Onion, 81 g	220	10	23
• Meat Lover's®, 85 g	280	16	22

• MOST HEALTHY • LEAST HEALTHY

WINGSTREET (cont.)

	Cal	Fat	Cbs
Pepperoni & Mushroom, 73 g	190	8	22
Pepperoni, 63 g	200	9	21
Spicy Sicilian, 81 g	220	10	22
Supreme, 88 g	240	12	23
Triple Meat Italiano, 76 g	240	12	22
• Veggie Lover's®, 86 g	180	6	23
12" Pizza Mia™ Pizza			
Cheese Only, 74 g	200	7	24
Pepperoni, 72 g	200	8	24
14" Large Stuffed Crust Pizza			
Cheese Only, 132 g	350	14	39
Dan's Original, 159 g	420	21	39
Ham & Pineapple, 143 g	340	13	41
Hawaiian Luau, 151 g	380	16	41
Italian Sausage & Red Onion, 153 g	390	18	40
• Meat Lover's®, 165 g	480	26	39
Pepperoni & Mushroom, 142 g	350	15	39
Pepperoni, 134 g	380	17	38
Spicy Sicilian, 153 g	400	19	40
Supreme, 163 g	420	21	40
Triple Meat Italiano, 151 g	420	21	39
• Veggie Lover's®, 155 g	330	13	40
9" Personal PANormous™ Pizza			
Cheese Only, 402 g	1100	45	124
Dan's Original, 477 g	1270	62	124
Ham & Pineapple, 421 g	1020	37	128
Hawaiian Luau, 446 g	1150	49	129
Italian Sausage & Red Onion, 464 g	1210	56	128
• Meat Lover's®, 491 g	1470	80	123
Pepperoni & Mushroom, 419 g	1050	42	123
Pepperoni, 387 g	1100	48	121
Spicy Sicilian, 463 g	1220	57	126
Supreme, 488 g	1270	62	125
Triple Meat Italiano, 447 g	1280	62	123
• Veggie Lover's®, 463 g	1010	38	127
Appetizers			
Baked Hot Wings (2 pieces), 44 g	100	6	1
Baked Mild Wings (2 pieces), 44 g	110	7	1
Breadsticks (each), 44 g	150	7	19
• Cheese Breadsticks (each), 56 g	180	7	20
• Marinara Dipping Sauce (3 oz), 85 g	60	0	12
Bone Out Wings			
• All American, 54 g	150	8	11
Buffalo Burnin Hot, 73 g	190	8	18
Buffalo Medium, 73 g	190	9	18
Buffalo Mild, 73 g	190	9	18

• MOST HEALTHY   • LEAST HEALTHY

WINGSTREET (cont.)

	Cal	Fat	Cbs
Cajun, 77 g	200	8	21
• Garlic Parmesan, 71 g	260	19	11
Honey BBQ, 82 g	220	8	27
Spicy Asian, 80 g	210	8	24
Spicy BBQ, 81 g	200	8	21
Crispy Bone In Wings			
• All American, 55 g	200	14	8
Buffalo Burnin Hot, 75 g	230	15	16
Buffalo Medium, 75 g	230	15	16
Buffalo Mild, 75 g	230	15	16
Cajun, 79 g	240	14	19
• Garlic Parmesan, 72 g	300	25	9
Honey BBQ, 83 g	260	14	24
Spicy Asian, 82 g	250	14	21
Spicy BBQ, 82 g	240	14	19
Desserts			
Cinnamon Sticks (2 pieces), 55 g	170	6	26
• Hershey's® Choco Dunkers® (2 pieces), 60 g	200	9	26
• Hershey's® Choco Sauce (1.5 oz), 43 g	120	3	24
White Icing Dipping Cup (2 oz), 57 g	170	0	44
P'Zone® Pizza			
Classic, 235 g	630	23	77
• Marinara Dipping Sauce (3 oz), 85 g	60	0	12
• Meaty, 246 g	710	31	76
Pepperoni, 219 g	630	24	76
Side items			
Apple Pie (2 pies), 87 g	330	17	40
• Fried Cheese Sticks (4 pcs), 119 g	380	24	29
• Wedge Fries (1/2 order), 123 g	320	18	35
Stuffed Pizza Rollers			
Marinara Dipping Sauce (3 oz), 85 g	60	0	12
Stuffed Pizza Rollers, 76 g	230	10	24
Traditional Wings			
• All American, 39 g	80	5	0
Buffalo Burnin Hot, 59 g	110	6	8
Buffalo Medium, 59 g	110	6	8
Buffalo Mild, 59 g	110	6	8
Cajun, 63 g	120	5	11
• Garlic Parmesan, 56 g	180	16	1
Honey BBQ, 67 g	140	5	16
Spicy Asian, 65 g	130	5	13
Spicy BBQ, 66 g	120	5	11
Tuscani Pastas			
• Bacon Mac N Cheese, 324 g	520	22	54
• Chicken Alfredo, 323 g	630	33	56
Lasagna, 321 g	600	33	43

• MOST HEALTHY   • LEAST HEALTHY

WINGSTREET (cont.)

	Cal	Fat	Cbs
Meaty Marinara, 315 g	520	24	50

YARD HOUSE

Appetizers

	Cal	Fat	Cbs
Bearnaise Sliders	1230	54	148
Blue Crab Cakes	1185	66	48
Buffalo Chicken Wings	1095	47	54
Chicken Nachos	1370	83	120
Chinese Garlic Noodles	1300	109	15
Coconut Shrimp	870	42	55
Edamame	585	34	142
Firecracker Chicken Wings	575	21	78
• Fried Calamari	1980	123	177
• Fried Chicken Strips w/ French Fries	300	9	88
Grilled Artichoke	1065	55	36
Grilled Korean BBQ Beef Ribs	1685	101	29
Jamaican Jerk Wings	530	45	27
Lettuce Wraps with Chicken	1125	75	72
Lettuce Wraps with Mushrooms	1065	56	37
Lettuce Wraps with Shrimp	1170	63	24
Lobster Pita & Chips	1175	52	80
Moo Shu Egg Rolls	945	53	55
Onion Ring Tower	1585	106	19
Pastrami Sliders	1455	101	94
Poke Stack	650	47	92
Seared Ahi Sashimi	875	66	92
Sliders	812	50	103
Spicy Tuna Roll	1965	141	92
Spinach Dip with Flat Bread	400	22	117
Turkey Burger Sliders	505	22	106

Desserts

	Cal	Fat	Cbs
Brownie with Caramel Ice Cream	1010	30	166
Brownie with Mint Chip Ice Cream	985	32	156
Brownie with Vanilla Ice Cream	870	31	131
Caramel Ice Cream	225	11	30
Chocolate Banana Crème Brulee	730	50	68
Chocolate Souffle	460	28	49
Kids Sundae	325	15	47
Kona Coffee Ice Cream	210	12	23
Kona Coffee Sundae	1160	60	159
Lemon Souffle	280	14	36
• Macadamia Nut Cheese Cake	1355	78	143
• Mango Sorbet	195	0	49
Peach Apple Cobbler	465	16	80
Trio Sampler	1205	58	165
Vanilla Ice Cream	210	12	23

• MOST HEALTHY   • LEAST HEALTHY

▶ YARD HOUSE (cont.)	Cal	Fat	Cbs
Dressings			
Thai Peanut Vinaigrette	45	2	5
Entrée Salads			
Ahi Crunchy Salad	810	50	58
• BBQ Chicken Salad	1665	108	109
• Caesar Salad	435	39	8
Caesar Salad with Ahi	570	42	8
Caesar Salad with Blackened Chicken	730	48	11
Caesar Salad with Breaded Chicken	795	55	10
Caesar Salad with Grilled Chicken	715	48	8
Caesar Salad with Shrimp	690	52	8
Grilled Hearts of Romaine	595	52	22
N.Y. Steak Salad	1280	96	41
Roasted Turkey Cobb Salad	1080	83	17
Thai Chicken Salad	935	28	99
Grilled Burgers			
Avocado Swiss Burger	1325	94	69
BBQ Cheddar Bacon Burger	1495	93	98
• Bearnaise Burger	2025	163	89
Bearnaise Sliders	1930	139	117
Classic Cheese Burger	1260	87	67
• Classic Sliders	1135	61	92
Hawaiian Burger	1485	94	104
Pastrami Sliders	1455	101	94
Pepper Crusted Gorgonzola Burger	1500	107	81
Pepper Jack Burger	1385	98	68
Surf & Turf Burger	1500	109	67
Turkey Burger	1255	81	83
Turkey Burger Sliders	1185	66	106
Healthy Dining Options			
Ahi Caesar Salad	260	10	14
Ahi Salad - Special Request	300	12	48
BBQ Chicken Pizza (2 slices)	315	12	19
Blackened Chkn Caesar Salad	420	16	69
• Caesar Salad - Special Request	130	7	17
California Roll	505	22	7
Grilled Chkn Caesar Salad	405	16	7
Hawaiian Fresh Fish w/Jasmine Rice	645	16	10
Margherita Pizza (2 slices)	285	13	7
Shrimp Caesar Salad	345	19	34
Spicy Tuna Roll (1/2 order)	295	17	32
Thai Chicken Pizza (2 slices)	330	14	32
• Thai Chicken Salad	675	14	71

YARD HOUSE (cont.)	Cal	Fat	Cbs
House Favorites			
Angel Hair Pasta	1535	113	96
Chicken Enchilada Stack	1820	127	73
Chicken Garlic Noodles	1440	95	87
Chicken Rice Bowl	1420	77	133
Jambalaya Pasta	1610	94	93
Jambalaya Rice	1600	94	96
Jerk Chicken with Shrimp Stack	1650	108	69
Macaroni and Cheese	1865	131	96
Maui Chicken	1270	62	117
Orange Peel Chicken	1820	85	197
Parmesan Crusted Chicken	1350	68	98
Penne with Chicken	1675	119	88
• Southern Fried Chicken Breast	1095	74	62
• Turkey Pot Pie	1940	118	133
Kids Klub			
Kids Buttered Noodles	720	49	59
Kids Cheeseburger	845	50	60
Kids Chicken Fingers	630	43	31
Kids Fish & Chips	1015	71	75
Kids Four Cheese Pizza	700	31	78
Kids Grilled Cheese	640	43	72
Kids Hamburger	760	43	60
• Kids Hot Dog	395	14	53
Kids Mac and Cheese	945	64	61
• Kids Pepperoni Pizza	1055	62	80
Kids Sides			
Broccoli with Cheese Sauce	165	13	5
• French Fries	555	35	54
• Fresh Fruit	105	1	26
Jasmine Rice	155	0	33
Kids Sundae	325	15	47
Parmesan Mashed Potatoes	185	14	3
Salad with Ranch Dressing	115	11	4
Lunch Specials			
BBQ Chicken Pizza	945	34	101
Beef Dip	695	34	52
Caesar Salad	185	17	5
Clam Chowder (6 oz.)	180	11	20
Crab Cake Hoagie	775	52	62
French Onion Soup (6 oz.)	365	30	15
Grilled Pastrami Snd	715	45	55
House Salad	170	9	20
Margherita Pizza	815	35	93
• Mixed Field Greens	115	9	8
• Pepperoni Pizza	1005	55	81

• MOST HEALTHY   • LEAST HEALTHY

▶ YARD HOUSE (cont.)	Cal	Fat	Cbs
Roasted Tkey Melt Snd	800	52	51
Tomato Bisque (6 oz)	190	13	18
Turkey Club Sandwich	710	38	76
Massachusetts & Texas Only			
Ahi Crunchy Salad	405	25	29
Angel Hair Pasta	820	58	57
BBQ Chicken Salad	865	57	57
• Caesar Salad	330	30	7
Cobb Salad	890	70	13
Jambalaya Pasta	770	47	55
Jambalaya Rice	775	46	59
• Macaroni and Cheese	975	65	56
Penne Chicken Pasta	900	60	52
Rice Bowl with Chicken	785	39	78
Rice Bowl with Shrimp	735	37	77
Thai Noodle Salad	510	15	58
Vodka Shrimp Pasta	670	38	46
Pizza			
BBQ Chicken Pizza	1260	46	135
Four Cheese Pizza	1100	52	106
• Ham & Pineapple Pizza	1055	40	116
Margherita Pizza	1135	50	128
• Pepperoni & Mushroom Pizza	1370	76	110
Thai Chicken Pizza	1320	55	129
Sandwiches			
• Ahi Steak Sandwich	980	64	55
Blue Crab Cake Hoagie	1220	79	95
Chicken and Avocado Sandwich	1270	82	70
Cuban Roast Pork Dip Sandwich	1710	117	93
Grilled Chz & Tom Bisque (w/o avocado & bacon)	1395	94	85
Grilled Pastrami Sandwich	1340	99	76
• N.Y. Steak Sandwich	1825	119	119
Portabello Burger	1105	80	82
Roast Beef Dip	1150	57	78
Roasted Turkey Melt Sandwich	1150	71	75
Spicy Chicken Breast Sandwich	1405	82	103
Turkey Club Sandwich	1055	57	111
Seafood			
Blackened Hawaiian Fresh Fish w/Jasmine Rice	1340	92	76
Crab Crusted Swordfish	1265	92	50
• Fish and Chips	1930	126	159
Ginger Crusted Salmon	1385	91	89
Grilled Hawaiian Fresh Fish w/Jasmine Rice	1210	78	74
Grilled Jumbo Shrimp	1335	76	107
• Hawaiian Fresh Fish Healthy Dining	645	16	71
Linguine and Clams	1585	106	82

• MOST HEALTHY   • LEAST HEALTHY

▷ YARD HOUSE (cont.)

	Cal	Fat	Cbs
Lobster Garlic Noodles	1165	66	85
Macadamia Nut Crust Hawaiian Fish w/Jasmine Rice	1360	119	76
Miso Glazed Sea Bass	1200	49	126
Orzo Scallops	1585	113	79
Pan Seared Ahi	980	40	89
Porcini Crusted Halibut	1265	99	38
Shrimp Rice Bowl	1420	79	135
Vodka Shrimp Pasta	1265	76	75

Sides, Dressings & Sauces

	Cal	Fat	Cbs
6 oz. blackened chicken breast	290	9	3
6 oz. breaded chicken	360	16	2
6 oz. grilled chicken breast	275	9	0
Apple Plum Sauce	20	1	2
Chipotle Ranch Dressing	50	5	1
• Cocktail Sauce	15	0	4
• French Fries (6 oz)	665	42	65
Potato Chips (3 cups)	440	25	50
Roasted Garlic Aïoli	70	7	2
Special Sauce	130	12	4
Thai Basil Pesto	135	12	6
Thai Peanut Vinaigrette	45	2	5

Starters

	Cal	Fat	Cbs
Caesar Salad	395	36	8
Chicken Tortilla Soup (cup)	558	45	20
Chopped Salad	470	35	31
• Clam Chowder (cup)	180	11	20
Classic Ranch Salad	370	28	19
French Onion Soup (cup)	365	30	15
Greek Salad	550	43	36
House Salad	380	20	46
Iceberg Wedge	550	51	20
Mixed Field Greens	390	33	22
Spinach Salad	640	55	25
• Summer Salad	815	66	57
Tomato Bisque (cup)	190	13	18
Walnut Pear Salad	660	53	40

Steaks, Ribs & Chops

	Cal	Fat	Cbs
BBQ Pork Tenderloin	1275	78	76
Grilled Ribeye Steak	1130	74	39
• New York Steak	2425	170	122
New Zealand Lamb Chops	1645	132	73
Peppercorn Crusted Filet	1390	105	52
St.Louis Style Ribs	2215	115	191
Steak & Grilled Shrimp	1345	86	40
Top Sirloin Steak	1005	53	47

• MOST HEALTHY   • LEAST HEALTHY

YOSHINOYA

	Cal	Fat	Cbs
Bowls			
• Chicken Only No Skin, 10 oz.	255	6	N/A
Combo Bowl Beef & Chicken	1220	36	171
Combo No Skin, 25 oz.	1043	28	N/A
Regular Beef Bowl	840	30	109
Regular Chkn Bowl (Teriyaki Or Spicy)	760	15	125
Regular Chicken No Skin, 17 oz.	608	7	N/A
Regular Vegetable Bowl	530	4	116
• Shrimp & Beef Bowl	1280	44	184
Shrimp & Chicken Combo Bowl	1260	35	191
Shrimp Bowl	910	29	143
Desserts			
Cheesecake	280	15	31
• Chocolate Cake	330	17	44
• Flan	230	7	35
Strawberry Shortcake	290	15	37
Side Orders			
Beef Only	370	28	6
Chicken and Vegetables Only	300	12	21
• Rice Only	460	3	104
• Vegetables Only	60	1	12

Z'TEJAS SOUTHWESTERN GRILL

	Cal	Fat	Cbs
• Grilled Chkn Breast w/ Fresh Vegetables	470	26	19
Grilled Cilantro Pesto-Rubbed Ruby Trout	530	25	31
• Grilled Miso Salmon	645	27	48
Grl Salmon w/ Fresh Veg & Cantaloupe Avocado Salad	480	28	20
Jerk Chicken Salad	515	24	27
Turkey Wrap	540	18	64
Voodoo Blackened Tuna	540	19	41

ZERO'S SUBS

	Cal	Fat	Cbs
Sandwich			
B.L.T., 6"	411	19	48
Cosmo Vegetarian Deluxe, 6"	488	25	48
Cosmo Vegetarian, 6"	469	23	46
• Grilled Veggie Sub, 6"	394	14	52
Grinder, 6"	557	31	48
Ham & Cheese, 6"	439	19	44
• Hot Italian Sausage, 6"	663	37	45
Meatball & Cheese, 6"	565	30	50
Pepperoni & Cheese, 6"	545	31	42
Philly Chicken & Cheese, 6"	402	10	48
Philly Steak & Cheese, 6"	492	21	49
Roast Beef & cheese, 6"	460	19	45

• MOST HEALTHY   • LEAST HEALTHY

ZERO'S SUBS (cont.)	Cal	Fat	Cbs
The Club, 6″	514	23	44
Tuna & Cheese, 6″	519	26	47
Turkey & Cheese, 6″	454	17	44

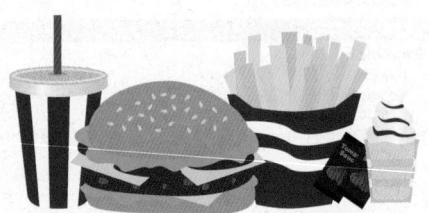

Popular Brands

POPULAR BRANDS

This chapter takes the guesswork out of grocery shopping and cooking by allowing you to quickly look up the calories, fat and carbs for hundreds of popular food brands. Look up items by category and find the most healthy entrées, sides, snacks, produce, dressings and ingredients to add to your shopping cart.

There is no need to spend an hour comparing product labels at the store. Bring this book with you and find the most and least healthy items in seconds.

Also, be aware that supermarkets place the least healthy items toward the center of the store, on aisle endcaps, and lining the checkout areas. Soda, cookies, chips, frozen pizzas and other high-calorie, high-fat foods are grouped near one another. Stick to the outer aisles where stores stock items such as fresh produce and dairy and you'll instantly be able to make smarter eating choices.

BAKERY & BREAD

	Cal	Fat	Cbs
BAGELS			
Lender's Bagels			
Blueberry, 4 oz.	300	3	61
Cinnamon Raisin, 4 oz.	310	4	60
Onion, 4 oz.	300	3	61
Plain, 4 oz.	310	3	62
Poppy Seed, 4 oz.	310	3	61
Sesame Seed, 4 oz.	310	3	60
• Stuffed Bagel w/ Plain Cream Chz, 4 oz.	320	11	46
Wheat, 4 oz.	310	2	61
Pepperidge Farm			
• 100% Whole Wheat, 1 bagel	250	2	49
Cinnamon Raisin, 1 bagel	270	1	57
Everything, 1 bagel	260	2	53
Plain, 1 bagel	260	1	54
Sesame, 1 bagel	280	3	53
Whole Grain White, 1 bagel	250	2	51
BREAKFAST LOAVES			
Pepperidge Farm			
Breakfast Bread Apple & Grains, 1 slice	90	2	18
Breakfast Bread Raisin & Grains, 1 slice	100	2	19
• Brown Sugar Cinnamon Swirl, 1 slice	110	0	21
• Cinnamon Swirl, 1 slice	80	2	15
Whole Grain Cinnamon Swirl, 1 slice	100	2	18
CHILLED AND FROZEN DOUGH			
New York Garlic Bread			
• 6 Carb Texas Garlic Toast, 28 g	120	8	8
Five Cheese Texas Toast, 48 g	180	9	20
Garlic Bread, 57 g	180	7	25
Garlic Breadsticks, 50 g	170	6	24
Lite Texas Garlic Toast, 40 g	130	5	18
Texas Cheese Toast, 48 g	170	10	16
Texas Garlic Toast, 40 g	150	9	15
Pepperidge Farm			
• Five Cheese Garlic Bread, 2.25" slice	190	8	24
Garlic Bread, 2.5" slice	170	7	24
Garlic Breadsticks, 1 stick	160	5	25
Texas Toast Garlic, 1 slice	150	7	18
Whole Grain Texas Toast, 1 slice	150	8	14
ENGLISH MUFFINS			
Pepperidge Farm			
100% Whole Wheat, 1 Muffin	140	2	26
Original English, 1 Muffin	130	2	25

• MOST HEALTHY   • LEAST HEALTHY

BAKERY & BREAD

	Cal	Fat	Cbs
HAMBURGER BUNS			
Pepperidge Farm			
Classic 100% Whole Wheat, 1 Bun	120	2	18
Classic Hamburger Buns, 1 Bun	120	2	22
• Clsc Onion Buns with Poppy Seeds, 1 Bn	150	3	28
Classic Buns with Sesame Seeds, 1 Bun	130	3	22
• Classic Whole Grain White, 1 Bun	100	1	18
HOT DOG BUNS			
Pepperidge Farm			
Classic Hot Dog Buns, 1 Bun	140	3	26
Classic Whole Grain White, 1 Bun	110	1	21
MUFFINS			
Bays English Muffins			
Honey Wheat, 57 g	130	2	25
Original, 57 g	140	2	27
Sourdough, 57 g	130	2	26
Zen Bakery			
Bran Muffins			
Apple Bran, 67 g	110	3	19
Blueberry Oat Bran, 68 g	135	3	23
Blueberry Raspberry Oat Bran, 68 g	135	3	23
Peach Bran, 68 g	110	3	21
Fiber Cakes			
• Apple Cranberry Fiber Cake, 57 g	80	2	22
• Banana Nut Muffin, 64 g	160	3	31
Blueberry Fiber Cake, 57 g	80	2	22
Carrot Cake Muffin, 60 g	110	2	23
PIZZA CRUST			
Boboli			
Pizza Crusts			
12" 100% Whole Wheat Thin Crust, 57 g	150	3	27
• 12" Original Crust, 50 g	140	3	24
12" Thin Crust, 57 g	170	4	28
Value Packs			
• 8" Original Crust Party Pack, 71 g	200	5	32
12" Original Crust Value Pack, 67 g	150	3	27
12" Thin Crust Value Pack, 85 g	190	4	33
ROLLS			
Pepperidge Farm			
• Farmhouse Premium Wheat Rolls, 1 Roll	220	5	36
Hot & Crusty French Rolls, 1 Roll	100	1	19
Hot & Crusty Sourdough Rolls, 1 Roll	100	1	21
• Parkerhouse Dinner Rolls, 1 Roll	80	2	14
Soft Country Style Dinner Rolls, 1 Roll	90	2	17

BAKERY & BREAD	Cal	Fat	Cbs
SANDWICH BREAD			
Pepperidge Farm			
Farmhouse Soft 100% Whl Wheat, 1 sl	110	2	19
Farmhouse Whole Grain White, 1 slice	110	2	21
Hot & Crusty Italian Bread, 2" slices	150	2	29
• Hot & Crusty Thin Sliced French, 2 slice	150	2	30
Italian Bread, 1 slice	90	1	17
• Oatmeal Bread, 1 slice	70	1	12
Original White Bread, 1 slice	70	1	13
Pumpernickel Bread, 1 slice	80	1	15
Very Thin Soft 100% Whole Wheat, 3 sl	110	2	20
Very Thin Whole Grain White Bread, 3 sl	110	2	21
White Sandwich Bread, 2 slices	130	3	23
Whole Grain 100% Whole Wheat, 1 slice	110	2	20
Whole Grain Rye with Seeds, 1 slice	70	1	14
Whole Grain White Bread, 2 slices	110	2	22

BAKING			
BAKING CHOCOLATE			
Baker's Chocolate and Coconut			
Chocolate - White Squares, 14 g	80	5	8
Chocolate - Semi-sweet, 14 g	40	5	8
Chocolate - Unsweetened Squares, 4 g	70	7	4
M&M's Bakery			
Milk Chocolate, 1 oz.	70	30	10
Semi-Sweet, 1 oz.	70	30	9
Nestle Toll House			
Baking			
• Choco Bake, 1/2 oz.	80	8	4
• Cocoa, 5 g	15	1	3
Unsweetened Choc Baking Bar, 1/2 oz.	70	7	4
Morsels			
Milk Choco and PB Swirled Morsels, 14 g	75	5	8
Milk Chocolate Morsels, 14 g	70	4	9
Semi-Sweet Chocolate Chunks, 12 g	60	4	8
BAKING COCONUT			
Baker's Chocolate and Coconut			
Coconut - Angel Flake Sweetened, 15 g	70	5	6
BAKING FLOUR			
Aunt Jemima			
Self Rising Flour, 1 oz.	90	0	20
BAKING MIX			
Aunt Jemima			
Coffee Cake, 1/4 cup	140	5	27
Corn Bread, 1/3 cup	140	5	24

BAKING

	Cal	Fat	Cbs
Betty Crocker			
Biscuits			
Complete Buttermilk Biscuits, 35 g	150	6	21
Heart Smart, 40 g	140	3	27
Original, 40 g	160	5	26
Bread			
Quick Bread Mix Banana, 1/12 Pckg	130	3	25
Quick Bread Mix Cinn. Streusel, 1/12 Pckg	160	4	28
Quick Bread Mix Cran Orange, 1/12 Pckg	150	3	29
Brownies			
• Brownie Mix Fudge Brownies, 1 oz.	100	1	22
Brownie Mix Lowfat Fudge, 1 oz.	130	3	27
• Warm Delights PB Fudge Brownie, 3 oz.	400	14	63
Cakes			
Angel Food White, 38 g	140	0	32
Pineapple Upside-Down Cake Mix, 102 g	350	9	65
SuperMoist White, 43 g	170	4	33
Cookies			
Pouch Mix Oatmeal Cookie Mix, 28 g	100	2	22
Pouch Mix Rainbow Cookie, 28 g	110	2	22
Pouch Mix Sugar Cookie Mix, 28 g	120	3	22
Muffins			
Muffin Mix Apple Streusel, 46 g	180	3	37
Muffin Mix Banana Nut, 37 g	150	4	27
Authentic Cornbread & Muffin Mix, 31 g	110	1	24
Pancakes			
Heart Smart, 40 g	140	3	27
Original, 40 g	160	5	26
Shake 'n Pour Buttermilk, 63 g	220	3	42
Bisquick			
Complete Buttermilk Biscuits, 35 g	150	6	21
Complete Cheese Garlic Biscuits, 37 g	160	7	22
Complete Three Cheese Biscuits, 36 g	160	7	22
Bruce Food Products			
Sweet Potato Biscuit Mix, 37 g	140	4	25
Sweet Potato Muffin Mix, 36 g	150	4	25
Sweet Potato Pancake Mix, 65 g	230	3	47
Martha White			
Biscuits			
Cheese Garlic, 1/3 cup	190	N/A	21
Extra Rich Butter Milk, 1/3 cup	190	N/A	22
Homestyle Butter, 1/3 cup	190	N/A	22
Brownies			
Fudge, 1/20 Package	130	N/A	27
Walnut, 1/20 Package	130	N/A	23

BAKING

	Cal	Fat	Cbs
Corn Meal			
Buttermilk, 31 g	110	1	22
Corn Meal White, 31 g	110	1	22
White Self-rising Oatmeal, 31 g	100	1	22
Yellow Cornmeal Mix, 31 g	110	1	22
Cornbreads			
Cornbreads Buttermilk, 34 g	130	N/A	23
Mexican Style, 28 g	110	N/A	18
Yellow Corn Bread, 37 g	140	N/A	25
Lowfat Varieties			
Lowfat Apple Cinnamon, 1/4 cup	130	N/A	27
Lowfat Blueberry, 1/4 cup	130	N/A	27
Lowfat Strawberry, 1/4 cup	130	N/A	27
Muffins			
Apple Cinnamon, 1/4 cup	140	N/A	24
Banana Nut, 1/4 cup	150	N/A	25
Honey Bran, 1/4 cup	140	N/A	26
Strawberry Cheesecake, 1/4 cup	150	N/A	22
Other Products			
Deep Pan Pizza, 1/5 Package	140	1	28
Flap Stax, 1/2 cup	240	N/A	44
Pizza Crust Mix, 1/4 Package	160	1	32
Whole Grain Varieties			
Whole Grain Apple Cinnamon, 1/4 cup	140	4	24
Wholegrain Banana Nut, 1/4 cup	150	5	25
Pillsbury			
Brownies - Chocolate Fudge, 39 g	112	6	24
Brownies - Triple Chocolate Chunk, 39 g	160	6	24
Simply Bake PB Choco Chunk Bars, 40 g	110	9	23
Simply Bake Turtle Supreme Bars, 40 g	110	9	23
Zatarain's			
Crab Cake Mix, 4 tbsp.	110	1	23
Salmon Cake Mix, 2 tbsp.	110	1	23
Tuna Cake Mix, 2 tbsp.	110	1	23
BREAD CRUMBS			
Progresso			
• Garlic & Herb, 28 g	110	2	20
Italian Style, 28 g	110	2	20
• Parmesan, 28 g	110	2	19
Plain, 28 g	110	2	20
CHILLED & FROZEN DOUGH			
Pillsbury			
Biscuits			
Buttermilk, 64 g	150	2	29
Flaky Layer, 64 g	160	4	28

• MOST HEALTHY   • LEAST HEALTHY

BAKING	Cal	Fat	Cbs
Golden Homestyle Buttermilk, 34 g	100	35	14
Golden Layers Honey Butter, 34 g	110	5	14
Bread Crusts			
Bread Country Italian Loaf, 47 g	110	2	21
Bread Crusty French Loaf, 52 g	120	2	24
Breadsticks Cornbread Twists, 41 g	140	6	18
Breadsticks, 52 g	240	3	25
Crescent Rolls			
Big N Buttery, 48 g	170	15	20
Big N Flaky, 48 g	180	15	20
Butterflake, 28 g	110	6	11
Original, 28 g	110	6	11
Reduced Fat, 28 g	90	5	12
Dinner Rolls - Freezer to Oven			
Dinner Rolls Butterflake, 48 g	160	7	21
Dinner Rolls Garlic, 38 g	140	6	17
Dinner Rolls Soft White, 35 g	110	4	17
• Dinner Rolls Whole Wheat, 35 g	90	1	17
Freezer to Oven Biscuits			
Buttermilk, 57 g	200	10	24
Cheddar Garlic, 59 g	190	9	22
Southern Style, 29 g	180	9	21
Grands! Biscuits			
Buttermilk Reduced Fat, 58 g	170	6	26
Buttermilk, 58 g	190	8	24
Extra Rich, 61 g	210	10	26
Homestyle, 58 g	190	3	24
Grands! Sweet Rolls			
Grands! Cinn w/ Cream Chz Icing, 99 g	310	9	54
Grands! Cinnamon with Icing, 99 g	310	9	54
Grands! Cinn w/ Buttercream Icing, 99 g	320	10	54
• Grands! Flaky Sprm w/ Choco Icing, 99 g	380	20	47
Sweet Rolls			
Caramel, 49 g	170	7	24
Cinnamon Rolls w/ Cream Chz Icing, 44 g	150	5	23
Cinnamon Rolls w/ Icing RedFat, 44 g	140	4	24
Cinnamon Rolls with Icing, 44 g	150	5	23
CONDENSED/POWDERED MILK			
Magnolia			
Dulce de Leche, 39 g	120	2	24
• Evaporated Milk, 30 ml.	40	2	3
• Sweetened Condensed Milk, 39 g	130	3	23
COOKIE DOUGH			
Nestle Toll House			
Chocolate Chip Cookie Dough, 1 oz.	130	6	18

• MOST HEALTHY   • LEAST HEALTHY

BAKING

	Cal	Fat	Cbs
Chocolate Chunk Cookie Dough, 1 oz.	120	6	15
Oatmeal Raisin Cookie, 1 oz.	160	6	24
Sugar Cookie Dough, 1 oz.	170	8	23
PB Choc. Chips & Chunks, 1 oz.	180	9	23
• Ultimates - White Choc. Mac. Nut, 1 oz.	190	10	22
• Walnut Chocolate Chip, 1 oz.	70	6	15

Pillsbury

Create 'n Bake Cookies

	Cal	Fat	Cbs
Chocolate Chip Cookies, 1 oz.	120	5	18
Gingerbread Cookies, 1 oz.	140	7	18
Oatmeal Chocolate Chip Cookies, 1 oz.	130	6	17
Peanut Butter Cookies, 1 oz.	130	6	16

Ready to Bake Cookies

	Cal	Fat	Cbs
Chocolate Chip, 1 oz.	170	9	22
Chocolate Chunk & Chip, 1 oz.	180	9	22
S'mores, 1 oz.	160	7	23
Shape Bunny or Snowman, 1 oz.	120	6	15
Sugar, 1 oz.	170	9	22

FLOUR

Gold Medal

	Cal	Fat	Cbs
• All Purpose Flour, 1 oz.	100	0	22
Harvest King Better for Bread, 1 oz.	110	0	22
Organic Flour, 1 oz.	100	0	22
Self-Rising Flour, 1 oz.	100	0	23
Unbleached All Purpose Flour, 1 oz.	100	0	22

Martha White

	Cal	Fat	Cbs
All Purpose Flour, 1 oz.	110	0	N/A
Self Rising Flour, 1 oz.	110	N/A	23

Purity Foods

	Cal	Fat	Cbs
Non-Organic White Spelt Flour, 1 oz.	100	1	21
Non-Organic Whole Grain Flour, 1 oz.	110	1	23
Organic White Spelt Flour, 1 oz.	100	1	21
• Organic Whole Grain Spelt Flour, 1 oz.	110	1	23

FROSTING & ICING

Betty Crocker

	Cal	Fat	Cbs
Frost Mix Homestyle Fluffy White, 1 oz.	100	0	24
• Frost Rich & Creamy Butter Cream, 1 oz.	140	5	23
• Frost Whipped Choc Mousse, 1 oz.	90	5	14
Frost Whipped Vanilla, 1 oz.	110	5	15

MARSHMALLOWS

Jet-Puffed

	Cal	Fat	Cbs
Chocomallows, 1 oz.	100	0	25
Marshmallows, 1 oz.	100	0	24
• Miniature, 1 oz.	90	0	23
Strawberrymallows, 1 oz.	100	0	24

• MOST HEALTHY   • LEAST HEALTHY

BAKING

	Cal	Fat	Cbs
• Toasted Coconut, 2 oz.	170	5	31

PIE CRUSTS & PASTRY SHELLS

Betty Crocker

	Cal	Fat	Cbs
Pie Crust Mix, 1 oz.	110	7	9

Honey Maid

	Cal	Fat	Cbs
• Pie Crust Graham Pie Crust, 1 oz.	150	8	18

Keebler

	Cal	Fat	Cbs
Chocolate 6 oz., 1 oz.	100	5	14
• Graham Cracker Crumbs, 1 oz.	70	2	13
Shortbread 6 oz., 1 oz.	110	5	14

Nilla Wafers

	Cal	Fat	Cbs
Nilla Pie Crust Pie Crust, 1 oz.	140	8	18

Oreo

	Cal	Fat	Cbs
Pie Crust, 1 oz.	130	7	19

Pillsbury

	Cal	Fat	Cbs
Pet-Ritz Pie Crsts Dp Dish All Veggie, 1 oz.	90	5	11
Pet-Ritz Pie Crusts Deep Dish, 1 oz.	90	5	11
Pie Crusts All Ready Rolled, 1 oz.	110	7	12

PIE FILLING

Libby's Pumpkin

	Cal	Fat	Cbs
Easy Pumpkin Pie Mix, 1/3 cup	90	1	20

Lucky Leaf

	Cal	Fat	Cbs
Coconut Creme, 1/3 cup	110	2	25
• Lite Apple, 1/3 cup	30	N/A	7
Peach, 1/3 cup	80	N/A	21
Premium Apple, 1/3 cup	90	N/A	22
Premium Cherry, 1/3 cup	100	N/A	24

Musselman's

	Cal	Fat	Cbs
Banana Creme, 1/3 cup	110	N/A	28
Blueberry, 1/3 cup	90	N/A	22
Cherries Jubilee, 1/4 cup	80	N/A	20
Cherry, 1/3 cup	100	N/A	24
Chocolate Creme, 1/3 cup	100	N/A	25
Coconut Creme, 1/3 cup	110	1	25

None Such

	Cal	Fat	Cbs
Classic Original Mincemeat, 4 oz.	200	0	48
Condensed Mincemeat, 2 oz.	150	1	36
• Mincemeat with Rum and Brandy, 4 oz.	200	1	47

ROLLS & PASTRY DOUGH

Pepperidge Farm

	Cal	Fat	Cbs
Puff Pastry Sheets, 1/6 sheet	170	11	14
Puff Pastry Shells, 1 shell	190	13	16

SHAKE & BAKE COATINGS

McCormick

	Cal	Fat	Cbs
• Cracker Meal Seafood Fry Mix, 2 tbsp.	130	1	24

• MOST HEALTHY   • LEAST HEALTHY

BAKING

	Cal	Fat	Cbs
Golden Dip® Breading Mix, 2 tbsp.	120	1	20
Golden Dip® Original Chkn Fry Mix, 1 tbsp.	50	0	9
Seafood Fry Mix, 1 tbsp.	60	0	13
Tempura Seafood Batter Mix, 2 tbsp.	100	0	21
Shake 'N Bake			
Extra Crispy, 1 tbsp.	35	1	7
Garlic & Herb, 1 tbsp.	35	0	7
Hot & Spicy, 1 tbsp.	40	1	7
Italian, 1 tbsp.	35	1	7
Original Chicken, 1 tbsp.	40	1	7
Original Pork, 1 tbsp.	40	0	8
• Ranch And Herb Crusted, 1 tbsp.	35	0	7
Zatarain's			
Crispy Seasoned Fish-Fri, 2 tbsp.	50	0	11
Garlic Fish-Fri, 1.5 tbsp.	40	0	9
Shrimp-Fri, 1.5 tbsp.	40	0	9
Wonderful Fish-Fri, 1 tbsp.	45	0	10

SUGAR & SWEETENERS

Equal

Equal Granular, 1 tsp.	0	0	1

BEVERAGES

FRUIT FLAVORED DRINKS & TEAS

Aquafina

Aquafina Alive Peach Mango, 8 fl.oz.	10	0	3
Sparkling Citrust Twist, 8 fl.oz.	0	0	0
Wild Berry Flavor Splash, 8 fl.oz.	0	0	0

Baskin Robbins

Medium

Berry Pomegranate Fruit Blast, 24 fl.oz.	211	0	128
• Strawberry Citrus Fruit Blast, 24 fl.oz.	480	1	122
Wild Mango Fruit Blast, 24 fl.oz.	470	2	116

Capri Sun

Fruit Punch Pouches, 200 ml.	70	0	19
Grape Pouches, 200 ml.	70	0	19
Orange Pouches, 200 ml.	100	0	27
Splash Cooler Pouches, 200 ml.	70	0	19
Wild Cherry Pouches, 200 ml.	70	0	19

Celestial Seasonings

African and Rooibos Teas

African Orange Mango Rooibos Tea, 2 g	0	0	0
Madagascar Vanilla Red Rooibos Tea, 2 g	0	0	0
Peach Apricot Honeybush Tea, 2 g	0	0	0
Red Safari Spice® Rooibos Tea, 2 g	0	0	0

• MOST HEALTHY   • LEAST HEALTHY

BEVERAGES	Cal	Fat	Cbs
Black Teas			
Canadian Vanilla Maple Decaf Black Tea, 2 g	0	0	1
Devonshire English Breakfast Black Tea, 2 g	0	0	1
Tuscany Orange Spice Black Tea, 2 g	0	0	1
Victorian Earl Grey Black Tea, 2 g	0	0	0
Chai Teas			
Chocolate Caramel Enchantment® Chai, 3 g	0	0	0
Decaf India Spice Chai, 2 g	0	0	0
India Spice Chai, 2 g	0	0	0
Vanilla Ginger Green Tea Chai, 2 g	0	0	0
Drink Mixes: Ciders			
Apple Caramel Kiss® Cider, 21 g	80	0	21
Harvest Apple Spice® Cider, 21 g	80	0	21
Honey Vanilla Apple Cider, 21 g	80	0	21
Green Teas			
Blueberry Breeze® Green Tea, 2 g	0	0	0
Decaffeinated Green Tea, 2 g	0	0	0
Green Tea, 2 g	0	0	0
Raspberry Gardens® Green Tea, 2 g	0	0	0
Herbal Tea			
Acaí Mango Zinger®, 2 g	0	0	1
Caffeine Free Herbal Tea, 2 g	0	0	0
Chamomile, 2 g	0	0	0
Honey Vanilla Chamomile, 2 g	0	0	0
Lemon Zinger®, 2 g	0	0	0
Iced Teas			
Blueberry Ice Cool Brew Iced Tea, 2 g	0	0	0
Lemon Ice Cool Brew Iced Tea, 2 g	0	0	0
Peach Ice Cool Brew Iced Tea, 2 g	0	0	0
Raspberry Ice Cool Brew Iced Tea, 2 g	0	0	0
White Teas			
China Pearl™ Decaf White Tea, 2 g	0	0	0
Perfectly Pear® White Tea, 2 g	0	0	0
Vanilla Apple White Organic Tea, 2 g	0	0	0
Coca-Cola			
Dasani			
Grape, 8 fl.oz.	1	N/A	0
Lemon, 8 fl.oz.	2	N/A	0
Raspberry, 8 fl.oz.	1	N/A	0
Nestea			
Citrus Green Tea, 8 fl.oz.	85	0	23
Diet Citrus Green, 8 fl.oz.	3	0	0
Diet Lemon, 8 fl.oz.	2	0	0
Diet White Tea Berry Honey, 8 fl.oz.	3	0	0
Sweetened, 8 fl.oz.	63	0	17

● MOST HEALTHY ● LEAST HEALTHY

BEVERAGES	Cal	Fat	Cbs
Unsweetened, 8 fl.oz.	2	0	0
Crystal Light			
Lemon Tea Sugar Free, 8 fl.oz.	5	0	0
Pink Lemon Hydration Sugar Free, 8 fl.oz.	5	0	0
Rasp. Ice Sugar Free, 8 fl.oz.	5	0	0
Sunrise Classic Orange, 8 fl.oz.	5	0	0
Sunrise - Ruby Red Grapefruit, 8 fl.oz.	5	0	0
Fruit 2 0			
Enhanced Water - Energy Rasp, 8 fl.oz.	0	0	0
E.W. - Hydration Strwbry Tang, 8 fl.oz.	0	0	0
Natural Cherry, 8 fl.oz.	0	0	0
Natural Peach, 8 fl.oz.	0	0	0
Lipton			
Black Tea			
Decaf Iced Tea, 2 g	0	0	0
Iced Tea, 2 g	0	0	0
Flavored Black Tea			
Honey & Lemon Black Tea, 2 g	0	0	1
Spiced Chai Black Tea, 3 g	0	0	0
Green Tea			
100% Natural Decaf Green Tea, 1 g	0	0	0
100% Natural Green Tea, 3 g	0	0	0
Herbal Tea			
Lemon Herbal Tea, 2 g	0	0	1
Quietly Chamomile Herbal Tea, 2 g	0	0	1
Traditional Tea			
Earl Gray, 2 g	0	0	0
English Breakfast, 2 g	0	0	0
Diet Raspberry Iced Tea, 2 g	5	0	1
Peach Iced Tea, 1 oz.	70	0	19
Sweetened Peach Iced Tea Mix, 1 oz.	80	0	19
Tuscan Lemon, 2 g	0	0	0
Paul Newman's Own			
Green Tea with Honey, 8 fl.oz.	70	0	18
Lightly Sweetened Lemonade, 8 fl.oz.	80	0	20
Orange Mango Tango, 8 fl.oz.	150	0	37
Razz-Ma-Tazz Raspberry, 8 fl.oz.	120	0	28
Snapple			
Acai Blackberry Juice Drink, 8 fl.oz.	120	0	30
Classic Black Tea Earl Grey, 8 fl.oz.	35	0	8
Classic Black Tea English Brkfst, 8 fl.oz.	40	0	10
Cranberry Raspberry Juice Drink, 8 fl.oz.	120	0	29
Decaf Tea, 8 fl.oz.	100	0	25
Diet Green Tea Original, 8 fl.oz.	0	0	0
Diet Lemon Tea, 8 fl.oz.	0	0	0

● MOST HEALTHY   ● LEAST HEALTHY

BEVERAGES	Cal	Fat	Cbs
Diet Lemonade Iced Tea, 8 fl.oz.	10	0	2
Fruit Punch 100% Juiced, 12 fl.oz.	170	0	42
Green Apple 100% Juiced, 12 fl.oz.	160	0	41
Green Tea Original, 8 fl.oz.	60	0	15
Lemonade Iced Tea, 8 fl.oz.	110	0	28
Peach Tea, 8 fl.oz.	100	0	26
Raspberry Peach Juice Drink, 8 fl.oz.	120	0	29
Raspberry Tea, 8 fl.oz.	100	0	26
Strawberry Lime 100% Juiced, 12 fl.oz.	180	0	45
Unsweetened Tea, 8 fl.oz.	0	0	0
Antioxidant Water			
Tropical Mango - Protect, 8 fl.oz	60	0	12
Dragonfruit - Awaken, 8 fl.oz	50	0	12
Raspberry Acerola - Defy, 8 fl.oz	45	0	11
Strawberry Acai - Awaken, 8 fl.oz	50	0	13
Special K			
Protein Water			
Lemon Twist, 16 fl.oz.	50	0	13
Mixed Berry, 16 fl.oz.	50	0	14
Strawberry Kiwi, 16 fl.oz.	50	0	13
Welch's			
Cocktails & Drinks			
Apple Cranberry Juice Cocktail, 8 fl.oz	180	0	45
Blueberry Kiwi Blast, 8 fl.oz	160	0	40
Cranberry Juice Cocktail, 8 fl.oz	140	0	35
Light Berry Juice Cocktail, 8 fl.oz.	70	0	17
Orange Pineapple Drink, 8 fl.oz	120	0	31
Pomegranate Pulse, 8 fl.oz	150	0	37
Strawberry Breeze Cocktail, 8 fl.oz	130	0	33
JUICE			
Alta Dena			
Apple Juice, 8 fl.oz.	120	0	28
Fruit Punch, 8 fl.oz.	110	0	28
Orange Juice, 8 fl.oz.	110	1	25
Apple Time			
Apple Juice, 8 fl.oz.	120	N/A	31
Cascadian Farm			
Juice Concentrate			
Apple Juice, 2 fl.oz.	120	0	29
Cranberry, 2 fl.oz.	120	0	32
Grape, 2 fl.oz.	150	0	38
Lemonade, 2 fl.oz.	110	0	28
Coca-Cola			
Fruitopia			
Cherry Vanilla Groove, 8 fl.oz.	110	0	30

● MOST HEALTHY   ● LEAST HEALTHY

BEVERAGES

	Cal	Fat	Cbs
Fruit Integration, 8 fl.oz.	110	0	30
Kiwiberry Ruckus, 8 fl.oz.	110	0	29
Raspberry Dragonfruit Reflection, 8 fl.oz.	110	0	29
Minute Maid Juices			
Apple Juice, 8 fl.oz.	110	0	28
Lemonade, 8 fl.oz.	100	0	28
• Light Lemonade, 8 fl.oz.	5	0	1
Light Orangeade, 12 fl.oz.	10	0	2
Strawberry Raspberry Blend, 8 fl.oz.	120	0	33
Country Fresh			
Apple Juice, 8 fl.oz	120	0	29
Cranberry Apple Juice, 8 fl.oz	120	0	30
Orange Juice, 8 fl.oz	110	0	25
Orange Juice with Calcium, 8 fl.oz	120	0	29
Dean's			
Apple Juice, 8 fl.oz	120	0	29
Cranberry Apple Juice, 8 fl.oz	120	0	30
Orange Juice, 8 fl.oz	110	0	25
Orange Juice with Calcium, 8 fl.oz	120	0	29
Del Monte			
Tomato Juice, 8 fl.oz	50	0	10
Dole			
Pineapple Juice, 6 fl.oz.	110	0	26
Pineapple Orange, 6 fl.oz.	100	0	24
Pineapple Orange Banana, 6 fl.oz.	100	0	25
Land O'Lakes			
Apple Juice, 8 fl.oz	120	0	29
Cranberry Apple Juice, 8 fl.oz	120	0	30
Orange Juice with Calcium, 8 fl.oz	120	0	29
Orange Juice, 8 fl.oz	110	0	25
Lucky Leaf			
Lucky Leaf Premium Apple Juice, 8 fl.oz.	120	N/A	31
Lucky Leaf Sparkling Apple Cider, 8 fl.oz.	150	N/A	36
Minute Maid			
Orange Juice & Blends			
Multi-Vitamin, 8 fl.oz.	120	0	27
Original, 8 fl.oz.	110	0	27
Pulp Free, 8 fl.oz.	110	0	27
Lemonade & Punches			
Cherry Limeade, 8 fl.oz.	120	0	34
Lemonade, 8 fl.oz.	110	0	31
Pink Lemonade, 8 fl.oz.	100	0	28
Tropical Punch, 8 fl.oz.	110	0	30
Low Calorie Beverages			
Light Orange Juice Beverage, 8 fl.oz.	50	0	13

• MOST HEALTHY   • LEAST HEALTHY

BEVERAGES	Cal	Fat	Cbs
Light Orange Tangerine, 8 fl.oz.	15	0	4
Light Orangeade, 8 fl.oz.	110	0	29
Variety Juices & Juice Drinks			
Cranberry Apple Raspberry, 8 fl.oz.	120	0	33
Cranberry Grape, 8 fl.oz.	150	0	39
Grapefruit Juice, 8 fl.oz.	100	0	25
Ruby Red Grapefruit, 8 fl.oz.	130	0	34
Musselman's			
Fresh Pressed Apple Cider, 8 fl.oz.	120	N/A	31
Ocean Spray			
Cranberry Blackcurrant, 8 fl.oz	165	0	34
Cranberry Classic, 8 fl.oz	124	0	31
Cranberry Light, 8 fl.oz	20	0	5
Ruby Red Grapefruit, 8 fl.oz	125	0	31
Sunny Delight			
Blends			
Orange Fused Mango, 8 fl.oz.	80	0	20
Orange Fused Peach, 8 fl.oz.	80	0	20
Orange Fused Pineapple, 8 fl.oz.	80	0	20
Orange Fused Strawberry, 8 fl.oz.	80	0	20
Original			
Fruit Punch, 8 fl.oz.	120	0	29
Mango, 8 fl.oz.	130	0	31
Smooth Style, 8 fl.oz.	130	0	32
SunnyD Reduced Sugar, 8 fl.oz.	60	0	15
SunnyD with Calcium, 8 fl.oz.	140	0	35
Tangy Original Style, 8 fl.oz.	120	0	29
Tropicana Juice			
Chilled Juices and Juice Beverages			
• Grape, 12 fl.oz.	230	0	58
Orchard Style Apple, 12 fl.oz.	170	0	43
Orchard Style Lemonade, 8 fl.oz.	120	0	31
Non-Refrigerated Juices & Juice Drinks			
100% Fruit Punch, 10 fl.oz.	170	0	40
100% Orange Juice, 8 fl.oz.	110	0	27
Grape, 8 fl.oz.	150	0	38
Light Apple, 10 fl.oz.	65	0	18
Light Mixed Berry, 10 fl.oz.	70	0	18
Pineapple Orange, 8 fl.oz.	130	0	32
Refrigerated Juice Drinks			
Fruit Punch, 8 fl.oz.	10	0	3
Light Fruit Punch, 8 fl.oz.	130	0	32
Tropicana Fruit Squeeze™			
Lime Raspberry, 8 fl.oz.	20	0	5
Pink Grapefruit, 8 fl.oz.	20	0	5

• MOST HEALTHY   • LEAST HEALTHY

BEVERAGES

	Cal	Fat	Cbs
Tropical Tangerine, 8 fl.oz.	20	0	5
Tropicana Pure™			
Pomegranate Blueberry, 8 fl.oz.	130	0	33
Valencia Orange, 8 fl.oz.	110	0	26
Tropicana Pure Premium®			
Light 'n Healthy, 8 fl.oz.	50	0	13
Orange Juice, 8 fl.oz.	110	0	26
Tropicana® Organics, 8 fl.oz.	120	0	28
V8			
Diet V8 Splash® Juice Drink			
Diet Berry Blend, 8 oz.	10	0	3
Diet Tropical Blend, 8 oz.	10	0	3
V8® 100% Vegetable Juice			
100% Vegetable Juice, 8 oz.	50	0	10
Low Sodium V8, 8 oz.	50	0	10
Organic V8, 8 oz.	50	0	10
Spicy Hot V8, 8 oz.	50	0	10
V8® VFusion™ Juice			
Acai Berry, 8 oz.	110	0	27
Light Peach Mango, 8 oz.	50	0	13
Pomegranate Blueberry, 8 oz.	100	0	25
Strawberry Banana, 8 oz.	120	0	28
V8 Splash® Juice Drink			
Berry Blend, 8 oz.	70	0	18
Fruit Medley, 8 oz.	70	0	19
Mango Peach, 8 oz.	80	0	20
Welch's			
100% Juice			
Fruit Punch, 8 fl.oz.	120	0	30
Orange Juice, 8 fl.oz.	120	0	30
Raspberry Lime Twist, 12 fl.oz.	200	0	49
Tropical Passion Fruit, 10 fl.oz.	190	0	46
White Grape Cherry, 8 fl.oz.	140	0	35
White Grape Peach, 8 fl.oz.	160	0	39
Concentrates			
100% Juice Concentrates, 2 fl.oz.	160	0	41
Fruit Juice Cocktail Concentrates, 2 fl.oz.	150	0	38
Juices and Drinks			
100% Grape Juice With Fiber, 8 fl.oz.	180	0	45
100% Grape Juice, 8 fl.oz.	170	0	42
100% White Grape Juice, 8 fl.oz.	160	0	39
Lighter Options			
Light Juice, 8 fl.oz.	70	0	17
Naturals, 10 fl.oz.	100	0	26
Orgnc 100% Concord Grape Jc, 10 fl.oz.	210	0	53

● MOST HEALTHY   ● LEAST HEALTHY

► BEVERAGES	Cal	Fat	Cbs
POWDERED DRINK MIXES			
Accelerade			
Powder Fruit Punch, 2 tbsp.	120	1	21
Powder Lemonade, 2 tbsp.	120	1	21
Powder Orange, 2 tbsp.	120	1	21
Celestial Seasonings			
Go Stix			
Fruit Punch Go Stix™, 14 g	60	0	14
Orange Citrus Punch Go Stix™, 14 g	60	0	14
Triple Berry Go Stix™, 14 g	60	0	14
Wild Cherry Go Stix™, 14 g	60	0	14
Zingers To Go			
Blueberry Splash™, 1 g	60	N/A	N/A
Peach Delight®, 1 g	60	N/A	N/A
Tangerine Orange Wave®, 1 g	60	N/A	N/A
Wild Berry Chill®, 1 g	60	N/A	N/A
Country Time Drink Mix			
Lemonade, 17 oz.	60	0	16
Lemonade Iced Tea Classic, 23 oz.	90	0	22
Lemonade Iced Tea Raspberry, 23 oz.	90	N/A	22
Lemonade Lite, 9 oz.	35	0	0
Pink Lemonade, 17 oz.	60	0	16
Pink Lemonade Lite, 9 oz.	35	0	8
Raspberry Lemonade, 21 oz.	80	0	19
Strawberry Lemonade, 22 oz.	80	0	20
Crystal Light			
Fruit Drinks - Fusion Fruit Punch, 1 g	5	0	0
Iced Tea - Peach Sugar Free, 1 g	5	0	0
Lemonade - Pink Lmnd Sugar Free, 2 g	5	0	0
On The Go - Lemonade Sugar Free, 2 g	5	0	0
On The Go - Peach Tea Sugar Free, 1 g	5	0	0
On The Go - Sunrise Classic Orange, 2 g	5	0	0
General Foods International Coffee			
Chai			
Chai Latte, 15 g	70	2	12
Sugar Free Chai Latte, 5 g	30	2	2
Vanilla			
Sugar Free Vanilla Creme, 6 g	35	3	3
Vanilla Creme, 14 g	60	3	11
Kool Aid			
Cherry Sugar-sweetened, 17 g	60	0	16
Grape Sugar Free, 1 g	5	0	0
• Lemonade Unsweetened, 1 g	0	0	0
Orange Unsweetened, 1 g	0	0	0
Strawberry Sugar-sweetened, 17 g	60	0	16

● MOST HEALTHY   ● LEAST HEALTHY

BEVERAGES

	Cal	Fat	Cbs
Tropical Punch Sugar Free, 1 g	5	0	0
Lipton			
Chocolate, 2 tbsp.	120	2	21
• Original, 2 tbsp.	120	2	21
Vanilla, 2 tbsp.	120	2	21
Nutrasweet			
Hot Cocoa Mix With Nutrasweet®, 1 tbsp.	50	N/A	9
Iced Tea Soft Drink Mix w/ Ntrswt®, 1 g	2	N/A	0
Red Punch Soft Drink Mix w/ Ntrswt®, 1 g	3	N/A	0
South Beach Living			
Strawberry Banana Drink Mix, 1 tbsp.	30	0	6
Tropical Breeze Drink Mix, 1 tbsp.	30	35	6
Special K			
Protein Water Mix Iced Tea, 17 fl.oz.	30	0	7
Protein Wtr Mix Pink Lemonade, 17 fl.oz.	30	0	6
Protein Wtr Mix Strawberry Kiwi, 17 fl.oz.	30	0	6
Tang			
Grape, 2 tbsp.	110	0	28
Orange, 2 tbsp.	90	0	23
Orange Pineapple, 2 tbsp.	100	0	24
Orange Strawberry, 2 tbsp.	24	0	27
Orange Sugar Free, 1 tbsp.	5	0	0
Wild Berry, 1 tbsp.	40	0	10
READY TO DRINK COFFEE			
General Foods International Coffee			
Chocolate			
• Sugar Free Suisse Mocha, 6 g	30	2	2
Suisse Mocha, 13 g	60	2	10
Swiss White Chocolate, 16 g	70	3	12
Coffee			
Cafe Vienna, 16 g	70	2	12
Creme Caramel, 15 g	60	2	12
Hazelnut Belgian Café, 16 g	70	2	12
Italian Cappuccino, 13 g	50	2	10
Vanilla			
DeCaf French Vanilla Café, 14 g	60	2	10
French Vanilla Café, 14 g	60	3	10
Sugar Free French Vanilla Café, 6 g	30	3	2
Starbucks Beverages			
Doubleshots			
Energy + Coffee Vanilla, 15 fl.oz.	210	2	25
• Energy + Coffee, 15 fl.oz.	210	2	26
Light, 15 fl.oz.	70	4	5
Regular, 15 fl.oz.	140	6	17

BEVERAGES

	Cal	Fat	Cbs
Frappuccino			
Caramel, 16 fl.oz.	200	3	31
Dark Chocolate Mocha, 16 fl.oz.	190	4	33
Mocha Lite, 16 fl.oz.	100	3	11
Mocha, 16 fl.oz.	180	3	31
Vanilla, 16 fl.oz.	200	3	31
SMOOTHIES			
Baskin Robbins			
Fruit Blast - Medium			
Berry Pomegranate Banana, 24 fl.oz.	710	1	172
Mango Fruit Blast, 24 fl.oz.	620	2	148
• Strawberry Banana, 24 fl.oz.	730	2	178
Clif Products			
Lime-ade Electrolyte Splash, 2 tbsp.	80	N/A	20
Watermelon Moons Energy Chews, 2 tbsp.	100	0	24
Dannon Light & Fit			
Berries & Cream, 7 fl.oz.	60	3	4
Mixed Berry, 7 fl.oz.	70	0	13
Peach Passion, 7 fl.oz.	70	0	13
Strawberry, 7 fl.oz.	70	0	13
Strawberry Banana, 7 fl.oz.	70	0	13
Strawberry Banana Cream, 7 fl.oz.	60	3	4
Strawberries & Cream, 7 fl.oz.	60	3	4
LightFull Foods			
Café Latte, 8 fl.oz.	90	1	37
Chocolate, 8 fl.oz.	90	1	36
Peachy Cream, 8 fl.oz.	90	0	37
Strawberry Bliss, 8 fl.oz.	90	0	37
Tropicana Juice			
Fruit Smoothies			
Mixed Berry, 11 fl.oz.	220	0	54
Strawberry Banana, 11 fl.oz.	220	0	53
Tropical Fruit, 11 fl.oz.	220	0	53
Twister®			
Cherry Berry Rev, 8 fl.oz.	70	0	16
Orange Strawberry Banana Blast, 8 fl.oz.	70	0	16
White Grape Kiwi Twist, 8 fl.oz.	70	0	16
V8			
• Strawberry Banana, 8 oz.	10	0	3
Tropical Colada, 8 oz.	100	0	21
SODA, COLA & TONIC			
7Up			
7Up Plus, 8 fl.oz.	10	0	2
7Up 100 % Natural Flavors, 8 fl.oz.	100	0	26
Diet 7Up, 8 fl.oz.	0	0	0

● MOST HEALTHY • LEAST HEALTHY

► BEVERAGES

	Cal	Fat	Cbs
Coca-Cola			
Seagram's Mixers			
• Club Soda, 8 fl.oz.	0	N/A	0
Diet Ginger Ale, 8 fl.oz.	2	N/A	0
Diet Tonic Water, 8 fl.oz.	3	N/A	0
Ginger Ale, 8 fl.oz.	90	N/A	24
Original Seltzer, 8 fl.oz.	0	N/A	0
Tonic Water, 8 fl.oz.	83	N/A	22
Soft Drink			
• Barq's Floatz, 8 fl.oz.	127	0	34
Barq's root beer, 8 fl.oz.	111	0	30
Coca-Cola classic, 8 fl.oz.	97	0	27
Diet Barq's root beer, 8 fl.oz.	1	0	0
Diet Coke, 8 fl.oz.	1	0	0
Fanta Orange, 8 fl.oz.	111	0	35
Fresca, 8 fl.oz.	2	0	0
Full Throttle Energy Drink, 8 fl.oz.	111	N/A	29
Pibb Xtra, 8 fl.oz.	97	0	26
Pibb Zero, 8 fl.oz.	2	0	0
Sprite Zero, 8 fl.oz.	2	0	0
Sprite, 8 fl.oz.	96	0	26
Mountain Dew			
AMP, 8 fl.oz.	110	0	29
Baja Blast, 8 fl.oz.	110	0	30
Diet Mountain Dew, 8 fl.oz.	0	0	0
Livewire, 8 fl.oz.	110	0	31
Mountain Dew, 8 fl.oz.	110	0	31
Mug Root Beer			
Cream Soda, 8 fl.oz	120	0	32
Diet Cream Soda, 8 fl.oz.	0	0	0
Diet Mug, 8 fl.oz	0	0	0
Mug, 8 fl.oz	100	0	29
Pepsi Drinks			
Diet Pepsi, 8 fl.oz.	0	0	0
Pepsi, 8 fl.oz.	100	0	28
SPORTS & ENERGY DRINKS			
Accelerade			
Accel Gel			
Citrus Orange, 41 g	100	0	20
Strawberry Kiwi, 41 g	100	0	20
Vanilla, 41 g	100	0	20
Ready to Drink			
Citrus Grape Fruit, 8 fl.oz.	80	0	15
Mountian Berry, 8 fl.oz.	80	0	15
Peach Mango, 8 fl.oz.	80	0	15

• MOST HEALTHY   • LEAST HEALTHY

BEVERAGES

	Cal	Fat	Cbs
Clif Products			
Clif Shot Electrolyte Drink			
Cran Razz, 20 g	80	0	19
Crisp Apple, 20 g	80	0	19
• Hot Apple Cider, 40 g	150	N/A	38
Lemonade, 1 Scoop	80	0	19
Clif Shot Gel			
Apple Pie, 32 g	100	0	25
Chocolate, 32 g	100	1	25
Double Expresso, 32 g	100	0	25
Strawberry, 32 g	100	0	25
Vanilla, 32 g	100	0	25
Clif Shot Recovery Drink			
French Vanilla, 1 Scoop	150	0	31
Hot Chocolate, 1 Scoop	140	2	23
Mango Orange, 1 Scoop	140	0	31
Coca-Cola			
Energy Drinks			
Full Throttle, 8 fl.oz.	111	0	29
Full Throttle Fury, 8 fl.oz.	112	0	29
Sugar Free Full Throttle, 8 fl.oz.	5	0	0
Tab Energy, 8 fl.oz.	6	0	0
Hybrid Energy Sodas			
Vault, 8 fl.oz.	119	0	32
• Vault Zero, 8 fl.oz.	4	0	0
Powerade			
Advance Cherry Lime, 8 fl.oz.	66	0	17
Arctic Shatter, 8 fl.oz.	64	0	17
Black Cherry Lime, 8 fl.oz.	64	0	17
Option Lemon, 8 fl.oz.	10	0	2
Gatorade			
AM, 8 fl.oz.	50	0	14
Fierce, 8 fl.oz.	50	0	14
Frost, 8 fl.oz.	50	0	14
Rain, 8 fl.oz.	51	0	14
X-Factor, 8 fl.oz.	50	0	1

BREAKFAST

BREAKFAST BARS

	Cal	Fat	Cbs
Post Cereal			
Banana Nut, 35 g	140	4	24
Cranberry Almond, 35 g	140	4	25
• Oatmeal Raisin, 35 g	130	3	25

BREAKFAST

	Cal	Fat	Cbs
South Beach Living			
High Protein Cereal Bar			
• Chocolate, 35 g	140	5	15
Cinnamon Raisin, 35 g	140	5	15
Cranberry Almond, 35 g	140	5	15
Peanut Butter, 35 g	140	5	15
CEREAL			
Cascadian Farm			
Cinnamon Raisin Granola, 55 g	210	3	42
Honey Nut Os, 30 g	120	2	24
Multi Grain Squares, 30 g	110	1	25
Oats & Honey Granola, 55 g	230	6	42
Purely O's, 30 g	110	2	22
Raisin Bran, 55 g	180	2	43
Chex			
Chocolate, 32 g	130	3	26
Corn, 31 g	120	1	26
Honey Nut, 32 g	120	1	28
Multi Bran, 47 g	160	2	39
Rice®, 27 g	100	1	23
Strawberry, 31 g	130	2	29
Wheat®, 47 g	160	1	38
Eggo			
French Toaster Sticks Original, 90 g	220	6	35
Stuffed French Sticks Maple Syrup, 59 g	150	4	27
General Mills Cereal			
Basic 4, 55 g	200	3	43
Boo Berry, 33 g	130	1	28
Cheerios, 28 g	100	2	20
Chex Corn, 31 g	120	1	26
Cinnamon Toast Crunch, 31 g	130	3	25
Cocoa Puffs, 27 g	110	2	23
Cookie Crisp, 26 g	100	1	22
• Fiber One, 30 g	60	1	25
French Toast Crunch, 31 g	130	1	24
Golden Grahams, 31 g	120	1	26
Kix, 30 g	110	1	25
Raisin Nut Bran, 49 g	180	3	38
Reese's Puffs, 29 g	120	3	22
Total Raisin Bran, 53 g	160	1	40
Total, 30 g	100	1	23
Trix, 32 g	120	2	28
Wheaties, 27 g	100	1	22
Kellogg's Cereal			
Corn Flakes, 1 oz.	100	0	24

BREAKFAST

	Cal	Fat	Cbs
Corn Pops®, 1 oz.	110	0	26
Cracklin' Oat Bran®, 2 oz.	200	7	35
Froot Loops®, 1 oz.	110	1	25
Froot Loops® Reduced Sugar, 1 oz.	120	1	28
Frosted Flakes®, 1 oz.	110	0	27
Frosted Mini-Wheats® Bite Size, 2 oz.	200	1	48
Honey Smacks®, 1 oz.	100	1	24
Lowfat Granola without Raisins, 2 oz.	190	3	40
Mini-Wheats® Unfrosted Bite Size, 2 oz.	200	2	46
Raisin Bran®, 2 oz.	190	2	45
Smart Start® Maple & Brown Sugar, 2 oz.	220	3	47
Life Cereal			
Cinnamon Life, 32 g	120	2	25
Honey Graham Life, 32 g	120	2	25
Life Cereal, 32 g	120	2	25
Life Chocolate Oat Crunch, 51 g	190	3	40
Life Vanilla Yogurt Crunch, 55 g	210	3	46
Malt O Meal			
Coco Roos, 30 g	120	2	26
Crispy Rice, 33 g	130	0	29
Frosted Flakes, 31 g	120	0	28
Golden Puffs, 27 g	110	0	24
Honey Buzzers, 29 g	110	1	26
Honey Graham Squares, 30 g	130	3	25
Mini Spooners, 55 g	190	1	45
Puffed Rice, 15 g	60	0	13
Raisin Bran, 59 g	220	2	49
Tootie Fruities, 32 g	130	1	28
Mom's Best			
Raisin Bran, 59 g	230	2	49
Toasted Wheat-fuls, 55 g	200	1	44
Toasted Whole Grain Oat Cereal, 30 g	120	2	23
Nature Valley			
Cereal Crunchy Cinnamon, 58 g	230	3	48
Cereal Crunchy Oats 'N Honey, 58 g	230	3	48
Organic Cereal Vanilla Nut, 50 g	190	2	41
Nutri-Grain			
Apple Cinnamon, 37 g	130	3	24
Blackberry, 37 g	130	3	24
Raspberry, 37 g	130	3	24
Strawberry, 37 g	130	3	24
Paul Newman's Own			
Flakes 'N Strawberries Cereal, 30 g	100	1	25
Honey Flax Flakes Cereal, 30 g	100	1	24
Honey Nut O's Cereal, 30 g	100	2	22

● MOST HEALTHY   ● LEAST HEALTHY

➤ BREAKFAST	Cal	Fat	Cbs
Wheat Puffs Cereal, 27 g	100	1	22
Post Cereal			
Honey Bunches of Oats			
Almond, 31 g	130	3	25
Banana, 31 g	120	2	26
Honey Roasted, 31 g	120	2	25
Strawberry, 31 g	120	2	26
Post Healthy Classic			
Bran Flakes, 30 g	100	1	24
Fruit & Bran, 55 g	200	3	42
Grape Nut O's, 32 g	120	0	28
Grape Nuts Flakes, 29 g	110	1	24
Grape Nuts Trail Mix Crunch, 48 g	180	3	37
Raisin Bran, 31 g	190	1	46
Shredded Wheat Family, 47 g	160	1	37
Post Kids Cereal			
Cocoa Pebbles, 30 g	110	2	26
Fruity Pebbles, 30 g	110	1	26
Golden Crisp, 31 g	110	0	25
Honeycomb, 32 g	120	1	27
Oreo O's, 27 g	110	2	22
Waffle Crisp, 30 g	120	3	25
Post Selects			
Cranberry Almond Crunch®, 51 g	200	4	39
• Banana Nut Crunch®, 59 g	240	6	44
Great Grains®-Raisins, 52 g	220	6	38
Maple Pecan Crunch®, 52 g	220	6	40
Purity Foods			
Vita-Spelt Toasted Flakes, 27 g	93	1	20
Red River Cereal			
Original, 40 g	154	3	27
Regular, 35 g	136	2	24
Maple & Brown Sugar, 40 g	153	2	29
Rice Krispies			
Berry Krispies™ cereal, 1 oz.	120	0	27
Cereal, 1 oz.	130	0	29
Cocoa Krispies® cereal, 1 oz.	120	1	27
Frosted Krispies® cereal, 1 oz.	110	0	27
Treats® Cereal, 1 oz.	120	2	26
South Beach Living			
Strawberry Harvest Crunch, 50 g	170	2	37
Vanilla Almond Crunch, 51 g	180	4	35
Special K			
Cereal, 1 oz.	120	1	22
Fruit & Yogurt cereal, 1 oz.	120	1	27

BREAKFAST	Cal	Fat	Cbs
Low Carb Lifestyle Protein Plus, 1 oz.	100	3	14
Vanilla Almond Cereal, 1 oz.	110	2	25
Total Cereal			
Cranberry Crunch, 58 g	190	2	44
Total Honey Clusters®, 48 g	170	2	38
Total Raisin Bran, 53 g	160	1	40
Total Whole Grain, 30 g	100	1	23
GRANOLA			
Purity Foods			
Granola - Apple Cinnamon Raisin, 50 g	220	8	33
Granola - Cranberry Vanilla Walnut, 50 g	220	9	33
South Beach Living			
• Cherry Almond Granola Clusters, 30 g	130	4	18
Mixed Berry Granola Clusters, 30 g	130	4	18
Sunridge Farms			
Apple Blueberry Granola, 55 g	230	7	36
Cranberry Craze Granola, 55 g	240	8	36
Golden Nut and Honey Granola, 55 g	230	9	33
Organic Crunchy Lite Granola, 55 g	220	6	38
Organic Grandma Dave's Granola, 55 g	210	5	35
Organic Magic Muesli, 55 g	210	6	35
Organic Rolled Oats, 45 g	170	3	30
• Super Nut Crunch Granola, 55 g	240	9	35
HOT CEREAL			
Malt O Meal			
Chocolate, 35 g	130	0	27
Creamy Hot Wheat, 35 g	130	0	27
• Maple & Brown Sugar, 45 g	170	0	37
Original, 35 g	130	1	27
Mom's Best			
Maple & Brown Sugar, 43 g	160	2	33
• Oats & Honey Blend, 30 g	120	2	25
Old Fashioned Oats, 40 g	150	3	27
TOASTER PASTRIES			
Eggo			
Cereal Cinnamon Toast, 1 oz.	130	3	26
• Cereal Maple Syrup, 1 oz.	110	2	25
French Toaster Sticks Cinnamon, 3 oz.	230	6	38
Mrs. Butterworth's			
French Toast Sticks - Original, 4 oz.	250	12	31
French Toast Sticks - Thin, 5 oz.	230	4	41
Pepperidge Farm			
Apple Dumplings, 1 dumpling	230	11	29
Apple Turnovers, 1 turnover	270	15	31
Peach Dumplings, 1 dumpling	250	11	34

• MOST HEALTHY • LEAST HEALTHY

BREAKFAST	Cal	Fat	Cbs
• Peach Turnovers, 1 turnover	280	15	34

Pillsbury

Toaster Scramble

	Cal	Fat	Cbs
Cheese, Egg & Bacon, 47 g	180	12	15
Cheese, Egg & Ham, 47 g	180	11	15
Reduced Fat Southwestern Style, 47 g	160	9	15

Toaster Strudel

	Cal	Fat	Cbs
Brown Sugar Cinnamon, 54 g	200	9	28
Cream Cheese, 54 g	200	11	23
Strawberry Banana, 54 g	180	9	24
Strawberry, 54 g	190	9	26

Turnovers

	Cal	Fat	Cbs
Turnovers Apple, 57 g	180	8	24
Turnovers Cherry, 57 g	180	8	24

Pop-Tarts

	Cal	Fat	Cbs
Apple Strudel, 50 g	200	6	35
Blueberry, 52 g	210	6	37
Brown Sugar Cinnamon, 50 g	210	8	33
Chocolate Chip, 52 g	220	7	36
Frosted Cookies & Creme, 50 g	200	5	35
Lowfat Frosted Strawberry, 52 g	190	3	39
Whole Grain Brown Sugar Cinn., 50 g	200	7	34
Whole Grain Strawberry, 50 g	190	5	35

WAFFLES AND PANCAKES

Aunt Jemima

	Cal	Fat	Cbs
Butter Milk Complete, 1/3 cup	160	2	31
Original, 1/3 cup	150	1	33
• Whole Wheat Blend, 1/4 cup	120	1	26

Eggo

Pancakes

	Cal	Fat	Cbs
Blueberry, 105 g	250	8	41
Buttermilk, 116 g	280	9	44
Jungle, 117 g	280	8	46
Minis, 110 g	260	8	42
Nutri-Grain® , 105 g	240	7	40

Waffles

	Cal	Fat	Cbs
Apple Cinnamon, 70 g	190	6	29
Buttermilk, 70 g	180	6	26
Chocolate Chip, 70 g	210	7	32
• Cinnamon Toast, 92 g	300	11	45
French Toast, 45 g	140	6	19
Homestyle Waffles, 70 g	190	7	27
Minis Homestyle Waffles, 93 g	260	10	38

Mrs. Butterworth's

	Cal	Fat	Cbs
Pancakes - Mini, 4 oz.	240	4	46

• MOST HEALTHY   • LEAST HEALTHY

BREAKFAST	Cal	Fat	Cbs
Pancakes - Original, 4 oz.	220	4	42
Waffles Jumbo Square, 3 oz.	200	6	32
Waffles Regular Square, 3 oz.	210	6	34
Pillsbury			
Pancakes Blueberry, 4 oz.	230	4	46
Pancakes Buttermilk, 4 oz.	240	4	47
Pancakes Maple Burst, 4 oz.	290	7	53
Pancakes Original, 4 oz.	250	4	49

CANDY

CHOCOLATE

Cadbury's	Cal	Fat	Cbs
Caramel Egg, 34 g	170	9	21
Caramello Candy Bar, 45 g	220	10	29
• Chocolate Egg, 34 g	150	5	25
Roast Almond, 39 g	210	13	21
Hershey Chocolates			
Cookies 'N' Créme Candy Bar, 34 g	170	9	21
Extra Creamy Chocolate & Caramel, 36 g	180	9	22
Hershey's Pretzel Bars, 20 g	100	5	13
Milk Chocolate, 43 g	210	13	26
Milk Chocolate With Almonds, 41 g	210	14	21
Special Dark Chocolate, 41 g	180	12	25
M&M's Bakery			
Almond, 1 oz.	200	100	21
Dark Chocolate, 2 oz.	240	100	33
M&M'S Minis, 1 oz.	150	60	21
Milk Chocolate, 2 oz.	240	90	34
Mint Crisp, 2 oz.	200	80	27
Peanut, 2 oz.	250	120	30
Peanut Butter, 2 oz.	240	120	26
Mauna Loa			
Candy Coated, 40 g	210	13	22
Dark Chocolate, 41 g	210	16	22
Milk Chocolate, 41 g	220	16	21
Snickers			
• Snickers, 2 oz.	280	14	35
Snickers Almond, 2 oz.	240	11	32
Snickers Dark, 2 oz.	250	13	30
Sorbee			
Chocolate Truffles, 40 g	180	12	22
Milk Chocolate Bar, 40 g	190	13	22
Peanut Butter Chocolates, 40 g	210	15	19
Peppermint Patties, 39 g	180	13	24

• MOST HEALTHY   • LEAST HEALTHY

CANDY

	Cal	Fat	Cbs
Stauffer's			
Almond, 1 oz.	230	15	19
Chocorooms, 1 oz.	160	8	20
Hello Panda Chocolate, 1 oz.	160	10	18
Pucca Regular Chocolate, 1 oz.	160	9	19
Sunridge Farms			
Chocolate Ginger, 40 g	170	7	28
Organic Chocolate Raisins, 40 g	160	6	27
Terry's			
Orange Dark, 44 g	240	13	28
Orange Milk, 44 g	230	12	27
Pure Milk, 44 g	230	12	27
Toblerone			
Swiss Choc w/ Honey & Almond Nougat, 33 g	170	9	21
Swiss Wt w/ Honey & Almond Nougat, 33 g	180	10	20
Truffle Peaks, 41 g	240	15	23
VARIOUS KINDS			
Sorbee			
Hard Candies			
• Chocolate Lites, 13 g	25	0	13
Coffee Lites, 13 g	25	0	13
Fruit Flavors Lites, 13 g	25	0	13
Soft Candy			
Bursts, 40 g	120	3	34
Sunridge Farms			
Black Licorice Chews, 40 g	140	2	27
Black Licorice Scotties, 40 g	130	0	33
Natural Licorice Raspberry Hearts, 40 g	140	0	35
Organic Jolly Beans, 40 g	150	0	37
Organic Sunny Bears, 40 g	30	0	9
Wonka			
Chewy Gobstopper®, 15 g	50	0	14
Chewy Runts®, 15 g	60	1	14
Laffy Taffy® Rope, 1 rope	80	1	19
Laffy Taffy® Stretchy & Tangy Taffy, 1 bar	165	4	33
Nerds® Rope , 1 rope	90	0	22
Sour Mixups®, 43 g	160	2	36
Sour Sweetarts Variety, 9 g	30	0	8
• Sweetarts Rope, 1 pkg	210	2	48
Sweetarts Squeeze, 1 tube	130	0	33

• MOST HEALTHY   • LEAST HEALTHY

CHEESE	Cal	Fat	Cbs
CHEESE			
Alouette			
Alouette® Baby Brie®			
Original, 1 oz.	110	10	1
With Herbs, 1 oz.	100	8	1
Alouette® Reserve™			
Baby Brie® Cheese, 1 oz.	100	8	1
Chevre Style Cheese, 1 oz.	80	7	1
Havarti, 1 oz.	90	0	0
Swiss Style Cheese, 1 oz.	100	7	1
Alta Dena			
Cheese			
Mild Cheddar Cheese, 1 oz.	110	9	1
Monterey Jack Cheese, 1 oz.	100	8	0
Whipped Cream Cheese, 1 oz.	80	7	1
Cottage Cheese			
Cottage Cheese w/ Pineapple, 4 oz.	120	2	14
Lowfat Cottage Cheese, 4 oz.	100	3	4
Small Curd Cottage Cheese, 1 oz.	120	5	3
Athenos			
Blue Cheese Crumbled Natural, 1 oz.	110	9	2
Crumbled Reduced Fat, 1 oz.	90	7	2
Crumbled Traditional, 1 oz.	80	6	1
Gorgonzola Crumbled Natural, 1 oz.	110	9	2
Breakstone's			
Cottage Cheese			
Liveactive Lowfat w/Mixed Bry, 4 oz.	120	2	18
Liveactive Lowfat With Pineapple, 4 oz.	110	2	17
Small Curd Fat Free, 4 oz.	80	0	8
Small Curd Lowfat 2% Milkfat, 4 oz.	90	3	6
Sm Curd Smooth & Crmy 4% Milkfat, 1 oz.	120	5	6
Cottage Doubles			
Blueberry Lowfat, 5 oz.	140	3	18
Raspberry Lowfat, 5 oz.	140	3	17
Strawberry Lowfat, 5 oz.	130	2	17
Country Fresh			
1% Lowfat Cottage Cheese, 4 oz.	90	2	5
2% Lowfat Cottage Cheese, 4 oz.	100	3	5
Cottage Cheese, 4 oz.	110	5	5
Fat Free Cottage Cheese, 4 oz.	80	0	5
Dean's			
1% Lowfat Cottage Cheese, 4 oz.	90	2	5
2% Lowfat Cottage Cheese, 4 oz.	100	3	5
Cottage Cheese, 4 oz.	110	5	5
Fat Free Cottage Cheese, 4 oz.	80	0	6

• MOST HEALTHY • LEAST HEALTHY

CHEESE

	Cal	Fat	Cbs
Deli Deluxe			
American 2% Milk Slices, 1 oz.	60	4	0
American Slices, 1 oz.	70	6	0
Colby Jack Slices, 1 oz.	90	7	0
Mild Cheddar Slices, 1 oz.	90	8	0
Mozzarella Slices Low Moisture, 1 oz.	60	4	0
Natural Swiss Slices, 1 oz.	80	7	0
Pepper Jack Spicy Slices, 1 oz.	90	7	0
Provolone Slices, 1 oz.	100	8	0
Sharp Cheddar 2% Milk Slices, 1 oz.	70	5	1
Sharp Cheddar Slices, 1 oz.	110	9	1
Swiss 2% Milk Reduced Fat Slices, 1 oz.	70	5	0
Swiss Slices, 1 oz.	90	7	1
Easy Cheese			
American, 1 oz.	90	6	2
Cheddar, 1 oz.	90	6	2
Cheddar 'N Bacon, 1 oz.	90	7	2
Sharp Cheddar, 1 oz.	80	6	2
Knudsen			
• Cottage Doubles Raspberry Lowfat, 5 oz.	150	3	20
Cottage Dbl Strawberry Lowfat, 5 oz.	140	3	19
Free Nonfat, 5 oz.	80	0	7
Lowfat & Pineapple, 5 oz.	120	2	15
Lowfat Small Curd, 5 oz.	100	3	6
Kraft Singles			
American 2% Milk, 1 oz.	50	3	2
American Fat Free, 1 oz.	30	0	2
Pepperjack 2% Milk, 1 oz.	50	3	2
Sharp Cheddar Fat Free, 1 oz.	30	0	2
Swiss Fat Free, 1 oz.	30	0	2
Swiss, 1 oz.	60	5	2
White American, 1 oz.	60	5	1
Land O'Lakes			
1% Lowfat Cottage Cheese, 4 oz.	90	2	5
2% Lowfat Cottage Cheese, 4 oz.	100	3	5
Cottage Cheese, 4 oz.	110	5	5
Fat Free Cottage Cheese, 4 oz.	80	0	6
Light N Lively			
Cottage Cheese - Fat Free, 4 oz.	80	0	8
Cottage Cheese - Lowfat, 4 oz.	80	1	5
Live Active			
Cottage Cheese - Breakstone's, 4 oz.	90	2	8
Cottage Cheese - Knudsen, 4 oz.	90	2	8
Natural Cheese			
Cheddar Bacon, 1 oz.	90	7	2

• MOST HEALTHY   • LEAST HEALTHY

CHEESE

	Cal	Fat	Cbs
Colby, 1 oz.	110	9	1
Medium Cheddar, 1 oz.	120	10	0
Monterey Jack, 1 oz.	110	9	0
Mozzarella Low-moisture, 1 oz.	80	6	1
Sharp Cheddar, 1 oz.	120	10	0
Polly O			
• Mozzarella Fat Free, 5 g	20	2	0
Mozzarella Part Skim, 64 g	70	3	3
Mozzarella Whole Milk, 28 g	80	7	0
Parmesan & Romano Grated, 43 g	120	10	0
Parmesan Grated, 5 g	20	2	0
Ricotta - Fat Free, 28 g	40	0	1
Ricotta - Lite, 28 g	60	3	1
Ricotta - Part Skim, 28 g	90	7	1
Ricotta Original, 63 g	110	6	2
Sargento			
Artisan Blends Shredded Cheese			
Mozzarella & Provolone, 1 oz.	90	9	0
Parmesan, 5 g	20	2	0
Swiss, 1 oz.	110	8	1
Bistro™ Blends Shredded Cheese			
Chipotle Cheddar Cheese, 1 oz.	100	8	1
Mozz & Asiago w/ Roasted Garlic, 1 oz.	80	5	2
Mozz w/ Sun-Dried Tomatoes & Basil, 1 oz.	90	6	1
Classic Fancy Shredded Cheese			
Cheddar Jack, 1 oz.	110	9	1
Mozzarella, 1 oz.	80	6	1
Sharp Cheddar, 1 oz.	110	9	1
Deli Style Sliced Cheeses			
Colby, 1 oz.	80	7	1
Colby-Jack Cheese, 1 oz.	70	6	0
Medium Cheddar, 1 oz.	80	6	0
Monterey Jack, 1 oz.	80	6	0
Mozzarella, 1 oz.	60	4	1
Muenster, 1 oz.	80	6	0
Pepper Jack Cheese, 1 oz.	80	6	0
Provolone, 1 oz.	70	6	0
Swiss, 1 oz.	70	5	1
Reduced Fat Deli Style Sliced Cheeses			
Reduced Fat Provolone, 1 oz.	50	4	0
Reduced Fat Swiss, 1 oz.	60	4	1
Reduced Fat Shredded Cheese			
4 Cheese Mexican, 1 oz.	80	6	1
Mild Cheddar, 1 oz.	80	6	1
Mozzarella, 1 oz.	80	5	1

▶ CHEESE	Cal	Fat	Cbs
Smart Balance			
Fat Free Slices, 1 oz.	25	0	N/A
Cheese Product Shreds, 1 oz.	80	5	1
South Beach Living			
Lowfat Cottage Cheese, 4 oz.	80	1	6
The Laughing Cow			
Mini Baby Bel			
Gouda, 1 oz.	80	6	0
Light, 1 oz.	50	3	0
Mild Cheddar, 1 oz.	70	5	0
Original, 1 oz.	70	6	0
Wedges			
Light Garlic & Herb, 1 oz.	35	2	1
Light Swiss Original,1 oz.	35	2	1
Original Creamy Swiss, 1 oz.	50	4	1
Velveeta			
2% Milk Cheese, 1 oz.	60	3	4
Mexican Mild Cheese, 1 oz.	80	6	3
Pepper Jack Cheese, 1 oz.	80	6	3
Regular Cheese, 1 oz.	80	6	3
CHEESE DIPS/SPREADS			
Alouette			
Crème Spreadable Cheese			
Crème de Brie®, Fine Herbs, 1 oz.	90	8	0
Crème de Havarti™, Garlic & Herb, 1 oz.	70	7	1
Crème de Swiss™, Original, 1 oz.	80	7	1
Elégante®			
Roasted Garlic & Pesto, 1 oz.	100	9	2
Roasted Peppers & Olive Tapenade, 1 oz.	100	9	2
Sundried Tomatoes & Garlic, 1 oz.	100	9	2
Reserve™ Spreadable Cheese			
Original, 1 oz.	70	6	1
Vidalia Onion, 1 oz.	70	6	2
Spreadable Cheese			
Light Garlic & Herbs, 1 oz.	50	4	2
Savory Vegetable, 1 oz.	70	6	1
Sundried Tomato & Basil, 1 oz.	80	7	1
Cheese Whiz			
Light, 1 oz.	80	4	6
Original, 1 oz.	90	7	4
Salsa Con Queso, 1 oz.	90	7	4
Philadelphia Cream Cheese			
Cream Cheese			
Cream Swirls Peaches 'N Cream, 1 oz.	91	7	5
Fat Free, 1 oz.	30	0	2

CHEESE	Cal	Fat	Cbs
Light, 1 oz.	70	5	2
Original, 1 oz.	100	10	1
Regular, 1 oz.	90	9	2
Salmon, 1 oz.	90	8	2
Whipped, 1 oz.	60	6	1
Rondele			
Bagel Temptations			
Garden Vegetable, 1 oz.	80	8	1
• Original Plain, 1 oz.	110	10	1
Strawberry, 1 oz.	90	8	4
Dairy Box			
Blue Cheese, 1 oz.	80	8	1
Garden Vegetable, 1 oz.	70	7	1
Lite Garlic & Herbs, 1 oz.	60	5	2
Deli Cup			
Garden Vegetable, 1 oz.	70	7	1
Garlic & Herbs, 1 oz.	70	7	1
Toasted Onion, 1 oz.	70	7	2
Pub Cheese			
Cheddar Horseradish, 1 oz.	70	7	1
Sharp Cheddar, 1 oz.	80	7	1
Zesty Salsa, 1 oz.	30	6	1
Smart Balance			
Light Cream Cheese Spread, 1 oz.	70	5	3
Regular Cream Cheese Spread, 1 oz.	90	6	2
SNACK DIP			
Athenos			
Artichoke & Garlic, 1 oz.	50	3	4
• Hummus Original, 1 oz.	50	3	5
Hummus Pesto, 1 oz.	50	3	5
• Roasted Eggplant, 1 oz.	45	2	5

CONDIMENTS, SPREADS & SPICES			
HORSERADISH			
Zatarain's			
Prepared Horseradish, 1 tbsp.	15	0	2
JALAPEÑOS AND PEPPERS			
B&G Foods			
Peppers			
• Hot Cherry Peppers Red & Green, 1 oz.	28	3	0
Hot Chopped Roasted Peppers, 1 oz.	5	0	1
Peperoncini, 1 oz.	10	0	2
Pepper Toppers			
• Sliced Hot Jalapeños, 1 oz.	0	0	1
Sweet Bell Pepper, 1 oz.	20	0	5

CONDIMENTS, SPREADS & SPICES	Cal	Fat	Cbs
Texas Pete			
Pepper Sauce, 1 tsp.	5	0	0
KETCHUP			
Annie's Naturals			
• Ketchup - Organic, 1 tbsp.	15	N/A	3
Del Monte			
Ketchup, 1 tbsp.	15	0	4
Quick Squeeze Ketchup, 1 tbsp.	15	0	4
Quick Squeeze Ketchup, 1 tbsp.	15	0	4
Heinz			
Ketchup 'With a Twist' Garlic, 4 oz.	97	0	22
Ketchup 'W/ a Twist' Sweet and Onion, 4 oz.	98	0	22
• Organic Tomato Ketchup, 4 oz.	113	0	26
Original Tomato Ketchup, 4 oz.	102	1	24
Reduced Sugar & Salt Tomato, 4 oz.	71	0	15
Muir Glen			
Tomato Ketchup, 1 tbsp.	20	0	4
MAYONNAISE			
Best Foods			
Mayonnaise			
Light Mayonnaise, 1 tbsp.	45	5	1
Real Mayonnaise, 1 tbsp.	90	10	0
Reduced Fat Dressing, 1 tbsp.	20	2	2
Other Favorites			
Tartar Sauce, 2 tbsp.	80	7	4
Hellman's			
Light Mayonnaise, 1 tbsp.	45	5	1
Lowfat Mayonnaise Dressing, 1 tbsp.	15	1	2
Mayonnaise w/ Ex. Virgin Olive Oil, 1 tbsp.	50	5	1
Real Mayonnaise, 1 tbsp.	90	10	0
Kraft Mayonnaise			
• Fat Free Dressing, 1 tbsp.	10	0	2
Light Mayonnaise, 1 tbsp.	40	4	2
• Real Mayonnaise Hot 'N Spicy, 1 tbsp.	100	11	0
Real Mayonnaise, 1 tbsp.	90	10	0
Smart Balance			
Omega Plus Light Mayonnaise, 1 tbsp.	50	5	2
MUSTARD			
Annie's Naturals			
Dijon Mustard - Organic, 1 tsp.	0	0	0
Honey Mustard - Organic, 1 tsp.	10	0	2
Yellow Mustard - Organic, 1 tsp.	0	0	0
Best Foods			
Deli Mustard, 1 tsp.	5	0	1
Dijonnaise™ Mustard, 1 tsp.	5	0	1

CONDIMENTS, SPREADS & SPICES

	Cal	Fat	Cbs
French's			
Bold N' Spicy Brown, 1 tsp.	5	0	0
• Classic Yellow®, 1 tsp.	0	0	0
Dijon, 1 tsp.	0	0	0
Sweet & Tangy Honey Mustard, 1 tsp.	10	0	1
Sweet 'N Zesty, 1 tsp.	5	0	1
Grey Poupon			
Country Dijon, 1 tsp.	5	0	0
Dijon, 1 tsp.	5	0	0
Hearty Spicy Brown, 1 tsp.	5	0	0
Mild & Creamy, 1 tsp.	0	0	1
Savory Honey, 1 tsp.	10	0	1
Hellman's			
Deli Mustard, 1 tsp.	5	0	1
Dijonnaise™ Mustard, 1 tsp.	5	0	1
Honey Mustard, 1 tsp.	10	0	2
Jack Daniel's			
Hickory Smoke Mustard, 1 tsp.	5	0	0
Honey Dijon, 1 tsp.	10	0	2
Horseradish Mustard, 1 tsp.	5	0	0
Olde No. 7 Mustard, 1 tsp.	5	0	0
Spicy Southwest Mustard, 1 tsp.	0	0	1
Stone Ground Dijon Mustard, 1 tsp.	5	0	0
Texas Pete			
• Honey Mustard, 3 tbsp.	45	0	11
Zatarain's			
Creole Mustard, 2 tsp.	10	1	1
PICKLES, RELISH & OLIVES			
B&G Foods			
Pickle Toppers			
Bread & Butter, 1 oz.	30	0	7
• Kosher Dill, 1 oz.	0	0	0
Pickles			
Dill, 1 oz.	0	0	0
Sweet Mixed, 1 oz.	35	0	9
Unsalted Kosher Dill, 1 oz.	10	0	2
Relish			
Dill Relish, 1 tbsp.	0	0	0
Sweet Relish, 1 tbsp.	15	0	4
Unsalted Relish, 1 tbsp.	20	0	5
Claussen Pickles			
Bread 'N Butter Chips, 2 tbsp.	20	0	4
Bread 'N Butter Slices, 2 tbsp.	5	0	5
Deli Style Kosher Dill Halves, 2 tbsp.	5	0	1

CONDIMENTS, SPREADS & SPICES	Cal	Fat	Cbs
Hearty Garlic Deli Style Slices, 2 tbsp.	5	0	1
Hearty Garlic Deli Style Wholes, 2 tbsp.	20	5	1
Pickle Relish - Sweet Squeeze, 1 tbsp.	10	0	3
Pickle Relish - Sweet, 1 tbsp.	15	0	3
Sweet Gherkins, 2 tbsp.	20	0	1
Del Monte			
Pickles			
Genuine Dill Halves, 2 tbsp.	5	0	1
Hamburger Dill Chips, 2 tbsp.	0	0	0
Sweet Pickle Chips, 2 tbsp.	40	0	10
• Sweet Pickles, 2 tbsp.	40	0	10
Tiny Kosher Dills, 2 tbsp.	5	0	1
Relish			
Hamburger Style Relish, 1 tbsp.	20	0	5
Hot Dog Style Relish, 1 tbsp.	15	0	4
Sweet Pickle Relish, 1 tbsp.	20	0	5
SALT & PEPPER			
Lawry's			
• Black Pepper Seasoned Salt, 1 g	0	0	0
Garlic Salt, 1 g	0	0	0
Lemon Pepper, 1 g	0	0	0
Seasoned Salt, 1 g	0	0	0
McCormick			
Asian Style Spiced Sea Salt, 1 g	0	0	0
Mediterranean Spiced Sea Salt, 1 g	0	0	0
Sicilian Sea Salt, 1 g	0	0	0
Pace Foods			
• Diced Green Chiles, 2 tbsp.	10	0	2
Jalapeños Nacho Sliced Peppers, 1 oz.	5	0	1
SANDWICH SPREADS			
Best Foods			
Sandwich Spread, 1 tbsp.	60	5	2
California Sun Dry			
Sun-Dried Tomato Spread, 2 tbsp.	50	3	N/A
Hellman's			
Sandwich Spread, 1 tbsp.	60	5	2
• Tartar Sauce, 2 tbsp.	80	7	4
Miracle Whip			
All-out Squeeze! Miracle Whip, 1 tbsp.	35	3	2
• Free Nonfat, 1 tbsp.	15	0	3
Light Super Easy Squeeze, 1 tbsp.	20	2	2
Super Easy Squeeze, 1 tbsp.	40	3	2

CONDIMENTS, SPREADS & SPICES	Cal	Fat	Cbs
SEASONING POWDER/MIXES			
Lawry's			
Meat Tenderizer			
• Original, 1 g	0	0	0
Seasoned, 1 g	0	0	0
Seasoning Mixes			
Enchilada Sauce, 6 g	20	0	4
Fajitas, 5 g	10	0	3
Guacamole, 2 g	0	0	1
Meat Loaf, 10 g	30	0	7
Sloppy Joes, 7 g	20	0	5
Taco, 5 g	15	0	3
McCormick			
Bag 'n Season			
Beef Stew, 5 g	15	0	1
Chicken, 6 g	20	0	3
Herb Roasted Pork Tenderloin, 3 g	5	0	0
Pot Roast, 3 g	10	0	1
Grill Mates			
Montreal Chicken Seasoning, 1 g	0	0	0
Montreal Steak Seasoning, 1 g	0	0	0
Salmon Seasoning, 1 g	0	0	0
Steamers			
Cheddar Cheese Veggie Steamers, 6 g	25	1	2
Garlic & Basil Veggie Steamers, 4 g	15	1	2
• Italian Herb Potato Steamers, 8 g	30	1	4
Rstd Garlic & Rosemary Potato Steamers, 8 g	30	1	4
Pace Foods			
Taco Seasoning Mix, 2 tbsp.	10	0	3
Taco Bell Home Originals			
Taco Seasoning Mix - Chipotle Flavor, 6 g	20	0	3
Taco Seasoning Mix - Original, 6 g	20	0	3
Zatarain's			
Boiled Seafood			
Crab & Shrimp Boil - Pro Boil, 1 oz	20	1	2
Seasoning and Spices			
Creole Seasoning, 1/4 tsp.	0	0	0
Pinto Bean Seasoning Mix, 1/2 cup prep	20	0	4
Red Bean Seasoning Mix, 1 tsp.	15	0	3
White Bean Seasoning Mix, 1 tsp.	15	0	3

DAIRY, FATS, & OILS			
BUTTER & MARGARINE			
Alta Dena			
• Salted Butter, 14 g	100	11	0

● MOST HEALTHY • LEAST HEALTHY

DAIRY, FATS, & OILS

	Cal	Fat	Cbs
Unsalted Sweet Butter, 14 g	100	11	0
Brummel & Brown			
• Spread, 14 g	45	5	0
Country Crock			
Limited Editions			
Cinnamon Apple, 11 g	60	6	2
Cinnamon Bluberry, 15 g	50	5	2
Cinnamon, 15 g	60	6	3
Maple, 15 g	60	6	3
Regular			
Churnstyle, 14 g	80	8	0
Plus Calcium And Vitamins, 14 g	50	5	0
Regular (Soft), 14 g	60	7	0
Spreadable Sticks, 14 g	60	7	0
Squeeze, 12 g	60	7	0
Spreads			
Omegaplus, 14 g	70	8	0
Spreadable Butter With Canolaoil, 11 g	80	9	0
Fleischmann's			
Light Margarine Sleeve, 1 tbs.	40	5	0
Olive Oil Sleeve, 1 tbs.	70	8	0
Original Margarine Sleeve, 1 tbs.	70	8	0
Parkay			
Light Margarine Sticks, 1 tbsp.	45	5	0
Margarine Sticks, 1 tbsp.	80	9	0
Soft Margarine Sleeve, 1 tbsp.	60	7	0
Smart Balance			
Butter Blends Sticks			
Stick Regular, 14 g	100	11	0
Unsalted with Omega-3, 14 g	100	11	0
Buttery Spreads With Flax Oil			
Light With Flax Oil, 14 g	45	5	0
Regular With Flax Oil, 14 g	80	9	0
Omega-3 Buttery Spreads			
Extra Virgin Olive Oil Light, 14 g	50	5	0
Extra Virgin Olive Oil, 11 g	60	7	0
Omega-3 Bundle Light, 14 g	50	5	0
Omega-3 Bundle, 13 g	80	9	0
Original Buttery Spreads			
37% Light Buttery Spread, 14 g	45	5	0
67% Buttery Spread, 14 g	80	9	0
Low Sodium Buttery Spread, 11 g	65	7	0
Organic Buttery Spread, 11 g	80	9	0

▶ DAIRY, FATS, & OILS

	Cal	Fat	Cbs
BUTTER ALTERNATIVES			
I Can't Believe It's Not Butter			
Calcium, 14 g	50	5	0
• Fat Free, 14 g	5	0	0
Light, 14 g	50	5	0
Mediterranean Blend Light, 14 g	50	5	0
Mediterranean Blend, 14 g	80	8	0
• Original, 14 g	80	8	0
COOKING OIL & SPRAYS			
American Roland Food Corporation			
• Grapeseed Oil, 14 g	130	14	0
Hazelnut Oil, 14 g	130	14	0
Olive Oil, 15 g	120	14	0
Sesame Oil, 14 g	120	14	0
Truffle Oil, 15 g	120	14	0
Annie's Naturals			
Basil Oil, 15 ml.	120	14	0
Dipping Oil (8.1 oz. Bottle), 15 ml.	40	14	0
Rstd Garlic Extra Virgin Olive Oil, 15 ml.	120	14	0
Canola Info			
Canola oil, 14 g	120	14	0
Pam			
Grilling Spray, 1/3 second spray	7	1	0
Olive Oil Spray, 1/3 second spray	7	1	0
Original Canola Spray, 1/3 second spray	7	1	0
• Vegetable Spray, 1/3 second spray	7	1	0
Planters			
Peanut Oil, 14 g	120	14	N/A
Smart Balance			
Cooking Spray, 1 g	0	0	0
Omega Cooking & Salad Oil, 14 g	120	14	0
Wesson			
Canola Oil, 1 tbsp.	120	14	0
Corn oil, 1 tbsp.	120	14	0
EGG NOG			
Alta Dena			
• Holiday Eggnog, 118 ml.	230	10	29
• Holiday Lite Eggnog, 118 ml.	170	4	29
Pumpkin Spice Eggnog, 120 ml.	230	10	29
EGGS			
Alta Dena			
• Eggs, 56 g	80	5	1
Egg Beaters			
• Egg Beaters Egg Whites, 46 g	25	0	1
Egg Beaters Original, 61 g	30	0	1

● MOST HEALTHY • LEAST HEALTHY

DAIRY, FATS, & OILS

	Cal	Fat	Cbs
Egg Beaters With Yolk, 61 g	40	2	1

HALF N HALF

Country Fresh

• Fat Free Half & Half, .5 oz.	20	0	3
Gourmet Half & Half, .5 oz.	35	4	1

Dean's

Fat Free Half & Half, 1 oz.	20	0	3
Gourmet Half & Half, 1 oz.	35	4	1

Land O'Lakes

Fat Half & Half, 1 oz.	20	0	3
Gourmet Half & Half, 1 oz.	35	4	1

LIGHT/REDUCED/FAT FREE SPREADS

Country Crock

Light (soft), 14 g	50	5	0
OmegaPlus Light, 14 g	50	5	0

MILK

Alta Dena

Chocolate Lowfat, 8 fl. oz.	200	3	32
• Chocolate Whole, 8 fl. oz.	260	9	37
Fat Free Milk, 8 fl. oz.	90	0	13
Half and Half, 1 fl. oz.	40	3	1
Reduced Fat Milk (2% Milkfat), 8 fl. oz.	130	5	13
Whole Milk, 8 fl. oz.	150	8	13

Carnation Milk

Evaporated Milk, 2 tbsp.	40	2	3
• Fat Free Evaporated Milk, 2 tbsp.	25	0	4
Instant Nonfat Dry Milk, 2 tbsp.	80	0	12
Lowfat 2% Evaporated Milk, 2 tbsp.	25	1	3
Sweetened Condensed Milk, 2 tbsp.	130	3	22

Country Fresh

1% Milk, 8 fl. oz.	100	3	13
1/2 % Milk, 8 fl. oz.	100	1	13
2% Milk, 8 fl. oz.	120	5	12
Skim Milk, 8 fl. oz.	90	0	13
Whole Milk, 8 fl. oz.	150	8	13

Dean's

1% Milk, 8 fl. oz..	100	3	13
2% Milk, 8 fl. oz.	120	5	12
Skim Milk, 8 fl. oz.	90	0	13
Whole Milk, 8 fl. oz.	150	8	12

Eagle Brand

Fat Free, 39 g	110	0	24
Lowfat Sweet Condensed Milk, 39 g	120	2	23
Original, 39 g	130	3	23

• MOST HEALTHY   • LEAST HEALTHY

DAIRY, FATS, & OILS

	Cal	Fat	Cbs
Land O'Lakes			
2% Milk, 8 fl. oz.	120	5	12
Skim Chocolate Milk, 8 fl. oz.	160	0	31
Skim Milk, 8 fl. oz.	90	0	13
Strawberry Milk, 8 fl. oz.	190	8	22
Whole Milk, 8 fl. oz.	150	8	12
Skinny Cow Milk			
2% Reduced Fat Choc Milk, 8 fl. oz.	150	0	26
Fat Free Whole Milk, 8 fl. oz.	110	0	17
Smart Balance			
1% Lowfat Choc Milk, 8 fl.oz.	150	1	26
1% Lowfat Milk, 8 fl.oz.	130	3	14
Lactose-Free Fat Free Milk, 8 fl.oz.	100	1	13
MILK ALTERNATIVES			
Blue Diamond Almonds			
Original Almond Breeze			
• Chocolate, 8 fl.oz.	110	3	22
Original, 8 fl.oz.	60	3	8
Vanilla, 8 fl.oz.	90	3	16
Unsweetened Almond Breeze			
Chocolate - Unsweetened, 8 fl.oz.	45	4	3
Original - Unsweetened, 8 fl.oz.	40	3	2
Vanilla - Unsweetened, 8 fl.oz.	40	3	2
Taste the Dream			
Almond Dream Original, 8 fl.oz.	50	3	6
• Almond Dream Unsweetened, 8 fl.oz.	30	3	1
NON DAIRY CREAMERS			
Cremora			
Original, 2 g	10	1	1
• Lite & Creamy, 2 g	10	0	1
International Delight			
Amaretto Bottles, 15 ml.	40	2	7
Chocolate Caramel, 15 ml.	45	2	7
Chocolate Cream, 13 ml.	35	2	6
Dulce de Leche, 15 ml.	45	2	7
French Vanilla Bottles, 15 ml.	45	2	7
• Vanilla Hazelnut, 15 ml.	45	2	7
Silk Soymilk			
French Vanilla, 15 ml.	20	1	3
Hazelnut, 15 ml.	20	1	3
Original, 15 ml.	15	1	1
RICE MILK			
Taste the Dream			
Rice Dream® Refrigerated			
• Enriched Original, 8 fl.oz.	120	3	23

• MOST HEALTHY • LEAST HEALTHY

DAIRY, FATS, & OILS	Cal	Fat	Cbs
Enriched Vanilla, 8 fl.oz.	130	3	26
Rice Dream® Shelf Stable			
• Enriched Chocolate, 8 fl.oz.	160	3	34
Original, 8 fl.oz.	120	3	24
Vanilla, 8 fl.oz.	130	3	27
SOUR CREAM			
Alouette			
Cuisine™, Crème Fraîche, 28 g	110	11	1
Reserve™, 28 g	100	8	1
Alta Dena			
• Creme Fraiche, 28 g	110	11	1
Light Sour Cream (2% Milkfat), 30 g	60	5	1
Sour Cream (4% Milkfat), 30 g	60	5	1
Breakstone's			
Sour Cream - All Natural, 30 g	60	5	1
Sour Cream - Free Fat Free, 32 g	30	0	5
Sour Cream - Reduced Fat, 31 g	40	3	2
Country Fresh			
Fat Free Sour Cream, 30 g	20	0	3
Light Sour Cream, 30 g	40	3	2
Sour Cream, 30 g	60	6	2
Dean's			
• Fat Free Sour Cream, 30 g	20	0	3
Light Sour Cream, 30 g	40	3	2
Sour Cream, 30 g	60	6	2
Knudsen			
Fat Free, 32 g	30	0	5
Hampshire 100% Natural, 30 g	60	6	1
Light, 31 g	30	2	2
Land O'Lakes			
Sour Cream			
Fat Free Sour Cream, 30 g	20	0	3
Light Sour Cream, 30 g	40	3	2
Sour Cream, 30 g	60	6	2
SOY MILK			
8-th Continent			
Fat Free			
Original, 8 fl.oz.	60	0	8
Vanilla, 8 fl.oz.	70	0	11
Light			
Chocolate, 8 fl.oz.	90	2	12
• Original, 8 fl.oz.	50	2	2
Vanilla, 8 fl.oz.	60	2	5
Original			
Chocolate, 8 fl.oz.	140	3	22

• MOST HEALTHY   • LEAST HEALTHY

DAIRY, FATS, & OILS	Cal	Fat	Cbs
Original, 8 fl.oz.	80	3	7
Vanilla, 8 fl.oz.	100	3	11
Silk Soymilk			
Light			
Light Chocolate, 8 fl.oz.	120	2	22
Light Plain, 8 fl.oz.	70	2	8
Light Vanilla, 8 fl.oz.	80	2	10
Unsweetened, 8 fl.oz.	80	4	4
Original			
Chocolate, 8 fl.oz.	140	4	23
Plain, 8 fl.oz.	100	4	8
Vanilla, 8 fl.oz.	100	4	10
Taste the Dream			
Soy Dream Refrigerated			
Classic Original, 8 fl.oz.	130	4	16
Enriched Original, 8 fl.oz.	100	4	9
Enriched Vanilla, 8 fl.oz.	120	4	14
Soy Dream Shelf Stable			
• Enriched Chocolate, 8 fl.oz.	150	4	21
Enriched Original, 8 fl.oz.	100	4	8
Enriched Vanilla, 8 fl.oz.	120	4	14
WHIPPED CREAM			
Alta Dena			
Heavy Whipping Cream, 6 g	50	5	0
• Whipped Light Cream, 6 g	15	1	1
Country Fresh			
Aersol Whipped Light Cream, 7 g	20	2	1
Heavy Whipping Cream, 7 g	50	5	0
Dean's			
Aersol Whipped Light Cream, 7 g	20	2	1
Heavy Wipping Cream, 7 g	50	5	0
Land O'Lakes			
Aerosol Whipped Light Cream, 7 g	20	2	1
• Heavy Whipping Cream, 7 g	50	5	0
YOGURT			
Alta Dena			
All Natural Yogurt			
Black Cherry, 8 oz.	220	2	41
Peach, 8 oz.	220	2	41
Strawberry Banana, 8 oz.	210	3	39
Lowfat Yogurt			
Plain, 8 oz.	170	5	20
Nonfat Yogurt			
Plain, 8 oz.	110	0	16
Strawberry, 8 oz.	181	0	36

DAIRY, FATS, & OILS

	Cal	Fat	Cbs
Vanilla, 8 oz.	160	0	30
Columbo Yogurt			
• Banana Strawberry, 8 oz.	230	2	47
Colombo Classic, 8 oz.	220	2	42
Fat Free Light Yogurt, 8 oz.	120	0	21
Lowfat Plain Flavour, 8 oz.	100	0	16
Lowfat Plain, 8 oz.	130	3	16
Lowfat French Vanilla, 8 oz.	180	3	32
Nonfat Vanila, 8 oz.	100	0	32
Strawberry, 8 oz.	190	3	33
Country Fresh			
Strawberry Lowfat Yogurt, 8 oz.	190	2	36
Strawberry Light Yogurt, 8 oz.	80	0	38
Dannon Light & Fit			
Carb & Sugar Control			
Blueberries & Cream, 4 oz.	60	3	3
Peaches & Cream, 4 oz.	60	3	3
Strawberries & Cream, 4 oz.	60	3	3
Vanilla & Cream, 4 oz.	60	3	3
Original			
• Blackberry, 6 oz.	60	0	10
Strawberry, 6 oz.	60	0	11
Vanilla, 6 oz.	60	0	10
White Chocolate Raspberry, 6 oz.	60	0	10
Land O'Lakes			
Strawberry Light Yogurt, 8 oz.	80	0	38
Strawberry Lowfat Yogurt, 8 oz.	190	2	36
Silk Soymilk			
Raspberry, 6 oz.	150	2	30
Strawberry, 6 oz.	160	2	31
Vanilla, 6 oz.	150	3	25

DELI FOODS

DELI MEATS

Empire Kosher

Deli Breasts			
Honey Smoked Turkey Breast, 2 oz.	45	0	3
Skinless All Natural Turkey Breast, 2 oz.	60	1	0
Smoked Turkey Breast, 2 oz.	45	0	0
Whole Turkey Pastrami, 2 oz.	70	4	0
Deli Slices			
Chicken Bologna, 2 oz.	80	6	1
Oven Prepared Turkey Breast, 2 oz.	50	0	1
Smoked Turkey Breast, 2 oz.	45	0	0
Turkey Salami, 2 oz.	90	5	0

• MOST HEALTHY   • LEAST HEALTHY

DELI FOODS

	Cal	Fat	Cbs
Farmer John			
• Premium Oven Roasted Turkey Brst, 1 oz.	25	0	1
Sliced Cotto Salami, 2 oz.	140	11	3
Sliced Thick Bologna, 2 oz.	160	14	2
Sliced Bologna, 2 oz.	160	14	2
Hebrew National			
Beef Bologna, 1 slice	90	8	0
• Beef Bologna Chubs, 2 oz.	180	17	0
Beef Salami, 2 oz.	160	15	0
Sliced Bologna, 1 slice	90	8	0
Sliced Salami, 3 slices	170	15	0
Oscar Mayer			
Bologna			
Bologna 98% Fat Free, 1 oz.	25	1	3
Bologna Beef, 1 oz.	90	8	1
Bologna Light, 1 oz.	60	4	2
Deli Fresh			
Chicken Breast Oven Roasted, 2 oz.	70	2	1
Ham Cooked, 1 oz.	30	1	0
Ham Honey Shaved, 2 oz.	50	1	2
Salami Beef Deli Thin, 2 oz.	150	13	1
Turkey Breast Smoked Shaved, 2 oz.	45	1	1
Turkey Breast Smoked, 2 oz.	60	1	0
Ham			
Ham Baked, 2 oz.	60	2	1
Ham Honey, 2 oz.	70	2	2
Ham Smoked 96% Fat Free, 2 oz.	50	1	0
Turkey			
Turkey Honey Smoked Lean White, 1 oz.	35	2	2
Turkey Oven Roasted White, 1 oz.	30	1	1
PACKAGED MEALS			
Carl Buddig			
Buddig Original Deli Pouches			
Beef, 2 oz.	90	5	1
Chicken, 2 oz.	110	7	1
Corned Beef, 2 oz.	90	5	1
Ham w/ Natural Juices, 2 oz.	120	7	1
• Honey Ham w/ Natural Juices, 2 oz.	120	7	3
Honey Turkey, 2 oz.	120	7	3
Oven-Roasted Turkey, 2 oz.	110	7	1
Pastrami, 2 oz.	90	5	1
Turkey, 2 oz.	110	7	1
Deli Cuts			
Baked Honey Ham, 2 oz.	80	3	3
Honey Roasted Cured Turkey Breast, 2 oz.	80	3	3

● MOST HEALTHY   • LEAST HEALTHY

DELI FOODS	Cal	Fat	Cbs
• Oven Roasted Cured Chicken Breast, 2 oz.	70	3	1
Oven Roasted Cured Turkey Breast, 2 oz.	70	3	1
Smoked Turkey Breast, 2 oz.	70	3	1
Original Big Pak Deli Pouches			
Beef, 2 oz.	90	5	1
Chicken, 2 oz.	85	5	1
Corned Beef, 2 oz.	90	5	1
Ham w/ NaturalJuices, 2 oz.	85	5	1
Honey Ham w/ Natural Juices, 2 oz.	90	5	2
Honey Turkey, 2 oz.	90	5	2
Oven-Roasted Turkey, 2 oz.	90	5	1
Turkey, 2 oz.	90	5	1
Value Pack Deli Pouches			
Beef, 2 oz.	90	5	1
Chicken, 2 oz.	85	5	1
Corned Beef, 2 oz.	90	5	1
Ham w/ Natural Juices, 2 oz.	85	5	1
Honey Ham w/ Natural Juices, 2 oz.	90	5	2
Honey Turkey, 2 oz.	90	5	2
Turkey, 2 oz.	90	5	1

SANDWICHES/WRAPS
Oscar Mayer
Deli Creations: Complete Sandwiches

	Cal	Fat	Cbs
• Oven Roasted Ham & Cheddar, 1 pk	460	16	51
Steakhouse Cheddar, 1 pk	430	140	47
Turkey & Cheddar Dijon, 1 pk	430	15	48
Turkey Monterey, 1 pk	450	17	50
Deli Creations: Flatbread Sandwich			
Buffalo Style Ranch Chicken, 1 pk	310	11	30
Chicken & Bacon Ranch, 1 pk	320	13	30
Fajita Beef & Salsa, 1 pk	280	9	34
Steakhouse Beef, 1 pk	330	14	30
Sun Dried Tomato Chicken, 1 pk	300	13	31

South Beach Living

	Cal	Fat	Cbs
Deli Ham & Turkey Ref. Wrap, 1 pk	220	10	23
Grilled Chicken Caesar Ref. Wrap, 1 pk	230	11	22
• Sesame Chicken Ref. Wrap, 1 pk	220	9	28
Southwestern Style Chkn Ref. Wrap, 1 pk	240	11	26
Turkey & Bacon Club Ref. Wrap, 1 pk	240	12	24

Tyson Chicken

	Cal	Fat	Cbs
Asiago Roast Beef Wrap , 1 pk.	320	14	30
South of the Border Chicken Wrap, 1 pk.	390	21	30
Turkey Club Wrap, 1 pk.	390	23	28

• MOST HEALTHY   • LEAST HEALTHY

DELI FOODS

SIDE DISHES	Cal	Fat	Cbs
Country Crock			
Seasonal Side Dishes			
Deluxe Cornbread Stuffing, 1/2 cup	150	5	22
Deluxe Homestyle Stuffing, 1/2 cup	150	5	22
Deluxe Mashed Sweet Potatoes, 1 cup	200	6	36
Side Dishes			
Deluxe Cheddar Broccoli Rice, 1 cup	270	11	35
• Deluxe Cinnamon Apples, 1/2 cup	130	3	26
• Deluxe Four Cheese Pasta, 1 cup	380	17	41
Deluxe Loaded Mashed Potatoes, 1 cup	200	11	22
Homestyle Mashed Potatoes, 1 cup	180	9	23

DESSERTS

CAKES	Cal	Fat	Cbs
Pepperidge Farm			
• Choco Coconut 3 Layer Cake, 1/8 cake	240	10	33
• Devil's Food 3 Layer Cake, 1/8 cake	220	9	34
Peppermint 3 Layer Cake, 1/8 cake	230	11	31
COOKIES			
100 Calorie Packs			
Cookie Crisps			
Alpha-bits Mini Cookies 6 Ct, 21 g	100	3	16
Chips Ahoy! 6 Ct, 23 g	100	3	18
Lorna Doone, 21 g	100	3	16
Planters Peanut Butter, 24 g	100	3	17
Variety Pack, 21 g	100	3	16
Chips Ahoy			
Big & Soft Chocolate Chunk, 39 g	170	7	27
Big & Soft Oatmeal Choc.Chunk, 39 g	180	8	26
Chewy Oatmeal Chocolate Chip, 27 g	120	6	18
Chewy, 27 g	120	6	18
Chocolate Chip Candy Blasts, 17 g	90	5	11
Chocolate Chip, 40 g	190	9	27
Chunky Chocolate, 17 g	80	5	11
Chunky White Fudge, 17 g	80	5	11
Mini Chocolate Chip Packs 2 Go!, 35 g	170	9	23
Peanut Butter Chunky, 17 g	90	5	10
Reduced Fat, 32 g	140	5	23
Famous Amos Cookies			
Chocolate Chip, 4 cookies	150	7	20
Oatmeal Raisin, 4 cookies	140	6	20
Peanut Butter Sandwich, 3 cookies	160	7	22
Vanilla Creme Sandwich, 4 cookies	170	7	25

DESSERTS	Cal	Fat	Cbs
Ginger Snaps			
Ginger Snaps, 28 g	120	3	23
Hershey Chocolates			
Caramel Cookies, 28 g	130	6	19
Hershey's With Almonds Cookies, 28 g	150	9	16
Sandwich Cookies, 28 g	130	6	1
Keebler			
Chips Deluxe			
Chocolate Lovers, 16 g	100	5	10
Original, 57 g	200	16	37
Peanut Butter Cups, 16 g	90	5	10
Soft 'n Chewy, 16 g	80	4	11
EL Fudge			
Double Stuffed, 35 g	180	9	24
Original, 18 g	90	4	13
Fudge Shoppe			
Caramel Filled, 30 g	160	8	20
Fudge Stripes, 21 g	150	7	21
Grasshopper, 29 g	140	7	19
Peanut Butter Filled, 30 g	170	10	16
Sandies			
Fudge Drops, 27 g	140	7	18
Simply Shortbread, 16 g	80	5	10
Vanilla Wafers			
Mini Vanilla Wafers, 30 g	140	6	21
Vanilla Wafers, 30 g	140	6	21
Mallomars			
Mallomars Cookies Pure Chocolate, 27 g	120	5	18
Mauna Loa			
Chocolate Chip, 28 g	150	9	17
Toffee Crunch, 28 g	150	9	17
Newtons			
Fig 100% Whole Grain, 37 g	130	3	26
Fig Newtons, 31 g	110	2	22
Fig Newtons Fat Free, 30 g	90	0	22
Fig Strawberry, 29 g	100	2	21
Nilla Wafers			
Mini, 30 g	140	6	21
Reduced Fat, 29 g	110	2	24
Wafers, 30 g	140	6	21
Nutter Butter			
Bites, 35 g	170	7	24
Bites - Milk Chocolate Covered PB, 36 g	180	9	24
Nutter Butter, 54 g	260	11	37
Sandwich Cookies, 28 g	130	6	19

● MOST HEALTHY   ● LEAST HEALTHY

DESSERTS

	Cal	Fat	Cbs
Oreo			
• Chocolate, 57 g	270	11	41
Double Stuffed, 42 g	210	10	30
Original Golden, 35 g	170	7	25
Original Oreo, 34 g	160	7	25
Pure White Fudge Covered, 20 g	100	5	13
Reduced Fat, 34 g	150	5	27
Pepperidge Farm			
Black & White Milano, 3 cookies	180	10	21
Chocolate Fudge Pirouettes, 2 wafers	120	4	18
Chocolate Petite Truffle, 5 cookies	180	12	15
Dark Chocolate Drenched Milano, 1 cookie	90	6	10
French Vanilla Pirouettes, 2 wafers	120	5	18
Geneva Cookies, 3 cookies	160	9	19
Milano Cookies, 3 cookies	180	10	21
Mini Butter Cookies, 9 cookies	140	6	21
Mint Brussels Cookies, 3 cookies	190	10	22
Orange Milano Cookies, 2 cookies	130	7	16
Soft Baked Milk Chocolate, 1 cookie	150	7	21
Sugar Free Milano, 3 cookies	170	9	21
Tahiti Cookies, 2 cookies	170	10	17
Sargento			
Chocolate Dip & Cookie Sticks, 28 g	130	6	18
S'mores, 22 g	110	6	14
Strawberry Dip & Cookie Sticks, 28 g	130	5	19
Snack Wells			
• Devil's Food Fat Free, 7 oz.	50	0	12
Cakes Chocolate Mint, 7 oz.	50	1	12
Cookies Creme Sandwich, 8 oz.	110	3	20
Lemon Creme Sugar Free, 7 oz.	130	6	23
Shortbread Sugar Free, 7 oz.	130	6	21
Sorbee			
Animal Cookies, 28 g	100	3	21
Chocolate Chip, 25 g	110	6	16
Chocolate Sandwich Cookies, 25 g	110	5	19
Lemon Sandwich Cookies, 25 g	120	5	18
Oatmeal, 25 g	110	4	10
Peanut Butter, 25 g	110	7	10
South Beach Living			
Hazelnut Crème Wafer Sticks, 22 g	100	6	10
Peanut Butter Wafer Sticks, 22 g	100	6	10
Stauffer's			
Breakfast Animal Cookies, 1 oz.	140	6	21
Chocolate Chip Animal Cookies, 1 oz.	140	5	22
Cotton Candy Animal Cookies, 1 oz.	140	4	23

● MOST HEALTHY   • LEAST HEALTHY

DESSERTS

	Cal	Fat	Cbs
Lightly Iced Animal Cookies, 1 oz.	130	2	23
Assorted Cookies			
Coconut Crisps, 1 oz.	140	5	22
Ginger Snaps Bag, 1 oz.	120	4	22
Iced Animal Cookies, 2 oz.	210	6	38
Shortbread Cookies, 1 oz.	150	7	20
Snickerdoodles Box, 1 oz.	130	5	19
Sandwich Cremes			
Banana Sandwich Crèmes, 1 oz.	150	6	23
Chocolate Sandwich Crèmes, 1 oz.	150	5	23
Peanut Butter Sandwich Crèmes, 1 oz.	130	5	21
Strawberry Sandwich Crèmes, 1 oz.	150	6	23
Vanilla Sandwich Crèmes, 1 oz.	160	6	24
Sugar Wafers			
Chocolate Sugar Wafers, 1 oz.	160	9	22
Strawberry Sugar Wafers, 1 oz.	140	8	17
Vanilla Sugar Wafers, 1 oz.	140	8	17

ICE CREAM CAKES & PIES

Baskin Robbins

	Cal	Fat	Cbs
Roll Ice Cream Cakes			
Mint Choc Chip Ice Crm/Choc, 4 oz.	290	14	36
• Vanilla Ice Crm/Choc, 4 oz.	270	14	39
Round Ice Cream Cakes			
• Choc Chip Cookie Dough Ice Crm/Devil's Food 6"	460	23	59
Pralines 'n Cream Ice Crm/Wht Sponge 9"	430	20	65
Vanilla & Choc Ice Crm/Fudge Crunch 9"	340	18	41
Sheet Ice Cream Cakes			
Pralines 'n Cream Ice Crm/Wht Sponge, 4 oz.	360	16	49
Vanilla & Choc Ice Crm/Fudge Crunch, 4 oz.	330	18	40
Very Strwbry Ice Crm/Wht Sponge, 4 oz.	310	13	44

ICE CREAM CONES & CUPS

Comet Ice Cream Cones

	Cal	Fat	Cbs
Ice Cream cups, 1 cup	20	0	4
Sugar Cones, 1 cone	50	0	11

Keebler

	Cal	Fat	Cbs
Fudge Shoppe Cups, 8 g	35	2	6
• Ice Cream Cups, 5 g	15	0	4
Sugar Cones, 13 g	50	1	10
Waffle Cones, 12 g	50	1	10

Oreo

	Cal	Fat	Cbs
• Chocolate Ice Cream Cones 12 Ct., 14 g	60	1	12

ICE CREAM, SORBET & SNACKS

Baskin Robbins

	Cal	Fat	Cbs
Cappuccino Blasts® (Medium)			
Caramel, 24 fl.oz.	720	24	121

• MOST HEALTHY   • LEAST HEALTHY

DESSERTS	Cal	Fat	Cbs
Mocha, 24 fl.oz.	240	18	87
Oreo® N' Cookies, 24 fl.oz.	800	31	118
Fruit Blast Bars			
Blue Raspberry Fruit Blast Bar, 1.75 fl.oz.	50	0	14
Mango Fruit Blast Bar, 1.75 fl.oz.	50	0	14
Strawberry Fruit Blast Bar, 1.75 fl.oz.	50	0	13
Grab-N-Go			
Choc Chip Cookie Dough Ice Crm, 3 oz.	200	10	23
Chocolate Ice Crm, 3 oz.	70	9	21
Jamoca® Almond Fudge Ice Crm, 3 oz.	180	10	21
Ice Cream: Classic Flavors			
French Vanilla Ice Cream, 4 oz.	280	18	26
Jamoca® Ice Cream, 4 oz.	240	13	26
Rocky Road Ice Cream, 4 oz.	290	15	36
Lighter Side: Lowfat, No Sugar Added			
Berries 'n Banana, 4 oz.	110	2	25
Chocolate Chocolate Chip, 4 oz.	150	5	31
Pineapple Coconut, 4 oz.	120	2	27
Nonfat Soft Serve Yogurt - No Sugar Added			
Truly Free® Cafe Mocha NF Sft Srv, 3 oz.	90	0	18
Truly Free® Chocolate, 3 oz.	80	0	15
Truly Free® Vanilla, 3 oz.	90	0	17
Shakes			
Chocolate Oreo® Shake Medium, 24fl.oz.	1350	69	172
Strawberry Shake Medium, 24fl.oz	650	19	104
Vanilla Shake Medium, 24 fl.oz.	980	45	125
Sherbet			
Rainbow Sherbet, 4 oz.	160	2	34
Rock 'n Pop Swirl Sherbet, 4 oz.	190	4	37
Wild 'N Reckless Sherbet, 4 oz.	160	2	33
Sundaes			
Banana Royale Sundae, 11 fl. oz.	630	27	91
Oreo® Sundae, 12 fl. oz.	1030	47	147
• Peppermint Brownie Sundae, 12 fl. oz	1580	75	221
Sundae cups			
Oreo® Sundae cup, 1 cup	330	15	45
Pralines 'n Cream Sundae Cup, 1 cup	330	16	43
Reese's® PB Sundae Cup, 1 cup	390	24	36
Ben & Jerry's			
Bars			
Cherry Garcia® Original Ice Cream, 1 bar	270	19	29
Vanilla Almond Original Ice Cream, 1 bar	340	23	30
Vanilla Original Ice Cream, 1 bar	300	20	26
Body & Soul™			
Cherry Garcia®, 1/2 cup	170	9	22

• MOST HEALTHY   • LEAST HEALTHY

DESSERTS

	Cal	Fat	Cbs
Choc Chip Cookie Dough, 1/2 cup	190	9	26
Chocolate Fudge Brownie™, 1/2 cup	180	7	25
Lowfat Frozen Yogurt			
Black Raspberry, 1/2 cup	140	2	28
Cherry Garcia®, 1/2 cup	170	3	32
Chocolate Fudge, 1/2 cup	190	3	35
Lowfat, 1/2 cup	170	3	33
Half Baked®, 1/2 cup	190	3	35
Vanilla Low, 1/2 cup	130	2	25
Novelties			
Wich Ice Cream Cookie Sandwich™	350	18	45
Organic Ice Cream			
Chocolate Fudge Brownie™, 1/2 cup	270	13	30
Strawberry, 1/2 cup	210	12	21
Sweet Cream & Cookies, 1/2 cup	250	15	24
Vanilla Organic Ice Cream, 1/2 cup	220	14	18
Original Ice Cream			
Black & Tan™, 1/2 cup	230	13	24
Chubby Hubby®, 1/2 cup	330	20	31
Oatmeal Cookie Chunk, 1/2 cup	270	15	31
Sorbet			
Berried Treasure™, 1/2 cup	110	0	29
Berry Berry Extraordinary™, 1/2 cup	100	0	27
Jamaican Me Crazy, 1/2 cup	130	0	33
Mango Lime, 1/2 cup	100	0	27
Strawberry Kiwi, 1/2 cup	110	0	27
Strawberry Kiwi Swirl, 1/2 cup	110	0	28
Blue Bunny Ice Cream			
Classics: Gelato			
Gelato Chocolate, 89 g	180	8	24
Gelato Hazelnut, 89 g	170	7	23
Gelato Italian Chocolate Chip, 64 g	130	7	16
Classics: Original			
Original Ice Cream Mint Chip, 66 g	140	7	17
Original Ice Cream Neapolitan, 66 g	130	6	16
Original Ice Cream Strawberry, 66 g	120	6	17
Classics: Premium			
All Natural Vanilla, 72 g	160	9	16
Double Strawberry, 74 g	140	6	20
Homemade Chocolate, 69 g	150	7	16
Lighter Options: Ice Cream			
Peanut Butter Fudge, 69 g	150	10	15
Rocky Road, 71 g	130	6	21
Vanilla, 69 g	110	5	16

● MOST HEALTHY   ● LEAST HEALTHY

▶ DESSERTS	Cal	Fat	Cbs
Lighter Options: Bars			
Sweet Freedom® Fudge Lites, 101 g	70	1	17
• Sweet Freedom® Sugar Free Pops, 53 g	15	0	7
Sweet Freedom® Supremes® PB cup, 55 g	160	11	17
Lighter Options: NSA, Fat Free Ice Cream			
Brownie Sundae, 74 g	90	0	23
Caramel Toffee Crunch, 71 g	90	0	24
Vanilla, 71 g	80	0	20
Lighter Options: No Sugar Added, Fat Free Bars			
FrozFruit® Chunky Strawberry, 90 g	35	0	15
Health Smart® Rasp. & Orange Crème Bars, 63 g	70	0	17
Sugar Free Bomb Pop®, 53 g	25	0	8
Lighter Options: Personals®			
Bunny Tracks®, 68 g	130	5	21
Double Strawberry, 69 g	100	2	19
Super Fudge Brownie®, 67 g	120	3	22
Lighter Options: 100 Calorie Bars			
English Toffee Ice Cream Bars, 39 g	100	8	10
Orange & Raspberry Ice Cream Bars, 1 Bar	100	1	19
Pecan Ice Cream Bars, 39 g	100	7	10
Lighter Options: Hi Lite			
Cookies & Cream, 65 g	130	4	21
Homemade Vanilla, 67 g	110	4	18
Vanilla, 65 g	100	3	17
Lighter Options: Fat Free: Novelties			
FrozFruit® Chunky Strawberry, 90 g	70	0	18
FrozFruit® Double Lime, 120 g	90	0	22
FrozFruit® Superfruit® Rspbry Acai, 90 g	60	0	15
Lighter Options: Fat Free: Frozen Yogurt			
Brownie Fudge Fantasy, 74 g	110	0	24
Homemade Vanilla, 74 g	100	0	19
Strawberry Cheesecake, 74 g	100	0	21
Yogurt Varieties: Light No Sugar Added			
Black Cherry Burst, 170 g	80	0	11
Blueberry Bliss, 170 g	80	0	12
Key Lime Pie, 170 g	80	0	11
Yogurt Varieties: Light Superfruit			
Black Currant, 170 g	100	0	14
Mango Pomegranate, 170 g	100	0	14
Pomegranate Cherry, 170 g	100	0	14
Yogurt Varieties: Light Omega 3			
Blackberry Crème, 113 g	80	1	14
Raspberry Crème, 113 g	80	1	14
Strawberry Patch, 113 g	80	1	14

• MOST HEALTHY   • LEAST HEALTHY

DESSERTS

	Cal	Fat	Cbs
Yogurt Varieties: Light			
Key Lime Pie, 170 g	100	0	15
Strawberry Sensation, 170 g	100	0	15
Vanilla Crème, 170 g	100	0	16
Country Fresh			
Ice Cream			
Light Vanilla Ice Cream, 65 g	100	3	17
Orange Sherbet, 90 g	130	2	28
Vanilla Ice Cream, 68 g	150	8	17
Dean's			
Light Vanilla Ice Cream, 65 g	100	3	17
Orange Sherbet, 90 g	130	2	28
Vanilla Ice Cream, 68 g	150	8	17
Dreyer's Ice Cream			
Dibs			
Rocky Road w/ Choc Almond Coating, 26 pcs	400	29	29
Strawberry w/ Choc Coating, 26 pcs	370	26	30
Vanilla w/ NESTLÉ CRUNCH® Coating, 26 pcs	370	26	30
Fruit Bars			
Creamy Coconut, 1 Bar	120	3	21
Grape, 1 Bar	80	0	20
Strawberry, 1 Bar	120	N/A	29
Grand			
Chocolate, 1/2 cup	150	8	17
Coffee, 1/2 cup	140	8	15
Mint Chocolate Chip, 1/2 cup	170	9	18
Vanilla, 1/2 cup	150	10	14
Light			
Double Fudge Brownie, 1/2 cup	120	4	120
French Vanilla, 1/2 cup	100	4	15
Peanut Butter cup, 1/2 cup	130	6	17
Strawberry, 1/2 cup	110	3	18
Loaded			
Butter Finger, 1/2 cup	130	5	19
Chocolate Chip Cookie Dough, 1/2 cup	130	5	21
Cookies 'N Cream, 1/2 cup	110	4	18
No Sugar Added			
Butter Pecan, 1/2 cup	120	5	15
French Vanilla, 1/2 cup	100	3	14
Neapolitan, 1/2 cup	90	3	13
Triple Chocolate, 1/2 cup	110	4	17
Sherbet			
Berry Rainbow, 1/2 cup	130	2	29
Orange Cream, 1/2 cup	120	2	23
Swiss Orange, 1/2 cup	150	3	30

● MOST HEALTHY   ● LEAST HEALTHY

DESSERTS	Cal	Fat	Cbs
Yogurt Blends			
Berry Granola Crunch, 1/2 cup	120	4	19
Cappuccino Chip, 1/2 cup	110	4	18
Chocolate Fudge Brownie, 1/2 cup	120	4	19
Peach, 1/2 cup	100	2	17
Edy's Ice Cream			
Grand			
French Vanilla, 1/2 cup	151	9	16
Real Strawberry, 1/2 cup	130	6	16
Rocky Road, 1/2 cup	170	10	19
Spumoni, 1/2 cup	120	5	19
Light			
Cookie Dough, 1/2 cup	130	5	20
French Vanilla, 1/2 cup	100	4	15
Raspberry Chip Royale, 1/2 cup	120	4	18
Strawberry, 1/2 cup	110	3	18
No Sugar Added			
Coffee, 1/2 cup	90	3	13
Cookies 'N Cream, 1/2 cup	120	5	16
French Vanilla, 1/2 cup	100	3	14
Triple Chocolate, 1/2 cup	110	4	17
Yogurt Blends			
Berry Granola Crunch, 1/2 cup	120	4	19
Cappuccino Chip, 1/2 cup	110	4	18
Strawberry, 1/2 cup	100	3	17
Eskimo Pie			
Nestle Crunch Crisp & Butterfinger, 2 bars	250	17	21
Vanilla & Chocolate Snack Pack, 2 bars	200	16	18
Vanilla with Dark Chocolate Coating, 1 bar	160	11	14
Vanilla with Nestle Crunch Coating, 1 bar	210	14	18
Haagen-Dazs			
Bar			
Raspberry Sorbet & Vanilla Yogurt, 71 g	100	0	21
Vanilla & Almonds, 87 g	320	12	22
Vanilla & Milk Chocolate, 83 g	290	21	22
Classic Flavor			
Chocolate Peanut Butter, 109 g	360	24	27
Dulce De Leche, 106 g	290	17	28
Pineapple Coconut, 95 g	230	13	25
Frozen Yogurt			
Vanilla, 106 g	200	5	31
Vanilla Raspberry Swirl, 108 g	170	3	32
Wildberry, 106 g	180	2	34
Light			
Caramel Cone, 110 g	250	8	39

● MOST HEALTHY   ● LEAST HEALTHY

DESSERTS	Cal	Fat	Cbs
Dutch Chocolate, 106 g	190	5	33
Mint Chip, 109 g	230	8	34
Reserve			
Brazilian Açaí Berry Sorbet, 106 g	120	2	25
Pom & Dk Choco Ice Cream Bars, 84 g	280	18	27
Tst Coconut Sesame Brittle Ice Crm, 102 g	300	18	31
Sorbet			
Coconut, 106 g	170	7	26
Mango, 114 g	120	0	37
Raspberry, 105 g	120	0	30

Healthy Choice

	Cal	Fat	Cbs
Lowfat Fudge Bar, 1 bar	90	2	15
Sorbet Cream Bar, 1 bar	90	1	17
Vanilla Ice Cream Sandwich, 1 Sandwich	130	2	25

Kool Aid

	Cal	Fat	Cbs
Kool Pops Freezer Bars - Variety, 85 g	50	0	13

Land O'Lakes

Ice Cream	Cal	Fat	Cbs
Light Vanilla Ice Cream, 65 g	100	3	17
Orange Sherbet, 90 g	130	2	28
Vanilla Ice Cream, 68 g	150	8	17

M&M's Bakery

M&M'S Brand Ice Cream	Cal	Fat	Cbs
Cookie Dough Ice Cream, 1/2 cup	180	90	20
Cookie Ice Cream Sandwiches, 1 Sndwch	260	110	34
Ice Cream Cake, 4 fl.oz.	240	120	28
Ice Cream Cone, 79 g	250	110	33
Ice Cream Treats, 49 g	190	130	13

Taste the Dream

Rice Dream® Non-Dairy Frozen Desserts - Novelties	Cal	Fat	Cbs
Chocolate Frozen Pies, 96 g	330	19	40
Mocha Frozen Pies, 96 g	330	19	40
Vanilla Bars with Chocolate Coating, 85 g	230	15	24
Rice Dream® Non-Dairy Frozen Desserts			
Strawberry, 80 g	160	8	Cbs
Vanilla Swiss Almond, 70 g	190	10	24
Vanilla, 70 g	150	6	23
Soy Dream® Non-Dairy Frozen Desserts			
Butter Pecan Pint, 70 g	150	9	19
Chocolate Quart, 70 g	120	6	17
Strawberry Swirl Quart, 70 g	140	7	20
Soy Dream® Non-Dairy Frozen Novelties			
Chocolate Lil' Dreamers, 40 g	100	5	15
Vanilla Lil' Dreamers, 40 g	100	4	15

● MOST HEALTHY   ● LEAST HEALTHY

DESSERTS	Cal	Fat	Cbs
Tropicana Juice			
Cherry Berry, 40 g	140	0	36
Orange Citrus, 40 g	140	0	36
Strawberry, 40 g	140	0	36
Smuckers			
Magic Shell			
Caramel, 34 g	220	17	14
Welch's			
Concord Grape No Sugar Added, 2 fl.oz.	30	0	8
Concord Grape, 3 fl.oz.	90	0	22
Strawberry Breeze - NSA, 2 fl.oz.	25	0	6
Strawberry Breeze, 2 fl.oz.	50	0	13
Wild Berry - No Sugar Added, 2 fl.oz.	25	0	6
Wild Berry, 2 fl.oz.	50	0	13
ICE CREAM TOPPINGS			
Smuckers			
Magic Shell			
• Caramel, 34 g	220	17	14
Chocolate, 34 g	210	16	17
Smores, 36 g	220	16	19
Turtle Delight, 34 g	210	15	17
Microwaveable Ice Cream Topping			
Chocolate Fudge, 40 g	130	2	28
Hot Fudge, 30 g	120	4	22
Specialty Ice Cream Topping			
Dove® Milk Chocolate, 38 g	130	4	21
Special Recipe Butterscotch Caramel, 42 g	140	1	31
Special Recipe Hot Fudge, 38 g	130	5	20
Special Recipe Triple Berry, 2 tbsp.	90	0	23
Spoonable Ice Cream Topping			
Butterscotch, 41 g	120	0	30
Dark Chocolate with Mint, 39 g	110	2	24
Dulce de Leche, 41 g	150	5	26
Hot Caramel, 41 g	140	4	27
Hot Fudge, 39 g	130	5	22
Light Hot Fudge, 39 g	90	0	23
Marshmallow, 40 g	110	28	28
Pecans in Syrup, 36 g	160	9	19
Strawberry, 40 g	100	0	26
Walnuts in Syrup, 36 g	150	7	20
Sugar Free Ice Cream Topping			
Caramel, 38 g	90	0	24
Hot Fudge, 38 g	90	0	24
• Strawberry, 33 g	25	0	9

• MOST HEALTHY   • LEAST HEALTHY

DESSERTS

	Cal	Fat	Cbs
PUDDING & GELATIN			
Snack Pack			
Banana Pudding, 1 pudding cup	110	4	19
Butterscotch Pudding, 1 pudding cup	120	4	21
Choco Butterscotch Pudding, 1 pud cup	130	5	22
Chocolate Pudding, 1 pudding cup	120	4	21
Fat Free Choco Pudding, 1 pudding cup	90	0	20
Fat Free Vanilla Pudding, 1 pudding cup	80	0	18
NSA Cherry Gels , 1 pudding cup	10	0	2
NSA Chocolate Pudding, 1 pudding cup	60	3	8
NSA Vanilla Pudding, 1 pudding cup	60	4	8
Strawberry Gelatin Gels, 1 Gel cup	5	0	2
• Strwbry Orange Gelatin Gels, 1 Gel cup	100	0	25
Tapioca Pudding, 1 pudding cup	120	4	20
Vanilla Pudding, 1 pudding cup	120	4	20
Swiss Miss			
Choco/vanilla Swirl Pudding, 1 cup	140	4	27
Classic Butterscotch Pudding, 1 cup	130	4	22
Creamy Milk Choco Pudding, 1 cup	150	4	27
Old Fashioned Tapioca Pudding, 1 cup	140	4	24
Triple Choco Dream Pudding, 1 cup	150	4	26
PUDDING & GELATIN MIX			
Uncle Ben's			
• Cinnamon & Raisins Rice Pudding, 42 g	160	1	37
• French Vanilla Rice Pudding, 33 g	120	0	28
WHIPPED TOPPINGS			
Cool Whip			
• Chocolate, 2 tbsp.	25	2	2
• French Vanilla, 2 tbsp.	25	2	2
Extra Creamy, 2 tbsp.	25	2	2
Regular, 2 tbsp.	25	2	2
Strawberry, 2 tbsp.	25	2	2
Sugar Free, 2 tbsp.	25	1	3
Topping - Lite, 2 tbsp.	20	1	3
Dream Whip			
• Whipped Topping Mix, 1 tbsp.	10	0	2

FROZEN MEALS

	Cal	Fat	Cbs
APPETIZERS & SIDES			
Cascadian Farm			
• Potatoes Country-Style Potatoes, 3 oz.	40	0	9
Potatoes Country-Style, 3 oz.	50	0	12
Potatoes Crinkle Cut French Fries, 3 oz.	130	4	21
Potatoes French Fries Straight Cut, 3 oz.	130	4	21
Potatoes Hash Browns, 3 oz.	60	0	14

• MOST HEALTHY   • LEAST HEALTHY

FROZEN MEALS	Cal	Fat	Cbs
Potatoes Oven Fries Wedge Cut, 3 oz.	110	3	21
Potatoes Shoe String Fries, 3 oz.	140	5	21
Potatoes Spud Puppies, 3 oz.	160	7	23
Empire Kosher			
Breaded Chicken Tenders, 3 oz.	220	3	26
Chicken Nuggets, 3 oz.	230	7	26
Frozen Appetizers			
Large Egg Rolls, 85 g	110	5	15
Mini Egg Rolls, 85 g	110	5	15
Mini Stuffed Cabbage, 113 g	90	2	9
Potato Pancakes, 56 g	120	5	19
Frozen Blintzes			
Apple Raisin Blintzes, 61 g	80	2	16
Blueberry Blintzes, 61 g	90	1	18
Cheese Blintzes, 61 g	80	2	13
Cherry Blintzes, 61 g	100	1	18
Potato Blintzes, 61 g	90	4	15
Green Giant			
Boxed Baby Brussels Sprouts & Butter, 4 oz.	60	1	9
Boxed Broccoli Spears & Butter, 4 oz.	40	2	6
Boxed Broccoli & Zesty Cheese, 4 oz.	60	2	8
Boxed Cheesy Rice & Broccoli, 4 oz.	270	5	50
Boxed Creamed Spinach, 4 oz.	70	3	9
Boxed Rstd Potatoes w/ Broccoli & Chz, 4 oz.	110	3	18
Boxed Shoepeg White Corn & Butter Sauce, 4 oz.	110	2	22
Jimmy Dean			
Pancakes & Ssg Minis: Blbry Sand, 72 g	260	18	19
Pancakes & Sausage Minis: Original, 72 g	260	18	19
Pancakes & Ssg On A Stick: Blbry, 71 g	230	13	23
Pancakes & Ssg On A Stick: Original, 71 g	220	13	21
Morningstar Farms			
New Products			
Asian Veggie Patties, 67 g	100	4	10
Ginger Teriyaki Veggie Cakes, 68 g	110	2	19
Southwestern Style Veggie Cakes, 68 g	130	3	21
Snacks			
Veggie Bites Broccoli Cheddar, 85 g	190	10	16
Veggie Bites Mushroom Mozzarella, 85 g	190	10	16
Veggie Bites Spinach Artichoke, 85 g	190	10	16
Mrs. Paul's			
Crab Cakes			
Deviled Crab Cakes, 82 g	220	12	12
Fish Sticks			
Crisp & Healthy Brded Fish Sticks, 104 g	140	1	24
Crunchy Breaded Sticks, 95 g	220	10	22

● MOST HEALTHY   ● LEAST HEALTHY

FROZEN MEALS	Cal	Fat	Cbs
Original Breaded Sticks, 95 g	220	10	22
X-Large Fish Sticks, 96 g	220	11	22
Fish Tenders			
Battered Fish Tenders, 4 oz.	210	10	22
Beer Battered Tenders, 4 oz.	230	11	22
Popcorn Fish, 4 oz.	220	12	18
Select Cuts			
Fried Clams - 8 oz, 3 oz.	270	13	29
Fried Scallops - 7oz, 4 oz.	260	11	28
Lightly Breaded Flounder, 4 oz.	150	7	12
Lightly Breaded Tilapia, 4 oz.	240	11	17
Shrimp+Calamari			
Beer Battered Shrimp, 4 oz.	200	6	22
Breaded Popcorn Shrimp, 4 oz.	260	11	30
Butterfly Shrimp, 4 oz.	250	11	27
Fried Calamari, 4 oz.	270	13	26
Sweet Potatoes			
Candied Sweet Potatoes - 12 oz, 5 oz.	300	1	73
Candied Sweet Potatoes - 20 oz, 5 oz.	300	1	73
SeaPak			
Maryland Style Crab Cakes, 4 oz.	240	13	19
Butterfly Shrimp			
Brd Butterfly Shrimp - Ready To Fry, 4 oz.	150	1	22
Butterfly Shrimp - Oven Crunchy, 3 oz.	210	10	20
Gourmet Brd Shrimp - Ready To Fry, 4 oz.	170	2	23
Jumbo Butterfly Shrimp - Oven Crunchy, 3 oz.	210	10	20
Wild Amer Butterfly Shrimp - Oven Crunchy, 3 oz.	210	10	20
Popcorn Shrimp			
Firecracker Shrimp, 3 oz.	210	10	20
Jumbo Popcorn Shrimp, 3 oz.	210	10	20
Popcorn Shrimp, 3 oz.	210	10	20
Shrimp Poppers, 3 oz.	220	12	18
Shrimp Scampi			
• Butter and Garlic, Tails Off, 4 oz.	350	29	2
Italian Parmesan, Tails Off, 4 oz.	330	29	2
Restaurant-Style, Tails On, 4 oz.	310	29	4
Wild American, Tails Off, 4 oz.	330	29	2
Specialty Shrimp			
Coconut Shrimp, 4 oz.	310	14	36
Crispy Light Shrimp, 3 oz.	190	10	13
Garlic Herb Marinated Shrimp, 4 oz.	130	4	3
Italian Garlic Shrimp, 3 oz.	180	11	11
Shrimp Alfredo, 3 oz.	210	15	5
Tempura Shrimp, 4 oz.	240	8	35

FROZEN MEALS

	Cal	Fat	Cbs
Simply Potatoes			
Homestyle Slices, 103 g	70	0	16
Red Potato Wedges, 81 g	50	0	10
Rosemary & Garlic Red Potato Wedges, 120 g	80	0	16
Tyson Chicken			
Frozen Bagged Items			
Any'tizers Pork Mini Ribs, 4 pieces	330	22	14
Fully Cooked Chicken Products			
Any'tizers BBQ Style Wings, 91 g	200	13	7
Any'tizers Buffalo Style Bnlss Wings, 84 g	150	7	8
Any'tizers Cheddar & Bacon Bites, 90 g	240	14	12
Any'tizers Homestyle Fries, 90 g	230	11	19
Any'tizers Mini Bites, 85 g	270	18	15
Buffalo Style Hot Wings, 96 g	220	15	1
Buffalo Style Popcorn Bites, 82 g	170	8	11
Chicken Nuggets, 92 g	280	18	16
Italian Style Meatballs, 84 g	180	11	6
Popcorn Bites™, 89 g	250	12	22
Southwest Seasoned Breast Strips, 84 g	110	3	2
Teriyaki Breast Fillets, 89 g	170	7	7
Teriyaki Flavored Wings, 90 g	200	12	4
Van de Kamp's			
Crisp Healthy			
C + H Breaded Fillets, 104 g	150	2	25
C + H Breaded Fish Sticks, 104 g	140	1	24
Fish Sticks			
Fish Sticks, 114 g	260	13	26
X-Large Sticks, 96 g	220	11	22
Shrimp + Calamari			
Beer Battered Shrimp, 113 g	200	6	22
Breaded Butterfly Shrimp, 113 g	250	11	27
Breaded Popcorn Shrimp, 113 g	260	11	30
Fried Calamari, 113 g	270	13	26
Tenders + Bites			
Battered Fish Tenders, 112 g	210	10	21
Breaded Popcorn Fish, 114 g	220	12	18
DINNERS & MEALS			
Banquet			
Crock Pot Classics			
Beef Stew, 2/3 cup	140	6	15
Herb Chicken & Rice, 2/3 cup	200	3	34
Stroganoff with Beef & Noodles, 2/3 cup	300	14	29
Dinners			
Pepperoni Pizza Meal, 1 Meal	550	29	57
Salisbury Steak Meal, 1 Meal	300	16	25

• MOST HEALTHY • LEAST HEALTHY

FROZEN MEALS	Cal	Fat	Cbs
Turkey Meal, 1 Meal	200	8	27
Hearty One			
Chicken Fried Steak, 1 Meal	750	42	66
Fried Chicken, 1 Meal	810	4	71
Turkey with Gravy, 1 Meal	430	16	43
Original			
Chicken Nuggets, 5 Nuggets	230	14	15
Crispy Chicken, 4 oz.	320	19	13
Pot Pies			
Beef Pot Pie, 1 Pie	450	27	36
Chicken Pot Pie, 1 Pie	370	21	34
Turkey Pot Pie, 1 Pie	390	21	36
Boca Meatless			
Wrap, Orig Sausage Egg Wh & Chz, 130 g	220	7	27
Wrap, S.W. Sausage Egg Wh & Chz, 130 g	200	7	25
Lasagna, Chky Tom & Hb w/ Boca Grd Bger, 298 g	290	5	42
Empire Kosher			
Chicken Continental, 177 g	300	10	38
Chicken Kiev, 117 g	590	43	24
Chicken Portobello, 177 g	370	17	27
Fully Cooked: Chicken			
Boneless Skinless Chicken Breasts, 84 g	250	7	26
Chkn Drumsticks & Thighs w/ Back Portions, 84 g	260	9	26
Split Chicken Breasts with Ribs, 84 g	250	7	26
Frozen Entrees			
Spaghetti & Meatballs, 369 g	400	13	48
Sweet & Sour Chicken Breast, 284 g	260	7	28
Teriyaki Turkey, 312 g	250	4	27
Turkey Meatloaf, 312 g	330	14	31
Frozen Meat Pies			
Frozen Chicken Pie, 227 g	460	23	43
Turkey Frozen Pie, 227 g	460	23	43
Farmer John			
Bacon, Egg & Cheese Burritos, 136 g	330	18	26
Sausage, Egg & Cheese Burritos, 136 g	350	21	28
S.W. Spicy Ssg, Egg & Chz Burritos, 136 g	350	21	28
Green Giant			
Boxed Rice Medley, 283 g	240	4	47
Boxed Rice Pilaf, 283 g	200	3	40
Boxed White & Wild Rice, 283 g	260	5	48
Complete Skillet Meal Chkn & Chsy Pasta, 227 g	250	5	39
Complete Skillet Meal Chkn Alfredo, 227 g	240	5	37
Complete Skillet Meal Garlic Chkn Pasta, 227 g	230	6	33
Create a Meal! Stir-Fry Sesame, 215 g	100	5	12
• Create A Meal! Stir-Fry Szechuan, 169 g	50	0	10

● MOST HEALTHY   ● LEAST HEALTHY

FROZEN MEALS	Cal	Fat	Cbs
Create A Meal! Stir-Fry Teriyaki, 170 g	50	0	11

Healthy Choice

	Cal	Fat	Cbs
Café Select Crmy Dill Salmon	240	6	26
Café Select Grl Basil Chkn	290	6	37
Café Select Rstd Chkn Chardonnay	270	6	30
Complete Select Country Breaded Chkn	370	9	53
Complete Select Lemon Pepper Fish	310	5	53
Complete Selections Meatloaf	300	8	40
Complete Select Sweet 'N Sour Chicken	430	9	69
Smpl Select Brded Chkn Brst Strip & Potatoes	200	3	31
Simple Select Chicken Enchilada	270	5	45
Simple Select Chicken Rigatoni	250	7	30
Simple Select Grilled Chkn With Potatoes	160	4	18
Simple Select Mandarin Chicken	240	3	39

Jimmy Dean

Breakfast Bowls

	Cal	Fat	Cbs
Eggs, Potato, & Ham, 227 g	390	23	23
Eggs, Potatoes, Bacon & Chdr Chz, 227 g	520	34	22
Eggs, Potatoes, Ssg & Chdr Chz, 227 g	490	34	20
Pancake and Sausage Links, 244 g	710	31	93

Omelets

	Cal	Fat	Cbs
Ham & Cheese, 122 g	250	19	4
Sausage & Cheese, 122 g	270	22	5
Three Cheese, 122 g	290	23	4
Western Style, 122 g	210	15	6

Sandwiches

	Cal	Fat	Cbs
D-lights Croissant: Trky Sge, Egg Wh & Chz, 136 g	300	12	32
D-lights Sdwiches: Ca Bcn, Egg Wh & Chz, 128 g	230	6	30
D-lights Sdwiches: Tky Sge, Egg Wh & Chz, 145 g	260	7	30

Skillets

	Cal	Fat	Cbs
Bacon, 127 g	230	13	14
Ham, 127 g	130	4	16
Smoked Sausage, 127 g	250	14	20
Southwest Style, 127 g	210	12	18

Kid Cuisine

	Cal	Fat	Cbs
All American Fried Chicken Meal	480	20	47
All Star Chicken Breast Nuggets Meal	440	17	53
Bug Safari Chicken Breast Nuggets Meal	450	15	58
Cheese Blaster Mac & Cheese Meal	390	9	64
Cheeseburger Builder Meal	390	12	56
Magical Cheese Stuffed Crust Pizza Meal	420	11	62
Pop Star Popcorn Chicken Meal	430	13	64

Lean Cuisine

Café Classics

	Cal	Fat	Cbs
Bow Tie Pasta & Chicken, 10 oz.	230	5	32

• MOST HEALTHY   • LEAST HEALTHY

FROZEN MEALS	Cal	Fat	Cbs
Chicken Carbonara, 9 oz.	270	7	33
Chicken Marsala, 8 oz.	140	4	12
Fiesta Grilled Chicken, 9 oz.	250	5	31
Glazed Chicken, 9 oz.	220	4	25
Parmesan Crusted Fish, 9 oz.	290	8	40
Shrimp Alfredo, 9 oz.	260	5	36
Steak Tips Portabello, 8 oz.	180	7	13
Sweet and Sour Chicken, 10 oz.	300	3	51
Teriyaki Steak, 11 oz.	280	6	37
Three Cheese Chicken, 8 oz.	210	10	10
Tortilla Crusted Fish, 8 oz.	330	9	45
Casual Eating™			
BBQ Recipe Chicken Pizza, 6 oz.	350	8	50
Chicken Philly Flatbread Melts, 7 oz.	330	8	41
Four Cheese Pizza, 6 oz.	360	8	55
Gourmet Mushroom Pizza, 6 oz.	320	7	49
Pepperoni French Bread Pizza, 5 oz.	290	8	43
Pepperoni Pizza, 6 oz.	370	9	50
Roasted Vegetable Pizza, 6 oz.	310	5	52
Steak, Cheddar & Mushroom Panini, 6 oz.	340	9	44
Comfort Classics			
Baked Chicken, 9 oz.	240	5	34
Glazed Turkey Tenderloins, 9 oz.	260	5	41
Herb Roasted Chicken, 8 oz.	180	4	20
Oven Roasted Beef, 9 oz.	210	8	18
Roasted Pork, 10 oz.	250	4	38
Roasted Turkey & Vegetables, 8 oz.	150	5	12
Salisbury Steak, 10 oz.	280	9	25
Dinnertime Selects™			
Balsamic Glazed Chicken, 12 oz.	350	9	43
Chicken Fettuccini, 12 oz.	400	8	48
Chicken Tuscan, 12 oz.	280	6	34
Grilled Chicken & Penne Pasta, 12 oz.	330	5	52
Orange Peel Chicken, 12 oz.	390	9	63
Salisbury Steak, 13 oz.	270	8	27
One Dish Favorites™			
Alfredo Pasta w/ Chkn & Broccoli, 10 oz.	250	6	33
Cheese Ravioli, 9 oz.	240	6	38
Chicken Fettuccini, 9 oz.	270	6	32
Chicken Florentine Lasagna, 10 oz.	290	6	37
Chicken Teriyaki Stir Fry, 10 oz.	300	5	49
Classic Five Cheese Lasagna, 12 oz.	320	8	44
Macaroni And Beef, 10 oz.	310	9	38
Spaghetti With Meatballs, 10 oz.	260	5	35
Stf Cabbage w/ Whpd Potatoes, 10 oz.	220	4	21

● MOST HEALTHY   ● LEAST HEALTHY

FROZEN MEALS

	Cal	Fat	Cbs
Spa Cuisine™ Classics			
Butternut Squash Ravioli, 10 oz.	350	9	56
Chicken In Peanut Sauce, 9 oz.	280	8	30
Chicken Pecan, 9 oz.	260	6	32
Ginger Garlic Stir Fry With Chkn, 10 oz.	290	4	46
Hunan Stir Fry With Beef, 9 oz.	270	7	37
Lemon Chicken, 9 oz.	300	9	40
Rosemary Chicken, 8 oz.	210	4	27
Salmon Mediterranean, 9 oz.	230	4	30
Salmon With Basil, 10 oz.	220	6	24
Marie Callender's			
• 1 Dish Classics Fettuccini Alfredo	870	51	76
1 Dish Classics Spaghetti w/ Meat Sauce	590	15	90
Beef Pot Pie, 1 cup	540	32	46
Beef Pot Roast	330	10	32
Beef Tips Dinner	360	12	35
Breaded Chicken Parmesan Dinner	650	29	66
Cheesy Chicken Pot Pie, 1 cup	600	37	46
Chicken Fried Beef	540	28	51
Chicken Pot Pie, 1 cup	530	31	48
Chicken Teriyaki	430	4	78
Chzy Chkn Breast, Rice w/ Broccoli	480	18	47
Country Fried Pork Chop	510	23	53
Creamy Mshr & Chkn Pot Pie, 1 cup	560	35	45
Fried Chicken Tenderloins	470	19	52
Golden Battered Filet Dinner	450	16	53
Herb Roasted Chicken	460	25	26
Lasagna with Meat Sauce, 1 cup	240	8	28
Roast Beef Dinner	370	13	37
Salisbury Steak Dinner	400	16	38
Stuffed Pasta Medley	440	15	55
Swedish Meatballs	580	30	48
Sweet & Sour Chicken	600	18	88
Michelina's			
Creamy Parmesan Chicken, 8 oz.	220	5	37
Enchilada Bake, 8 oz.	300	8	47
Layered Lasagna with Meat Sauce, 8 oz.	310	6	49
Macaroni and Cheese, 8 oz.	270	4	47
Mandarin Chicken, 8 oz.	260	3	46
Meatloaf, 8 oz.	180	6	21
Penne Primavera, 8 oz.	280	6	43
Roasted Sirloin Supreme, 8 oz.	230	5	34
Santa Fe Style Rice and Beans, 8 oz.	330	9	55
Shrimp Scampi, 8 oz.	290	6	45

FROZEN MEALS

	Cal	Fat	Cbs
Morningstar Farms			
Breakfast Starters Classic Scramble, 78 g	60	1	8
Veggie Bites Country Scramble, 85 g	180	8	17
Veggie Bites Eggs Florentine, 85 g	180	8	17
Patio			
Beef Enchilada	380	12	55
Beef Tamale and Enchilada	460	14	69
Cheese Enchilada	390	13	58
Chicken Burrito	280	8	42
Chicken Enchilada	380	11	57
Hot Beef & Bean Burrito with Red Chili	310	11	42
Pepperidge Farm			
Chili w/ Beans & Cornbread 1 Dish Meal, 1 cup	360	17	40
Crmy Alfredo Chkn & Broc Premium Pot Pie, 1 cup	500	32	40
Roasted White Meat Chkn Pot Pie, 1 cup	510	32	43
Roasted White Meat Tkey Pot Pie, 1 cup	501	33	38
Rosetto Pasta			
All Natural			
Beef Ravioli	220	4	39
Cheese Ravioli	210	5	34
Whole Wheat Cheese Ravioli	200	5	33
Classic			
Beef Ravioli	240	4	40
Cheese Manicotti	270	11	30
Cheese Ravioli	230	4	37
Cheese Stuffed Shells	260	11	27
Cheese Tortellini	240	5	41
Chicken & Herb Ravioli	210	2	36
Gourmet			
Butternut Squash Ravioli	240	3	45
Pesto Ravioli with Walnuts	300	8	44
Steam 'n Eat			
Medium Square Cheese Ravioli	230	4	37
Eat Small Round Cheese Ravioli	230	4	36
SeaPak			
Artichoke Pesto Tilapia, 6 oz.	300	8	31
Herb Butter Salmon, 5 oz.	350	26	3
South Beach Living			
Caprese Style Chicken, 266 g	240	8	10
Chicken Fettuccini Alfredo, 263 g	240	7	20
Chkn in Roasted Red Pepper Sauce, 266 g	280	12	25
Garlic Herb Chicken, 232 g	240	10	10
Garlic Parmesan Chicken, 286 g	270	10	22
Garlic Sesame Beef, 255 g	210	9	15
Kung Pao Chicken, 235 g	250	9	14

● MOST HEALTHY   ● LEAST HEALTHY

FROZEN MEALS	Cal	Fat	Cbs
Meatloaf with Gravy, 255 g	210	9	17
Roasted Turkey, 269 g	240	9	27
Savory Pork, 266 g	230	9	13
Tyson Chicken			
Meals and Entrees			
Chicken Cordon Bleu, 168 g	380	24	20
Chicken Kiev, 168 g	480	37	19
Chkn w/ Broccoli and Cheese, 168 g	310	16	23
Refrigerated			
Chkn Brst Medals in Italian Hrb Sauce, 140 g	120	2	7
Chkn Brst Medals in Sesame Teriyaki Sauce, 140 g	190	3	22
Chkn Brst Medals in Wh Wine & Grlc Sauce, 140 g	140	6	3
Van de Kamp's			
Battered Fillets, 100 g	190	9	20
Battered Haddock Fillets, 104 g	210	11	21
Beer Battered Fish Fillets, 60 g	120	6	12
Breaded Fish Fillets, 99 g	230	13	21
Lightly Breaded Tilapia, 113 g	240	11	17
Zatarain's			
Blackened Chkn & Yellow Rice	460	13	67
Blackened Chicken Alfredo	500	25	46
Chicken Jambalaya	400	5	69
Red Beans & Rice w/ Sausage	510	20	68
Sausage Jambalaya	480	14	77
FROZEN PIZZA			
California Pizza Kitchen			
Crispy Thin			
Crust BBQ Chicken Recipe, 139 g	290	9	35
Crust Garlic Chicken, 119 g	290	11	31
Crust Margherita, 121 g	290	13	31
Crust Sicilian Recipe, 120 g	310	14	30
Original			
BBQ Chicken, 122 g	270	2	33
BBQ Recipe Chicken, 132 g	310	9	38
Five Cheese & Tomato, 129 g	350	15	Cbs
Hawaiian, 123 g	260	4	31
Sausage, Pepperoni & Mshr, 118 g	290	13	30
Thai Recipe Chicken, 132 g	310	11	38
Digiorno Pizza			
Cheese Stuffed Crust Four Chz, 150 g	360	14	41
• Digiorno For 1, Garlic Bread Crust Pep, 274 g	840	44	81
Digiorno For 1, Thn Crst Grl Chkn & Veg 240 g	520	17	64
For One Traditional Crust Supreme, 283 g	790	36	85
Garlic Bread Pizza Supreme, 121 g	290	13	31
Half & Half Rising Crust Pep & Chz, 150 g	390	18	40

• MOST HEALTHY   • LEAST HEALTHY

FROZEN MEALS	Cal	Fat	Cbs
Harvest Wheat Thin Crispy Crust Supreme, 133 g	250	8	32
Rising Crust Supreme, 135 g	320	14	35
Rising Crust Supreme, 155 g	370	15	41
Thin Crispy Crust Supreme, 141 g	300	12	36
U S w/ Rst Veggie-parm Focaccia Crust, 151 g	390	19	43
Ultimate Supreme Thin Crust, 150 g	360	17	34
Empire Kosher			
• Bagel Cheese Pizzas, 64 g	103	3	19
Four Cheese Pizza, 104 g	210	6	32
Mushroom Pizza, 104 g	210	4	32
Vegetable Supreme Pizza, 132 g	250	5	38
Healthy Choice			
French Bread Cheese Pizza, 1 Pizza	350	5	55
French Bread Pepperoni Pizza, 1 Pizza	350	5	54
French Bread Supreme Pizza, 1 Pizza	340	4	53
Jack's Pizza			
Half & Half Pepperoni/cheese, 170 g	440	23	38
Half & Half Sausage/pepperoni, 125 g	290	14	29
Naturally Rising The Works, 144 g	330	12	42
Naturally Rising Three Meat, 137 g	330	12	41
Original Cheese, 142 g	320	13	38
Original Pepperoni, 142 g	370	18	36
Original Sausage, 120 g	290	13	29
Original Spicy Italian Sausage, 158 g	380	17	38
Pizza Bursts - Pepperoni, 85 g	260	15	25
Pizza Bursts - Supreme, 85 g	260	14	25
Michelina's			
Five Cheese Pizza, 142 g	290	7	42
Pepperoni Pizza Snacks, 85 g	200	8	24
Pepperoni Pizza, 142 g	300	9	41
South Beach Living			
Deluxe, 192 g	340	11	37
Four Cheese, 178 g	340	11	37
Grilled Chicken & Vegetable, 192 g	330	10	37
Pepperoni, 178 g	350	12	36
Tombstone Pizza			
Brickoven Style Cheese, 151 g	350	15	38
Brickoven Style Deluxe, 134 g	280	12	30
Brickoven Style Supreme, 136 g	320	16	29
Garlic Bread Cheese, 130 g	350	14	40
Garlic Bread Pepperoni, 131 g	370	17	40
Half & Half Cheese/Sausage, 115 g	270	11	30
Half & Half Pepperoni & Cheese, 159 g	410	21	37
Half & Half Pepperoni/Sausage, 147 g	370	18	37
Harvest Wheat Thin Crust Supreme, 131 g	260	10	29

FROZEN MEALS	Cal	Fat	Cbs
Light Veggie, 131 g	230	6	31
Original Deluxe, 124 g	270	12	29
Original Pepperoni, 113 g	280	14	28
Original Supreme, 130 g	300	14	31
Thin Crust Pepperoni, 128 g	320	18	28
Thin Crust Three Cheese, 134 g	310	15	28

Totino's Pizza Rolls

Totino's Party Pizzas

	Cal	Fat	Cbs
Cheese, 139 g	320	15	34
Combination, 152 g	380	21	34
Sausage, 153 g	360	19	34

Totino's Pizza Rolls

	Cal	Fat	Cbs
Cheese, 85 g	190	6	26
Combination, 85 g	220	11	24
Pepperoni, 85 g	210	10	25
Mega Pizza Rolls Ultimate Pep, 93 g	230	11	25

FRUITS

FRUITS, CANNED

Del Monte

Apricots

	Cal	Fat	Cbs
Apricot Halves, 127 g	100	0	26
Lite Apricot Halves, 122 g	60	0	16

Cherries Products

	Cal	Fat	Cbs
Chunky Mixed Fruit in 100% Juice, 124 g	60	0	15
Dark Sweet Cherries, 120 g	100	0	24
Very Cherry Mixed Fruit, 124 g	90	0	22

Citrus Fruit Products

	Cal	Fat	Cbs
Citrus Fruit Salad, 126 g	80	0	20
Mandarin Oranges, 126 g	80	0	19
Red Grapefruit, 126 g	90	0	21
SunFresh® Wh Grapefruit in Real Fruit Juice, 126 g	45	0	11

Fruit Cocktail Products

	Cal	Fat	Cbs
Fruit Cocktail, 127 g	100	0	24
Lite Fruit Cocktail, 124 g	60	0	15

Peaches Products: Freestone Peaches

	Cal	Fat	Cbs
Freestone Slices, 127 g	100	0	24
Lite Freestone Slices, 124 g	60	0	14

Pear Products

	Cal	Fat	Cbs
Cinnamon Flavored Pear Halves, 126 g	80	0	21
Lite Pear Halves, 124 g	60	0	15
Pear Halves, 127 g	100	0	24

Pineapple Products

	Cal	Fat	Cbs
Pineapple Slices in Its Own Juice, 114 g	60	0	16
Pineapple Slices in Heavy Syrup, 117 g	90	0	23

• MOST HEALTHY   • LEAST HEALTHY

⬗ FRUITS	Cal	Fat	Cbs
Tropical Fruit Products			
Fruit Naturals® Tropical Medley, 124 g	70	0	18
SunFresh® Trop Mxd Frt in Lt Syrup, 126 g	80	0	21
Tropical Fruit Salad, 122 g	60	0	16
Yellow Cling Peaches			
Lite Peach Halves, 124 g	60	0	15
Peach Halves, 127 g	100	0	24
Dole			
Dates, 40 g	120	0	33
Diced Peaches, 113 g	70	0	18
Diced Pears, 113 g	80	0	19
Mandarin Oranges, 113 g	70	0	18
Mandarin Oranges, 122 g	80	0	19
Pineapple in 100% Juice, 114 g	60	0	15
Pineapple in Heavy Syrup, 123 g	90	0	24
Pineapple, 113 g	60	0	16
Prunes, 40 g	110	0	26
Raisins, 40 g	130	0	31
Tropical Mixed Fruit, 122 g	90	0	21
Luck's			
Fried Apples with Cinnamon, 1/2 cup	100	0	25
Fried Apples, 1/2 cup	110	0	29
Lucky Leaf			
Apple Sauce, 4 oz.	80	N/A	20
• Dutch Baked Apples, 1/2 cup	170	N/A	41
Lemon Creme Pie Filling, 1/3 cup	130	1	31
Lemon Pie Filling, 1/3 cup	120	1	29
Lite Strawberry Fruit 'N Sauce, 4 oz.	60	N/A	14
Unsweetened Apple Sauce, 1/2 cup	50	N/A	13
Musselman's			
Lite Mixed Berry Fruit'N Sauce, 4 oz.	60	N/A	14
Lite Strawberry Fruit'N Sauce, 4 oz.	60	N/A	14
Sesame Street Grape Apple Sauce, 4 oz.	80	N/A	20
Sesame Street Green Apple Sauce, 4 oz.	80	N/A	21
Sesame Street Watermelon Apple Sauce, 4 oz.	70	N/A	17
Sliced Apples, 1/2 cup	50	N/A	12
Ocean Spray			
• Jellied Cranberry Sauce, 10 g	16	0	4
Whole Berry Cranberry Sauce, 10 g	16	0	4
FRUITS, DRIED			
Ocean Spray			
Craisins®, 40 g	130	0	33
Sun-Maid			
Raisins			
California Apricots, 40 g	100	0	26

● MOST HEALTHY   ● LEAST HEALTHY

FRUITS	Cal	Fat	Cbs
Cape Cod Cranberries, 30 g	120	4	22
Chocolate Yogurt Raisins, 30 g	130	5	21
Fruit Bits, 40 g	130	0	33
Jumbo Raisins, 40 g	130	0	31
Milk Chocolate Covered Raisins, 39 g	170	6	25
Peaches, 40 g	100	0	23
Pitted Plums, 40 g	100	0	26
Raisins, 40 g	130	0	31
Variety Pack			
Chopped Dates, 40 g	120	0	33
Goldens and Cherries, 40 g	130	0	31
Mixed Fruit, 40 g	100	0	26
Pitted Dates, 40 g	110	0	30
Sun-Maid Raisins, 28 g	90	0	22
Tropical Trio, 40 g	140	0	34
Vanilla Yogurt Raisins, 28 g	120	5	20
Sunridge Farms			
• Banana Chips, 40 g	210	13	23
California Pitted Prunes, 40 g	100	0	26
Dried Cranberries, 40 g	120	1	33
Fancy Apricots, 40 g	100	0	25
Pineapple Rings, 40 g	170	5	30
Tropical Fruit Mix, 40 g	130	1	32
Welch's			
Berry Medley, 40 g	135	0	32
Cranberries & Spiced Apples, 40 g	135	0	34
Dried Cherries, 40 g	140	0	32
• Dried Fruit Variety Packs, 26 g	90	0	20
Dried Mixed Fruit, 40 g	140	0	32
FRUITS, FROZEN & FRESH			
Cascadian Farm			
Blackberries, 140 g	80	1	22
Blueberries, 140 g	70	1	17
Sliced Peaches, 140 g	50	0	14
• Strawberries, 140 g	45	0	13
Sweet Cherries, 140 g	90	0	22
Dole			
Blackberries,140 g	90	0	22
Blueberries, 140 g	70	1	17
• Dark Sweet Cherries, 140 g	90	4	22
Mango Chunks, 140 g	90	0	24
Mango Slices, 140 g	90	0	24
Mixed Berries, 140 g	70	0	17
Mixed Fruit, 140 g	60	0	16
Organics, 140 g	90	0	24

• MOST HEALTHY   • LEAST HEALTHY

▶ FRUITS	Cal	Fat	Cbs
Raspberries, 140 g	70	0	16
Whole Strawberries, 140 g	50	0	13
Wild Blueberries, 140 g	70	0	17

FRUITS, JARRED

Apple Time

Natural Apple Sauce, 4 oz.	50	N/A	12

FRUITS, PACKAGED FRESH

Chiquita

Bananas, 126 g	110	0	29
Cantaloupe, 134 g	50	0	12
Grapefruit, 154 g	60	0	16
Grapes, 138 g	90	1	24
Honeydew Melons, 134 g	50	0	13

Other Fruits and Vegetables

Apples, 154 g	80	0	22
Apricots, 114 g	60	1	11
Avocados, 60 g	55	5	3
Cherries, 140 g	00	1	22
Kiwifruit, 148 g	100	1	24
Nectarines, 140 g	70	1	16
Peaches, 98 g	40	0	10
Pears, 166 g	100	1	25
Plums, 132 g	80	1	19
Tangerines, 109 g	50	1	15

Dole

Apples, 154 g	80	0	22
Apricots, 114 g	60	1	11
Avocados, 30 g	55	5	3
Bananas, 126 g	110	0	29
Cantaloupe, 134	50	0	12
Cherries, 140 g	90	0	22
Coconuts, 50 g	180	17	8
Cranberries, 55 g	30	0	7
Goji Berries, 30 g	110	0	22
Grapes, 138 g	30	1	24
Honeydew Melons, 134 g	50	0	13
Mangoes, 104 g	70	0	17
Oranges, 154 g	70	0	21
Peaches, 98 g	40	0	10
Pears, 166 g	100	1	25
Pineapples, 112 g	60	0	16
• Plantains, 200 g	232	0	62
Plums, 66 g	40	0	10
Raspberries, 125 g	50	0	17
Strawberries, 147 g	45	0	12

FRUITS

	Cal	Fat	Cbs
Sunkist			
Grapefruit, 154 g	60	0	15
• Lemons, 58 g	15	0	5
Limes, 67 g	20	0	7
Oranges, 154 g	80	0	19
Tangerines, 109 g	50	0	13

GRAINS, PASTA & BEANS

CANNED BEANS	Cal	Fat	Cbs
Allens			
Baked Beans			
Barbeque Baked Beans, 128 g	150	1	29
Homestyle Baked Beans, 128 g	140	1	29
Maple Cured Bacon Baked Beans, 128 g	140	1	27
Onion Baked Beans, 128 g	140	2	25
Original Baked Beans, 129 g	150	1	29
Vegetarian Baked Beans, 128 g	140	0	28
Black Beans			
Black Beans, 128 g	100	1	19
Blackeyed Peas			
Blackeyed Peas with Bacon, 128 g	120	2	20
Blackeyed Peas with Snaps, 126 g	120	1	20
Blackeyed Peas, 126 g	120	1	21
Dry Blackeye Peas, 126 g	110	1	18
Butter Beans			
Baby Butter Beans, 129 g	120	1	22
Garbanzo Beans, 125 g	120	3	19
Large Butter Beans, 128 g	120	1	20
Kidney Beans			
Dark Red Kidney Beans, 128 g	130	1	22
Light Red Kidney Beans, 129 g	120	1	22
Lima Beans			
Green & White Lima Beans, 128 g	110	1	20
Medium Green Lima Beans, 128 g	120	0	23
Northern Beans			
Great Northern Beans, 128 g	100	1	19
Navy Beans, 129 g	110	1	19
Red Beans, 128 g	100	1	19
Pinto Beans			
Pinto Beans, 128 g	110	1	20
Refried Beans			
Refried Beans, 128 g	150	3	24
Refried Black Beans No Fat Added, 121 g	120	0	23
American Roland Food Corporation			
Beans, Black, 130 g	120	0	21

• MOST HEALTHY   • LEAST HEALTHY

GRAINS, PASTA & BEANS

	Cal	Fat	Cbs
Beans, Garbanzo, 130 g	110	1	20
Beans, Red Kidney, 130 g	110	0	18
Beans, Spicy Black, 130 g	110	2	0
Campbell's Soups			
Bkd Beans Brwn Sugar & Bcn Flvrd Beans, 1/2 cup	160	3	30
Pork and Beans, 1/2 cup	140	2	25
Luck's			
Blackeye Peas, 1/2 cup	120	2	20
Fat Free Lima Beans, 1/2 cup	120	0	22
Fat Free Pinto Beans, 1/2 cup	110	0	21
Giant Lima Beans, 1/2 cup	130	2	22
Great Northern Beans, 1/2 cup	130	2	20
Mixed Bean & Pork, 1/2 cup	130	2	21
Pinto Beans, 1/2 cup	130	2	21
Red Kidney, 1/2 cup	110	0	22
Progresso			
Beans Black, 1/2 cup	100	1	17
Beans Cannellini, 1/2 cup	110	0	20
Beans Chick Peas, 1/2 cup	100	2	17
Beans Red Kidney, 1/2 cup	110	0	20
Ranch Style			
Beans, 1/2 cup	130	3	20
Beans with Jalapeño, 1/2 cup	120	3	19
Beans with Onion, 1/2 cup	130	3	19
Black Beans, 1/2 cup	100	1	19
Jalapeño Beans, 1/2 cup	130	3	21
Kidney Beans, 1/2 cup	110	0	21
Original Beans, 1/2 cup	130	3	19
Rosarita			
Fat Free Refried Beans, 1/2 cup	100	0	19
Traditional Refried Beans, 1/2 cup	120	2	18
Vegetarian Refried Beans, 1/2 cup	120	2	19
Van Camp's			
Baked Beanee Weenees, 1 can	290	8	42
BBQ Beanee Weenees, 1 can	260	8	35
Beanee Weenees with Chili, 1 can	240	9	26
• Dark Red Beans, 1/2 cup	90	0	19
Hickory & Bacon Baked Beans, 1/2 cup	150	1	32
Homestyle Baked Beans, 1/2 cup	170	1	33
Original Baked Beans, 1/2 cup	140	1	30
• Original Beanee Weenees, 1 can	340	11	39
DRY BEANS			
Bush's Beans			
Baked Beans			
Barbecue, 130 g	150	1	32

GRAINS, PASTA & BEANS

	Cal	Fat	Cbs
Bold & Spicy, 130 g	110	1	24
• Honey Baked, 130 g	160	1	32
Original, 130 g	140	1	29
Vegetarian, 130 g	130	0	29
Other Varieties of Beans			
Black Beans, 130 g	110	1	23
Blackeye Peas, 130 g	100	0	15
Butter Beans – Baby, 130 g	120	1	19
Chili Beans, 130 g	120	1	20
• Field Peas with Snaps, 130 g	80	0	16
Garbanzo Beans, 130 g	105	2	20
Great Northern Beans, 130 g	80	0	17
Kidney Beans – Dark Red, 130 g	105	0	22
Navy Beans, 130 g	80	0	17
Pinto Beans, 130 g	110	0	19
Purple Hull Peas, 130 g	90	0	19
Red Beans, 130 g	110	1	19

GRAINS

Purity Foods

	Cal	Fat	Cbs
Non-Organic Spelt Kernel, 46 g	130	1	32
• Organic Spelt Kernel, 46 g	130	1	32
• Organic Wheat Kernels (Berries), 47 g	160	1	34

PASTA

Purity Foods

	Cal	Fat	Cbs
• White Vita-Spelt Elbows, 2 oz.	210	1	42
White Vita-Spelt Lasagna, 2 oz.	210	1	42
White Vita-Spelt Spaghetti, 2 oz.	210	1	42
Whole Grain Vita-Spelt Elbows, 2 oz.	190	2	40
Whole Grain Vita-Spelt Lasagna, 2 oz.	190	2	40
Whole Grain Vita-Spelt Spaghetti, 2 oz.	190	2	40

Ronzoni Healthy Harvest

7 Grain Pasta

	Cal	Fat	Cbs
• 7 Grain Fussilli, 2 g	180	2	40
7 Grain Spaghetti, 2 g	180	2	40

Whole Wheat Blend Pasta

	Cal	Fat	Cbs
Lasagna, 2 g	180	2	41
Linguine, 2 g	180	2	41
Penne Regate, 2 g	180	2	41
Rotini, 2 g	180	2	41
Spaghetti, 2 g	180	2	41

RICE

American Roland Food Corporation

	Cal	Fat	Cbs
Basmati Rice, 50 g	180	2	37
Jasmine Rice, 100% Natural, 45 g	160	0	36
Sushi Rice - Calrose, 45 g	160	0	36

GRAINS, PASTA & BEANS	Cal	Fat	Cbs
Wild Rice, 100% Natural, 45 g	170	0	35
Carolina Enriched Rice			
Brown Rice Whole Grain, 42 g	150	1	32
Gold (Parboiled), 47 g	160	0	37
Aromatic Rice			
Indian Basmati, 45 g	160	0	36
Thai Jasmine, 45 g	160	0	36
Goya Foods			
Brown, 98 g	108	1	22
Regular White, 79 g	103	0	22
Parboiled, 88 g	100	0	22
• Precooked White, 83 g	81	0	18
Mahatma Rice			
Aromatic Rice			
Indian Basmati, 45 g	160	0	36
Thai Jasmine, 45 g	160	0	36
Regular Rice			
Brown Rice (Whole Grain), 42 g	150	1	32
Gold (Parboiled), 47 g	160	0	37
Valencia (Short Grain), 46 g	160	0	36
White Rice, 45 g	150	0	35
Minute Rice			
Boil-In-Bag, 50 g	180	0	41
Brown Rice, 43 g	150	2	34
Minute Ready To Serve Brown Rice, 125 g	170	5	28
Minute Ready To Serve Brown Rice, 125 g	190	4	34
Minute Ready To Serve White Rice, 125 g	190	4	34
Premium White Rice, 50 g	190	0	41
White Rice, 55 g	200	0	45
Uncle Ben's			
White Rice			
Boil-In-Bag Rice, 58 g	190	1	44
Instant Rice, 52 g	190	1	43
Original Converted, 49 g	170	0	38
Whole Grain Brown Rice			
Fast & Natural™ Instant Brown Rice, 47 g	170	1	36
Natural Whole Grain Brown Rice, 47 g	170	2	35
• Ready Rice® Whole Grain Brown, 140 g	220	4	41

MEAT			

BACON

Butterball

Original Bacon Style Turkey, 30 g	70	6	1
Salt Reduced Bacon Style Turkey, 30 g	70	6	1

• MOST HEALTHY   • LEAST HEALTHY

▶ MEAT

	Cal	Fat	Cbs
Farmer John			
• Dry Salt Pork, 56 g	250	24	1
Premium Low Sodium Bacon, 16 g	80	7	0
Premium Regular Smoked Bacon, 16 g	70	5	0
Premium Thick Sliced Bacon, 12 g	60	4	0
Jimmy Dean			
• Hardwood Smkd Trky Premium Bacon, 14 g	25	2	0
Lower Sodium Premium Bacon, 10 g	50	4	0
Original Premium Bacon, 10 g	50	4	0
Thick Slice Premium Bacon, 14 g	80	6	0
Oscar Mayer			
Bacon Lower Sodium, 14 g	70	6	0
Bacon Natural Smoked Uncured, 15 g	60	5	0
Bacon Ready To Serve, 16 g	70	6	0
Tyson Chicken			
Fully Cooked Hickory Bacon, 15 g	90	7	0
Ready to Cook Hickory Bacon, 15 g	90	7	0
Ready To Cook Thick Cut Hickory Bacon, 24 g	140	11	0
BEEF			
Libby's			
• Corned Beef, 2 oz.	120	7	0
• Corned Beef Hash, 1 cup	420	24	33
Hawaiian Corned Beef, 2 oz.	120	7	0
Potted Meat, 1/4 cup	121	9	0
Tyson Chicken			
Country Fried Steak, 90 g	310	23	15
Seasoned Beef Strips, 84 g	130	6	1
Steak Fingers, 71 g	250	18	14
HAM			
Farmer John			
Bone-In Ham			
Gold Trad Prem Brwn Sugar & Hny Half Ham, 56 g	70	1	3
Gold Trad Prem Original Smkd Half Ham, 56 g	110	7	3
Maple Ham Steak, 56 g	60	1	1
Original Ham Steak, 56 g	50	1	2
• Premium Ham Sliced Ham Steaks, 84 g	160	11	4
Premium Spiral Sliced Whole Hams, 56 g	90	4	3
Whole Hams, 56 g	110	7	3
Sliced Ham			
• Premium Black Forest Sliced Ham, 38 g	35	1	1
Premium Brown Sugar & Honey Sliced Ham, 38 g	45	1	2
Premium Sliced Ham, 57 g	50	2	1

▶ MEAT

HOT DOGS & FRANKS	Cal	Fat	Cbs
Ball Park Franks			
Ball Park Franks			
Ball Park Cheese Franks, 57 g	190	16	3
Ball Park Franks, 56 g	180	16	3
Better For You Franks			
Bun Size Smkd White Tkey Franks, 50 g	45	0	5
Fat Free Franks, 50 g	40	0	4
Lite Franks, 50 g	100	7	3
Bun Size Franks			
Bun Size Franks, 56 g	180	16	3
Bun Size Smkd White Tkey Franks, 50 g	45	0	5
Grillmaster®			
Deli Style Beef, 81 g	250	23	3
Hearty Beef Franks, 81 g	250	23	3
Butterball			
Biggies Turkey Smokies, 75 g	150	12	2
Turkey Franks, 56 g	120	8	5
Empire Kosher			
Chicken Franks, 57 g	100	7	0
Turkey Franks, 57 g	100	8	0
Farmer John			
Official Dodger Dogs®, 76 g	240	22	2
Premium Jumbo Meat Wieners, 57 g	170	17	0
Premium 1/4 Pounder Beef Franks, 113 g	350	31	5
Premium Meat Wieners, 46 g	140	13	0
Hebrew National			
Beef Knockwurst, 2 oz.	180	17	0
• Dinner Franks, 1 Frank	360	33	1
Franks in a Blanket, 5 Pieces	300	24	12
Light Bologna, 4 Slices	80	5	1
Light Salami, 4 Slices	90	5	0
Oscar Mayer			
Beef Franks			
Jumbo, 57 g	170	15	1
Light, 45 g	90	6	2
Regular, 45 g	130	12	1
Fast Franks			
Beef, 96 g	300	8	21
Fast Franks, 96 g	290	19	21
Little Wieners Little Smokies			
Little Smokies Cheese, 57 g	190	17	2
Little Smokies, 57 g	170	15	1
Little Wieners, 57 g	180	17	1

• MOST HEALTHY   • LEAST HEALTHY

▶ MEAT	Cal	Fat	Cbs
Smokies			
Beef, 50 g	150	13	1
Sausage, 50 g	150	13	1
Wieners			
• 98% Fat Free, 50 g	40	0	3
Jumbo, 57 g	170	16	0
Light, 45 g	90	7	1
Regular, 45 g	130	12	1
MEAT ALTERNATIVES			
Boca Meatless			
• Boca In A Bun Chik'n & Swiss Snds, 143 g	350	14	44
Bratwurst Sausage, 71 g	140	7	6
Breakfast Links, 45 g	70	3	5
Brkfst Patties Made w/ Organic Soy, 38 g	70	3	5
• Breakfast Patties, 38 g	60	3	5
Bruschetta Tomato Basil Parm Pattie, 71 g	70	2	9
Cheeseburger, 71 g	100	5	5
Garden Vegetable Burger, 71 g	130	3	9
Grilled Vegetable, 71 g	80	1	7
Original Chik'n Nuggets, 87 g	180	7	17
Savory Mshr Mozzarella Pattie, 71 g	100	3	11
Spicy Chik'n Patties, 71 g	160	6	15
Gardenburger			
Black Bean Chipotle, 71 g	80	3	13
California Burger, 71 g	90	4	5
Flame Grilled, 71 g	90	4	5
Garden Vegan, 71 g	100	1	12
Portabella, 71 g	90	3	15
Sun-Dried Tomato Basil, 71 g	100	3	15
The Original, 71 g	100	4	14
Veggie Medley, 71 g	90	3	15
Morningstar Farms			
Veggie Bacon Strips, 16 g	60	5	2
Veggie Sausage Links, 45 g	80	3	3
Veggie Sausage Patties, 38 g	80	3	3
Burgers			
Grillers Prime® Veggie Burgers, 71 g	170	9	4
Grillers® Original, 64 g	130	6	5
Grillers® Original, 71 g	100	3	7
Philly Cheese Steak Burgers, 64 g	120	6	6
Chik'n			
Buffalo Wings Veggie Wings, 85 g	200	8	20
Chik'n Nuggets, 86 g	190	7	18
Chik'n Patties® Original, 71 g	150	6	16
Chik'n Patties® Parmesan Ranch, 71 g	170	7	17

• MOST HEALTHY   • LEAST HEALTHY

MEAT	Cal	Fat	Cbs
Dogs			
America's Original Veggie Dog® Links, 57 g	80	1	6
Mini Veggie Corn Dogs, 76 g	160	5	21
Veggie Corn Dogs, 71 g	150	4	22
Meal Starters			
Meal Starters™ Chik'n Strips, 85 g	140	4	6
Meal Starters™ Grillers® Recipe Crumbles, 55 g	80	3	4
Meal Starters™ Veggie Steak Strips, 85 g	150	4	8
Organic and Natural			
Breakfast Pattie, 38 g	80	3	4
Classic Burger, 64 g	150	6	9
Thai Burger, 67 g	100	4	7
Vegan Burger, 71 g	90	2	8
Veggie Corn Dogs, 71 g	170	5	22
Veggie Medley Burger, 67 g	120	4	11
Soy Boy			
Baked Tofu			
Smoked Tofu, 2 oz.	100	5	3
Tofu Lin, 2 oz.	100	5	4
Meat Alternatives			
Not Dogs, 2 oz.	95	3	10
Okara Courage Burger, 3 oz.	130	5	8
Vegetarian Franks, 2 oz.	65	2	2
SoyBoy Organic Tofu			
Organic Tofu Extra Firm, 3 oz.	110	6	1
Organic Tofu Firm, 3 oz.	90	5	1
PORK			
Farmer John			
California Natural Fresh Pork			
Boneless Pork Butt, 112 g	210	13	0
Boneless Pork Sirloin, 112 g	220	14	0
Extra Lean Ground Pork, 4 oz.	180	4	0
• Tenderloins, 112 g	120	3	0
Jimmy Dean			
Fully Cooked			
Original Sausage Links, 272 g	240	22	1
Original Sausage Patties, 34 g	240	23	1
Turkey Sausage Links, 272 g	120	7	1
Turkey Sausage Patties, 34 g	120	7	1
Heat N' Serve			
Sausage Links Hot, 55 g	230	22	2
Sausage Links Maple, 55 g	250	25	2
Sausage Links, 55 g	250	24	2
Sausage Patties, 51 g	190	18	1

• MOST HEALTHY • LEAST HEALTHY

MEAT

	Cal	Fat	Cbs
Links & Patties			
Maple Links, 56 g	170	14	2
Maple Patties, 53 g	170	14	2
Original Links, 53 g	170	14	1
Original Patties, 69 g	240	23	1
Tyson Chicken			
Fresh Boneless Loin Roast, 112 g	190	12	0
Fresh Loin Back Ribs, 112 g	250	20	0
Fresh Pork Chops, 112 g	200	13	0
Fresh Pork Roasts, 112 g	130	5	0
Fresh Sirloin Roast, 112 g	140	6	0
• Fresh Spareribs, 112 g	290	24	0
Fresh Tenderloin, 112 g	120	4	0
SAUSAGE			
Butterball			
Bratwurst, 94 g	160	10	3
Hardwood Smoked, 94 g	160	10	4
Monterey Jack Cheese, 94 g	150	10	4
Spicy Chipotle Peppers, 94 g	170	10	6
Empire Kosher			
• Mushroom Garlic Sausages, 71 g	80	2	3
Sun Dried Tomato Basil Sausages, 71 g	80	2	3
Sweet Apple & Cinnamon Sausages, 71 g	80	2	3
Farmer John			
Breakfast Sausage			
Old-Fashioned Maple Skinless Links, 37 g	150	13	2
Original Skinless Links, 37 g	140	12	1
Premium Original Chorizo, 75 g	220	19	2
Premium Sausage Patties Lowfat, 39 g	110	8	1
Dinner Sausage			
Premium Beef Rope Sausage, 56 g	150	12	3
Premium Polish Sausage, 56 g	170	16	1
Premium Pork Rope Sausage, 56 g	160	14	0
Red Hots Ext Hot! Prem Smkd Ssg, 85 g	270	24	2
Hebrew National			
Polish Sausage, 1 link	240	22	2
Jimmy Dean			
All Natural Hot, 12 oz.	210	17	1
Premium Pork Italian, 16 oz.	190	17	1
Premium Pork Light, 12 oz.	140	11	1
Premium Pork Mild Country, 16 oz.	200	21	1
Premium Pork Regular, 12 oz.	180	16	1
Johnsonville			
Brats			
Cheddar Bratwurst Links, 85 g	170	22	3

• MOST HEALTHY • LEAST HEALTHY

▶ MEAT	Cal	Fat	Cbs
Johnsonville Grilling Chorizo, 85 g	280	22	3
• Natural Casing Stadium Style Brats, 102 g	330	30	2
Original Bratwurst, 85 g	270	22	2
Smoked Brats, 76 g	240	21	2
Breakfast Sausage			
Brown Sugar & Honey Links, 55 g	170	13	4
Home-style Breakfast Patties, 43 g	140	11	0
Original Breakfast Links, 55 g	180	14	2
Original Breakfast Patties, 65 g	210	17	2
Italian Sausage			
All Natural Ground Mild Italian Ssg, 2 oz.	170	13	1
Heat & Serve Italian Sausage, 2 oz.	280	24	3
Mild Italian Links, 2 oz.	270	22	3
Smoked Sausage			
Beef Summer Sausage, 2 oz.	170	15	1
Hot Links, 2 oz.	230	20	2
New Orleans Brand Smkd Sausage, 2 oz.	230	20	2
Original Summer Sausage, 2 oz.	170	15	1
Polish Sausage, 2 oz.	240	21	2
Smoked Turkey Sausage, 2 oz.	110	6	4
Libby's			
BBQ Vienna Sausage, 3 links	140	12	4
Oscar Mayer			
Beef Summer Sausage, 28 g	90	7	1
Hard Salami, 27 g	100	8	1
Summer Sausage, 46 g	140	12	0
Perdue Farms			
Lean Tkey Ssg Links, Sweet Italian, 3 oz.	150	8	4
Tkey Breakfast Sausage, 2 oz.	80	5	0
Tkey Brkfst Sausage, Sweet Italian, 2 oz.	90	5	2

▶ POULTRY			
CHICKEN			
Bumblebee Tuna			
Prime Fillet® Chkn Brst w/ BBQ Sauce, 4 oz.	170	2	10
Prime Fillet® Chkn Brst w/ Garlic & Herbs, 4 oz.	110	2	1
Prime Fillet® Chkn Brst w/ S.W. Seasonings, 4 oz.	120	1	1
Empire Kosher			
Chicken Burgers, 112 g	150	9	1
Chicken Thighs, 112 g	220	16	0
Fresh Boneless Skinless Breasts, 112 g	180	9	0
Fresh Ground Chicken, 112 g	150	9	1
Fresh Leg Quarters, 113 g	210	14	0
Fresh Whole Broiler, 112 g	240	17	0
Roasters, 112 g	220	15	0

• MOST HEALTHY   • LEAST HEALTHY

POULTRY	Cal	Fat	Cbs
Rock Cornish Broiler, 112 g	165	10	0

Oscar Mayer

	Cal	Fat	Cbs
Breast Cuts - Honey Roasted, 85 g	130	3	3
Breast Cuts Oven Roasted, 85 g	130	3	1
Breast Strips - Grilled, 84 g	110	3	1
Breast Strips - Italian, 84 g	110	3	1
Breast Strips- Breaded Restaurant Style, 84 g	170	6	14

Perdue Farms

Cooked Chicken

	Cal	Fat	Cbs
Carved Chicken Breast, 71 g	100	2	2
Carved Chicken Breast, Grilled, 71 g	90	2	1
Carved Chkn Breast, Original Rstd, 71 g	90	2	0

Fit & Easy® Chicken

	Cal	Fat	Cbs
Bnlss, Skinless Chkn Breast Tenderloins, 4 oz.	120	1	0
Boneless, Skinless Chkn Breasts, 4 oz.	110	1	0
Boneless, Skinless Chkn Thighs, 4 oz.	140	6	0

Fresh Baked Breaded Chicken

	Cal	Fat	Cbs
Breast Cutlets, Homestyle, 3 oz.	160	7	12
Breast Pattie, 4 oz.	230	12	14
Breast Tenderloins, 3 oz.	170	7	15
Nuggets w/ Whole Grain Breading, 3 oz.	160	7	13

Fresh Breaded Chicken

	Cal	Fat	Cbs
Chicken Breast Cutlets, Original, 3 oz.	210	12	13
Chkn Breast Nuggets, Dinosaur Shapes, 3 oz.	180	9	12
Chicken Breast Nuggets, Original, 3 oz.	200	12	14
Chicken Breast Strips, Original, 3 oz.	180	11	11

Fresh Chicken Parts

	Cal	Fat	Cbs
• Boneless, Skinless Chkn Thighs, 3 oz.	70	9	0
Chicken Drumsticks, 2 oz.	110	6	0
Chicken Thighs, 3 oz.	240	19	0
Chicken Wings, 3 oz.	210	15	0

Frozen Breaded Chicken

	Cal	Fat	Cbs
Breast Nuggets, 4 oz.	230	14	14
Breast Tenders, 4 oz.	240	14	14
Strips, Buffalo Style, 3 oz.	180	7	14
Strips, Homestyle, 3 oz.	230	9	21

Ground Chicken

	Cal	Fat	Cbs
Fresh Grnd Chkn Filet of Breast Meat, 4 oz.	100	1	0
Fresh Ground Chicken, 4 oz.	180	12	0
Ground Chicken Patties, 4 oz.	170	11	0

Perfect Portions® Chicken

	Cal	Fat	Cbs
Boneless, Skinless Chicken Breasts, 5 oz.	130	2	0
Bnlss, Sknlss Chkn Brsts, All Natural, 5 oz.	140	2	0
Bnlss, Sknlss Chkn Brsts, Teriyaki, 5 oz.	160	2	7

• MOST HEALTHY • LEAST HEALTHY

POULTRY

	Cal	Fat	Cbs
Tyson Chicken			
Fresh Bnlss, Skinless Chkn Brsts, 112 g	110	3	0
Fresh Chicken Breast Tenders, 112 g	100	1	0
Fresh Chicken Drumsticks, 112 g	150	9	0
Fresh Chicken Leg Quarters, 112 g	190	13	0
Fresh Chicken Thighs, 112 g	220	17	0
Fresh Family Roaster, 112 g	210	15	0
Fresh Split Chkn Breasts w/ Ribs, 112 g	170	10	0
• Fresh Young Chicken, 112 g	250	19	0
TURKEY			
Butterball			
Roast 'n Slice Bnlss Stuffed Tkey, 100 g	140	7	5
Fresh Whole Turkey			
Fresh - 5 to 7 kilos, 100 g	160	9	0
Fresh - 7 to 9 kilos, 100 g	210	14	0
Fresh - Over 9 kilos, 100 g	190	12	0
Fresh- Under 5 kilos, 100 g	160	9	0
Frozen Specialty Roasts - Cook from Frozen			
Boneless Light & Dark Tkey Roast, 100 g	90	2	0
Boneless Stuffed Turkey Breast, 100 g	120	4	7
Boneless Turkey Breast, 100 g	80	1	0
Stuffed Turkey Breast with bone, 100 g	150	6	11
Turkey Breast with bone, 100 g	100	3	0
Frozen Whole Turkey - Plump & Juciy			
5 to 7 kilos, 100 g	120	5	0
7 to 9 kilos, 100 g	120	4	1
9 to 11 kilos, 100 g	220	17	1
Over 5 kilos, 100 g	160	9	2
Under 5 kilos, 100 g	150	8	1
Stuffed Whole Turkey			
Frozen- 5 to 7 kilos, 100 g	160	7	12
Frozen- 7 to 9 kilos, 100 g	170	10	9
Turkey Chicken Trio			
Smoked Ham Style Turkey, 33 g	40	2	1
• Smoked Turkey Breast, 33 g	30	1	1
Empire Kosher			
Fresh White Ground Turkey, 112 g	140	5	0
Fresh Whole Turkey Breast, 112 g	210	1	0
Fresh Whole Turkey, 112 g	180	9	0
• Frozen Ground Turkey, 112 g	230	17	0
Frozen Whole Breast, 112 g	160	7	0
Frozen Whole Turkey, 112 g	180	10	0
Turkey Burgers, 112 g	220	15	0
Turkey Tenders, 112 g	120	1	0

• MOST HEALTHY • LEAST HEALTHY

POULTRY	Cal	Fat	Cbs
Perdue Farms			
Cooked Turkey			
Carved Turkey Breast, Oven Roasted, 71 g	90	1	2
FIT & EASY® Turkey			
Boneless, Skinless Tkey Brst Fillets, 4 oz.	120	1	0
Bnlss, Skinless Tkey Brst Tendoin, 4 oz.	120	1	0
Bnlss, Sknlss Tkey Brsts, Thin-Slice, 3 oz.	100	1	0
Ground Turkey			
Turkey Breast, 4 oz.	120	2	0
Turkey Patties, 4 oz.	160	8	0
Turkey, 4 oz.	230	17	0
Ground Turkey, 4 oz.	160	8	0
Turkey Parts			
Fresh Turkey Drumsticks, 3 oz.	130	5	0
Fresh Turkey Thighs, 3 oz.	190	12	0
Fresh Turkey Wings, 3 oz.	160	8	0
Fresh Whole Turkey Breast, 3 oz.	170	8	0
Whole Turkey			
Fresh Turkey (Roasted Dark Meat), 3 oz.	190	11	0
Fresh Turkey (Roasted White Meat), 3 oz.	150	7	0

PREPACKAGED MEALS & SIDES			
BABY FOOD			
Beech-Nut Baby Food			
DHA Plus			
Banana Supreme, 1 jar	110	0	25
• Carrots, 1 jar	45	0	10
• Whole Wheat Pasta Parmesan, 1 jar	230	5	37
New Beverages			
G.M. Chiquita Banana Juice w/ Yogurt, 6 fl.oz.	110	1	25
Good Evening Veggie Delight Juice, 6 fl.oz.	130	1	27
Yogurt Blends w/ Juice-mixed Berry, 6 fl.oz.	90	1	20
Stage 2			
Apples & Bananas, 1 jar	70	0	16
Corn & Sweet Potatoes, 1 jar	90	0	18
Good Evening Turkey Tetrazzini, 1 jar	130	3	23
Wholesome New			
G.E. Whole Wheat Pasta In Tomato Sauce, 1 jar	100	2	19
G.E. Whole Wheat With Raisins Cereal, 15 g	50	0	10
Whole Wheat Pasta Parm, 1 jar	230	5	37
BOXED SALAD MIXES			
South Beach Living			
• Cranberry Walnut Chicken Salad Kit, 6 oz.	290	13	25
Santa Fe Style Chicken Salad Kit, 7 oz.	240	6	24

● MOST HEALTHY   • LEAST HEALTHY

PREPACKAGED MEALS & SIDES	Cal	Fat	Cbs
Tyson Chicken			
• Premium Chunk Chkn Salad Kit, 108 g	210	9	15
CANNED MEALS			
Bush's Beans			
Bush Chunky Chili, 246 g	260	10	28
Bush Hot Chili, 246 g	250	10	26
Bush No Bean Chili, 246 g	240	14	16
Bush Original Chili, 246 g	250	10	26
Chef Boyardee			
2 Cheese Pizza, 1 cup	250	4	45
Beef Ravioli, 1 cup	250	8	32
Beefaroni, 1 cup	240	9	30
Big Beefaroni, 1 cup	260	9	32
Cheese Ravioli, 1 bowl	200	5	31
Cheese Ravioli, 1 cup	240	7	32
Cheesy Burger Macaroni, 1 cup	200	5	30
Cheesy Burger Ravioli, 1 cup	250	6	38
Cheesy Nacho Twistaroni, 1 cup	220	7	32
Chili Mac, 1 cup	260	13	26
Fat Free Beef Ravioli, 1 cup	170	2	33
Mini Bites Beef Ravioli, 1 cup	280	13	31
Mini Bites Pasta Shells, 1 bowl	210	8	27
Mini Bites Ravioli, 1 cup	250	9	35
Mini Bites Spaghetti & Meatballs, 1 cup	250	10	30
Overstuffed Beef Ravioli, 1 cup	270	6	42
Rice with Chicken, 1 bowl	230	9	30
Rings with Meatballs, 1 cup	240	9	30
• Sauce with Meat, 1/2 cup	80	4	10
Tomato & Beef Twistaroni, 1 cup	230	5	38
Twistaroni Chili Cheese Do, 1 cup	220	6	32
Dennison's			
Chili Con Carne, 1 cup	350	15	31
• Chili Con Carne with Beans, 1 cup	360	14	38
Chunky Chili with Beans, 1 cup	300	10	32
Fat Free Chili with Beans, 1 cup	210	2	29
Hot Chili with Beans, 1 cup	350	14	11
Hot Chunky Chili with Beans, 1 cup	300	10	32
Turkey Chili, 1 cup	210	3	29
Vegetarian Chili, 1 cup	190	2	34
Luck's			
Chicken Dumplings, 1 cup	170	5	21
DINNER MIXES			
Betty Crocker			
Chicken Helper Jambalaya, 45 g	150	2	30
• Comp Meals Chkn & Buttermilk Biscuits, 155 g	280	11	37

• MOST HEALTHY   • LEAST HEALTHY

PREPACKAGED MEALS & SIDES	Cal	Fat	Cbs
Hamburger Helper Chdr Chz Melt, 36 g	130	1	26
Tuna Helper Tetrazzini, 40 g	140	1	29
Bumblebee Tuna			
Chunk Light Tuna in Water, 3 oz.	70	1	0
• Fat Free Tuna Salad with Crackers, 3 oz.	70	0	10
Regular Keebler Crackers, 1 oz.	90	5	12
Sensations® EZ Pl Bowls Lmn & Crckd Pepper, 5 oz.	130	4	2
Sensations® EZ Pl Bowls Spicy Thai Chili, 5 oz.	190	8	11
Tuna Salad Original w/ Crackers, Crackers, 1 oz.	90	5	12
Tuna Salad Original w/ Crackers, Tuna Salad, 3 oz.	190	16	6

LUNCH/DINNER MEALS

Campbell's Soups	Cal	Fat	Cbs
Herb Chicken With Rice, 1/7 Box	160	2	33
Lemon Chicken With Herb Rice, 1/7 Box	160	2	34
SW-style Chkn w/ Rice, 1/6 Box	150	1	32
Traditional Rst Chkn w/ Stuffing, 1/6 Box	160	3	29
Chef Boyardee			
Cheese Pizza Kit Single, 1/4 Package	260	5	45
Pepperoni Pizza Mix, 1/4 Package	290	8	44
Hamburger Helper			
Cheesy Baked Potato, 36 oz.	130	2	27
Cheesy Hashbrowns, 48 oz.	170	1	37
• Crunchy Taco, 42 oz.	140	3	26
Double Cheese Quesadilla, 46 oz.	160	1	36
Lunchables			
Chkn Dunks - w/ 100% White Meat, 1 pk.	310	6	52
Cracker Stackers - Ham & Cheddar, 1 pk.	400	20	40
Cracker Stackers - Tkey & Cheddar, 1 pk.	400	13	59
Mini - Tacos Beef, 1 pk.	410	10	61
Mini Hot Dogs - Hot Dogs, 1 pk.	380	11	61
• Pizza - Pizza & Treatza, 1 pk.	460	10	79
Starkist Tuna			
StarKist Lunch To-Go®, 1 Kit	210	9	27
Taco Bell Home Originals			
Soft Taco Dinner - Flour Tortillas & Sauce, 93 g	230	5	40
Taco Dinner - Chz Double Decker, 67 g	230	9	30
Taco Dinner - Sauce & Taco Shells, 60 g	250	5	20
Tyson Chicken			
Beef Chuck Roast Kit w/ Vegs, 113 g	320	21	14
Beef Fajitas Meal Kit, 107 g	140	4	17
Beef Pot Roast in Gravy, 140 g	170	8	2
Beef Steak Quesadilla, 1 kit	270	14	19
Beef Stew Kit with Vegetables, 194 g	240	13	20
Beef Tips in Gravy, 140 g	200	12	5
Pork Roast Kit with Vegetables, 113 g	190	4	18

• MOST HEALTHY   • LEAST HEALTHY

PREPACKAGED MEALS & SIDES	Cal	Fat	Cbs
Seasoned Beef Meatloaf, 140 g	320	23	16
Zatarain's			
Ready-to-Serve			
Blackened Chkn w/ Yellow Rice, 1 pkg	300	5	52
Dirty Rice with Pork, 1 cup	280	5	54
Red Beans & Rice with Sausage, 1 cup	350	7	57
Sausage & Chicken Gumbo, 1 pkg	150	7	16
MICROWAVE MEALS			
Betty Crocker			
Bowl Appetit Cheddar Broccoli Rice, 74 g	290	7	51
Bowl Appetit Herb Chkn Veg Rice, 68 g	260	5	49
• Bowl Appetit Three-Cheese Rotini, 88 g	360	10	55
Campbell's Soups			
Microwavable Bowls			
Chicken Noodle Soup, 1 cup	70	2	10
Creamy Tomato Soup, 1 cup	160	5	25
Tomato Soup, 1 cup	110	0	24
Vegetable Beef Soup, 1 cup	80	1	15
Vegetable Soup, 1 cup	110	0	22
Chunky™ Microwavable Bowls			
Beef w/ Country Vegetables Soup, 1 cup	150	3	21
New England Clam Chowder, 1 cup	180	8	20
Sirloin Burger w/ Country Vegs Soup, 1 cup	160	4	18
Healthy Request® Chunky™ Microwavable Bowls			
Classic Chicken Noodle Soup, 1 cup	110	3	15
Grilled Chicken & Sausage Gumbo, 1 cup	130	3	20
Healthy Request® Select™ Microwavable Bowls			
Italian Wedding Soup, 1 cup	120	3	15
Mexican Style Chicken Tortilla, 1 cup	130	3	19
Select™ Microwavable Bowls			
98% FF New England Clam Chowder, 1 cup	110	2	16
Chicken with Egg Noodles Soup, 1 cup	90	2	12
Mexican Style Chkn Tortilla Soup, 1 cup	130	3	18
Minestrone Soup, 1 cup	100	1	19
Soup at Hand®			
• Chicken & Stars Soup, 1 container	60	2	10
Creamy Chicken Soup, 1 container	130	9	13
Creamy Tomato Soup, 1 container	190	4	34
Velvety Potato Soup, 1 container	161	7	21
Chef Boyardee			
Microwave Beef Ravioli Bowl, 1 cup	60	7	32
Microwave Beefaroni Bowl, 1 cup	250	9	31
Microwave Mini Beef Bowl, 1 cup	240	8	33
Healthy Choice			
Chkn Noodle Soup Mcrowv Bowl, 1 cup	110	2	17

• MOST HEALTHY   • LEAST HEALTHY

PREPACKAGED MEALS & SIDES	Cal	Fat	Cbs
Chkn w/ Rice Soup Mcrowv Bowl, 1 cup	90	0	13
Kraft Macaroni and Cheese			
Easy Mac Macaroni & Cheese			
Bacon Microwave cup, 2 oz.	220	5	38
Extreme Cheese Microwavable, 2 oz.	230	4	42
Original Microwavable, 2 oz.	230	4	42
Original Microwave cup, 2 oz.	220	3	39
Triple Cheese Microwave cup, 2 oz.	220	5	39
Luck's			
Microwave Chicken Dumpling, 1 Bowl	160	4	21
Progresso			
Beef Vegetable, 250 g	100	2	15
Chicken Noodle Soup, 240 g	80	2	10
Italian-Style Wedding Soup w/ Meatballs, 239 g	120	4	14
Lentil Soup, 241 g	130	3	21
Minestrone Soup, 240 g	90	2	17
PASTA MIXES			
Betty Crocker			
• Chkn Helper Creamy Chkn & Noodles, 28 g	90	1	19
Hamburger Helper Salisbury, 34 g	120	1	25
Tuna Helper Creamy Broccoli, 47 g	170	1	34
Chef Boyardee			
Lasagna Kit, 5 oz.	210	4	35
Hamburger Helper			
Bacon Cheeseburger, 49 g	190	3	34
Beef Pasta, 31 g	110	1	22
Cheddar Cheese Melt, 36 g	130	1	26
Cheeseburger Macaroni, 31 g	110	1	23
Double Cheeseburger Macaroni, 33 g	130	2	25
Four Cheese Lasagna, 38 g	130	1	28
Italian Sausage, 39 g	130	1	29
Hamburger Helper Lasagna, 35 g	120	1	26
Philly Cheesesteak, 37 g	140	4	24
Knorr-Lipton			
Fiesta Sides			
Beef Lo Mein, 62 g	230	4	14
Jalapeño Jack Pasta, 62 g	230	4	15
Nacho Pasta, 63 g	230	4	15
Teriyaki Noodles, 66 g	250	5	15
Thai Sesame Noodles, 62 g	230	5	14
Grain Sides			
Alfredo, 60 g	300	17	14
Chicken, 62 g	270	12	15
Pasta Sides			
Alfredo Broccoli, 63 g	250	9	13

• MOST HEALTHY   • LEAST HEALTHY

PREPACKAGED MEALS & SIDES	Cal	Fat	Cbs
Alfredo, 62 g	240	9	13
Cheesy Cheddar, 59 g	220	3	14
Parmesan, 60 g	230	7	13
Stroganoff, 56 g	210	3	13
Kraft Macaroni and Cheese			
Bistro Deluxe - Crmy Portabello Mshr, 98 g	310	11	40
Bistro Deluxe - Sundried Tomato Parm, 98 g	300	11	40
Bistro Deluxe - Three Chz Italiano, 98 g	310	11	40
Mac & Chz Deluxe w/Org Chdr Chz Sauce, 98 g	320	10	45
Mac & Chz Premium Thick 'N Crmy, 56 g	250	2	50
Mac & Chz Dinner - The Cheesiest, 70 g	260	4	48
Rice-A-Roni and Pasta Roni			
Classic Favorites			
Angel Hair Pasta with Herbs, 2 oz.	190	3	38
Fettuccine Alfredo, 3 oz.	250	6	44
White Cheddar & Broccoli, 2 oz.	200	4	36
Nature's Way			
Creamy Parmesan, 2 oz.	200	3	38
Mushrooms in Cream Sauce, 2 oz.	200	3	37
Olive Oil & Italian Herb, 2 oz.	200	3	38
Soy Boy			
Original Tofu Ravioli, 100 g	180	3	31
Ravioli Rosa, 100 g	180	3	29
Velveeta			
• Rotini & Cheese - Broccoli, 126 g	400	16	49
Shells & Cheese - 2% Milk, 112 g	330	5	58
Shells & Cheese - Bacon, 112 g	360	14	45
Shells & Cheese - Original, 112 g	360	12	49
Zatarain's			
Alfredo Pasta Mix, 36 g	140	4	22
Gumbo Pasta Dinner Mix, 1 cup	120	1	23
Scampi Pasta Dinner, 35 g	110	1	21
POTATO MIXES			
Betty Crocker			
• Potatoes Specialty Four Chz Mashed, 25 g	80	0	19
Specialty Deluxe 3 Chz Mashed Potato Bake, 45 g	150	5	24
• Sweet Potato Casserole, 44 g	210	5	39
Campbell's Soups			
Cheesy Chicken with pasta, 1/7 box	150	3	24
Creamy Stroganoff Sauce w/ pasta, 1/6 box	190	4	33
Garlic Chicken with pasta, 1/7 box	190	2	36
Martha White			
Hush Puppy Mix, 1/4 cup	120	N/A	25
Spud Flakes, 1/3 cup	80	N/A	17

• MOST HEALTHY   • LEAST HEALTHY

PREPACKAGED MEALS & SIDES	Cal	Fat	Cbs
Simply Potatoes			
Country Style Mashed Potatoes, 141 g	110	2	20
Mashed Sweet Potatoes, 141 g	100	1	21
Sour Cream and Chive Mashed Potatoes, 141 g	130	5	18
Velveeta			
Cheesy Au Gratin, 58 g	180	6	26
Cheesy Bacon Scalloped, 60 g	190	7	26
Cheesy Mashed, 42 g	140	5	19
Zatarain's			
Hush Puppy Mix, 3 tbsp.	100	1	23
RICE MIXES			
Carolina Enriched Rice			
Authentic Spanish, 2 oz.	180	0	42
Black Beans & Rice, 2 oz.	200	2	39
Broccoli & Cheese, 2 oz.	200	3	39
Chicken & Rice, 2 oz.	190	0	42
Classic Pilaf, 2 oz.	190	1	43
Long Grain & Wild, 2 oz.	200	1	43
Red Beans & Rice, 2 oz.	190	1	41
Saffron Yellow, 2 oz.	190	0	43
Spicy Yellow, 2 oz.	180	1	41
Knorr-Lipton			
Chicken Broccoli, 63 g	270	11	15
Chipotle Rice, 72 g	260	2	18
Mexican Rice, 68 g	250	2	17
• Sesame Chicken, 70 g	300	14	17
Spanish Rice, 67 g	240	2	17
Taco Rice, 68 g	250	2	17
Asian Sides			
Chicken Fried Rice, 66 g	240	2	16
Teriyaki Rice, 65 g	240	2	17
Cajun Sides			
Dirty Rice, 68 g	250	2	17
Garlic Butter Rice, 67 g	260	6	16
New Orleans Style Chicken Rice, 67 g	240	2	17
Red Beans and Rice, 80 g	290	2	21
Rice Sides			
Chicken, 65 g	250	5	16
Creamy Chicken, 68 g	270	8	16
Mushroom, 67 g	240	2	17
Rice Medley, 62 g	230	3	15
Rice Pilaf, 61 g	220	2	15
Mahatma Rice			
Authentic Spanish, 2 oz.	180	0	42
Broccoli & Cheese, 2 oz.	230	4	43

PREPACKAGED MEALS & SIDES	Cal	Fat	Cbs
Classic Pilaf, 2 oz.	190	1	43
Long Grain & Wild, 2 oz.	200	1	43
Saffron Yellow, 2 oz.	190	0	43
Minute Rice			
Ready To Serve			
Chicken Rice Mix, 125 g	190	4	35
Long Grain & Wild Rice Mix, 125 g	190	4	34
Yellow Rice Mix, 125 g	190	4	35
Rice-A-Roni and Pasta Roni			
Classic Favorites			
Broccoli Au Gratin, 3 oz.	260	6	46
Chicken & Broccoli, 3 oz.	240	3	47
Long Grain & Wild Rice, 2 oz.	190	1	42
Nature's Way			
Italian Cheese & Herb, 3 oz.	270	6	50
Long Grain & Wild Rice, 2 oz.	190	1	43
Parmesan & Romano Cheese, 2 oz.	210	3	40
Savory Whole Grain Blends			
Chicken & Herb Classico, 2 oz.	190	2	41
Roasted Garlic Italiano, 2 oz.	210	3	41
Spanish, 2 oz.	200	2	42
Uncle Ben's			
Country Inn®			
Broccoli Rice Au Gratin, 57 g	200	2	43
Chicken & Broccoli Rice, 57 g	190	1	42
Chicken & Wild Rice, 57 g	200	1	42
Oriental Fried Rice, 57 g	200	1	42
Long Grain & Wild Rice			
Butter & Herb, 57 g	190	1	40
Roasted Garlic & Olive Oil, 54 g	180	1	39
Vegetable Pilaf, 57 g	180	1	40
Ready Rice			
Creamy Four Cheese Flavored, 160 g	230	4	44
Long Grain & Wild, 153 g	220	3	43
Rice Pilaf, 155 g	220	4	42
Spanish Style, 144 g	200	3	41
Ready Whole Grain Medley™			
Brown & Wild, 146 g	220	4	42
Santa Fe, 160 g	220	3	42
Vegetable Harvest, 153 g	220	3	44
Zatarain's			
Reduced Sodium			
Dirty Rice, 38 g	130	0	29
Jambalaya, 38 g	130	0	29
Red Beans & Rice, 57 g	190	0	40

PREPACKAGED MEALS & SIDES	Cal	Fat	Cbs
Rice Mixes			
Caribbean Rice Mix, 45 g	160	2	34
Chicken Flavored Rice, 45 g	210	1	44
Dirty Rice Mix, 46 g	130	0	29
Long Grain & Wild Rice, 33 g	230	1	49
Red Beans & Rice, 28 g	190	0	40
Spanish Rice, 26 g	180	0	41
• Yellow Rice Mix, 25 g	110	0	23

STUFFING
Butterball

	Cal	Fat	Cbs
• Homestyle Stuffing, 75 g	190	9	25

Pepperidge Farm

	Cal	Fat	Cbs
Cornbread Stuffing, 3/4 cup	170	2	33
Country Style Stuffing, 3/4 cup	140	1	27
Herb Seasoned Stuffing, 3/4 cup	170	2	33
Sage & Onion Stuffing, 3/4 cup	140	1	26

Stove-Top

	Cal	Fat	Cbs
Stuffing Mix - Chicken One Step, 28 g	150	3	20
Stuffing Mix - Traditional Sage, 28 g	110	1	21
Stuffing Mix - Turkey, 28 g	110	1	20

Zatarain's

	Cal	Fat	Cbs
Cornbread Stuffing, 1/2 cup prepared	100	1	21
• Creole Chicken Stuffing, 1/2 cup prepared	100	1	20
French Bread Stuffing, 1/2 cup prepared	100	1	20

SALAD DRESSING & TOPPINGS

CROUTONS & TOPPINGS
Betty Crocker

	Cal	Fat	Cbs
Bacos Bits, 2 tsp.	30	2	2
Bacos Chips, 2 tsp.	30	2	2

French's

	Cal	Fat	Cbs
French Fried Onions, 2 tsp.	45	4	3

McCormick

	Cal	Fat	Cbs
Bac'n Pieces™ Bacon Flavored Bits, 2 tsp.	30	2	2
Bac'n Pieces™ Bacon Flavored Chips, 2 tsp.	30	2	2
Salad Toppins™ Garden Vegetable, 2 tsp.	35	2	3
Salad Toppins™, 2 tsp.	35	2	2

Pepperidge Farm

	Cal	Fat	Cbs
• Classic Caesar Croutons, 6 croutons	30	1	5
Four Chz and Garlic Croutons, 6 croutons	30	1	5
Seasoned Croutons, 6 croutons	30	1	5
Zesty Italian Croutons, 6 croutons	30	1	5

Sargento

Potato Finishers	Cal	Fat	Cbs
All American, 39 g	130	9	3

SALAD DRESSING & TOPPINGS	Cal	Fat	Cbs
Au Gratin, 39 g	130	9	5
Cheddar Broccoli, 39 g	140	10	2
Salad Finishers			
Bistro Chicken, 44 g	110	7	2
• Cheddar Bacon, 36 g	160	9	9
Cheddar Chicken, 53 g	150	8	9
Chicken Caesar, 41 g	100	4	6
Cranberry Pecan, 33 g	140	10	9

DRESSING MIX

Good Seasons

	Cal	Fat	Cbs
Cheese Garlic, 2 oz.	5	0	1
• Garlic & Herb, 2 oz.	5	0	1
• Gourmet Caesar, 4 oz.	15	0	2
Mild Italian, 4 oz.	10	0	2

SALAD DRESSINGS

Annie's Naturals

	Cal	Fat	Cbs
Dressings			
Balsamic Vinaigrette, 2 tbsp	100	10	3
Goddess Dressing, 2 tbsp	130	13	2
• Strawberry & Balsamic Dressing, 2 tbsp	10	0	2
Organic Dressings			
Buttermilk Dressing - Organic, 2 tbsp	70	7	1
Caesar Dressing - Organic, 2 tbsp	120	12	1
Red Wine & Olive Oil Vinaigrette, 2 tbsp	160	17	1

Bernsteins

	Cal	Fat	Cbs
Fat Free			
Cheese and Garlic Italian, 2 tbsp	10	0	2
Light Fantastic			
Cheese Fantastico, 2 tbsp	25	2	3
Parmesan Garlic Ranch, 2 tbsp	50	3	6
Roasted Garlic Balsamic, 2 tbsp	45	4	3
Regular			
Chunky Blue Cheese, 2 tbsp	120	13	2
Creamy Caesar, 2 tbsp	120	13	1
Italian Dressings & Marinade, 2 tbsp	110	12	1

Betty Crocker

	Cal	Fat	Cbs
Suddenly Salad Caesar, 3 tbsp	170	1	34
Suddenly Salad Chipotle Ranch, 3 tbsp	140	1	28
• Suddenly Salad Classic, 3 tbsp	180	1	37

California Sun Dry

	Cal	Fat	Cbs
Sun-Dried Tomato Salad Dressing, 2 tbsp	20	13	N/A

Good Seasons

	Cal	Fat	Cbs
Asian Sesame With Ginger, 2 tbsp	110	9	7
Cls Balsamic Vinaigrette w/ Ex Virgin Olive, 2 tbsp	90	8	4
Creamy Caesar w/ Aged Parmesan, 2 tbsp	100	9	3

SALAD DRESSING & TOPPINGS	Cal	Fat	Cbs
Red Rspbry Vinaigrette w/ Poppyseed, 2 tbsp	60	4	5
Kraft Salad Dressings			
Creamy Italian, 2 tbsp	100	11	2
French Style Fat Free, 2 tbsp.	45	0	11
Honey Dijon Fat Free, 2 tbsp.	50	0	12
Italian Fat Free, 2 tbs.	20	0	4
Light Done Right Caesar, 2 tbsp.	60	5	3
Light Done Right Creamy French, 2 tbsp	80	5	10
Ranch Garlic, 2 tbsp	120	12	3
Special Collection Greek Vinaigrtte., 2 tbsp	110	12	2
Special Collection Parm Romano, 2 tbsp	140	14	2
Marzetti			
1000 Island Dressing, 2 tbsp	150	15	5
Buttermilk Ranch Dressing, 2 tbsp	160	17	1
Caesar Dressing, 2 tbsp	140	15	1
Ginger Mango Dressing, 2 tbsp	120	9	8
Light Caesar Dressing, 2 tbsp	70	7	2
Light Honey Dijon Dressing, 2 tbsp	90	6	8
Lite Ranch Dressing, 2 tbsp	80	8	2
Strawberry Chardonnay Dressing, 2 tbsp	110	9	7
Sweet Italian Dressing, 2 tbsp	150	14	8
Ultimate Blue Cheese Dressing, 2 tbsp	160	17	1
Paul Newman's Own			
Lighten Up			
Balsamic Vinaigrette Dressing, 2 tbsp	45	4	1
Light Cranberry Walnut, 2 tbsp	70	4	8
Lowfat Sesame Ginger Dressing, 2 tbsp	135	2	5
Sun Dried Tomato Dressing, 2 tbsp	60	4	5
Organic			
Organic Creamy Caesar Dressing, 2 tbsp	170	18	1
Organic Light Balsamic Dressing, 2 tbsp	45	4	3
Organic Lowfat Asian Dressing, 2 tbsp	35	2	5
Organic Tuscan Italian Dressing, 2 tbsp	100	11	1
Regular			
Balsamic Vinaigrette Dressing, 2 tbsp	90	9	3
Caesar Dressing, 2 tbsp	150	16	1
Family Recipe Italian Dressing, 2 tbsp	120	13	1
Parm & Roasted Garlic Dressing, 2 tbsp	110	11	2
Two Thousand Island Dressing, 2 tbsp	140	14	4
Salad Mist			
Asian Sesame Natural Salad Mist, 10 sprays	10	1	1
Balsamic Natural Salad Mist, 10 sprays	15	1	2
Tuscan Italian Natural Salad Mist, 10 sprays	10	1	1
Seven Seas Salad Dressing			
Creamy Italian, 2 tbsp	110	12	2

● MOST HEALTHY   ● LEAST HEALTHY

SALAD DRESSING & TOPPINGS

	Cal	Fat	Cbs
Green Goddess, 2 tbsp	130	13	2
Red Wine Vinaigrette Fat Free, 2 tbsp	15	0	3
Red Wine Vinaigrette, 2 tbsp.	90	9	2
Viva Italian, 2 tbsp	90	9	2
Viva Italian Reduced Fat, 2 tbsp.	45	4	2
South Beach Living			
Balsamic Vinaigrette Dressing, 2 tbsp	50	4	4
Italian Dressing, 2 tbsp	30	4	3
Ranch Dressing, 2 tbsp	70	7	2

VINEGAR
Progresso
	Cal	Fat	Cbs
Vinegar Balsamic, 3 tsp.	10	0	2

SAUCES & MARINADES

BARBECUE SAUCE
Annie's Naturals
	Cal	Fat	Cbs
Annie's Original BBQ Sauce - Organic, 2 tbsp.	45	1	9
Consorzio BBQ Sauce, 2 tbsp.	45	0	11
Smokey Maple BBQ Sauce - Organic, 2 tbsp.	45	1	9
Cattleman's Sauces			
Cattlemen's Classic, 2 tbsp.	60	0	15
Cattlemen's Gold, 2 tbsp.	60	0	14
Cattlemen's Hot & Spicy, 2 tbsp.	45	0	11
Cattlemen's Original, 2 tbsp.	40	0	9
Cattlemen's Smoky, 2 tbsp.	40	0	9
Cattlemen's Sweet & Bold, 2 tbsp.	60	0	14
• Honey BBQ Sauce, 2 tbsp.	70	0	17
Texas Pete			
• Original BBQ Sauce, 1 tsp.	5	0	0

GRAVY & GLAZES
Campbell's Soups
Campbell's™ Gravies
	Cal	Fat	Cbs
Beef Gravy, 1/4 cup	25	1	3
• Country Style Sausage Gravy, 1/4 cup	70	5	4
• Fat Free Beef Gravy, 1/4 cup	15	0	3
Turkey Gravy, 1/4 cup	25	1	3

Campbell's™ Microwavable Gravies
	Cal	Fat	Cbs
Beef Gravy, 1/4 cup	25	1	3
Chicken Gravy, 1/4 cup	40	3	3
Turkey Gravy, 1/4 cup	25	1	3

Franco-American Gravies
	Cal	Fat	Cbs
Fat Free Slow Roast Beef Gravy, 1/4 cup	20	0	3
Fat Free Slow Roast Chkn Gravy, 1/4 cup	20	0	4
Fat Free Slow Roast Tkey Gravy, 1/4 cup	20	0	4
Slow Roast Beef Gravy, 1/4 cup	25	1	3

• MOST HEALTHY   • LEAST HEALTHY

SAUCES & MARINADES	Cal	Fat	Cbs
Slow Roast Chicken Gravy, 1/4 cup	20	1	3
Slow Roast Turkey Gravy, 1/4 cup	25	0	4
McCormick			
Homestyle Gravy Mix, 1 tsp.	25	1	4
Mushroom Gravy Mix, 1 tsp.	20	1	2
Original Country Gravy Mix, 1 tsp.	50	4	4
Peppered Country Gravy Mix, 1 tsp.	45	3	4
HOT SAUCE			
Del Monte			
Chili Sauce, 1 tbsp.	20	0	5
Frank's Red Hot Sauces			
Buffalo Sandwich Sauce, 1 tbsp.	5	0	1
Buffalo Wing Sauce, 1 tbsp.	5	0	1
• Chile 'N Lime™ Hot Sauce, 1 tsp.	0	0	0
• Gold Fever™ Zing Sauce, 2 tbsp.	40	5	8
Original Cayenne Pepper Sauce, 1 tsp.	0	0	0
Xtra Hot Cayenne Pepper Sauce, 1 tsp.	0	0	0
Taco Bell Home Originals			
Hot, 1 tsp.	0	0	0
Mild, 1 tsp.	0	0	0
Texas Pete			
Buffalo Style Chkn Wing BBQ Sauce, 1 tbsp	30	1	5
Hot Sauce, 1 tsp.	0	0	0
MARINADES			
Annie's Naturals			
Mango Cilantro Marinade - Organic, 1 tbsp.	20	1	3
Organic Steak Marinade, 2 tbsp.	50	4	5
• Smokey Tomato Marinade - Organic, 2 tbsp.	60	6	1
Lawry's			
Herb & Garlic, 3 tsp.	10	0	2
• Mesquite, 3 tsp.	5	0	1
Sesame Ginger, 3 tsp.	30	0	7
Tequila Lime, 3 tsp.	15	0	4
Teriyaki, 3 tsp.	20	0	5
Paul Newman's Own			
Herb & Roasted Garlic Marinade, 3 tsp.	20	1	3
Lemon Pepper Marinade, 3 tsp.	15	0	3
Teriyaki Marinade, 3 tsp.	25	0	6
MEAT & STEAK SAUCE			
A-1 Steak Sauce			
A1 Original Steak Sauce, 3 tsp.	30	0	8
A1 Zesty Steak Sauce, 3 tsp.	12	0	3
Del Monte			
Hickory Flavor, 5 tbsp.	60	0	14
Hickory Flavor, 5 tbsp.	60	0	14

● MOST HEALTHY   • LEAST HEALTHY

SAUCES & MARINADES	Cal	Fat	Cbs
Original Recipe, 5 tbsp.	50	0	11
Original Recipe, 5 tbsp.	50	0	11

French's
• Worcestershire Sauce Tabletop, 1 tsp.	0	0	0

Manwich
BBQ Sloppy Joe Sauce, 1/4 cup	50	0	13
• Bold Sloppy Joe Sauce, 1/4 cup	60	1	13
Original Sloppy Joe Sauce, 1/4 cup	30	0	7
Sloppy Joe Sauce, 1/4 cup	30	0	7

McCormick

Beef
Beef Stew Seasoning Mix, 5 g	15	0	2
Sloppy Joes Seasoning Mix, 5 g	20	0	3
Swedish Meatballs Seasoning & Sauce Mix, 11 g	45	1	4

Chicken
Hickory BBQ Buffalo Wings Seasoning Mix, 8 g	25	0	5
Original Buffalo Wings Seasoning Mix, 8 g	30	0	5

Pace Foods
Enchilada Sauce, 1/4 cup	25	0	5
Taco Sauce, 2 tbsp.	10	0	2

Paul Newman's Own
All-Natural Steak Sauce, 17 g	20	1	4

Taco Bell Home Originals
Taco Sauce - Medium, 31 g	10	0	2

Texas Pete
Chili, 14 g	10	0	0
Worcestershire Sauce, 4 g	5	0	0

SEAFOOD SAUCES

Del Monte
Seafood Cocktail Sauce, 78 g	100	0	24

McCormick

Cocktail & Tartar Sauces
Fat Free Tartar Sauce for Seafood, 32 g	32	0	7
Original Cocktail Sauce for Seafood, 67 g	100	0	18
Original Tartar Sauce for Seafood, 28 g	160	15	3

Seafood Sauces & Marinades
• Cajun Seafood Sauce, 32 g	15	0	3
Lemon Butter Dill Seafood Sauce, 29 g	100	9	4
Lemon Herb Seafood Sauce, 30 g	140	15	1
Mediterranean Seafood Sauce, 32 g	20	0	4
• Scampi Seafood Sauce, 28 g	160	17	0

Texas Pete
Seafood Cocktail, 60 g	50	1	11

▶ SAUCES & MARINADES	Cal	Fat	Cbs
Zatarain's			
Cocktail Sauce, 1/4 cup	70	0	17
PASTA SAUCE			
California Sun Dry			
Sun-Dried Tomato Pesto, 1/4 cup	130	13	N/A
Del Monte			
Italian Herb Chunky Spaghetti Sauce, 124 g	60	1	12
Spaghetti Sauce w/ Grn Pepper & Mshrms, 125 g	80	1	16
Spaghetti Sauce w/ Tomatoes & Basil, 125 g	70	1	16
Spaghetti Sauce with Meat, 125 g	60	1	14
Healthy Choice			
Garlic Herb Pasta Sauce, 1/2 cup	60	0	12
Traditional Pasta Sauce, 1/2 cup	60	0	13
Zesty Gumbo Soup, 1 cup	100	2	16
Hunt's			
Paste			
Tomato Paste Basil, Garlic & Oregano, 2 tbsp.	25	0	6
Tomato Paste No Salt Added, 2 tbsp.	30	0	6
Sauce			
Tom Sauce Basil, Garlic & Oregano Sauce, 1/4 cup	15	0	3
Tomato Sauce No Salt Added, 2 tbsp.	30	0	6
Tomato Sauce Roasted Garlic, 1/4 cup	15	0	3
McCormick			
Creamy Garlic Alfredo Sauce Mix, 1 tbsp.	90	6	4
Four Cheese Sauce Mix, 1 tbsp.	40	2	5
Italian-Style Spaghetti Sauce Mix, 1 tbsp.	35	0	7
• Pesto Sauce Mix, 1 tsp.	10	0	1
Muir Glen			
Pasta Sauces			
Fire Roasted Tomato, 1/2 cup	70	2	11
Four Cheese, 1/2 cup	80	3	11
Garden Vegetable, 1/2 cup	60	1	10
Portobello Mushroom, 1/2 cup	50	0	10
Tomato Sauces, Pastes and Purees			
Chunky Tomato Sauce, 1/4 cup	15	0	4
Pizza Sauce, 1/4 cup	40	2	6
Tomato Paste, 1/8 cup	30	0	6
Tomato Puree, 1/4 cup	25	0	6
Paul Newman's Own			
Organic			
Marinara Sauce, 1/2 cup	70	2	12
Tomato Basil Sauce, 1/2 cup	91	5	12
Traditional Herb Sauce, 1/2 cup	90	4	13
Original			
Bombolina Sauce, 1/2 cup	40	5	13

• MOST HEALTHY   • LEAST HEALTHY

SAUCES & MARINADES

	Cal	Fat	Cbs
Five Cheese Sauce, 1/2 cup	80	3	10
Italian Sausage & Peppers Sauce, 1/2 cup	90	4	11
Marinara Sauce, 1/2 cup	70	2	12
Roasted Garlic & Peppers Sauce, 1/2 cup	70	3	11
Sweet Onion & Rst Garlic Pasta Sauce, 1/2 cup	60	2	12
Vodka Sauce, 1/2 cup	110	5	11

Prego Sauces

Chunky Garden Italian Sauce

	Cal	Fat	Cbs
Garden Combo, 1/2 cup	70	2	13
Mushroom Supreme, 1/2 cup	90	3	13
Tomato, Onion & Garlic, 1/2 cup	90	3	13

Classic Italian Sausage

	Cal	Fat	Cbs
Flavored with Meat, 1/2 cup	130	5	19
Fresh Mushroom, 1/2 cup	90	3	14
Marinara, 1/2 cup	100	5	11
Mini Meatball, 1/2 cup	110	5	13
Onion & Garlic, 1/2 cup	100	5	12
Roasted Garlic & Herb, 1/2 cup	00	4	13
Roasted Garlic Parmesan, 1/2 cup	70	1	13
Tomato, Basil & Garlic, 1/2 cup	80	3	12
Traditional, 1/2 cup	80	3	13

Heart Smart Italian Sauces

	Cal	Fat	Cbs
Mushroom Italian Sauce, 1/2 cup	100	3	15
Traditional Italian Sauce, 1/2 cup	90	3	13

Organic Italian Sauces

	Cal	Fat	Cbs
Mushroom Italian Sauce, 1/2 cup	70	3	13
Tomato & Basil Italian Sauce, 1/2 cup	80	3	13

Progresso

	Cal	Fat	Cbs
Pasta Sauce Red Clam, 1/2 cup	60	1	8
• Pasta Sauce White Clam, 1/2 cup	130	10	5
Tomato Puree, 1/4 cup	25	0	5
Tomatoes Whole Peeled Italian w/ Basil, 1/2 cup	20	0	4

PIZZA SAUCE

Boboli

	Cal	Fat	Cbs
Sauces, 1/3 cup	50	0	10

Chef Boyardee

	Cal	Fat	Cbs
• Pizza Sauce, 1/8 package	280	7	440

Contadina

	Cal	Fat	Cbs
• Four Cheese Pizza Sauce 15 oz., 1/3 cup	30	0	3
Italian Bread Crumbs 10 oz., 2 tbsp.	100	2	19
Pizza Sauce-Original 8 oz., 1/3 cup	30	0	6
Sweet & Sour Sauce 16 oz., 2 tbsp.	40	1	8

SEAFOOD	Cal	Fat	Cbs
CRAB & LOBSTER			
Bumblebee Tuna			
Lump Crabmeat, 2 oz.	40	1	0
Pink Crabmeat, 2 oz.	35	1	0
White Crabmeat, 2 oz.	40	1	0
Chicken of the Sea			
Fancy Crabmeat, 6. oz., 2 oz.	40	0	2
• Pink Crab Meat, 6 oz., 2 oz.	30	0	1
Premium Imitation Crab Pouch, 3 oz.	40	0	6
White Crabmeat, 6 oz., 2 oz.	30	0	1
Louis Kemp Seafood			
Crab Delight			
Crab Delights® Chunk Style, 85 g	70	0	10
• Crab Delights® Easy Shreds, 85 g	80	0	12
Crab Delights® Flake Style, 85 g	70	0	10
Lobster Delights			
Lobster Delights® Chunk Style, 85 g	70	0	10
Lobster Delights® Salad Style, 85 g	70	0	10
FISH			
Bumblebee Tuna			
Prime Fillet® Salmon Steaks			
Pink Salmon, 2 oz.	90	5	0
Red Salmon, 2 oz.	110	7	0
Teriyaki Salmon, 4 oz.	160	3	8
Sardine Mackerel			
Sardines in Hot Sauce, 160 g	170	12	1
Sardines in Oil, 75 g	130	9	0
Sardines in Water, 75 g	120	7	0
Tuna			
Coral® Chunk Light Tuna in Oil, 2 oz.	110	6	0
Coral® Chunk Light Tuna in Water, 2 oz.	60	1	0
Prime Fillet® Solid White Albacore in Water, 2 oz.	70	1	0
Sensations® EZ Peel Bowls Spicy Thai Chili, 5 oz.	190	8	11
Chicken of the Sea			
Albacore Tuna			
Genova Solid White Tuna in Olive Oil, 2 oz.	110	6	0
Genova Solid White Tuna in Water, 2 oz.	70	1	0
Solid White Albacore Tuna in Oil, 2 oz.	90	3	0
Solid White Albacore Tuna in Spring Water, 2 oz.	70	1	0
Light Tuna			
Chunk Light Tuna in Oil, 2 oz.	110	6	0
• Chunk Light Tuna in Spring Water, 2 oz.	60	1	0
Genova Tonno in Olive Oil, 2 oz.	130	8	0
Genova Tonno in Water, 2 oz.	70	1	0

• MOST HEALTHY   • LEAST HEALTHY

▷ SEAFOOD	Cal	Fat	Cbs
Mackerel			
Jack Mackerel in Tomato Sauce, 1/4 cup	70	3	2
Jack Mackerel in Water, 1/3 cup	90	4	0
Salmon			
Prem Sknlss & Bnlss Pink Salmon Pouch, 2 oz.	60	2	0
Skinless & Boneless Pink Salmon, 2 oz.	60	2	0
Traditional Red Salmon, 2 oz.	110	7	0
Sardines			
Fish Steaks in Hot Sauce, 2 oz.	70	3	1
Sardines in Mustard Sauce, 1 can	150	8	2
Sardines in Tomato Sauce, 1 can	130	6	2
Sardines in Water, 1 can	100	4	2
• Smoked Sardines in Oil, 1 can	190	14	2
Progresso			
Tuna Albacore in Olive Oil, 56 g	90	3	0
Tuna Light in Olive Oil, 56 g	120	6	0
Starkist Tuna			
Chunk Light Tuna, 2 oz.	60	5	0
Gourmet Choice Tuna Fillet, 2 oz.	60	1	0
Low Sodium Tuna, 2 oz.	60	5	0
Solid White Albacore Tuna, 2 oz.	70	1	0
StarKist Flavor Fresh Pouch®, 2 oz.	90	1	0
StarKist Select®, 2 oz.	60	1	0
StarKist Tuna Creations™, 2 oz.	60	1	0
OYSTERS, CLAMS & SCALLOPS			
Bumblebee Tuna			
Clam			
• Chopped Clams, 2 oz.	25	0	2
Fancy Whole Baby Clams, 2 oz.	50	1	2
Smoked Clams, 2 oz.	130	9	1
Oyster			
Smoked Oysters, 2 oz.	120	7	6
Whole Oysters, 2 oz.	70	3	3
Chicken of the Sea			
Clams			
Chopped Clams, 1/4 cup	30	0	2
Minced Clams, 1/4 cup	30	0	2
Premium Whole Baby Clams Pouch, 3 oz.	40	1	1
Oysters			
Oysters, 2 oz.	80	3	6
• Smoked Oysters in Oil, 1 can	170	8	8
Smoked Oysters in Water, 1 can	120	3	10
SHRIMP & PRAWNS			
Bumblebee Tuna			
• Deveined Medium Shrimp, 2 oz.	40	0	0

SEAFOOD

	Cal	Fat	Cbs
Regular Broken Shrimp, 2 oz.	40	0	0
Regular Medium Shrimp, 2 oz.	40	0	0

Chicken of the Sea

Frozen Shrimp

	Cal	Fat	Cbs
Premium Cooked, 3 oz.	80	1	0
Premium Raw, 4 oz.	120	2	1
• Ready to Cook Medium, 4 oz.	120	2	1
Ready to Eat Medium, 3 oz.	80	1	0

Shrimp

	Cal	Fat	Cbs
Medium Deveined Shrimp, 2 oz.	45	1	1
Medium Shrimp, 2 oz.	45	1	1
Premium Shrimp Pouch, 3 oz.	55	1	1
Tiny Shrimp, 2 oz.	45	1	1

SNACKS

CHIPS & CRISPS

100 Calorie Packs

	Cal	Fat	Cbs
Tst Chips - Baked Snack Crackers, 21 g	100	3	16
Toasted Chips - Ritz Minis Original, 22 g	100	3	17
Toasted Chips - Ritz Snack Mix, 22 g	100	3	16
Tst Chips - Wheat Thins Minis Multi-grain 6 Ct, 22 g	100	3	16

Bugles

	Cal	Fat	Cbs
Bugles Nacho Cheese, 30 g	160	9	18
Bugles Original, 30 g	160	9	18

Cheetos

	Cal	Fat	Cbs
Asteroids® 100 Calorie Mini Bites Chz, 1 pkg	100	6	9
Baked! Crunchy 100 Calorie Mini Bites Chz, 1 pkg	100	4	14
Baked! Crunchy Cheese Flavored Snacks	130	5	19
Baked! Flamin' Hot® Chz Flavored Snacks	130	5	19
Cracker Trax Chzy Cheddar, 30 g	140	5	21
Cracker Trax Spicy Cheddar, 30 g	140	5	21
• Crunchy Chdr Jalapeño Flavored Snacks	170	11	15
Crunchy Cheese Flavored Snacks	160	10	15
Fantastixi Chili Chz, 1 pkg	130	5	19
Flamin' Hot® Cheese Flavored Snacks	170	11	15
Flamin' Hot® Limon Chz Flavored Snacks	160	11	15
Jumbo Puffs Cheese Flavored Snacks	160	10	13
Jumbo Puffs Flamin' Hot Chz Flavored Snacks	150	10	14
Mix & Move Cheese Flavored Snacks	160	11	14
Natural White Cheddar Puffs Chz	150	9	16
Puffs Cheese Flavored Snacks	160	10	15
Twisted Cheese Flavored Snacks	160	10	13
Xxtra Flamin' Hot Chz Flavored Snacks	170	11	15

Flat Earth

	Cal	Fat	Cbs
Apple Cinnamon Grove Fruit Crisps, 1 oz.	130	5	21

▷ SNACKS

	Cal	Fat	Cbs
Farmland Cheddar Veggie Crisps, 1 oz.	130	5	19
Garlic & Herb Field Veggie Crisps, 1 oz.	130	5	19
Peach Mango Paradise Fruit Crisps, 1 oz.	130	5	21
Tangy Tomato Ranch Veggie Crisps, 1 oz.	130	5	19
Wild Bry Patch Flavored Baked Fruit Crisps, 1 oz.	130	5	21
Garden Harvest			
Apple Cinnamon, 28 g	120	3	22
Tomato Basil, 28 g	120	4	20
Vegetable Medly, 28 g	120	4	20
Lays			
Baked! BBQ Flavored Potato Crisps, 1 oz.	120	3	22
Baked! Cheddar & Sour Cream Crisps, 1 oz.	120	4	21
Baked! Original Potato Crisps, 1 oz.	110	2	23
Classic Potato Chips, 1 oz.	150	10	15
Cracker Crisps Delightfully Crispy, 1 package	100	4	17
Hot 'N Spicy BBQ Flavored Potato Chips, 1 oz.	160	10	15
Kettle Cooked Original Potato Chips, 1 oz.	150	8	18
Kettle Cooked Reduced Fat, 1 oz.	140	6	19
Light BBQ Flavored Potato Chips, 1 oz.	75	0	17
Light Original Potato Chips, 1 oz.	75	0	17
Sour Cream & Onion Potato Chips, 1 oz.	160	10	15
Wavy Ranch Flavored Potato Chips, 1 oz.	150	10	16
Wavy Regular Potato Chips, 1 oz.	150	10	15
Pringles			
Extreme			
Blazin' Buffalo Wing, 1 oz.	150	10	14
Kickin' Cheddar, 1 oz.	150	11	14
Flavors			
Original, 1 oz.	160	11	14
Sour Cream & Onion, 1 oz.	150	10	14
Select			
Cheddar Jack, 1 oz.	130	8	16
Cinnamon Sweet Potato, 1 oz.	150	9	16
Smart Snacking			
• Fat Free Original, 1 oz.	70	0	15
Smart Flavors Original, 1 oz.	140	8	17
Stix			
Stix Pizza, 1 oz.	90	4	11
Snyder's of Hanover			
Baked Pita Chips Sundried Tom & Herb, 28 g	140	5	17
Cheddar Baked Crunchies, 28 g	130	6	18
French Onion Sunflower Chips, 28 g	140	6	20
White Cheddar Puffs, 30 g	130	6	19
Chips			
BBQ Potato Chip, 1 oz.	150	6	20

• MOST HEALTHY   • LEAST HEALTHY

SNACKS	Cal	Fat	Cbs
Original Potato Chip, 1 oz.	150	7	19
Salt & Vinegar Potato Chip, 1 oz.	140	6	19
Sour Cream & Onion Potato Chip, 1 oz.	150	6	20
SunChips			
Cinnamon Flavor Multigrain Snacks, 1 oz.	130	6	18
Frn Onion Flavor Multigrain Snacks, 1 oz.	140	6	18
Garden Salsa Flavor Multigrain Snacks, 1 oz.	140	6	19
Original Flavor Multigrain Snacks, 1 oz.	140	6	18
COOKIES			
100 Calorie Packs			
Chewy Granola Bars - Nutter Butter, 28 g	100	2	21
Chewy Granola Bars - Oreo, 28 g	100	2	21
CRACKERS			
100 Calorie Packs			
Cookie Crisps - Barnum's Animals Choco , 22 g	100	3	17
Cookie Crisps - Cheese Nips, 21 g	100	3	15
American Roland Food Corporation			
Rice Crackers - Nori Seaweed, 30 g	110	0	25
Rice Crackers - Original, 30 g	110	0	25
Rice Crackers - Wasabi, 30 g	110	0	25
Arrowroot			
• National Biscuit, 5 g	20	1	4
Barnum's Animal Crackers			
Animal Crackers, 2 oz.	120	4	22
Blue Diamond Almonds			
Nut Thins® Almond, 16 crackers	130	3	23
Nut Thins® Hazelnut, 16 crackers	130	3	23
Nut Thins® Pecan, 16 crackers	130	4	23
Cheese Nips			
Cheddar Reduced Fat, 30 g	150	6	1
Cheddar, 35 g	170	7	22
Crackers - Cheddar, 30 g	150	6	19
Four Cheese, 30 g	150	7	18
Flavor Originals			
Better Cheddars Baked, 31 g	160	8	18
Chicken In A Biskit, 31 g	160	8	19
Sociables Baked Savory Crackers, 14 g	70	4	9
Vegetable Thins Crackers, 30 g	150	7	20
Handi-Snacks			
Oreo Cookie Sticks 'N Creme, 28 g	140	7	20
Premium Breadsticks 'N Cheeez, 31 g	110	5	13
Ritz Crackers 'N Cheez, 27 g	100	6	10
Honey Maid			
Grahams Chocolate, 31 g	130	3	24
Grahams Cinnamon, 31 g	130	3	25

• MOST HEALTHY • LEAST HEALTHY

SNACKS	Cal	Fat	Cbs
Grahams Honey, 31 g	130	4	24
Grahams Squares, 27 g	120	4	20
Keebler			
Club Crackers			
Club® & Cheddar Cracker, 36 g	190	10	23
Original, 14 g	70	3	9
Puffed Original, 30 g	140	6	20
Reduced Fat, 16 g	70	3	12
Snack Sticks Original, 29 g	130	6	19
Grahams			
Honey, 31 g	140	4	23
Lowfat Honey, 27 g	110	2	22
Original, 29 g	130	4	22
On The GO			
Animals Variety Pack, 28 g	180	6	30
Cinnamon Snack Pack, 28 g	120	4	20
Right Bites® Variety Pack, 28 g	100	4	17
Variety Snack Pack, 28 g	140	5	23
Sandwich Crackers			
Cheese & Peanut Butter, 39 g	200	10	23
Club® & Cheddar, 36 g	190	10	23
Toast & Peanut Butter, 39 g	200	10	23
Wheat & Cheddar, 36 g	190	10	23
Toasteds			
Buttercrisp, 16 g	80	4	10
Organic, 29 g	130	6	20
Wheat, 16 g	80	4	10
Townhouse			
Original, 16 g	80	5	10
Reduced Fat, 15 g	60	2	11
Toppers Original, 14 g	70	3	9
Wheatables			
Multigrain, 30 g	140	6	20
Original Golden Wheat, 30 g	140	6	20
Reduced Fat, 31 g	140	4	22
Pepperidge Farm			
Baby Cheddar Goldfish, 89 pieces	140	5	20
• Cinnamon Goldfish Graham Snacks, 1 pk	210	8	32
Original Goldfish, 55 pieces	150	6	20
Parmesan Goldfish, 60 pieces	130	4	20
Pizza Goldfish, 55 pieces	140	5	20
Premium			
Fat Free, 15 g	60	0	12
Low Sodium, 14 g	60	2	11
Multigrain, 14 g	60	2	10

• MOST HEALTHY   • LEAST HEALTHY

> SNACKS	Cal	Fat	Cbs
Original, 15 g	60	2	11
Toasted Onion, 15 g	60	2	11
Purity Foods			
Cajun Spelt Sesame Sticks, 28 g	150	9	15
Garlic Spelt Sesame Sticks, 28 g	150	9	15
Whole Grain Spelt Sesame Sticks, 28 g	150	9	14
Wild Rice Spelt Sesame Sticks, 28 g	140	0	17
Ritz			
Real Cheese, 39 oz.	200	12	22
Low Sodium, 16 oz.	80	4	10
Peanut Butter, 39 oz.	190	9	24
Sargento			
Cheese Dip & Cheddar Sticks , 28 g	100	6	11
Cheese Dip & Crackers , 27 g	100	5	10
Social Tea			
Biscuits, 31 g	140	4	24
Stauffer's			
All Natural Animal Crackers			
Chocolate, 1 oz.	130	3	23
Original & Chocolate, 1 oz.	120	3	25
Original, 1 oz.	120	2	24
Animal Crackers			
Chocolate, 1 oz.	120	3	23
Chocolate Graham Crackers, 1 oz.	120	3	23
Cinnamon, 1 oz.	110	2	21
Cinnamon Graham Crackers, 1 oz.	110	2	21
Original, 1 oz.	120	2	24
Assorted Crackers			
Cheese, 1 oz.	140	7	17
Chicken Flavored, 1 oz.	150	8	19
Stauffer's Oyster, 1 oz.	120	3	22
Whales Baked, 2 oz.	210	9	27
Sunridge Farms			
Organic Japanese Rice Crackers, 30 g	110	0	26
Teddy Grahams			
Chocolate, 30 g	130	5	22
Cinnamon, 35 g	150	5	26
Honey, 30 g	130	4	23
Oatmeal, 30 g	130	4	23
Triscuit			
Baked Whole Grain Deli-style Rye, 28 g	120	5	19
Baked Whole Grain Thin Crisps, 30 g	130	5	21
Wheat Thins			
Low Sodium, 31 g	150	6	22
Multi-Grain, 30 g	140	5	22

● MOST HEALTHY   ● LEAST HEALTHY

SNACKS	Cal	Fat	Cbs
Original, 31 g	140	6	21
Ranch, 29 g	130	6	20
Reduced Fat, 29 g	130	4	21
Zwieback			
Stay Fresh Crackers, 8 g	35	1	6
FRUIT SNACKS			
Betty Crocker			
Fruit By The Foot Tropical Tango, 21 g	80	1	17
• Fruit Gushers Watermelon Blast, 25 g	90	1	20
• Fruit Roll-Ups Strawberry, 14 g	50	1	12
Tropicana Juice			
Cherry, 19 g	70	0	17
Strawberry, 19 g	70	0	17
JERKY			
Pemmican			
Natural Hickory Smkd Beef Jerky, 1 bag	140	2	6
Natural Sweet & Hot Beef Jerky, 1 bag	150	2	9
• Original Beef Jerky, 1 bag	70	1	4
Original Steak Tips, 1 oz.	70	2	7
Shredded Peppered Beef Jerky, 1 oz.	80	2	3
Teriyaki Shredded Beef Jerky, 1 oz.	80	2	3
Slim Jim			
Beef Jerky Canister, 7 pcs	130	8	3
• Classic Handipack, 1 box	210	19	3
Giant Jerk, 1 pkg	80	5	2
Giant Jerk Caddy, 1 pkg	80	5	2
Giant Pepperoni Caddy, 1 pkg	150	13	3
Mild Canister, 4 pcs	170	15	2
Natural Peppered Beef Jerky, 1 oz.	80	2	4
Original Canister, 4 pcs	170	15	2
Pepperoni Canister, 4 pcs	170	15	2
NUTS & TRAIL MIX			
American Almond			
Almonds, 1 oz.	167	15	6
Hazelnuts, 1 oz.	179	19	4
Macadamias, 1 oz.	199	21	4
Peanuts (Unsalted), 1 oz.	166	14	6
Pecans, 1 oz.	189	19	5
Walnuts, 1 oz.	182	18	5
Blue Diamond Almonds			
Honey Roast Almonds, 28	170	14	8
Jordan Almonds, 40	180	8	28
Oven Roasted No Salt, 1 oz.	170	15	5
Chex			
Mix Bold Party Blend, 30 g	140	6	20

• MOST HEALTHY   • LEAST HEALTHY

➤ SNACKS	Cal	Fat	Cbs
Mix Cheddar, 30 g	130	4	22
Mix Hot 'n Spicy, 30 g	130	4	20
Mix Peanut Lovers, 30 g	140	5	19
Mix Select - Chocolate PB, 33 g	150	5	24
Mix Select - Chocolate Turtle, 33 g	150	5	24
Mix Select - Dark Chocolate, 30 g	140	5	23
Mix Sweet 'n Salty Caramel Crunch, 30 g	130	4	23
Mix Sweet 'n Salty Honey Nut, 30 g	130	4	22
Mix Sweet 'n Salty Trail Mix, 32 g	140	5	22
Mix Traditional, 30 g	130	4	22
Simply Chex Cheddar, 30 g	130	4	22
Corn Nuts			
Barbecue, 48 g	220	8	34
Chile Picante, 48 g	210	8	33
Nacho Cheese, 28 g	130	5	19
Original, 28 g	120	5	20
Ranch, 48 g	220	8	33
Salsa Jalisco, 48 g	220	8	34
David Seeds			
BBQ Sunflower Seed Kernels, 1/4 cup	190	15	5
• In Shell Sunflower Seeds, 1/4 cup	260	21	7
Jalapeño & Hot Salsa In Shll Snflwr Seeds, 1/4 cup	180	14	6
Nacho In Shell Snflwr Seeds, 1/4 cup w/o Shell	170	14	5
Pumpkin Seeds, 1/4 cup	160	12	4
Red Sodium Snflwr Seeds, 1/4 cup w/o Shell	190	14	7
Sunflower Seeds, 1/4 cup	190	15	5
Fisher Nuts			
Almonds, 1 oz.	170	14	6
Butter Toffe Peanuts, 1 oz.	130	6	17
Dry Roasted Peanuts, 1 oz.	170	14	6
Honey Roasted Peanuts, 1 oz.	170	13	7
Jumbo Cashews, 1 oz.	170	15	8
Mixed Nuts, 1 oz.	180	16	5
Oil Roasted Peanuts, 1 oz.	170	15	5
Pecans, 1 oz.	200	20	4
Walnuts, 1 oz.	200	20	3
Mauna Loa			
Mauna Loa Macadamias			
Honey Roasted, 28 g	180	16	9
Maui Onion & Garlic, 14 g	100	11	2
Salted Dry Roasted, 28 g	230	24	4
Unsalted Dry Roasted, 28 g	230	24	4
Mauna Loa Mix			
Island Nut & Fruit, 30 g	150	10	16
Macadamias & Almonds, 28 g	180	17	4

● MOST HEALTHY   • LEAST HEALTHY

SNACKS

	Cal	Fat	Cbs
Mixers			
Snack Mix - Cheddar, 28 g	130	5	19
Snack Mix - Traditional, 30 g	130	5	21
Nature Valley			
Trail Mix Bars Apple Cinnamon, 35 g	140	4	25
Trail Mix Bars Fruit & Nut, 35 g	140	4	25
Trail Mix Bars Mixed Berry, 35 g	140	4	26
Planters			
Cashew Halves & Pieces			
Lightly Salted, 28 g	170	14	8
Regular, 28 g	170	14	8
Chocolate Covered Almonds			
Chocolate Lovers, 41 g	220	17	18
Deluxe & Select Mixed Nuts,			
Deluxe Regular, 28 g	170	15	6
Select Cashew, Almond & Pecan, 28 g	170	16	6
Select Macadamia, Cashew & Almond, 28 g	180	17	6
Cocktail Peanuts			
Honey Roasted, 28 g	160	13	8
Lightly Salted, 28 g	170	15	5
Regular, 28 g	170	14	6
Unsalted, 28 g	170	14	6
Dry Roasted Peanuts			
Honey Roasted, 28 g	150	12	7
Lightly Salted, 28 g	160	14	5
Regular, 28 g	170	14	5
Unsalted, 28 g	170	14	5
Fruit & Raisin Mixes			
Fruit & Nut, 28 g	140	9	14
Mixed Nuts & Raisins, 29 g	150	11	10
Nuts, Seeds & Raisins, 31 g	160	12	11
Lovers' Mixes			
Cashew, 28 g	180	17	6
Macadamia, 28 g	190	19	4
Pecan, 28 g	180	17	6
Pistachio, 28 g	160	13	7
Mixed Nuts			
Honey Roasted, 28 g	160	12	9
Lightly Salted, 28 g	170	15	5
Regular, 28 g	170	15	5
Unsalted, 28 g	170	15	5
More Cashews			
Chocolate Lovers, 42 g	230	16	20
Dry Roasted, 19 g	160	12	9
Jumbo, 28 g	171	14	8

• MOST HEALTHY   • LEAST HEALTHY

SNACKS	Cal	Fat	Cbs
Other Nuts			
Nutrition Salted, 28 g	170	15	6
Nutrition Smoked, 28 g	170	15	6
Spanish Peanuts, 28 g	180	14	5
Sweet n' Crunchy Peanuts, 28 g	140	7	16
Sweet & Salty Mixes			
Energy Mix, 42 g	240	19	14
Honey Nut Medley, 32 g	160	10	16
Nut & Chocolate, 33 g	160	10	16
Sweet & Nutty, 30 g	150	10	14
Whole Cashews			
Honey Roasted, 28 g	150	12	11
Lightly Salted, 28 g	170	14	8
Regular, 28 g	170	14	8
Poppycock			
Cashew Lovers, 30 g	140	6	21
Original, 31 g	160	8	20
Pecan Delight, 30 g	150	8	20
Sunridge Farms			
Organic Cranberry Harvest, 30 g	140	9	13
• Oriental Cracker Mix, 30 g	110	0	27
Oriental Party Mix, 30 g	160	11	12
Sesame Sticks, 30 g	170	12	14
Super Deluxe Trail Mix, 30 g	150	11	11
Tropical Trail Mix, 30 g	140	9	13
Wasabi Peas, 30 g	120	1	20
Nuts and Seeds			
Almonds, Roasted, No Salt, 30 g	180	15	6
California Almonds Supreme, 30 g	190	15	5
Fancy Mixed Nuts, 30 g	180	15	5
Honey Mixed Nuts, 30 g	170	14	9
Natural Pumpkin Seeds, 30 g	160	14	5
Natural Sunflower Seeds, 30 g	170	14	6
Pecan Halves, 30 g	220	20	4
Walnut Halves, 30 g	200	21	4
POPCORN			
Act II Microwave Popcorn			
94% Fat Free Butter Popcorn, 3 tbsp.	130	3	28
Butter Lovers Popcorn, 2 tbsp.	170	12	16
Butter Popcorn, 2 tbsp.	160	10	18
Extreme Butter Popcorn, 2 tbsp.	180	13	15
Movie Theater Butter Popcorn, 2 tbsp.	170	12	16
Healthy Choice			
Butter Popcorn, 3 tbsp.	130	3	28
Natural Popcorn, 3 tbsp.	130	3	28

• MOST HEALTHY • LEAST HEALTHY

▶ SNACKS

	Cal	Fat	Cbs
Jiffy Pop			
Butter Popcorn, 2 tbsp.	140	7	19
Orville Redenbacher's			
Movie Theater			
Butter Light Popcorn, 2 tbsp.	120	5	19
Butter Popcorn, 2 tbsp.	170	12	16
Popcorn			
• Butter Popcorn, 2 tbsp.	210	14	20
Light Butter Popcorn, 2 tbsp.	120	5	19
Popcorn Cakes			
• Caramel Popcorn Cakes, 1 cake	45	0	11
White Cheddar Popcorn Cakes, 2 cakes	60	1	14
Smart Pop			
Movie Theater Butter Popcorn, 2 tbsp.	130	3	28
Popcorn, 1 bag	110	2	240
Paul Newman's Own			
94% Fat Free Microwave Popcorn, 30 g	110	2	20
Butter Microwave Popcorn, 30 g	130	5	18
Light Butter Microwave Popcorn, 30 g	120	4	19
White Kernel Popcorn, 30 g	130	5	18
Pop Secret			
1-Step Cheddar, 3 tbsp.	180	13	17
94% Fat Free Butter, 3 tbsp.	120	2	26
Butter, 3 tbsp.	180	12	17
Extra Butter, 3 tbsp.	180	13	17
Homestyle, 3 tbsp.	170	12	17
Kettle Corn, 3 tbsp.	180	13	15
Light Butter, 3 tbsp.	140	5	24
Smart Balance			
Light Butter Popcorn, 28 g	120	5	18
Smart 'n Healthy Popcorn, 31 g	120	2	24
Smart Movie Style Popcorn, 32 g	170	11	16
PRETZELS			
Gardetto's			
Deli-Style Mustard Pretzel Mix, 30 g	130	2	24
Italian Cheese Blend, 30 g	140	5	20
Original, 30 g	150	6	20
Reduced Fat Original, 30 g	130	4	20
Roasted Garlic Rye Chips, 30 g	160	10	16
Purity Foods			
Spelt Pretzels, 1 oz.	110	2	21
Vita Spelt Low Sodium Pretzels, 1 oz.	110	2	21
Vita Spelt Organic Sourdough Pretzels, 1 oz.	110	1	23

• MOST HEALTHY • LEAST HEALTHY

SNACKS	Cal	Fat	Cbs
Snyder's of Hanover			
Multigrain			
Honey Mustard & Onion Nibblers, 30 g	140	5	20
Lightly Salted Pretzel Sticks, 30 g	120	2	23
Olde Tyme Pretzel Twists, 30 g	120	2	22
Pretzel Crackers			
Butter Sesame Pretzel Crackers, 30 g	120	3	23
Original Pretzel Crackers, 30 g	120	3	23
Pumpernickel & Onion Pretzel Crackers, 28 g	120	3	22
Pretzels			
Garlic Bread Nibblers, 1 oz.	130	3	24
Homestyle Pretzels, 1 oz.	120	1	25
Honey Mustard & Onion Nibblers, 1 oz.	130	3	23
Honey Wheat Sticks, 1 oz.	120	2	24
Mini Pretzels, 1 oz.	110	1	25
• Thins, 1 oz.	100	0	23
Sunridge Farms			
• Yogurt Pretzels, 40 g	190	7	29
SNACK BARS			
100 Calorie Packs			
Chewy Granola Bars - Chips Ahoy!, 28 g	100	2	22
Balance Bar			
Balance 100 Calories			
Chocolate Caramel Crisp, 28 g	100	4	14
Peanut Butter Crisp, 28 g	100	5	14
Vanila Crisp, 28 g	100	4	15
Balance Bar Original			
Almond Brownie, 50 g	200	6	22
Chocolate, 50 g	200	6	23
Peanut Butter, 50 g	200	6	22
Balance Carbwell			
Caramel N Chocolate, 50 g	190	7	23
Chocolate Fudge, 50 g	190	6	23
Chocolate Peanut Butter, 50 g	200	8	22
Balance Gold			
Chewy Chocolate Chip, 20 g	210	7	25
Cookies N Crème Crunch, 50 g	210	6	22
Triple Chocolate Chaos, 50 g	210	7	24
Balance Organic			
Apricot Mango Crisp, 45 g	180	7	23
Cranberry Pomegranate Crisp, 45 g	180	7	23
Cherry Almond Crisp, 45 g	180	7	23
Cascadian Farm			
Chewy Granola Bars Chocolate Chip, 35 g	140	3	25
Chewy Granola Bars Fruit & Nut, 35 g	140	4	24

SNACKS	Cal	Fat	Cbs
Chewy Granola Bars Harvest Bry, 35 g	130	2	27
Chewy Granola Bars Multi Grain, 35 g	130	2	27
Clif Products			
Clif Bar			
Apricot, 68 g	230	3	45
Carrot Cake, 68 g	240	4	46
Chocolate Almond Fudge, 68 g	250	5	44
Oatmeal Raisin Walnut, 68 g	240	5	43
Clif Builders			
Chocolate, 68 g	270	8	30
• Chocolate Mint, 68 g	270	8	31
Cookies N Cream, 68 g	270*	8	30
Clif Kid Twisted Fruit			
• Grape, 20 g	70	0	16
Pineapple, 20 g	70	0	16
Luna, 20 g	70	0	16
Sour Apple, 20 g	70	0	16
Clif Kid Zbar			
Apple Cinnamon, 36 g	120	2	23
Blueberry, 36 g	120	3	23
Honey Graham, 36 g	130	2	26
Peanut Butter, 36 g	140	5	20
Clif Minis			
Mini Chocolate Brownie, 28 g	100	2	18
Mini Chocolate Chip, 28 g	100	2	18
Mini Crunchy Peanut Butter, 28 g	100	3	17
Clif Mojo			
Fruit Nut Crunch, 45 g	190	7	24
Honey Roasted Peanut, 45 g	200	10	20
Mixed Nuts, 45 g	210	11	19
Peanut Butter Pretzel, 45 g	200	9	21
Clif Mojo Dipped			
Chocolate Peanut, 45 g	210	10	22
Fruit & Nut, 45 g	200	8	24
Peanut Butter and Jelly, 45 g	220	11	21
Clif Nectar			
Apple Cinnamon, 45 g	160	6	30
Cherry Pomegranate, 45 g	150	5	29
Cranberry Apricot Almond, 45 g	170	6	29
Lemon Vanilla Cashew, 45 g	160	6	27
Clif Nectar Cacao			
Dark Chocolate Mocha, 45 g	160	6	27
Dark Chocolate Raspberry, 45 g	150	5	29
Dark Chocolate Walnut, 45 g	160	6	27

SNACKS	Cal	Fat	Cbs
Clif Shot Bloks			
Black Cherry, 30 g	100	0	24
Cola, 30 g	100	0	24
Piña Colada, 30 g	100	0	24
Strawberry, 30 g	100	0	24
Luna Bar			
Berry Almond, 48 g	180	4	27
Chai Tea, 48 g	180	5	25
Cookies N Cream Delight, 48 g	180	5	26
Peanut Butter Cookie, 48 g	180	6	23
Luna Sport			
Blueberry Moons Energy Chews, 30 g	100	0	24
Dark Chocolate Recovery Smoothie, 1 oz.	120	N/A	21
Strwbry Banana Recovery Smoothie, 1 oz.	120	N/A	21
Luna Sunrise			
Apple Cinnamon, 48 g	180	5	27
Blueberry Bliss, 48 g	170	5	26
Strawberry Crumble, 48 g	170	5	26
Vanilla Almond, 48 g	180	5	29
Luna Teacakes			
Berry Pomegranate, 40 g	140	2	30
Mint Chocolate, 40 g	130	3	25
Orange Blossom, 40 g	130	2	30
Vanilla Macadamia, 40 g	150	4	28
Honey Maid			
Snack Bars - Oatmeal, 34 g	150	6	24
Snack Bars Oatmeal Raisin, 34 g	150	6	24
Nature Valley			
Chwy Granola Bars Blueberry Yogurt, 35 g	140	4	26
Granola Bars Apple Crisp, 42 g	180	6	29
Granola Bars Vanilla Nut, 42 g	190	7	28
Healthy Heart Granola Bars Honey Nut, 40 g	160	4	28
Roasted Nut Bars - Almond Crunch, 35 g	200	14	11
Nutri-Grain			
Fruit & Nut Bars - Berry & Almond, 32 g	120	4	22
Fruit & Nut Bars - Cran, Raisin & Pnt, 32 g	120	4	22
Yogurt Bars - Strawberry, 37 g	140	4	25
Yogurt Bars - Vanilla, 37 g	140	4	26
Philadelphia Cream Cheese			
Snack Bars - Classic Cheesecake, 42 g	190	11	20
Snack Bars - Marble Brownie, 42 g	170	9	20
Snack Bars - Strwbry Cheesecake, 42 g	180	9	22
Snack Bites - Choco Covered Strwbry, 28 g	130	7	15
Pop-Tarts			
Go-Tarts!™ Frstd Bwn Sugr Cinn Snack Bars, 35 g	140	4	24

• MOST HEALTHY   • LEAST HEALTHY

▸ SNACKS™	Cal	Fat	Cbs
Go-Tarts!™ Frstd Choco Chip Snack Bars, 35 g	140	5	24
Go-Tarts!™ Frstd Choco Fudge Snack Bars, 35 g	140	4	24
Go-Tarts!™ Frstd Strwbry Snack Bars, 35 g	140	4	25
Rice Krispies			
Treats® Chocolatey PntBtr bars, 22 g	100	4	15
Treats® Mini-Squares, 44 g	180	5	34
Treats® Original, 22 g	90	3	17
Treats® Rainbow, 22 g	90	3	17
Solo GI			
Berry Bliss Bar, 50 g	200	6	25
Chocolate Charger Bar, 50 g	200	7	26
Mint Mania Bar, 50 g	200	7	26
Peanut Power, 50 g	200	8	23
South Beach Living			
Caramel Peanut Crispy Meal Bar, 60 g	210	7	26
Chocolate Caramel Meal Bar, 50 g	180	5	22
Chocolate Crispy Meal Bar, 60 g	210	6	26
Chocolate Mint Snack Bar Delights, 28 g	100	4	15
Nut Medley Sweet Nut Creations, 35 g	150	7	18
Peanut Butter Snack Bar Delights, 28 g	100	4	14
Roasted Pnut Sweet Nut Creations, 35 g	150	7	18
Vanilla Crème Crispy Meal Bar, 60 g	220	7	26
Special K			
Bar Chocolatey Drizzle, 22 g	90	2	17
Bar Strawberry, 23 g	90	2	18
Bliss™ Bar Orange, 22 g	90	2	17
Bliss™ Bar Raspberry, 22 g	90	2	17
Protein™ Meal Bar Double Choco, 45 g	180	5	25
Protein™ Meal Bar Strawberry, 45 g	180	5	24
Protein™ Snack Bar Choco Peanut, 26 g	110	4	15
SNACK DIPS & SPREADS			
California Sun Dry			
Sun-Dried Tomato Salsa, 2 tbsp.	20	3	N/A
Country Fresh			
French Onion Dip, 30 g	80	8	3
Veggie Dip, 31 g	60	6	2
Dean's			
French Onion Dip, 30 g	80	8	3
Veggie Dip, 31 g	60	6	2
McCormick			
• Ranch Dip Mix, 2 g	5	0	0
Spinach Dip Mix, 2 g	10	0	1
Vegetable Dip Mix, 2 g	5	0	0
Muir Glen			
Salsa Black Bean & Corn Medium, 31 g	20	0	4

● MOST HEALTHY   ● LEAST HEALTHY

> SNACKS	Cal	Fat	Cbs
Salsa Medium, 31 g	10	0	3
Salsa Mild, 31 g	10	0	3
Pace Foods			
Mexican 4 Chz Salsa con Queso, 2 tbsp.	90	7	5
Picante Sauce, 2 tbsp.	10	0	2
Pico De Gallo, 2 tbsp.	10	0	3
Salsa Verde, 2 tbsp.	15	1	2
Tequila Lime Salsa, 2 tbsp.	15	0	3
Thick & Chunky Salsa, 2 tbsp.	10	0	2
Paul Newman's Own			
All-Natural Bandito Chunky Salsa Peach, 32 g	25	0	6
All-Natural Bandito Salsa Mild, 32 g	10	0	2
All-Natural Bandito Salsa Tequila Lime, 31 g	15	0	3
Farmer's Garden Salsa, 32 g	15	0	4
Mango Salsa, 32 g	20	0	5
Organic Chunky Medium Salsa, 31 g	10	0	3
Snyder's of Hanover			
• Fire Roasted Salsa, 1 oz.	150	6	20
Garden Style Sweet Salsa, 2 tbsp.	20	0	5
Salsa Con Queso, 2 tbsp.	35	2	4
Tres Bean Dip, 2 tbsp.	25	0	5
Taco Bell Home Originals			
Bean Con Queso - Home Originals, 31 g	35	2	2
Chili Con Queso - Home Originals w/ Meat, 31 g	40	2	3
Salsa - Thick 'N Chunky Medium, 31 g	15	0	3
Salsa - Thick 'N Chunky Mild, 31 g	15	0	3
TORTILLA/CORN CHIPS			
Azteca Foods			
Chips			
Fried White Corn Tortilla Chips, 1 oz.	140	6	19
Fried Yellow Corn Tortilla Chips, 1 oz.	140	6	19
Unfried Corn Tortilla Chips, 1 oz.	80	1	15
Salad Shells			
• Salad Shells, 59 g	280	16	29
Tortillas			
Pressed Flour Tortillas, 2 oz.	153	3	27
• White Corn Tortillas, 1 oz.	75	1	15
Yellow Corn Tortillas, 1 oz.	75	1	15
Doritos			
Baked! Nacho Chz® Flavored Chips, 1 oz.	120	4	21
Cool Ranch® Flavored Chips, 1 oz.	140	7	18
Fiery Habanero Flavored Chips, 1 oz.	130	7	16
Light Nacho Chz® Flavored Chips, 1 oz.	100	2	19
Nacho Cheese® Flavored Chips, 1 oz.	140	8	17
Salsa Verde Flavored Chips, 1 oz.	140	7	19

• MOST HEALTHY   • LEAST HEALTHY

SNACKS

	Cal	Fat	Cbs
Smokin' Chdr BBQ Flavored Chips, 1 oz.	150	8	17
Spicy Nacho Flavored Chips, 1 oz.	140	7	18
Toasted Corn Chips, 1 oz.	140	7	18
Fritos			
BBQ Flavored Corn Chips, 1 oz.	150	10	16
Chili Cheese Flavored Corn Chips, 1 oz.	160	10	15
Original Corn Chips, 1 oz.	160	10	15
SCOOPS!® Corn Chips, 1 oz.	160	10	16
Tangy Rstd Corn Flav Corn Chips, 1 oz.	160	1	16
Snyder's of Hanover			
Restaurant Style Tortillas, 1 oz.	130	5	20
Savory Blue Tortillas, 1 oz.	140	7	17
White Corn Tortillas, 1 oz.	140	5	23
Yellow Corn Tortillas, 1 oz.	140	5	23
Tostitos			
Baked! Scoops!® Tortilla Chips, 1 oz.	120	3	22
Flour Tortilla Chips, 1 oz.	140	7	19
Light Restaurant Style Tortilla Chips, 1 oz.	90	1	20
Multigrain Tortilla Chips, 1 oz.	150	8	18
Restaurant Style Tortilla Chips, 1 oz.	140	7	19
Scoops!® Tortilla Chips, 1 oz.	140	7	18

SOUPS & BROTHS

BOUILLON/BROTHS

	Cal	Fat	Cbs
Allens			
Allens Chicken Broth, 1 cup	10	0	0
Campbell's Soups			
Beef Broth, 1/2 cup	15	0	1
Chicken Broth, 1 cup	25	1	1
• Scotch Broth, 1/2 cup	70	2	9
College Inn			
Beef Broth			
Beef Broth, 1 cup	25	1	0
French Onion, 1 cup	15	0	0
Chicken Broth			
Chicken Broth, 1 cup	15	1	0
• Chicken Fat Free, 1 cup	5	0	0
Chicken Light, 1 cup	15	1	0
Lemon Herb, 1 cup	15	1	0
Roasted Garlic, 1 cup	20	0	3
Roasted Veggies and Herb, 1 cup	20	0	3
Garden Vegetable Broth			
Garden Veg, 1 cup	25	0	6
Turkey Broth, 1 cup	20	0	0

• MOST HEALTHY   • LEAST HEALTHY

SOUPS & BROTHS	Cal	Fat	Cbs
Swanson Broth			
Beef Broth, 1 cup	15	0	1
Certified Organic Beef Broth, 1 cup	15	1	1
Certified Organic Chicken Broth, 1 cup	15	1	1
Chicken Broth, 1 cup	10	1	1
Seasoned Beef Broth, 1 cup	20	1	2
Seasoned Chkn Broth w/ Rstd Garlic, 1 cup	20	1	2
Vegetable Broth, 1 cup	15	0	3
CANNED SOUP			
Campbell's Soups			
Beef Noodle Soup, 1/2 cup	70	2	8
Cream of Broccoli Soup, 1/2 cup	90	4	12
Cream of Onion Soup, 1/2 cup	100	6	10
French Onion Soup, 1/2 cup	45	2	6
Tomato Soup, 1/2 cup	90	0	20
Vegetable Beef Soup, 1/2 cup	90	1	15
Chunky™ Soups			
Hearty Beef Barley Soup, 1 cup	170	3	26
Hearty Chkn w/ Vegetables Soup, 1 cup	90	2	13
Hold the Beans Chili, 1 cup	240	10	20
New England Clam Chowder, 1 cup	210	9	25
Chunky™ Fully Loaded Soups			
Beef Stew Soup, 1 cup	160	4	20
Rigatoni & Meatballs Soup, 1 cup	220	8	24
• Stroganoff-Style Beef Soup, 1 cup	250	14	18
Turkey Pot Pie Soup, 1 cup	200	8	21
Healthy Request® Chunky™ Soups			
Beef Barley Soup, 1 cup	140	2	21
Chicken Noodle Soup, 1 cup	120	3	15
Old Fashioned Veggie Beef Soup, 1 cup	110	2	17
Healthy Request® Condensed Soups			
Chicken Noodle Soup, 1/2 cup	60	2	8
Tomato Soup, 1/2 cup	90	2	17
Vegetable Soup, 1/2 cup	100	1	19
Healthy Request® Select™ Soups			
Chicken w/ Egg Noodles, 1 cup	100	3	13
Italian-Style Wedding, 1 cup	120	3	15
Mexican Style Chicken Tortilla, 1 cup	130	3	20
Savory Chkn and Long Grain Rice, 1 cup	110	2	18
Low Sodium Soups			
Chicken with Noodles Soup, 1 can	160	5	17
Cream of Mushroom Soup, 1 can	160	8	19
Select™ Gold Label Soup			
Creamy Tomato Parmesan, 1 cup	200	9	25
Italian Tomato with Basil & Garlic, 1 cup	90	0	19

• MOST HEALTHY   • LEAST HEALTHY

SOUPS & BROTHS

	Cal	Fat	Cbs
Southwestern Corn Soup, 1 cup	190	8	26
Select™ Soups			
98% FF New England Clam Chowder, 1 cup	110	2	18
Creamy Chicken Alfredo Soup, 1 cup	180	7	18
New England Clam Chowder, 1 cup	160	8	15
Potato Broccoli Cheese Soup, 1 cup	120	4	18
Healthy Choice			
Bean & Ham Soup, 1 cup	180	2	29
Chicken & Dumplings Soup, 1 cup	140	3	21
Chicken Noodle Soup, 1 cup	100	2	13
Chicken Rice Soup, 1 cup	110	2	17
Country Vegetables Soup, 1 cup	110	1	19
Hearty Chicken Soup, 1 cup	130	2	20
New England Clam Chowder, 1 cup	110	1	19
Split Pea & Ham, 1 cup	140	2	22
Vegetable Beef Soup, 1 cup	130	1	22
Muir Glen			
Classic Minestrone, 1 cup	110	2	19
Creamy Tomato, 1 cup	170	6	26
Garden Vegetable, 1 cup	80	1	16
Hearty Tomato, 1 cup	130	2	25
Homestyle Split Pea, 1 cup	170	1	35
Progresso			
Low-Fat/Low-Carb			
Light Homestyle Veg and Rice, 1 cup	60	0	14
Light Italian-Style Vegetable, 1 cup	60	0	14
Light Savory Vegetable Barley, 1 cup	60	0	14
Light Southwestern-Style Veg, 1 cup	60	0	12
Healthy Favorites 50% Less Sodium			
Chicken Gumbo, 1 cup	110	2	18
Chicken Noodle, 1 cup	90	2	12
Garden Vegetable, 1 cup	100	0	22
Minestrone, 1 cup	120	2	24
Rich & Hearty			
Chicken & Homestyle Noodles, 1 cup	110	2	14
Chicken Corn Chowder, 1 cup	210	9	23
Chicken Pot Pie Style, 1 cup	170	6	21
Creamy Chicken Wild Rice, 1 cup	150	8	13
New England Clam Chowder,1 cup	190	9	22
Savory Beef Barley Vegetable, 1 cup	130	1	22
Slow Cooked Vegetable Beef, 1 cup	120	1	20
Steak & Roasted Russet Potatoes, 1 cup	140	2	23
Traditional			
Carb Monitor Chkn Chz Enchilada, 1 cup	170	12	8
Manhattan Clam Chowder, 1 cup	100	2	17

● MOST HEALTHY   ● LEAST HEALTHY

SOUPS & BROTHS

	Cal	Fat	Cbs
Chicken Noodle, 1 cup	100	3	12
Chicken Sausage Gumbo, 1 cup	130	4	18
Minestrone with Chicken, 1 cup	120	4	16
New England Clam Chowder, 1 cup	190	10	20
Potato Broccoli & Chz Chowder, 1 cup	180	10	18
Soup Turkey Noodle, 1 cup	80	2	12
Vegetable Classics			
99% Fat Free Minestrone, 1 cup	100	1	19
Creamy Mushroom, 1 cup	130	10	9
• French Onion, 1 cup	50	2	8
Green Split Pea with Bacon, 1 cup	170	1	28
Hearty Penne in Chicken Broth, 1 cup	80	1	14
Lentil, 1 cup	150	2	28
Macaroni & Bean, 1 cup	160	4	25
Tomato Basil, 1 cup	160	3	30

SOUP MIX

Campbell's Soups

• Onion Soup Mix, 1 tbsp.	15	0	4

Top Ramen

Beef, 1/2 cup	83	4	11
Chicken, 1/2 cup	83	4	11
Oriental, 1/2 cup	83	4	11
Pork, 1/2 cup	83	4	11

Uncle Ben's

• Hearty Soup Broccoli Chz & Rice, 1/2 cup	110	2	43

SYRUP, JAMS, NUT BUTTERS

FRUIT SPREADS

Apple Time

Apple Butter, 1 tbsp.	30	N/A	8

Brummel & Brown

• Simply Strawberry® Creamy, 12 g	50	4	3

Cascadian Farm

Apricot, 19 g	40	0	10
Blackberry, 19 g	45	0	11
Blueberry, 19 g	45	0	11
Strawberry, 19 g	40	0	10

Knott's Berry Farm

Light Strawberry Jam, 1 tbsp.	20	0	5
Strawberry Jam, 1 tbsp.	50	0	13

Lucky Leaf

Lucky Leaf Apple Butter, 1 tbsp.	30	N/A	8

Smuckers

Fruit Butter

Cider Apple Butter, 19 g	45	0	11

● MOST HEALTHY   • LEAST HEALTHY

SYRUP, JAMS, NUT BUTTERS	Cal	Fat	Cbs
Spiced Apple Butter, 19 g	45	0	11
Jam			
Blackberry, 20 g	50	0	13
Concord Grape, 20 g	51	0	13
Raspberry, 20 g	50	0	13
Jelly			
Apple, 20 g	50	0	13
Blackberry, 20 g	50	0	13
Mixed Fruit, 20 g	50	0	13
Low Sugar			
Apricot, 17 g	21	0	6
Strawberry, 17 g	25	0	6
Sweet Orange Marmalade, 17 g	25	0	2
Preserves			
Boysenberry, 20 g	50	0	13
Cherry, 20 g	50	0	13
Peach, 20 g	50	0	13
Simply Fruit			
Black Cherry, 19 g	40	0	10
Blueberry, 19 g	40	0	10
Red Raspberry, 19 g	40	0	10
Sugar Free			
• Boysenberry Preserves w/ Splenda, 17 g	10	0	5
Concord Grape Jam with Splenda, 17 g	10	0	5
Strawberry with NutraSweet, 17 g	10	0	5
Welch's			
Jelly, Jam & Spread Jars, 20 g	50	0	13
NUT BUTTER			
Jif			
Reduced Fat Jif Creamy, 36 g	190	12	15
Reduced Fat Jif Crunchy, 36 g	190	12	15
Regular Jif Creamy, 32 g	190	16	7
Regular Jif Extra Crunchy, 32 g	190	16	7
Nutella			
Hazelnut Spread w/ Skim Milk & Cocoa, 37 g	200	11	23
Peter Pan			
Creamy Peanut Butter, 2 tbsp.	190	17	6
Crunchy Peanut Butter, 2 tbsp.	190	16	6
• Whipped Creamy Peanut Butter, 2 tbsp.	140	12	5
Skippy Peanut Butter			
Creamy, 32 g	190	16	7
Natural, 32 g	180	17	6
Reduced Fat Creamy, 36 g	180	12	15
Reduced Fat Super Chunk, 35 g	180	12	15
Roasted Honey Nut Creamy, 32 g	190	16	7

• MOST HEALTHY   • LEAST HEALTHY

SYRUP, JAMS, NUT BUTTERS	Cal	Fat	Cbs
Roasted Honey Nut Super Chunk, 32 g	190	16	6
Super Chunk®, 32 g	190	16	7
Smart Balance			
Chunky, 32 g	200	17	6
Creamy, 32 g	200	17	6
Smuckers			
Goober PB & J			
• Grape, 53 g	240	13	24
Strawberry, 53 g	240	13	24
Natural Peanut Butter			
Chunky, 32 g	210	16	6
Creamy, 32 g	210	16	6
Honey, 33 g	200	16	9
SYRUP			
Aunt Jemima			
Lite, 1/4 cup	100	0	26
Original, 1/4 cup	210	0	52
Eggo			
Butter Pecan Syrup, 1/4 cup	220	0	55
Buttery Syrup, 1/4 cup	160	0	41
Lite Syrup, 1/4 cup	110	0	27
Original Syrup, 1/4 cup	240	0	60
Karo Syrup			
Dark Corn Syrup, 1/8 cup	120	0	31
Light Corn Syrup, 1/8 cup	120	0	31
• Pancake Syrup, 1/4 cup	240	0	63
Knott's Berry Farm			
Blueberry Syrup, 1/4 cup	210	0	52
Boysenberry Syrup, 1/4 cup	210	0	52
Mrs. Butterworth's			
Original Syrup, 1/4 cup	220	0	55
Smuckers			
Blackberry, 1/4 cup	210	0	52
Blueberry, 1/4 cup	210	0	52
Red Raspberry, 1/4 cup.	210	0	52
Strawberry, 1/4 cup	210	0	52
Sugar Free Breakfast Syrup, 1/4 cup	20	0	8
Sorbee			
Blueberry Syrup, 2 tbsp.	10	0	4
Chocolate Syrup, 2 tbsp.	15	0	4
• Strawberry Syrup, 2 tbsp.	5	0	2

▷ VEGETABLES	Cal	Fat	Cbs
VEGETABLES, CANNED			
Allens			
Carrots			
Tiny Sliced Carrots, 127 g	35	0	8
Green Beans			
Cut Green Beans, 120 g	30	0	6
French Style Green Beans, 119 g	25	0	4
Green Bean Casserole, 120 g	40	1	6
Green Beans No Salt, 120 g	15	0	3
Whole Green Beans, 124 g	30	0	6
Greens			
Collard Greens No Salt, 116 g	30	1	5
Kale Greens No Salt, 116 g	30	1	3
Mixed Greens No Salt, 121 g	30	1	8
Mustard Greens No Salt, 118 g	30	1	5
Seasoned Collard Greens, 118 g	35	1	5
Seasoned Kale Greens, 118 g	35	1	5
Seasoned Mixed Greens, 110 g	45	1	0
Seasoned Mustard Greens, 118 g	45	1	6
Ssn Turnip Greens w/Diced Turnips, 118 g	35	1	5
Seasoned Turnip Greens, 118 g	35	1	5
Turnip Greens No Salt, 121 g	25	1	3
Turnip Greens w/ Diced Turnip No Salt, 119 g	30	1	5
Hominy			
Golden Hominy, 128 g	120	1	27
Pepi Golden Hominy, 128 g	120	1	27
White Hominy, 127 g	100	1	22
Okra			
Cut Okra & Tomatoes, 114 g	30	0	5
Cut Okra, 124 g	30	0	6
Cut Okra, Tomatoes & Corn, 117 g	30	0	6
Peas			
Allens Field Peas with Snaps, 128 g	120	1	21
Crowder Peas, 127 g	110	1	19
Purple Hull Peas, 126 g	120	1	21
American Roland Food Corporation			
Artichokes			
Bottoms, 130 g	50	0	10
Hearts, Marinated, 30 g	20	2	2
Hearts, Small, 126 g	35	0	6
Asparagus			
Spears, Green, 130 g	20	0	3
Spears, White, 135 g	30	0	5
Bamboo Shoots			
Sliced, 130 g	25	0	3

VEGETABLES	Cal	Fat	Cbs
Strips, 130 g	25	0	3
Carrots			
Baby Carrots, 120 g	35	0	7
Julienne Strips, 120 g	45	0	9
Peas & Carrots, 120 g	90	0	17
Celery			
Hearts, 120 g	15	0	2
Knob Strips, 120 g	45	0	10
Chestnuts			
Cream - Creme de Marrons, 30 g	80	0	18
In Water - Marrons, 30 g	30	0	7
Natural Chestnuts - Marrons, 30 g	50	0	11
Corn			
Baby Corn, Cut, 130 g	25	0	4
Baby Corn, Medium Whole, 130 g	25	0	4
White Corn, Organic, 100 g	110	1	23
Eggplant			
Eggplant Appetizer, 142 g	140	10	11
Stuffed Eggplants, 101 g	80	4	11
Mushrooms			
Mushrooms, Whole, 120 g	25	0	4
Mushrooms, Wild Forest, 120 g	85	0	1
Shiitake, Dried, 9 g	30	0	5
Onions			
Baby Whole, 130 g	24	0	5
Cocktail, 14 g	0	0	0
• Whole, 130 g	25	0	5
Peas			
Peas & Carrots, 120 g	90	0	17
Peas, Green Extra Fine, 120 g	120	0	21
Peas, Pigeon, 130 g	80	0	15
Sundried Tomatoes			
Sundried Tomatoes, 5 g	15	0	3
Sundried Tomato Strips w/ Herbs, 15 g	35	1	6
Sundried Tomatoes in Olive Oil, 8 g	25	2	3
• Sweet Dried Tomatoes, 40 g	130	0	31
Bush's Beans			
Greens			
Chopped Collard Greens, 130 g	30	0	4
Chopped Kale Greens, 130 g	30	0	4
Chopped Mixed Greens, 130 g	25	0	3
Chopped Mustard Greens, 130 g	25	0	3
Chopped Turnip Greens, 130 g	25	0	3
Hominy			
Golden Hominy, 130 g	60	0	13

• MOST HEALTHY   • LEAST HEALTHY

▷ VEGETABLES

	Cal	Fat	Cbs
White Hominy, 130 g	70	1	14
California Sun Dry			
Julienne Cut Sun-Dried Tom in Oil, 1 tbsp.	45	3	N/A
Sun-Dried Tomato Garlic, 2 tbsp.	90	7	N/A
Sun-Dried Tomato Halves in Oil, 1 tbsp.	45	3	N/A
Sun-Dried Tomato Sun-Cups, 1 oz.	15	0	N/A
Contadina			
Recipe Ready Tomatoes			
Crushed Tomatoes 28 oz, 61 g	20	0	4
Crsh Tomatoes w/ Italian Herbs 28 oz, 61 g	20	0	3
Crsh Tomatoes w/ Rst Garlic 28 oz, 61 g	20	0	3
Diced Tomatoes - Marinara 15 oz, 122 g	70	2	13
Diced Tomatoes 15 oz, 122 g	30	0	6
Diced Tomatoes w/ Itln Herbs 15 oz, 122 g	45	0	10
Stewed Tomatoes			
Italian Style Stewed Tom 15 oz, 122 g	35	0	8
Stewed Tomatoes 15 oz, 122 g	35	0	9
Tomato Paste			
Tomato Paste 6 oz, 33 g	30	0	6
Italian Paste w/ Italian Ssn 6 oz, 33 g	35	1	7
Tomato Paste 12 oz, 33 g	30	0	6
Tomato Puree			
Tomato Puree 15 oz, 63 g	20	0	4
Tomato Sauce			
Tomato Sauce 8 oz, 61 g	15	0	3
Extra Thick & Zesty Tom Sc 15 oz, 62 g	20	0	3
Garlic & Onion Tomato Sauce 15 oz, 61 g	20	0	4
Tomato Sauce 29 oz, 61 g	15	0	3
Del Monte			
Asparagus			
Asparagus Cuts & Tips, 124 g	20	0	3
Asparagus Spears, 124 g	20	0	3
Extra Long Asparagus Spears, 124 g	20	0	3
Beans			
Lima Beans, 126 g	80	0	15
Wax Beans, 121 g	20	0	4
Carrots			
Honey Glazed Carrots, 130 g	70	0	18
Peas & Carrots, 128 g	60	0	11
Sliced Carrots, 123 g	35	0	8
Corn			
Corn in Butter Sauce, 126 g	90	3	14
Sweet Corn Cream Style, 125 g	60	1	14
White Corn, 125 g	60	1	11
White Corn Cream Style, 125 g	100	1	21

● MOST HEALTHY   ● LEAST HEALTHY

VEGETABLES

	Cal	Fat	Cbs
Diced Tomatoes			
Diced Tomatoes, No Salt Added, 126 g	25	0	6
Diced w/ Basil, Garlic and Oregano, 126 g	50	0	11
Diced w/ Green Pepper and Onion, 126 g	40	0	9
Diced with Mushroom and Garlic, 126 g	45	0	10
Green Beans			
Cut Green Beans, 121 g	20	0	4
Cut Italian Beans, 121 g	30	0	6
French Style Green Beans, 121 g	20	0	4
Whole Green Beans, 121 g	20	0	4
Mixed Vegetables			
Homestyle Vegetable Medley, 120 g	70	3	11
Mixed Vegetables, 124 g	40	0	8
Peas & Carrots, 128 g	60	0	11
Peas			
Peas & Carrots, 128 g	60	0	11
Sweet Peas, 125 g	60	0	13
Very Young Small Sweet Peas, 125 g	60	0	10
Petite Cut Diced Tomatoes			
Diced Tomatoes, 126 g	25	0	6
With Garlic and Olive Oil, 126 g	45	1	10
With Zesty Jalapeños, 126 g	30	0	6
Potatoes			
Diced New Potatoes, 122 g	45	0	11
Mixed Vegetables with Potatoes, 125 g	45	0	10
Potatoes Au Gratin, 124 g	80	3	13
Whole New Potatoes, 158 g	60	0	13
Sauerkraut			
Sauerkraut, 30 g	0	0	0
Bavarian Sauerkraut, 30 g	15	0	4
Spinach			
Chopped Spinach, 115 g	30	0	4
Whole Leaf Spinach, 115 g	30	0	4
Stewed Tomatoes			
Italian Recipe, 126 g	30	0	8
Mexican Recipe, 126 g	35	0	9
Original Recipe, 126 g	35	0	9
Wedges			
Tomato Wedges, 126 g	35	0	9
Zucchini			
Zucchini with Tomato Sauce, 121 g	30	0	7
Green Giant			
Asparagus, 123 g	20	0	3
Cream Style Sweet Corn, 127 g	90	1	19
Cut Green Beans, 120 g	20	0	4

• MOST HEALTHY   • LEAST HEALTHY

VEGETABLES	Cal	Fat	Cbs
Mushrooms Whole, 120 g	25	0	4
Sweet Peas, 122 g	60	0	12
Whole Kernel Sweet Corn, 124 g	60	1	11
Hunt's			
Diced			
Original Tomatoes, 1/2 cup	20	0	5
Tomatoes in Sauce, 1/2 cup	30	0	7
Tomatoes with Roasted Garlic, 1/2 cup	30	0	6
Tomatoes with Sweet Onions, 1/2 cup	45	0	10
Stewed			
Tomatoes, 1/2 cup	30	0	7
Tomatoes No Salt Added, 1/2 cup	40	0	9
Whole			
Tomatoes No Salt Added, 1/2 cup	20	0	4
Tomatoes, 1/2 cup	20	0	4
Libby's Pumpkin			
Libby's 100% Pure Pumpkin, 1/2 cup	40	1	9
Muir Glen			
Crushed Tomatoes with Basil, 65 g	25	0	5
Ground Peeled Tomatoes, 65 g	20	0	4
Stewed Tomatoes, 128 g	30	0	6
Whole Peeled Tomatoes, 122 g	25	0	5
Progresso			
Artichoke Hearts Marinated, 32 g	60	5	2
Artichoke Hearts, 130 g	30	0	7
Ro*Tel			
Chunky Tomatoes w/ Green Chilis, 1/2 cup	20	0	4
Diced Tomatoes, 1/2 cup	25	0	5
Hot Diced Tomatoes, 1/2 cup	20	0	4
Italian Diced Tomatoes, 1/2 cup	30	0	6
Mexican Fiesta Diced Tomatoes, 1/2 cup	30	0	6
Tomatoes with Green Chilis, 1/2 cup	20	0	4
VEGETABLES, DRIED			
California Sun Dry			
Sun-Dried Tomato Cello Bags, 1 oz.	15	0	N/A
VEGETABLES, FROZEN & FRESH			
Cascadian Farm			
Gourmet Boxed			
Broccoli Florets, 85 g	25	0	4
Cut Spinach, 85 g	25	0	3
French Green Beans w/ Almonds, 105 g	70	3	8
Winter Squash, 130 g	70	0	19
Premium Bagged			
Broccoli Florets, 85 g	20	0	4
Peas & Carrots, 85 g	50	0	10

● MOST HEALTHY ● LEAST HEALTHY

VEGETABLES	Cal	Fat	Cbs
• Sweet Corn, 85 g	90	1	19
Sweet Peas, 85 g	70	0	12
Premium Blends			
California-Style Blend, 85 g	25	0	5
Chinese Stirfry, 85 g	25	0	6
Gardener's Blend, 85 g	50	0	11
Mixed Vegetables, 85 g	60	0	12
Thai Stirfry, 85 g	25	0	5
Green Giant			
Corn On The Cob			
Extra Sweet, 62 g	60	1	11
Nibblers, 61 g	70	1	14
Bagged			
Broccoli & Carrots w/ Garlic Herbs, 112 g	40	1	7
Garden Vegetable Medley, 120 g	70	1	14
Plain Chopped Broccoli, 79 g	25	0	4
Plain Mixed Vegetables, 84 g	50	0	11
Plain Sweet Peas, 89 g	70	0	12
Select Sugar Snap Peas, 79 g	40	0	9
Select Whole Green Beans, 83 g	30	0	5
Boxed - Simply Steam			
Baby Veggie Medley Seasoned, 103 g	40	1	9
Broccoli and Carrots, 131 g	60	3	8
Garden Vegetable Medley, 99 g	50	1	11
• No Sauce Asparagus Cuts, 86 g	20	0	3
No Sauce Baby Lima Beans, 76 g	80	0	15
VEGETABLES, PACKAGED FRESH			
Chiquita			
Bell Peppers, 148 g	30	0	7
Cucumbers, 99 g	15	0	3
Tomatoes, 48 g	35	1	7
Dole			
Fresh Vegetables			
Artichokes, 56 g	25	0	6
Asparagus, 93 g	25	0	4
Broccoli, 148 g	45	0	8
Brussels Sprouts, 84 g	40	0	6
Butter Lettuce, 85 g	10	N/A	N/A
Carrots, 78 g	35	0	8
Cauliflower, 99 g	25	0	5
Celery, 110 g	20	0	5
Green Cabbage, 92 g	20	N/A	N/A
Green Leaf Lettuce, 90 g	15	N/A	3
Iceberg Lettuce, 89 g	15	0	3
• Mushrooms, 35 g	9	0	1

• MOST HEALTHY   • LEAST HEALTHY

VEGETABLES

	Cal	Fat	Cbs
Romaine Lettuce, 85 g	20	0	3
Packaged Salads			
Baby Spinach, 85 g	20	0	3
Butter & Red Leaf, 85 g	10	0	3
Classic Cole Slaw, 85 g	25	0	5
European, 85 g	15	0	3
Field Greens, 100 g	150	11	10
Italian, 85 g	15	0	3
Leafy Romaine, 85 g	15	0	3
Light Caesar Kit, 85 g	15	0	3
Mediterranean, 85 g	100	7	8
Romano Kit, 85 g	15	0	3
Shredded Carrots, 85 g	40	0	9
Spinach, 85 g	150	12	9
Fresh Express			
Complete Salad Kits			
Caesar Lite, 10 oz.	100	7	8
• Caesar Supreme, 8 oz.	170	14	8
Caesar, 8 oz.	150	13	8
Crispy Lettuces			
Green & Crisp w/ Double Carrots, 3 oz.	20	0	4
Original Iceberg Garden Salad, 3 oz.	15	0	3
Premium Romaine, 3 oz.	15	0	3
Flavorful Whole Baby Blends			
Baby Spinach, 3 oz.	20	0	0
Sweet Baby Greens, 3 oz.	10	0	2
Veggie Spring Mix, 3 oz.	20	0	5
Organics			
Baby Spinach, 3 oz.	35	0	9
Hearts of Romaine, 3 oz.	15	0	2
Italian, 3 oz.	15	0	3
Tender Lettuce Mixes			
Fancy Field Greens™, 3 oz.	20	0	3
Hearts of Romaine, 3 oz.	15	0	3
Italian, 3 oz.	15	0	2
Veggie Lovers Salad, 3 oz.	20	0	4
River Ranch			
Cut Vegetables			
Broccoli Florets, 3 oz.	25	0	4
Broccoli Stir Fry, 3 oz.	30	0	5
Cauliflower Florets, 3 oz.	20	0	4
Vegetable Medley Blend, 3 oz.	25	0	6
Salads			
Caesar Salad Kit, 4 oz.	150	12	7
Chopped Romaine, 3 oz.	10	0	2

• MOST HEALTHY   • LEAST HEALTHY

VEGETABLES	Cal	Fat	Cbs
Cole Slaw Mix, 3 oz.	25	0	5
European Salad Blend, 3 oz.	10	0	2
Garden Salad, 3 oz.	15	0	3
Italian Salad Blend, 3 oz.	15	0	2
Raspberry Vinaigrette Salad Kit, 4 oz.	130	8	13
Shredded Carrots, 3 oz.	35	0	9
Soy Boy			
Organic 5 Grain Tempeh, 3 oz.	130	3	15
Organic Soy Tempeh's, 3 oz.	160	6	9

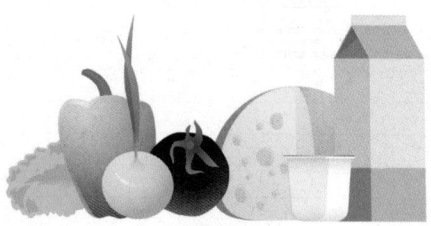

• MOST HEALTHY   • LEAST HEALTHY